Lameness in Horses

Lameness in Horses

O. R. Adams, D.V.M., M.S.

Professor, Department of Clinical Sciences, College of Veterinary
Medicine, Colorado State University, Fort Collins, Colorado.
Charter Diplomate, American College of Veterinary Surgeons.

Third Edition

530 Illustrations

LEA & FEBIGER   PHILADELPHIA

Dedicated to NAN
for her encouragement and patience
and to
GAIL, KENT, LYNNE, GARY, *and* ROBERT
for their love of horses

Library of Congress Cataloging in Publication Data
Adams, Ora Robert.
Lameness in horses.

1. Lameness in horses. 2. Horseshoeing.
I. Title. [DNLM: 1. Horse diseases. SF959.L25
A216L 1974]
SF959.L25A3 1974 636.1′08′9758 73-16030
ISBN 0-8121-0474-9

First Edition, 1962
Reprinted December 1962, August 1963, March 1965

Second Edition, 1966
Reprinted September 1967, June 1969, January 1972, September 1972

Third Edition, 1974

Reprinted January, 1976

PRINTED IN THE UNITED STATES OF AMERICA

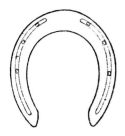

Preface

Interest in equine lameness has increased steadily since the first edition of this book in 1962, necessitating this third edition to present current information. Although proliferation of literature and the length of the publication process make it impossible to be completely up-to-date, I have made every effort to present the reader with the latest information available. I have included many new references for use by those who wish to review individual articles, even though I may not have used them.

The acceptance of this text has again exceeded all expectations, and the cooperation of colleagues worldwide in aiding with corrections and additional material is hereby recognized.

I have not changed all anatomical terminology to some of the latest terms because I believe they are not yet generally accepted, but I have used some of the newer terms.

The preparation of this book would have been impossible without the cooperation of faculty, interns, and students in the Veterinary Clinic at Colorado State University. In addition, practitioners and faculty from other institutions have generously aided me with suggestions and illustrations.

Mrs. Pat Dietemann has again designed the cover and has drawn new illustrations for this edition, and her talent is greatly appreciated.

This edition has a section on evaluation of stallion semen in Chapter 3 that will be of great aid to practitioners doing breeding soundness examination in stallions. I am indebted to Dr. Bill Pickett for this work. Dr. J. P. Morgan has revised his chapter on Radiology, giving a more complete treatise on this subject that will be useful to all equine practitioners.

As usual, Lea & Febiger has given me complete cooperation and encouragement in preparation of this edition.

I hope that this book will be useful to all who take the time to read it and that I will continue to receive your cooperation in making corrections and suggested additions for future revisions.

O. R. Adams

Fort Collins, Colorado

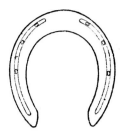

Contents

The Relationship between Conformation and Lameness

The conformation of a horse is the key to his method of progression. The horse is a working animal, and his value is determined by the condition of his limbs and feet. Poor conformation of limbs contributes to certain lamenesses and may actually be the cause of lameness in some cases. The proportions of the body conformation, as compared with the limb conformation, may determine whether or not there will be any type of interference of the limbs during progression. Conformation, a major factor in soundness of the limbs, often determines the useful lifetime of a horse. Very few horses have perfect conformation, but in the selection of breeding stock, conformation should be considered carefully, and animals with serious weaknesses should be eliminated.

Inheritable conformation predisposing to navicular disease, bone spavin, carpal bone fracture, curb, and upward fixation of the patella is prevalent. Conformation of the limb leading to deviation of the foot in flight is also inheritable and should be considered undesirable either when purchasing a horse or when considering a stallion or mare for mating. Whenever possible, the stallion or mare should be mated in the hope of correcting difficulties found in the sire or dam so that the offspring will be improved in conformation.

In the evaluation of conformation of horses, there are other factors that make it difficult to always evaluate a horse accurately. It has been said that "the best conformation of a horse is speed," and of course speed is important. If a horse has speed but also has bad conformation, he is apt to be a short-term race horse. If he has speed, plus good conformation that does not predispose him to interference and lameness, he is more apt to be a long-term race horse. Another factor is that called "heart." This could be properly termed "desire," and some horses definitely have more of a sense of competition than others. This desire often permits a horse that is suffering pain from certain types of lamenesses to compete successfully and win. It is also very evident in some working rodeo horses, who will do their jobs and then limp out of the arena. The best combination of all is good conformation, speed, and heart.

CONFORMATION OF THE BODY (Fig. 1–1)

Conformation of the body varies among different breeds, and this factor must be

1

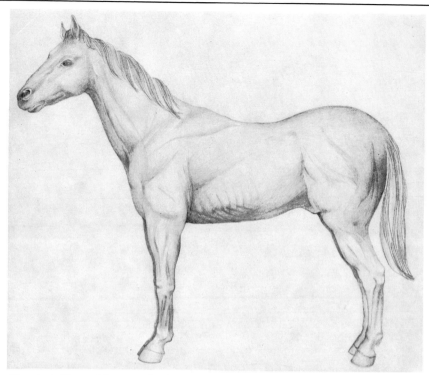

FIG. 1–1. Normal horse. The body and limbs should be well proportioned.

considered in the evaluation of the horse. For example, an Arabian has a short back in comparison with a Thoroughbred; a Quarter Horse of certain blood lines has a shorter, heavier body and shorter legs than a Thoroughbred. In some Quarter Horse blood lines the outcrossing with Thoroughbred breeding has been extensive enough to make the offspring nearly indistinguishable from a pure Thoroughbred. Even in the Thoroughbred breed there are conformational differences among American, English, and French blood lines. Therefore, the evaluation of body conformation must be based on individual breed specifications. Long-backed horses may develop a swing in the gait that materially alters the movement of the limbs. Such horses are prone to speedy-cutting and to cross-firing. Short-backed horses, with legs too long for the body, may be prone to over-reaching, forging, and scalping.

Certain requirements are essential to all breeds, and the veterinarian must famil-iarize himself with the ideal body characteristics. The body should be in pleasing balance with the limbs and should have good proportion. Body conformation is not a common cause of lameness, so further discussion in this book will pertain to limb conformation.

CONFORMATION OF THE LIMBS

To evaluate limb conformation, the horse should be observed from a distance as well as close at hand. The limbs should be studied at rest and in motion. The veterinarian should determine whether abnormal conformation in the horse develops low in the limb or whether it actually begins at the hip and/or shoulder joints. The limbs should be well suited to the height, depth, and length of the body. The drive of the hindlimbs affects the forelimbs, so overall balanced conformation is very important.

Conformation of the limbs also determines the shape of the feet, the wear of the feet, distribution of weight, and the flight of the feet. Faulty limb conformation is not an unsoundness in itself (curby conformation being the exception); however, it may be considered a warning or sign of weakness, and it predisposes the horse to many lamenesses that would not occur had he been born with good conformation.

One can often determine the interference that occurs among the limbs by observing the walking and trotting gaits. In the rapid gaits, interference is difficult to perceive because the eye cannot follow the feet at high speed. Race horses seldom have limb contact problems if they have good overall conformation; however, if slight conformational abnormalities are present, interference of the limbs may occur that would not develop if the horse were used less strenuously (see Chapter 4, page 97). Contact problems may occur in a horse with good conformation when he is used for events that require rapid turning, such as barrel racing, cutting, pole bending, and reining.

In studying limb conformation of horses, it is important to not form rash opinions based on observation of the horse in a standing position only. The horse should be observed during movement on a hard surface, so that the feet can be studied as they leave the ground, during flight, and as they land. This study cannot be made on a soft surface or in grass. Prejudging the conformation before studying the horse in motion may cause errors in evaluation.

The Forelimbs

The forelimbs bear some 60 to 65 percent of the weight of the horse. This amount can vary according to the conformation of the horse, whose head, neck, abdomen, and croup can present very diverse proportions. This means the forelimbs are subjected to more injuries from concussion and trauma than the rear

limbs because the forelimbs not only bear the weight of the body in movement, but also aid the hindlimbs in propelling the body. Ideal or perfect conformation means proper length of bone as well as proper angulation between these bones. The horse may have good conformation from one view and poor conformation from another or may be good in one forelimb and not the other.

Examination for conformation of the forelimbs should be done while the horse is standing with the weight well distributed between the fore and hind feet and then again while the horse is in motion. When the horse is standing quietly, observe him from a distance, and then examine the limbs from a closer view. Ideal conformation of the forelimb does not put excess strain on any structure of the limb.

Anterior View (Fig. 1–2A)

Both limbs should bear weight equally. The legs should be straight. A line dropped from the point of the shoulder (middle of the scapulo-humeral joint)

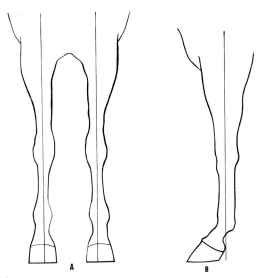

A   B

FIG. 1–2. Anterior and lateral views of normal forelimbs. *A*, Line dropped from the point of the shoulder joint bisects the limb. *B*, Line from the tuber spinae of the scapula bisects the limb as far as the fetlock and drops at the heel.

should bisect the leg. The chest should be well developed and well muscled. The toes should point straight forward, and the feet should be as far apart on the ground as the limbs are at their origin in the chest. Deviations from a straight limb will cause strain to be placed on the collateral ligaments of the hinge joints in the forelimb. The carpal joints should be balanced and should not deviate toward, or away from, one another. The cannon bone should be centered under the carpus and not to the lateral side (Bench knees) (Fig. 1–18).

Lateral View (Figs. 1–1 and 1–2B)

The shoulder should be sloping. A line dropped from the tuber spinae, on the spine of the scapula, should bisect the leg to the fetlock joint and then carry to a point just behind the heel. The carpus should not deviate anteriorly or posteriorly. The musculature of the forearm should be well developed and balance the limb. The area just distal to the carpus

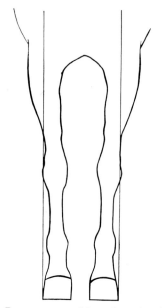

FIG. 1–3. Base narrow. Note that the distance between the center lines of the limbs at their origin is greater than the distance between the center lines of the feet on the ground.

should not be cut in on the anterior or posterior surface (Cut out under the knees, Tied-in knees, Fig. 1–19). The hoof wall should slope at the same angle as the pastern.

The angle of the scapula with the body will vary from 55 to 78 degrees and there is an angle of 85 to 100 degrees between the scapula and the humerus at the point of the shoulder. An angle of about 120 to 138 degrees is present between the humerus and radius at the elbow joint, and the angle between the third metacarpal bone and the first phalanx is about 125 to 135 degrees. The angle between the ground surface of the foot and the anterior line of the hoof wall and pastern (foot axis) should be approximately 45 to 50 degrees. These angles vary among different breeds, e.g., Arabians ordinarily have more sloping shoulders and pasterns than do Quarter Horses.

Faults of Conformation in the Forelimb

Base Narrow (Fig. 1–3)

In base-narrow conformation, the distance between the center lines of the feet at their placement on the ground is less than the distance between the center lines of the limbs at their origin in the chest when viewed from the front. This is found most often in horses having large chests and well-developed pectoral muscles, such as the Quarter Horse. This conformation may be accompanied by a toe-in (pigeon-toed) or toe-out (splay-footed) conformation.

This type of conformation (base narrow) inherently causes the horse to bear more weight on the outside of the foot than on the inside. The base-narrow condition makes it impossible for the weight to be borne in any other way. Consequently, whether the foot toes in or toes out, the outside of the foot will land first,

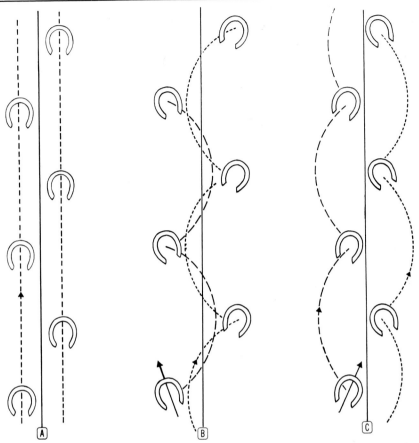

FIG. 1–4. How toe-in and toe-out affects foot path. *A*, Normal foot path. *B*, Foot path of a horse with toe-out conformation. *C*, Foot path of a horse with toe-in conformation.

and most of the weight will be taken on this area. Because of this, the outside of the foot and limb is subjected to more strain, causing the lateral aspect of the limb to be under constant tension. Articular windpuffs of the fetlock joint, lateral ringbone, and lateral sidebone are common pathological conditions resulting from this conformation. In nearly all cases, base-narrow conformation forces the horse to land on the outside wall of the hoof, regardless of whether the feet toe in or toe out. This requires that the inside wall be trimmed to level the foot.

Base Wide (Fig. 1–8)

In this conformation, the distance between the center lines of the feet on the ground is greater than the distance between the center lines of the limbs at their origin in the chest, when viewed from the front. This condition is found most commonly in narrow-chested horses such as the American Saddlebred and the Tennessee Walking Horse. In base-wide conformation, the horse often is affected with toe-out (splay-footed) position of the feet. Base-wide, toe-out conformation usually causes "winging" to the inside (Figs. 1–4B and 1–9).

Base-wide conformation forces the horse to bear more weight on the inside of the foot than the outside of the foot. Since the weight is distributed in this fashion, the horse will usually land on the inside of the foot, a situation opposite to that seen in base-narrow conformation.

Consequently, the inside of the limb takes the most strain in base-wide conformation, causing the medial aspect of the fetlock and pastern joints to be under constant tension. Articular windpuffs of the fetlock joint, medial ringbone, and medial sidebone are common pathological conditions resulting from this conformation. In nearly all cases, base-wide conformation forces the horse to land on the inside wall of the hoof, regardless of whether the feet toe in or toe out. This requires that the outside wall be trimmed to level the foot.

Toe-In or Pigeon-Toed
(Figs. 1–7 and 1–10)

Toe-in is a position of the feet in which the toes point toward one another when viewed from the front. It is congenital, and the limb may be crooked as high as its origin at the chest, or as low as the fetlock down. It is usually accompanied by a base-narrow conformation but rarely is present when the horse is base-wide. In the young foal, the condition may be par-

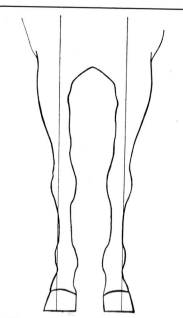

FIG. 1–6. Base-narrow, toe-out conformation.

tially corrected by proper trimming of the feet, and young horses may be correctively shod to prevent a worsening of the condition (see Chapter 9). When the affected horse moves, there is a tendency to "paddle" with the feet (Figs. 1–4C and 1–5). This is an outward deviation of the foot during flight. The foot breaks over the outside toe and lands on the outside wall. If a horse toes in, he will usually "paddle" whether he is base-narrow or base-wide. If there is inward deviation of the pastern and foot from the fetlock down, the horse may carry the foot to the inside instead of the outside. This complication of base-narrow, toe-in conformation can cause interference, especially at the fetlock joint, causing damage to the medial sesamoid bone.

Toe-Out or Splay-Footed
(Figs. 1–6 and 1–11)

When viewed from the front, the toes point away from one another. The condition is usually congenital and is usually due to legs that are crooked from their origin down. In some cases, however, the

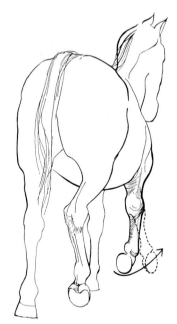

FIG. 1–5. Paddling. This accompanies toe-in conformation.

condition is aggravated by a twisting at the fetlock. It may be accompanied by either base-wide or base-narrow conformation. As with a toe-in conformation, it may be controlled or partially corrected by corrective trimming or corrective shoeing in the young horse (Chapter 9). The flight of the foot goes through an inner arc when advancing and may cause interference with the opposite forelimb (Figs. 1–4B and 1–9). A horse that toes out will usually "wing" to the inside, whether it is base-narrow or base-wide. When toe-out attitude of the feet occurs with base-narrow conformation, there is a greater likelihood of limb interference and plaiting (Fig. 1–12A).

Base-Narrow, Toe-In Conformation (Fig. 1-7)

Base-narrow, toe-in conformation causes excessive strain on the lateral collateral ligaments of the fetlock and pastern joints. Articular windpuffs, lateral ringbone, and lateral sidebone are common pathological conditions with this conformation; they result from the me-

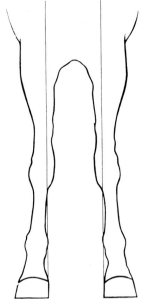

FIG. 1–8. Base-wide conformation. Note that the distance between the center lines of the feet is wider than the distance between the center lines of the limbs at the chest.

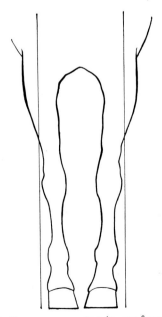

FIG. 1-7. Base-narrow, toe-in conformation.

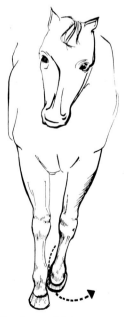

FIG. 1–9. Winging, which may cause interference, is caused by a toe-out position of the feet.

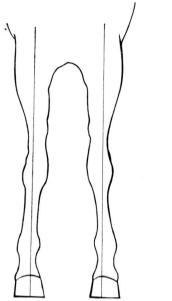

FIG. 1–10. Base-wide, toe-in position of feet.

chanical strains caused by the base-narrow conformation and an excess of body weight on the outside hoof wall. Examination of the foot will show that it is worn low on the outside because the foot lands on the outside wall, causing excessive wear in this area. Trimming the inside wall is required to level the foot. Base-narrow, toe-in conformation usually causes "paddling" (Figs. 1–4C and 1–5). This is a common type of conformational abnormality; corrective shoeing is discussed in Chapter 9.

Base-Narrow, Toe-Out Conformation (Fig. 1–6)

Base-narrow, toe-out conformation is one of the worst types of conformation in the forelimb. Horses having this conformation seldom can shoulder the strain of heavy work. The closely placed feet, combined with a tendency to "wing" inwardly from the toe-out position, commonly cause limb interference. The base-narrow attitude of the limb places the weight on the outside wall, as with base-narrow, toe-in conformation. The hoof breaks over

the outside toe, swings inward and lands on the outside wall. This causes great strain on the limb below the fetlock. Plaiting (Fig. 1–12A) may be evident. Corrective shoeing is very similar to base-narrow, toe-in conformation since the foot lands on the outside wall. One should study the foot closely in flight to make sure of the corrections necessary (Fig. 1–12B). These usually involve lowering the inside wall and toe to level the foot.

Lesions on the medial aspect of the third metacarpal bone, fractures of the second metacarpal bone and an occasional fracture of the medial sesamoid may result from the interference. Diagnosis of interference is discussed on page 97. Corrective shoeing is discussed in Chapter 9.

Base-Wide, Toe-Out Conformation (Fig. 1–11)

When a horse is base-wide, the usual attitude of the feet is to toe out. The base-wide conformation places the greatest stress on the inside of the limb. This

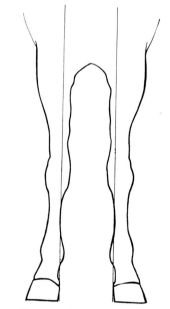

FIG. 1–11. Base-wide, toe-out position of the feet.

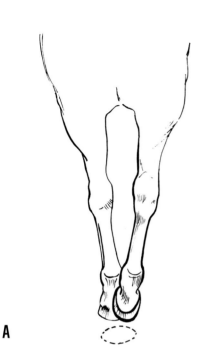

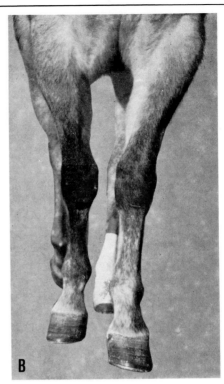

Fig. 1–12A. Plaiting. Plaiting is most often found in a horse with base-narrow, toe-out conformation. After the foot travels an inward arc it lands more or less directly in front of the opposite forefoot. In some cases this leads to stumbling as a result of interference. B, Base-narrow, toe-out conformation. Note left forefoot landing on the outside wall, typical of this type of conformation. There is also a degree of plaiting.

means that there is greater strain on the medial collateral ligament of the metacarpophalangeal (fetlock) and proximal interphalangeal (pastern) joints. In addition, medial sidebone and ringbone are common. With this conformation, the foot usually breaks over the inside toe, deviates ("wings") to the inside, and lands on the inside hoof wall. This means that the correction is just the opposite of that for base-narrow, toe-out conformation. When one studies the foot, it will be seen that the outside wall must be lowered to level the foot. Blemishes on the medial aspect of the third metacarpal bone, medial splints, and fracture of the second metacarpal bone occur with this conformation because of interference. Corrective shoeing is discussed in Chapter 9, page 404.

Base-Wide, Toe-In
Conformation (Fig. 1–10)

This type of conformation is unusual, but it does occur. The base-wide attitude of the limbs throws the greatest stress on the inside of the limb, with the same resulting pathological changes as for base-wide, toe-out conformation. In most cases, the horse affected with base-wide, toe-in conformation will "paddle" to the outside even though he breaks over the inside toe and lands on the inside wall.

There is always the possibility that other conformational abnormalities of the limb, especially from the fetlock down, may change the path of the foot so it does not correspond to the above descriptions. These abnormalities include twisting of the fetlock so that the base-narrow, toe-in horse actually "wings" to the inside. These variations are rare, and since they all cannot be listed, there will be no discussion of them here. The principles of corrective shoeing and trimming can be applied to the variations when accurate observation of the foot flight has been made. In every case, the veterinarian should study the progression of the foot closely to see how it lands, so that he can make proper recommendations about correction.

Plaiting (Fig. 1–12A)

Some horses, especially those with base-narrow, toe-wide conformation, tend to place one forefoot directly in front of the other. This is an undesirable characteristic, since it can produce interference and stumbling resulting from an advancing forelimb hitting the one placed in front of it.

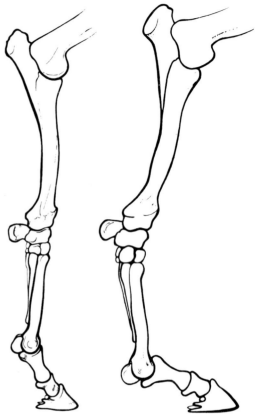

FIG. 1–14. Example of normal (left) and calf-kneed (right) position of the forelimb. (Courtesy Dr. W. Berkley.)

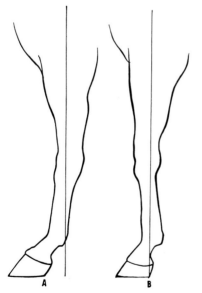

FIG. 1–13. Examples of poor conformation. Compare with Figure 1–2B. A, Calf knees—a posterior deviation of the carpus. B, Bucked knees—an anterior deviation of the carpus.

Posterior Deviation of the Carpal Joint (Calf Knees or Sheep Knees) (Figs. 1–13A and 1–14)

Posterior deviation of the carpal joint is a weak conformation, and the legs seldom remain sound under heavy work. This conformation places a strain upon the inferior check ligament, the anterior aspect of the carpal bones, the volar annular ligament of the carpus, and the volar aspect of the carpal joint capsule. Chip fractures from the third, radial, and intermediate carpal bones are common (Figs. 1–14, 1–15, and 1–22). Small chip fractures from the radius may also occur (see Chap. 6).

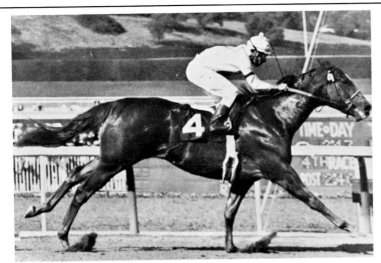
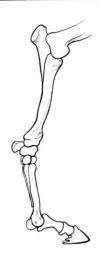

FIG. 1–15. Photograph of a Thoroughbred near the finish of a race. Note the backward deviation of the carpus, predisposing to chip fracture of the carpal bones. If a horse has a backward deviation of the carpus before limb fatigue forces it into this position, there is even greater possibility of carpal fracture. (Courtesy Dr. W. Berkley.)

Anterior Deviation of the Carpal Joint (Bucked Knees or Knee Sprung) (Fig. 1–13B)

This condition may also be called "goat knees" or "over in the knees." It is an anterior deviation of the carpus, but it causes less trouble than the calf-knee condition described above. Anterior deviation of the carpus is caused by contraction of the carpal flexors, i.e., ulnaris lateralis, flexor carpi ulnaris, and flexor carpi radialis. Extra strain is placed on the sesamoid bones, the superficial flexor tendon, the extensor carpi radialis, and the suspensory ligament. The condition is often present at birth, but if it is not severe, it usually disappears by six months of age. Congenital forms are nearly always bilateral and may be accompanied by a knuckling of the fetlocks resulting from contraction of the superficial digital flexor tendon (for a complete discussion, see Chapter 6, p. 168). Anterior deviation of the carpal joints may be present in rickets and may be accompanied by an enlarged epiphysis of the radius (see Chapter 5, p. 125).

Medial Deviation of the Carpal Joints (Knock Knees or Knee-Narrow Conformation) (Fig. 1–16B)

This is a medial deviation of the carpal joints toward each other. A strain is put on the inferior check ligament and suspensory apparatus, the capsule of the carpal joint medially, the medial collateral ligaments of the carpus, and the lateral aspect of the carpal bones (for complete discussion, see Chap. 6, p. 171).

Lateral Deviation of the Carpal Joints (Bow Legs or Bandy-Legged Conformation) (Fig. 1–16A)

Bow legs cause an outward deviation of the carpal joints when viewed from the front of the horse. It may be accompanied

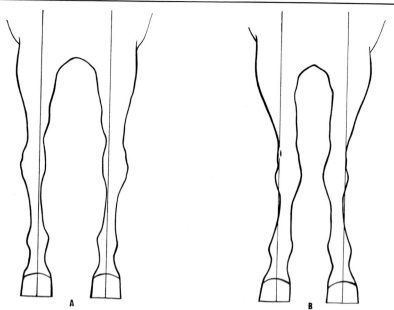

Fig. 1–16. Examples of poor conformation. Compare with Figure 1–2A. A, Bow legs. B, Knock knees.

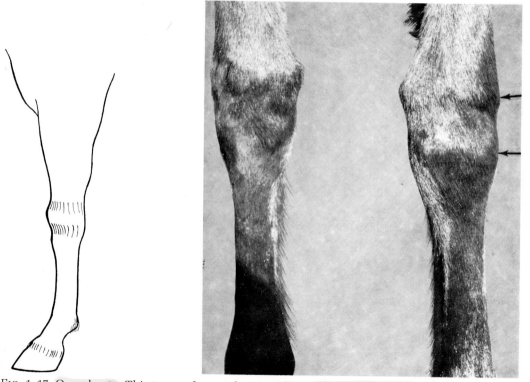

Fig. 1–17. Open knees. This term refers to the irregular profile of the carpal joint when viewed from the side. It is due to the enlarged distal epiphysis of the radius and enlargement in the area of the carpometacarpal joint. It is usually the result of a mineral imbalance and becomes less obvious as the horse grows to maturity.

by a base-narrow, toe-in conformation. This condition causes excessive strain on the lateral collateral ligament of the carpus, the medial side of the carpal bones, and the lateral portion of the carpal joint capsule (for complete discussion, see Chap. 6, p. 171).

Open Knees

The term refers to an irregular profile of the carpal joint when viewed from the side (Fig. 1–17). This irregularity gives the impression that the carpal joints are not fully closed. This conformation is usually found in young horses (1 to 3 years of age) before full maturity and is often accompanied by epiphysitis (Chap. 5, p. 125) resulting from mineral imbalance. As the horse matures, the joints usually become more pleasing in appearance. Most people regard this as a weak conformation subject to carpal injury. On the basis of experience, this is probably so. Radiographically, this irregularity in the carpal joints does not show outstanding changes.

Lateral Deviation of the Metacarpal Bones (Offset Knees or Bench Knees) (Fig. 1–18)

Offset knee is a conformation in which the cannon bone is offset to the lateral side and does not follow a straight line from the radius. It is evident when the limbs are viewed from the front. It is congenital in origin and should be considered a weak conformation. The medial splint bone is under greater stress than normal, and medial splints are common (Fig. 6–42, p. 208). The medial splint bone normally carries more weight than the lateral splint bone because the medial splint bone has a flat articulation, and the lateral splint bone an oblique articulation. In offset knees, there is even more direct weight bearing on the medial splint bone, which in turn carries more weight to the interosseous ligament, increasing the possibility of splints.

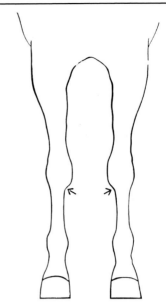

FIG. 1–18. Offset knees (bench knees). Note that the metacarpal bones are set too far laterally.

Tied-In Knees (Fig. 1–19B)

Viewed from the side, the flexor tendons appear to be too close to the cannon bone just below the carpus. This is poor conformation and inhibits free movement. A heavy fetlock may give the appearance of "tied-in knees" even though the condition is not actually present.

Cut Out under the Knees (Fig. 1–19A)

Viewed from the side, this condition causes a "cut out" appearance just below the carpus on the anterior surface of the cannon bone. It is a fundamentally weak conformation.

Standing Under in Front (Fig. 1–20A)

This is a deviation in which the entire forelimb from the elbow down is placed back of the perpendicular and too far under the body when the animal is viewed from the side. This may be brought about by disease and not be caused by conformation.

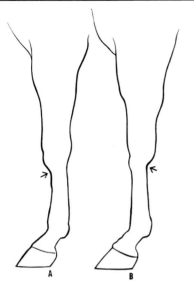

FIG. 1-19. Examples of poor conformation. Compare with Figure 1-2B. *A*, Cut out under the knees, as indicated by arrow. *B*, Tied-in knees, as indicated by arrow.

With this conformation, the base of support is shortened, overloading the forelimbs and limiting the anterior phase of the stride by overburdening the forelimb left on the ground. The limb in motion must come down sooner and there-

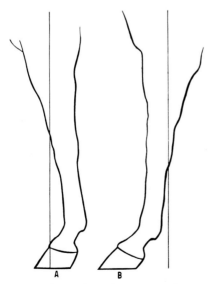

FIG. 1-20. Examples of poor conformation. Compare with Figure 1-2B. *A*, Standing under in front. *B*, Camped in front.

fore has a low arc of foot flight. The steps are more frequent, the arc of foot flight is low, and the foot is carried too close to the ground, predisposing to stumbling. Overall, it causes excessive wear and fatigue of bones, ligaments, and tendons. There is a diminution of speed, and the horse is predisposed to falling.

Camped in Front (Fig. 1-20B)

This is a condition opposite to that described above. The entire forelimb, from the body to the ground, is too far forward when viewed from the side. This limb attitude may be present in certain pathological conditions, such as bilateral navicular disease and laminitis.

Short Upright Pastern (Fig. 1-21B)

The short upright pastern increases the effect of concussion on the metacarpophalangeal (fetlock) joint, the proximal interphalangeal (pastern) joint, and the navicular bone (see pastern axis, p. 22). A horse with this conformation has increased predisposition to osselets (traumatic arthritis of the metacarpophalangeal joint), ringbone of the proximal interphalangeal joint, and navicular disease. This type of conformation is often associated with a base-narrow, toe-in conformation and is most often present in the horse with short legs and powerful body and leg musculature. A straight shoulder usually accompanies this type of conformation.

Long Sloping Pastern (Fig. 1-32B)

A long sloping pastern is one characterized by a normal or subnormal angulation of the forefoot (45 degrees or under) with a pastern that is too long for the length of the limb (see pastern axis, p. 22). This type of conformation predisposes to injury of the flexor tendons (tendosyno-

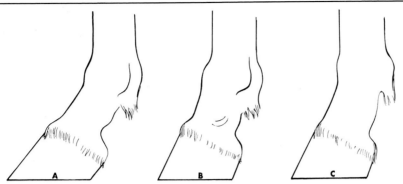

FIG. 1-21. Examples of pastern conformation. *A,* A normal angulation of hoof and pastern. *B,* A short upright pastern predisposing to injuries of the fetlock joint, ringbone of the pastern joint, and navicular bursitis. *C,* Long upright pastern predisposes to injuries of the fetlock joint and navicular bursa. This type of conformation does not seem to predispose to ringbone as often as does B.

vitis), sesamoid bones (sesamoiditis and fractures), and the suspensory ligament (desmitis).

Long Upright Pastern (Fig. 1–21C)

A long upright pastern predisposes the metacarpophalangeal joint and the navicular bursa to injury. Concussion to these areas is increased, because the normal anticoncussion mechanism of a normally sloping pastern is not present (*see* pastern axis, p. 22). Osselets (traumatic arthritis) and navicular disease are common findings with this type of conformation, and both types of lameness may be present at the same time. The stresses are very similar to those found in the short upright pastern (Fig. 1–21B), but pathology of the proximal interphalangeal (pastern) joint is not so common.

Pressure on the navicular bursa is often increased by efforts of the horseshoer to produce a normal angulation of the hoof wall. This causes a break between the pastern and foot axes at the coronary band (Fig. 1–23). This conformation is most commonly seen in Thoroughbreds and racing Quarter Horses.

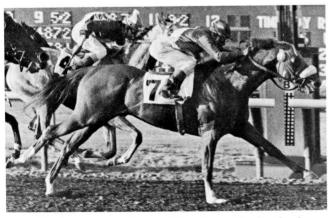

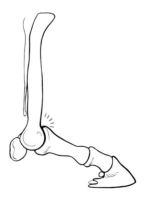

FIG. 1-22. Photograph of a Thoroughbred near the finish of a race. Note the backward deviation of the carpus and the extreme dropping of the fetlock. When the fetlock is in this position there is a possibility of chip fracture of the proximal end of the first phalanx. (Courtesy Dr. W. Berkley.)

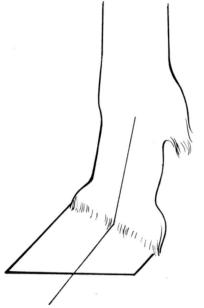

FIG. 1–23. A long upright pastern with a broken foot and pastern axis caused by lowering of the heels in an attempt to produce normal angulation of the hoof wall. This puts even greater stress on the navicular bursa by forcing the deep flexor tighter against the navicular bone, and is a common example of improper trimming in an attempt to force normal angulation of the pastern.

The Hind Limbs (Figs. 1–1, 1–24 and 1–25)

It is important to understand what constitutes normal conformation of the hind limb, even though there is less lameness there than in the forelimb. Conformation does play an important role in curb, upward fixation of the patella, and some forms of spavin.

Rear View

Viewed from behind, the limb should have a pleasing, well-balanced appearance. The hocks should be large enough to hold the weight of the animal, but smooth. The musculature on the inside of the thigh should carry down into the medial side of the gaskin so that the tibial

area does not appear too thin. A line dropped from the point of the tuber ischii should divide the leg into equal parts (Fig. 1–24). This gives equal distribution of weight, equal bone pressure and equal strain on collateral ligaments.

Lateral View

Viewed from the side, the limb should have a well-balanced appearance. The musculature should not end abruptly at the stifle joint, but should carry down onto the tibia and taper gradually to the hock. The angle of the stifle and hock should be neither too straight nor too angulated. A stifle and hock that are too straight may cause bog spavin of the hock and upward fixation of the patella. Excessive angulation of the hock (sickle hock)

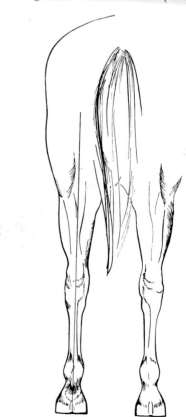

FIG. 1–24. Normal hind limbs. A line dropped from the point of the tuber ischii bisects the limb.

Faults of Conformation in the Hind Limbs

Base Narrow (Fig. 1–26)

Base-narrow conformation in the hind limbs means that when the animal is viewed from behind, the distance between the center lines of the feet is less than the distance between the center lines of the limbs in the thigh region. This is most commonly evident in heavily muscled horses where there is excessive strain on the lateral aspect of the limb in the bones, ligaments, and joints. The feet may toe-in or have straight toes. Base-narrow conformation is often accompanied by "bow legs" or a condition in which the hocks are too far apart. The legs may ap-

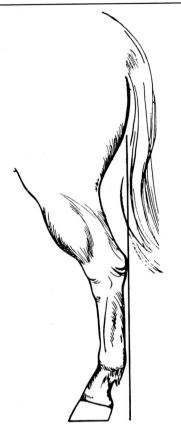

FIG. 1–25. Normal hind limbs from side view. A line dropped from the tuber ischii follows the metatarsus.

may cause curb and bone or bog spavin. If the stifle is too straight or too angulated, the hock will also be too straight or too angulated because of the reciprocal apparatus. A line dropped from the tuber ischii should hit the point of the hock, go down the posterior aspect of the metatarsal area, and then should strike 3 to 4 inches behind the heel (Fig. 1–25). A line dropped from the hip joint should strike halfway between the heel and toe. These angles cannot be changed by corrective shoeing or other measures.

In judging the hind limbs from the front of the animal, the limbs appear to be in base-narrow position because of the perspective. One must check the horse from behind before evaluating the position of the hind limbs.

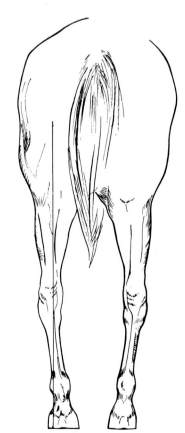

FIG. 1–26. Base narrow behind. This is often accompanied by bow legs, as shown. Compare with Figure 1–24.

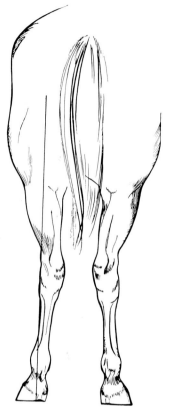

FIG. 1-27. Cow hocks accompanied by base-wide conformation. Such horses are usually base-narrow as far as the hocks, but base wide from the hocks down. Compare with Figure 1-24.

pear fairly straight to the hock and then deviate inward. When a horse has good conformation in front, and is base narrow behind, many types of interference can occur between the fore and hind limbs.

Base Wide (Fig. 1-27)

Base wide means that when viewed from behind, the distance between the center lines of the feet at their placement on the ground is greater than the distance between the center lines of the limbs in the thigh region. Base-wide conformation is not so frequent in the hind limbs as in the forelimbs. The most common form of base-wide conformation is cow hocks.

Medial Deviation of the Hock Joints (Cow Hocks) (Fig. 1-27)

"Cow hocked" means that the limbs are base narrow to the hock, and base wide from the hock to the feet. Cow hocked conformation is a common defect. The hocks are too close, point toward one another, and the feet are widely separated. Viewed laterally, the horse may be sickle-hocked. Cow hocks is one of the worst hind limb conformations because there is excessive strain on the medial side of the hock joint, which may cause bone spavin.

Excessive Angulation of the Hock Joints (Sickle Hocks) (Fig. 1-28)

When viewed from the side, the angle of the hock joint is decreased so that the

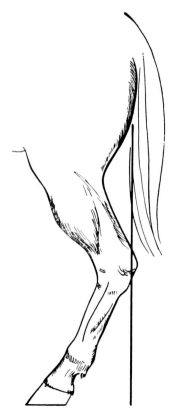

FIG. 1-28. Sickle hocks. Note the excessive angle of the hock joints. Compare with Figure 1-25.

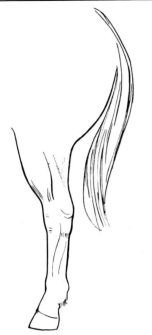

FIG. 1–29. Too straight behind. There is too little angulation of the hock and stifle joints.

horse is standing under from the hock down. The plantar aspect of the hock is under a greater strain, especially the plantar ligament. A horse so affected is predisposed to curb. This is called "curby conformation," because it predisposes the animal to injury of the plantar ligament.

Base Narrow from Fetlocks Down

This conformation places stress on the lateral collateral ligaments of the fetlock, pastern, and coffin joints and similar strain on the bones and tendons in this area.

Excessively Straight Legs or "Straight Behind" (Fig. 1–29)

When viewed from the side there is very little angle between the tibia and femur, and the hock joint is correspondingly straight. This predisposes the horse particularly to bog spavin and upward fixation of the patella. The straight

hock places increased tension on the anterior aspect of the joint capsule, causing irritation and chronic distention of the joint capsule with synovia. This type of leg is easily injured by heavy work. It is not uncommon to find upward fixation of the patella accompanying this conformation. The pasterns will also be too straight.

Standing Under Behind (Fig. 1–30)

Viewed from the side, the entire limb is placed too far forward, or sickle hocks are present. A perpendicular line from the hip joint would hit the ground at the heel or behind the heel instead of halfway between the heel and toe.

Camped Behind (Fig. 1–31)

Camped behind means that the entire limb is placed too far posteriorly, when viewed from the side. A perpendicular

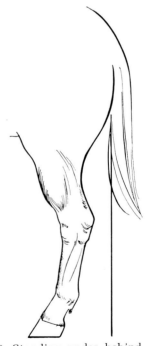

FIG. 1–30. Standing under behind. Compare with Figure 1–25.

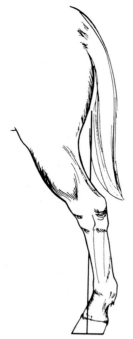

FIG. 1–31. Camped behind. Compare with Figure 1–25.

line dropped from the hip joint would hit at the toe, or in front of it, instead of halfway between the toe and heel. This condition is often associated with upright pasterns behind.

Evaluation of Limb Conformation for Judging Purposes

In judging horses, one must decide when the good qualities exceed the bad or vice versa. Only by understanding the fundamentals of conformation can good judgment be formed in a rapid examination.

When judging one undesirable conformation characteristic of the limbs against another, the following factors should be considered:

Forelimb

1. *Base-Narrow, Toe-Out Conformation.* Base-narrow, toe-out conformation

will consistently cause more locomotion problems than other types of abnormal conformation. The tendency to interfere, resulting in lesions on the medial aspect of the third metacarpal bone, possible fracture of the second metacarpal bone, and occasional fracture of the medial sesamoid bone from trauma by the opposite hoof wall, makes this type of conformation most undesirable.

2. *Base-Wide, Toe-Out Conformation.* This type of conformation also predisposes to interference, but the base-wide foundation keeps the feet farther apart and acts as a mechanical separation. However, the foot still travels inward, and contact often occurs, with the same results as in base-narrow, toe-out conformation. Either of these two types of conformation should be considered less desirable than base-narrow, toe-in conformation.

3. *Base-Narrow, Toe-In Conformation.* Although this type of conformation is not good, it is not as undesirable as the above two types. The foot usually travels in an outward arc (paddling) and causes no contact problems. There is greater stress on lateral ligaments, lateral articulations, and the lateral collateral cartilage of the foot.

4. *Anterior Deviation of the Carpal Joint (Buck Knees).* When slight bilateral anterior deviation of the carpal joints occurs, it is usually the result of contraction of the carpal flexors as a foal. If the condition is slight, it causes only minor stresses on the limbs. If the deviation is marked, it is quite undesirable because of the stresses described above. Unilateral anterior deviation is objectionable because of probable pathologic changes in the limb. Slight bilateral anterior deviation of the carpal joints is not so undesirable as posterior deviation (calf knees) of the carpal joints.

5. *Posterior Deviation of the Carpal Joints (Calf Knees).* This is a poor type of conformation because of the tendency to

produce carpal fractures when the limb is stressed. It is more objectionable than slight anterior deviation of the carpal joints (buck knees).

6. *Lateral Deviation of the Metacarpal Bones (Bench Knees).* This type of conformation is undesirable in that it tends to increase the possibility of medial splints. Uneven pressures on the carpal bones also are present.

Hind Limb

1. *Straight Hind Leg.* The straight hind leg predisposes to bog spavin and upward fixation of the patella. Straight hind legs are somewhat less objectionable than sickle hocks.

2. *Sickle Hocks.* Sickle hocks are thought to predispose to bone spavin. In addition, curb may result from stress on the plantar ligament caused by the excessive angulation of the hock. Sickle hocks are usually accompanied by cow hocks and together constitute the most undesirable conformation of the hind limbs.

3. *Cow Hocks.* Cow hocks are usually present to some degree in most horses; when mild and unaccompanied by other undesirable conditions, they do not constitute a serious problem. When the condition is excessive, it should be considered undesirable, and when both cow hocks and sickle hocks are present, the conformation should be considered very undesirable.

CONFORMATION OF THE FOOT

Good conformation of the foot is essential to normal activities of the horse. No matter how good the conformation of other areas, if the foot is weak, the horse is not a useful animal. This fact, perhaps, gives rise to the adage: "No frog, no foot—no foot, no horse." To have good foot conformation, a horse must have rea-sonably good limb conformation, since the foot reflects poor conformation of the limbs.

Much variation in quality of structure exists in the feet of horses. Ideally, the wall should be thick enough to bear the weight of the horse without excessive wear, resistant to drying, be pliable and should have normal growth qualities. The sole should be thick enough to resist bruising and should shed normally. The bars should be well developed, and the frog should be large, strong, and should divide the sole evenly, with its apex pointing directly to the toe of the hoof wall. A hoof wall that contains pigment is preferable to a white hoof wall, since a white hoof wall is subject to drying and cracking and is not as resistant to trauma as a pigmented hoof.

In some breeds of horses—e.g., show stock of the American Saddlebred and Tennessee Walking Horse breeds—the foot is forced into an abnormal conformation. Because of the artificial action that these horses are forced to use, the wall is allowed to grow excessively long. This removes frog pressure, and contraction of the heel results. These horses are subject to tendon injuries, thrush, and contraction of the hoof wall around the third phalanx or "hoof bound." This artificial foot conformation also aggravates basic conformation weaknesses, such as base-wide, toe-out position of the feet, and a high incidence of ringbone and sidebone results. It is very difficult to maintain such horses in a sound condition, since fundamental principles of foot health are violated.

Quarter Horses and Thoroughbreds often have feet that are too small to bear the weight of the animal. This is brought about by selective breeding, and, although it gives the horse a pleasing appearance, it subjects the foot to greater concussion, because the shock is distributed over a smaller area. As a result, such lamenesses as navicular disease are more frequent.

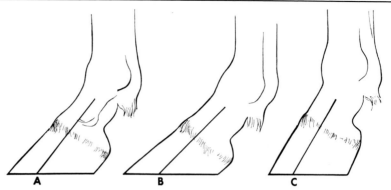

FIG. 1–32. Side view of foot and pastern axis. *A*, Normal front foot and pastern axes (approximately 47 degrees). *B*, Foot and pastern axes less than normal (less than 45 degrees in front or less than 50 degrees behind). *C*, Foot and pastern axes greater than normal (greater than 50 degrees in front or greater than 55 degrees behind).

Foot Axis and Pastern Axis

The pastern axis, as viewed from the front and side, is an imaginary line passing through the center of the pastern. This line should divide the first and second phalanges into equal parts, from both views (Figs. 1–32*A* and 1–33).

The foot axis, as viewed from the side, should be continuous with the pastern axis and should follow the same angle.

The foot axis, as viewed from the front, is an imaginary line passing through the center of the toe of the hoof wall. It extends from the coronary band to the ground surface of the toe and blends

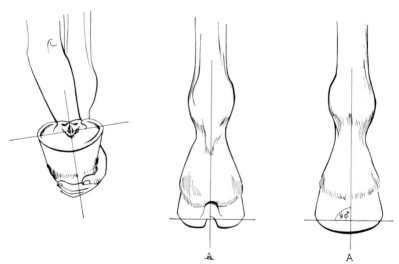

FIG. 1–33. Line *A* shows the foot and pastern axes as viewed from in front and from behind. This line should be straight with no deviation of the limb from the fetlock down. The line crossing the foot axis at the ground surface is a line indicating foot level. If the foot is level, these two lines form 90-degree angles when viewed from in front or behind the foot (*left*). When observing the foot after it has been picked up, an imaginary line should be projected down the foot and pastern; this line should cross another imaginary line on the ground surface of the wall at the quarters. If two 90-degree angles are not formed when these lines are projected, the foot is off level, and proper correction should be made.

above with the pastern axis. The pastern and foot axes are continuous lines from both front and side views, and ideally they should blend at the same angles (Figs. 1–32A and 1–33). The angle formed by the ground surface of the hoof wall and dorsal surface of the toe will be the same angle as the foot axis when viewed from the side. When viewing from the side, the normal foot axis in front should be 45 to 50 degrees; in the hind feet, it should be 50 to 55 degrees. The angle of the hoof can be measured with a foot protractor (Fig. 1–34). The length of hoof wall between the coronary band and the bearing surface can be measured with a caliper at the toe; this length varies among breeds (Fig. 8–7, p. 396).

If the foot and pastern axes are too sloping or too steep, pathological changes may occur. Ideally, the slope of the pastern and the slope of the anterior surface of the hoof wall will be identical when viewed from the side (Fig. 1–32). If the foot and pastern axes are too sloping or too steep, but the angles of the pastern

axis and of the foot axis are identical and appear as a smooth continuous line, the foot should not be trimmed or shod to change these angles (Fig. 1–32B and C). Radical changes to bring the foot and pastern to a theoretically normal axis will usually produce pathological changes (Fig. 1–23). However, if the angle of the pastern and the angle of the hoof wall are not identical, then correction by trimming or shoeing is indicated to make the slope of the pastern and the slope of the hoof wall identical (Fig. 1–35).

The Foot Level

A level foot indicates that the medial and lateral walls are of the same length. To determine foot level, the limb is held so that the ground surface of the foot can be viewed along the longitudinal axis (Fig. 1–36). An imaginary line dividing the longitudinal axis of the cannon bone, fetlock and pastern, crossed by a transverse line that touches the ground surface of each heel should result in two 90-degree angles

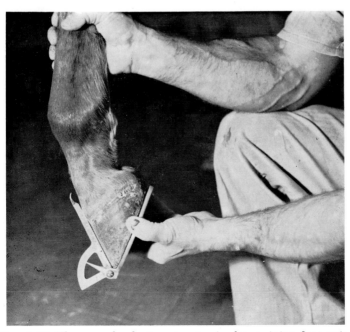

FIG. 1–34. The use of a foot protractor in determining foot axis.

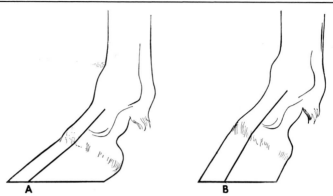

FIG. 1–35. Examples of broken foot and pastern axis. *A,* Broken foot axis with toe too long and heel too low. *B,* Broken foot axis with toe too short and heel too high.

at the junction of these lines (Fig. 1–36). A level foot indicates that the horse is wearing the foot evenly. A horse that lands on the inside wall will have a low inside wall, while a horse that lands on the outside wall will be low on the outside wall. The foot can be flat enough to shoe and yet be off level. Off-level shoeing is a poor method, and foot level should be maintained even if one wall has to be shimmed with leather.

Effect of Foot Conformation on Stride and Way of Going

On the lateral view, the foot should break squarely over the toe, and the flight of the foot should have a normal, even

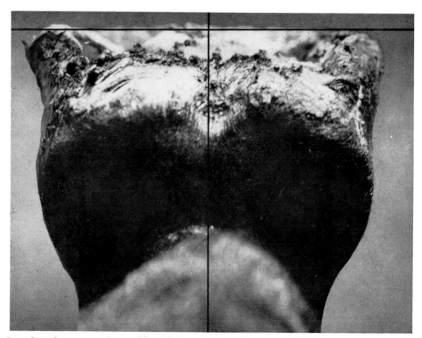

FIG. 1–36. Graphic demonstration of foot level. An imaginary line bisecting the limb longitudinally and a transverse line across the heels should give two 90 degree angles at their intersection. If the transverse line is tilted either way, the foot is off level.

arc, with the horse landing squarely upon the foot. The heels should land just before the toe and the center of weight should be located at the point of the frog. In the normal foot, the hoof reaches the peak of the flight arc as it passes the opposite supporting limb (Fig. 1–37A).

If the horse has a long toe and low heel, this usually means that there is less than a 45-degree angle to the hoof wall (Fig. 1–32B). A long toe will cause the foot to delay the breakover, since it acts as a long leverage point. This delayed breakover causes the foot to reach the peak of the flight arc before it passes the opposite supporting limb (Fig. 1–37B). If this conformation is accompanied by identical angulation of the pastern and of the anterior hoof wall, the horse will usually have a sloping shoulder. Sloping shoulders and pastern usually indicate that the horse will give a smooth ride.

With a long toe and low heel, the center of the weight is anterior to the point of the frog. The added effort required to force the foot to break over the long fulcrum causes the horse to have a long sweeping stride, longer than the stride of a horse with a normal foot axis and normal toe length. The toe is sometimes lengthened on trotting and pacing horses for this increased length of stride. Longer toe length increases the strain on the flexor tendons, suspensory ligament, and proximal sesamoid bones.

When the horse has a short toe and high heel, the foot breaks over quickly and reaches the peak of the flight arc after passing the opposite supporting member (Fig. 1–37C). The foot comes to the ground at a sharp angle and causes a disagreeable ride. A steep foot axis is usually accompanied by a steep angle of the shoulder.

With short toe and high heel, the center

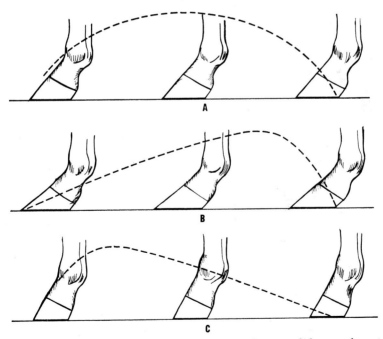

FIG. 1–37. Examples of foot flight. *A*, Flight of a foot with normal foot and pastern axis. The peak of the arc occurs as the foot passes the opposite supporting foot. *B*, Flight of a foot with foot and pastern axis less than normal: long toe, low heel. The peak of the arc occurs before the foot reaches the opposite supporting foot. *C*, Flight of foot with foot axis greater than normal: short toe and high heel. The peak of the arc occurs after the foot passes the opposite supporting foot.

of the weight is posterior to the point of the frog. There is little strain on the flexor tendons or sesamoid bones in this conformation; however, there is increased concussion, which is a factor conducive to ringbone, navicular disease, and traumatic arthritis of the fetlock. The stride of a horse with a short toe and high heel is shorter than that of a normal horse or one with a long toe and short heel.

The center of weight should not be confused with the center of gravity. The center of gravity lies approximately at a crossing of a horizontal line separating the middle from the ventral (inferior) third of the body and a vertical line through the xyphoid cartilage.

The Forefoot (Fig. 1–38)

Ideally, the forefoot should be round and wide in the heels, and the size and shape of the heels should correspond to the size and shape of the toe. The bars should be well developed. The wall should be thickest at the toe and should thin gradually toward the heels; the inside wall should be slightly straighter than the outside wall.

The sole should be slightly concave medial to lateral and anterior to posterior, but an excessive concavity is evidence of a chronic foot disease. There should be no primary contact between the ground and the sole, as it is not a weight-bearing structure.

The foot and pastern axes in the forefoot should be between 45 and 50 degrees. The angle of the heel should correspond to the angle of the toe, and there should be no defects in the wall. The foot should show that the animal is breaking squarely over the center of the toe, and not over the medial or lateral portion of the toe. The wall should show that it is wearing evenly.

The frog should be large and well developed with a good cleft, have normal consistency, elasticity, and show no moisture. It should divide the sole into two nearly equal halves, and the apex should point to the center of the toe. Unequal size of the two halves may indicate a base-wide or base-narrow conformation.

The Hind Foot (Fig. 1–39)

The hind foot should present a more pointed appearance at the toe than does the forefoot. It should show evidence of

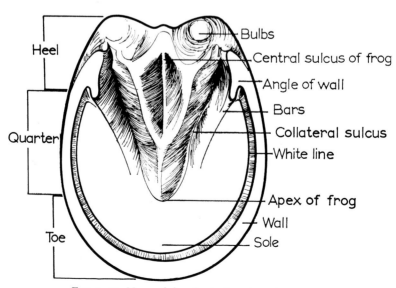

FIG. 1–38. Normal forefoot showing structures.

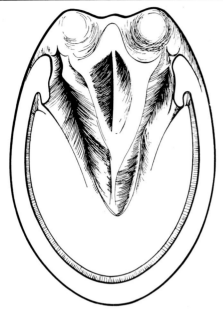

FIG. 1–39. Normal hind foot. Compare with Figure 1–38. The toe of the hind foot is more pointed than that of the forefoot.

breaking straight over the toe, and the frog should divide the sole into equal halves. The foot axis should be 50 to 55 degrees, and there should be no defects in the wall. The walls should show normal wear on the medial and lateral sides, and the sole should be slightly concave medial to lateral and anterior to posterior. The sole of the hind foot is normally more concave than that of the forefoot.

ABNORMAL CONFORMATION OF THE FOOT

Flat Feet

A flat foot lacks the natural concavity in the sole; it is not a normal condition in light horses, but is present in some draft breeds. Flat feet may be heritable and are much more common in the forefeet than in the hind. The horse will often land on the heels in order to avoid sole pressure with this condition. Sole bruising, and the lameness that results, are common se-

quelae of flat feet. No remedy will cure a flat foot, but corrective shoeing can be done to prevent aggravation of the condition. Corrective shoeing is discussed in Chapter 9, page 419.

Dropped Sole or "Pumiced Foot"

When the sole has dropped to, or beyond, the level of the bearing surface of the hoof wall, the condition is called dropped sole (Fig. 6–81, page 252). The sole is flat and has no concavity; in extreme cases it may be convex. Dropped sole is a sequel to chronic laminitis; it is accompanied by heavy rings in the hoof wall that are characteristic of chronic laminitis (Fig. 1–40).

In addition to being flat, the sole in this disorder is very thick and is composed of heavy flakes. Removal of these flakes will usually bring a pink-colored sole in view. This color is produced by proximity to blood. In some cases the accumulation of this flaky sole will harbor an infection similar to thrush that may actually penetrate into the sensitive laminae.

Dropped sole is usually accompanied by a rotation of the third phalanx (Fig. 1–41). It may be found after removal of the excess sole that the tip of the third

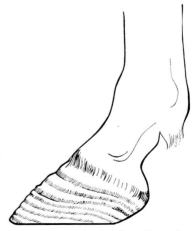

FIG. 1–40. Rings in the hoof wall produced by chronic laminitis.

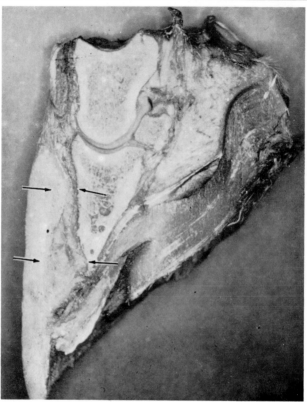

FIG. 1–41. Rotation of the third phalanx. Note the greater distance between the two lower arrows than between the two top arrows. This represents a discrepancy produced by rotation of the third phalanx as a result of chronic laminitis.

phalanx is protruding through the sole. If there is a protrusion of the sole below the wall at the toe, this area should be carefully trimmed to prevent exposure of the third phalanx.

Dropped sole is always a serious condition, and, in most cases, the horse is useless for work on hard surfaces. When the third phalanx has protruded through the sole, or there is infection that has penetrated through the sole, treatment is often useless. Corrective shoeing is discussed in Chapter 9, page 419 (see Laminitis, Chap. 6).

Contracted Foot or Contracted Heels (Fig. 1–42)

Contracted foot is a condition in which the foot is narrower than normal. This is especially true of the posterior half of the foot. This condition is much more common in the front feet than in the hind feet, and it may be unilateral or bilateral. Local or coronary contraction of the foot is a contraction at the heels confined to the horn immediately below that occupied by the coronary cushion. This term merely reflects an arbitrary subdivision of contracted foot.

One should bear in mind that certain breeds of horses normally have a foot that more closely approaches an oval than a circle in form. A narrow foot is not necessarily a contracted foot, and donkeys and mules normally have a foot shape that would be called contracted on a horse. Foot contraction is often present in the Tennessee Walking Horse and American Saddlebred when these horses are used for show stock; the hoof wall is allowed to grow excessively long, and no frog pressure is present.

Contraction of the foot is always due to lack of frog pressure, which may be induced by improper shoeing and by shoeing a horse unnecessarily, preventing contact of the frog with the ground. Lameness in the limb from any cause can prevent the horse from pressing the foot firmly to the ground, and this also results in foot contraction from lack of frog pressure. It is also possible that heredity plays a part in some cases of contracted feet. Excessive dryness of the foot, especially in those horses that have been confined in moist pastures and then moved to a dry lot, may predispose the animal to contraction of the foot in hot weather.

True contraction of the foot should be considered pathological in all cases. It may take a year or more to overcome contraction of the foot or heels that may have resulted from one or two months of disuse.

Foot contraction is usually accompanied by a "dished sole," or an increased concavity of the sole, both anterior to posterior and medial to lateral. If the hoof wall contracts sufficiently around the heels, it may press so firmly against the third phalanx that lameness results. This lameness is called a "hoof-bound" condition.

The diagnosis is based on the appearance of the foot, which shows narrowing, especially at the heel, and the frog is recessed and atrophied. The feet should be compared with one another to determine contraction, but keep in mind that conditions such as bilateral navicular disease or poor shoeing will cause contraction of both forefeet.

The most important factor in diagnosis of this condition is determination of the cause. Contraction can be produced by improper shoeing over a period of time, in which case lameness is usually not present. If lameness is present, though, the

cause should be determined and corrected so that frog pressure can be re-established, since the frog will be small and obviously not in contact with the ground. In severe cases the bars may actually touch each other. Thrush may be present in the atrophied frog. Long-continued disuse of the foot will cause the wall, sole, and frog to become hard and dry, and trimming is difficult.

In long-standing cases of contraction of the foot the os pedis may become deformed and lose its circular shape. The digital cushion will atrophy and become less resilient. This neutralizes the protective action of the digital cushion in the area of the deep flexor tendon and navicular bone and could conceivably aid in the production of navicular disease. The coronary cushion is affected in the same manner. Corrective shoeing is discussed on page 410.

Unilateral Contracted Foot

In some horses, a unilateral contraction of one forefoot is present. This is often

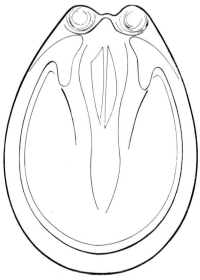

FIG. 1–42. Contracted foot. Note narrowing of the heels and quarters. Compare with Figure 1–38.

congenital, and it is not known whether there is an inheritable tendency for this abnormality. The contracted foot may or may not eventually show lameness, but it should be regarded as an undesirable feature.

Brittle Feet

Brittle feet are usually associated with dryness of the atmosphere and lack of moisture in the soil, and are more apt to occur in unpigmented or white feet. Complications of toe or quarter cracks and fractures of the wall resulting from brittleness may occur. Brittleness requires almost daily treatment with a nondrying agent such as lanolin, fish oils, pine tar, olive oil, or a good proprietary hoof dressing. Shoeing may be required to prevent fractures of the hoof wall. Feeding gelatine may improve the quality of the hoof wall.

Bull-Nosed Foot (Fig. 1-43)

A foot that has been rasped down in front to fit the shoe is called a bull-nosed foot. If an animal is continually shod in this fashion, pathological changes often result.

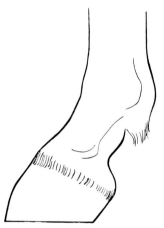

FIG. 1-43. Bull-nosed foot.

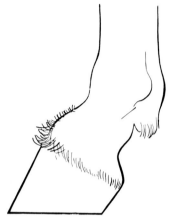

FIG. 1-44. Buttress foot.

Buttress Foot (Figs. 1-44, 6-69 and 6-70, page 239)

Buttress foot is an exostosis on the extensor process of the third phalanx. This exostosis may be a low ringbone or the result of a fracture of the extensor process of the third phalanx (Fig. 1-45). A swelling on the anterior surface of the hoof wall at the coronary band results. A squaring of the toe from the coronary band to the ground surface, a result of deformed hoof growth, is caused by chronic inflammation. Corrective shoeing for this condition is discussed in Chapter 9, page 412.

Rings in the Wall of the Foot

Some rings are normal and indicate changes of seasons or planes of nutrition. Laminitis is the most common cause of pathological rings (Fig. 1-40). Large, single rings may be the result of a past febrile reaction to a systemic disease such as pneumonia, but blistering of the coronary band with iodine or other preparations will also produce lines in the foot. Wavy lines on the heels and quarters may indicate a chronic foot disease. Low ringbone may also produce rings in the foot. Dietary changes, inflammatory processes of the foot or coronary band, and systemic rise of temperature over a period of several days may also produce lines in the hoof wall. No treatment is indicated for the lines alone, although the hoof is sometimes dressed to eliminate them. However, this removes the protective outer layer and makes the wall more subject to drying.

Thin Wall and Sole

Thin walls and sole accompany one another and are inheritable. The conformation of the foot may appear to be normal, but the hoof wall either wears away too rapidly or does not grow fast enough to avoid sole pressure. This condition is especially noticeable at the heels, where the foot axis may be broken by the tendency of the heel to be too low (Fig. 1-35A).

The sole is easily bruised and lameness is common following hoof trimming. Examination of the sole with a hoof tester may show it to be easily compressible and very thin. Flinching over bruised areas results when the sole is compressed by the hoof tester.

Treatment includes making the hoof wall grow more rapidly and proper shoeing to prevent excessive wear. Mild irritants, such as tincture of iodine, used on the coronary band may stimulate growth of the wall. If the horse is allowed to go unshod, as much wall as possible should be left. Seldom will the wall ever become too long, since it wears too rapidly. Occasionally, shoe pads of leather or neolite are necessary to prevent lameness resulting from sole bruising. Building up the heels with leather shims under the shoe may be necessary to re-establish proper foot axis.

A horse's foot may be toughened by turning him onto rough ground unshod. Over a period of time the foot will become more resistant to injury even though it has a thin wall and sole. Six months' time on rough ground will greatly increase the resistance of the foot to lame-

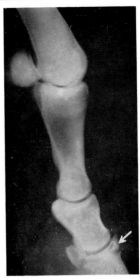

FIG. 1-45. Fracture of the extensor process of the third phalanx (arrow). This fracture cannot be seen on the anteroposterior view. (Carlson, *Veterinary Radiology*, Lea & Febiger.)

ness from bruising and breaking of the hoof wall. Feeding gelatine may improve the quality of the hoof wall.

Club Foot

A club foot is one that has a foot axis of 60 degrees or more. When club foot is unilateral, it is due to some injury that has prevented proper use of the foot. When it is bilateral, it may be inheritable or due to nutritional deficiency. The condition is accompanied by contraction of the superficial digital flexor tendon, and occasionally the deep flexor and suspensory ligament are shortened. When a horse is immature, nutritional deficiencies can cause club feet. Injury causes club foot by disuse contraction of the tendons.

Horses affected with club feet are usually unfit for saddle use because of an undesirable, rough gait. Stumbling may occur in these cases due to contraction of the superficial digital flexor tendon. Nutritional causes should be corrected, as discussed in the section on nutritional deficiencies of foals (Chap. 5). If the condition is thought to be inheritable, the brood stock should be considered unfit for breeding.

Coon-Footed (Fig. 1–46)

The pastern of the coon-footed horse slopes more than does the anterior surface of the hoof wall. In other words, the foot and pastern axis is broken at the coronary band. It may occur in either the fore or hind feet, and it causes strain on the flexor tendons, sesamoid bones, and distal sesamoid ligaments. There may also be strain on the common digital extensor tendon. Very little can be done for correction, except to modify the angle of the foot by trimming the heel as much as possible, while still retaining normal foot axis. The foot axis should not be trimmed to below 45 degrees.

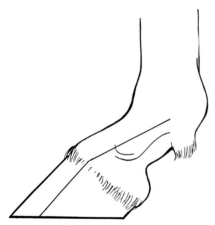

Fig. 1–46. Broken angle between hoof and pastern axis—(coon-footed). The foot axis is steeper than the pastern axis.

REFERENCES

Axe, J. W. 1906. The Horse in Health and Disease. Vol. I and II. London: Gresham Publishing Co.

Beeman, G. M. 1972. Conformation. Part 1. Amer. Quarter Horse J. 25(3): 82–128.

Beeman, G. M. 1973. Conformation. Part 2. Amer. Quarter Horse J. 25(4): 46–88.

Britton, John W. 1961. Conformation and lameness. Calif. Thoroughbred 33(6): 502.

Churchill, E. A. 1968. Lameness in the standardbred, p. 794. In Care and Training of the Trotter and Pacer. Columbus, Ohio: U.S. Trotting Association.

Davidson, A. H. 1970. Some relationships of conformation to lameness and the evaluation of potential. Proc. 16th Ann. AAEP, pp. 399–404.

Goldschmidt, S. G. 1933. An Eye for a Horse. New York: Chas. Scribner and Sons.

Haughton, W. R. 1968. Selecting the yearling, p. 74. In Care and Training of the Trotter and Pacer. Columbus, Ohio: U.S. Trotting Association.

Knezevic, P. 1966. Measuring of strain in the hoof capsule of the horse. Proc. AAEP, pp. 293–295.

McKillip, M. H. 1918–1919. Lameness, consideration of predisposing causes as an aid in diagnosis. Amer. J. Vet. Med. 14: 270.

Russell, W. 1907. Scientific Horseshoeing. 10th ed. Cincinnati: C. J. Krenbiel & Co.

Pritchard, C. C. 1965. Relationships between conformation and lameness in the equine foot. Auburn Vet. 22(1): 11–14.

Simpson, J. F., Sr. 1968. The theory of shoeing and balancing, p. 292. In Care and Training of the Trotter and Pacer. Columbus, Ohio: U.S. Trotting Association.

Smith, F. 1921. A Manual of Veterinary Physiology. 5th ed. Chicago: Alex Eger and Co., Inc.

Stump, J. E. 1967. Anatomy of the normal equine foot, including microscopic features of the laminar region. JAVMA 151(12): 1588–1598.

Taylor, A. M., et. al. 1966. Action of certain joints in the legs of the horse measured electrogoniometrically. Amer. J. Vet. Res. 27(116): 85–89.

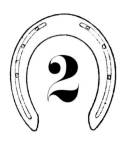

Anatomy and Physiology of the Foot

ANATOMY OF THE FOOT

By definition, the foot of the horse includes the hoof and all structures contained therein, including the sole and frog. The hoof is only the cornified epidermis of the foot (wall, sole, and frog), is non-vascular in structure, and has no nerve supply. Nutrition for the hoof is obtained from the combined coria. The hoof is composed of the following structures:

The Wall (Fig. 1-38, page 26)

The hoof wall is approximately 25 percent water and is a modified cornified epithelium. It is composed of keratinized epithelial cells that are solidly cemented with keratin. The keratinized cells are arranged in tubules that result from their formation by the papillae of the coronary corium. These tubules run perpendicularly from the coronary band to the ground surface of the wall and parallel one another. The center of the tubule is composed of keratin and dead cells.

The hoof wall is a cornified epidermis and is composed of three layers:

a. The first or outer layer is the periople and stratum tectorium. The periople extends about three fourths of an inch below the coronary band, except at the heels, where it caps the bulbs of the heels. The stratum tectorium is a thin layer of horny scales that gives the glossy appearance to the outside of the wall below the periople. It helps protect the wall from evaporation.

b. The second or middle layer composes the bulk of the hoof wall and is the densest portion of the wall. This is the layer that contains the pigment in pigmented feet.

c. The third or inner layer is the laminar layer that forms the epidermal laminae of the hoof. This laminar layer is concave from side to side and bears about 600 thin primary laminae. Each of these primary laminae bears 100 or more secondary laminae on its surface. These laminae intermesh with the dermal laminae covering the dorsum of the third phalanx and firmly attach the hoof wall to the third phalanx. These combined laminae bear much of the weight of the horse.

The ground surface of the hoof wall is divided into areas called the toe, quarters, and heel (see Fig. 1-38). Growth of the wall is quite slow: it grows approximately $\frac{1}{4}$ inch per month, and it normally takes from nine to twelve months for the toe of the hoof wall to grow out. The wall grows more slowly in cold winter months and in cold climates. Slower growth also is apparent in dry weather when adequate moisture is not present in the wall. The hoof wall grows evenly below the coronary band so that the youngest portion of the wall is at the heel (Fig. 2-1). Since this is the youngest wall, it is also the most

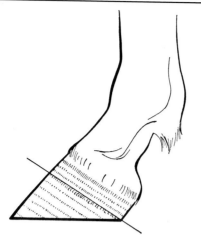

FIG. 2-1. Diagram illustrating the method of hoof wall growth. This demonstrates that the youngest hoof wall is at the heel.

elastic, which aids in heel expansion during movement. The wall is thickest at the toe and gradually reduces in thickness so that the thinnest portion of the wall is at the heels; however, it thickens slightly at the angles where the bars are formed. This junction of the wall and bar is commonly called the "buttress" of the foot.

The Bars (Fig. 1-38)

At the heels the wall turns anteriorly to form the bars that converge toward one another and parallel the collateral sulci of the frog. The sole conforms to the inner curvature of the wall and to the angles formed by the wall and the bar.

The Sole (Fig. 1-38)

The sole, comprising most of the ground surface of the hoof, is approximately 33 percent water. The structure is similar to that of the wall, and the tubules run vertically as formed by the papillae of the sole corium. These tubules curl near the ground surface, which accounts for the self-limiting growth of the sole and causes shedding. The sole should not bear weight from the ground surface, but it is designed

to bear internal weight. If the sole is allowed to contact the terrain, lameness will often develop from sole bruising. That portion of the sole that conforms to the angle formed by the wall and bars is called the angle of the sole. It is in this area that corns usually develop (Chapter 6, p. 283).

The Frog (Fig. 1-38)

The frog is a wedge-shaped mass that occupies the angles bounded by the bars and the sole. It is quite soft because it is approximately 50 percent water. The frog is divided into (1) apex—which is the anterior angle of the frog; (2) base—which is the posterior aspect; and (3) frog stay—which is the central ridge of the internal surface (Fig. 2-2).

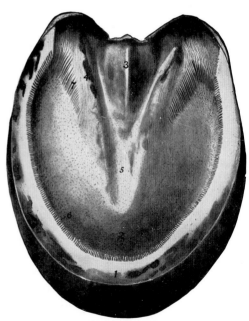

FIG. 2-2. Section of hoof of horse. The section is cut just above the ridges of the frog and bars parallel with the ground surface. 1, Wall; 2, sole; 3, spine of frog or "frog-stay"; 4, ridge formed by junction of frog and bar; 5, central furrow over apex of frog; 6, laminae of wall; 7, laminae of bar. (Sisson and Grossman, *Anatomy of Domestic Animals*, courtesy of W. B. Saunders Company.)

WEIGHT-BEARING STRUCTURES
OF THE FOOT

The wall, bars, and frog are the weight-bearing structures of the foot. The sole should not bear weight except for a strip about $\frac{1}{4}$ inch wide, or less, inside of the white line (see below). The bars should bear weight and in shoeing should not be removed but lowered only enough to allow fitting of the shoe. The bearing surface of the wall should be level with the frog for even distribution of the weight.

OTHER STRUCTURES
OF THE FOOT

The White Line

This is the junction of the wall and the sole. It is visible as a white line following the circumference of the wall at the junction of the sole and hoof wall (Fig. 1-38). The white line is the junction between the laminae of the wall and the tubules of the sole. It is only as deep as the inner layer of the sole and is not a specially secreted structure.

The Corium or Dermal Layer

The corium is a modified vascular tissue that furnishes nutrition to the hoof. It is divided into five parts, each part nourishing the corresponding part of the hoof.

1. *Perioplic Corium* is a narrow band lying in the perioplic groove above the coronary border of the wall. It is continuous with the corium of the skin and is marked off below by a groove from the coronary corium. It bears fine short papillae that furnish the perioplic structures around the top of the hoof wall.

2. *Coronary Corium* (Fig. 2-3) occupies the coronary groove and, with the perioplic corium, forms the "coronary band." It is composed of villiform papillae on the convex surface. It furnishes the bulk of

nutrition to the hoof wall and is responsible for growth of the wall. It is very vascular, and lacerations cause profuse hemorrhage.

3. *Laminar Corium* is attached to the dorsal surface of the third phalanx by a modified periosteum. It bears primary, secondary, and tertiary dermal laminae that intermesh with the epidermal laminae of the hoof wall (Fig. 2-4). The laminar corium nourishes the dermal laminae, the epidermal laminae of the wall, and the interlaminar horn of the white line.

There is some confusion in the use of the term "sensitive laminae" and "dermal laminae." They are not synonymous. When the horny hoof is removed by maceration, the cornified and uncornified layer of the epidermis separate. The stratum germinativum is left on the dermal laminae, and together they make up the sensitive laminae (Trautman and Febiger, 1962). Therefore, the sensitive laminae comprise the dermal laminae and the stratum germinativum of the epidermal laminae. The insensitive laminae comprise all the layers of the epidermis except the stratum germinativum.

4. *Sole Corium* (Fig. 2-3) is composed of the fine hair-like papillae over the entire inner surface of the sole. The papillae originate from the modified periosteum of the third phalanx that attaches the corium to the third phalanx. These papillae project into cavities in the horny tissues of the sole and furnish nourishment and growth for the sole proper.

5. *Frog Corium* is similar in structure to the sole corium, and furnishes nourishment and growth for the frog. The deep face blends with the digital cushion.

Digital Cushion (Fig. 2-3)

This is a fibroelastic, fatty, pale yellow, relatively avascular, and yielding pyramidal structure containing islands of cartilage in the posterior half of the foot. The primary purpose of this structure is to

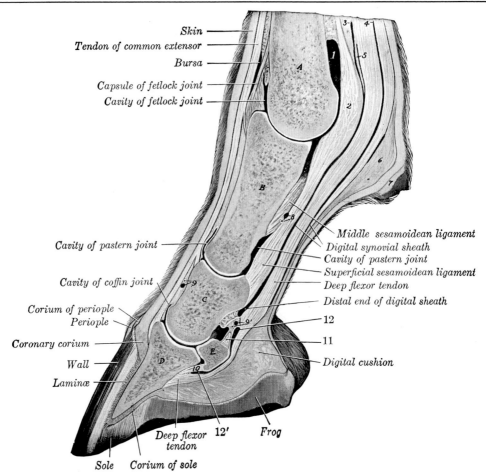

Skin
Tendon of common extensor
Bursa
Capsule of fetlock joint
Cavity of fetlock joint

Cavity of pastern joint

Cavity of coffin joint

Corium of periople
Periople

Coronary corium

Wall

Laminæ

Middle sesamoidean ligament
Digital synovial sheath
Cavity of pastern joint
Superficial sesamoidean ligament
Deep flexor tendon
Distal end of digital sheath
12
11
Digital cushion

Deep flexor 12'
tendon

Frog

Sole   Corium of sole

FIG. 2-3. Sagittal section of digit and distal part of metacarpus of horse. *A*, Metacarpal bone; *B*, first phalanx; *C*, second phalanx; *D*, third phalanx; *E*, distal sesamoid bone. *1*, volar pouch of capsule of fetlock joint; *2*, intersesamoidean ligament; *3,4*, proximal end of digital synovial sheath; *5*, ring formed by superficial flexor tendon; *6*, fibrous tissue underlying ergot; *7*, ergot; *8,9,9'*, branches of digital vessels; *10*, distal ligament of distal sesamoid bone; *11*, suspensory ligament of distal sesamoid bone; *12,12'*, proximal and distal ends of navicular bursa. The superficial flexor tendon (behind *4*) is not marked. (Sisson and Grossman, *Anatomy of Domestic Animals*, courtesy of W. B. Saunders Company.)

reduce concussion to the foot. It is bounded laterally and medially by the cartilages of the third phalanx, below by the frog, and above by the second phalanx and the deep digital flexor tendon. Posteriorly, it is subcutaneous and forms the bulbs of the heels.

Coronary Cushion

The coronary cushion is the elastic portion of the coronary corium; it aids

slightly in reducing concussion. It fits into the groove formed at the proximal part of the hoof wall. The cushion is widest at its center and narrows as it joins the heels. At the proximal aspect of the heels, it blends with the digital cushion.

Lateral Cartilages (Fig. 2-5)

These are part fibrous tissue and part hyaline cartilage. They slope upward and backward from the wings of the third

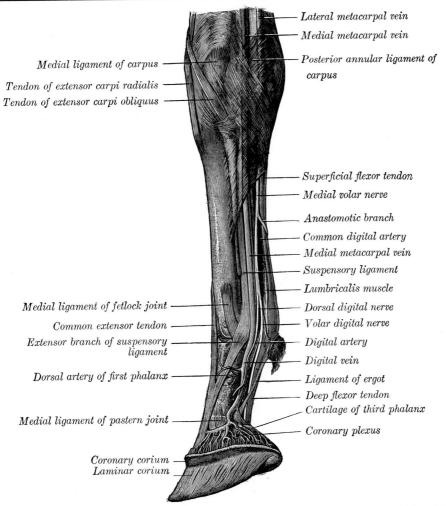

Lateral metacarpal vein
Medial metacarpal vein
Posterior annular ligament of carpus

Medial ligament of carpus
Tendon of extensor carpi radialis
Tendon of extensor carpi obliquus

Superficial flexor tendon
Medial volar nerve
Anastomotic branch
Common digital artery
Medial metacarpal vein
Suspensory ligament
Lumbricalis muscle
Dorsal digital nerve
Volar digital nerve
Digital artery
Digital vein
Ligament of ergot
Deep flexor tendon
Cartilage of third phalanx
Coronary plexus

Medial ligament of fetlock joint
Common extensor tendon
Extensor branch of suspensory ligament
Dorsal artery of first phalanx
Medial ligament of pastern joint

Coronary corium
Laminar corium

FIG. 2–4. Dissection of right carpus, metacarpus, and digit of horse; medial view. (After Schmaltz, *Atlas d. Anat. d. Pferdes*; Sisson and Grossman, *Anatomy of Domestic Animals*, courtesy of W. B. Saunders Company.)

phalanx, and reach above the margin of the coronary band, where they may be palpated. Ossification of these cartilages is called "Sidebones"; *see* Chap. 6, p. 245.

Coronary Band

The coronary band is the combined perioplic corium, coronary corium, and coronary cushion; it is the primary growth and nutritional source for the bulk of the hoof wall. Injuries to this structure are serious and usually leave a permanent defect in the growth of the hoof wall.

Bulbs of the Heel

These are located in the posterior aspect of the foot where the perioplic corium covers the angles of the posterior aspect of the hoof wall. They are supported by the digital cushion.

BLOOD SUPPLY TO THE FOOT
(Figs. 2–4 and 2–6)

The blood supply to the foot is furnished by the medial and lateral digital arteries, which are formed by the bifurca-

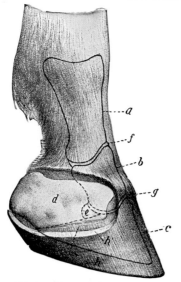

FIG. 2-5. Digit of horse showing surface relations of bones and joints. The cartilage is largely exposed. *a*, First phalanx; *b*, second phalanx; *c*, third phalanx; *d*, cartilage; *e*, distal sesamoid or navicular bone; *f*, pastern joint; *g*, coffin joint; *h'*, cut edge of wall of hoof (*h*); *i*, laminar corium. (After Ellenberger, in *Leisering's Atlas*; Sisson and Grossman, *Anatomy of Domestic Animals*, courtesy of W. B. Saunders Company.)

tion of the common digital artery in the distal fourth of the metacarpus. The digital arteries diverge and pass over the abaxial surface of the sesamoid bones of the fetlock and descend parallel to the borders of the deep flexor tendon to the volar grooves of the third phalanx. Here the vessels enter the volar foramina of the third phalanx to form the terminal arch (Fig. 2-6). This arch gives off branches through the dorsal surface of the bone that supply the corium of the wall and the sole of the hoof. In the area of the pastern, the vein passes anterior to the artery and the posterior digital nerve just behind the artery.

NERVE SUPPLY
TO THE FOOT (Fig. 2-4)

The nerve supply to the foot is furnished by the medial and lateral palmar (volar) nerves. These nerves bifurcate above the fetlock joint, forming the anterior and posterior digital nerves. Commonly, a third, or middle digital, branch is present.

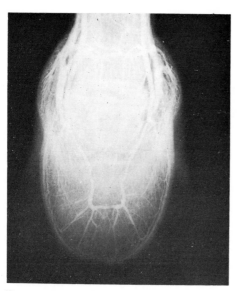

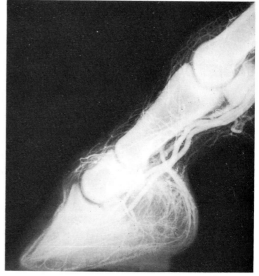

FIG. 2-6. X-ray of circulatory system of equine foot after injection with radiopaque material.

In almost half of the horses examined by me, some variation of the classically described nerve anatomy is present. In many cases, there are small subcutaneous branches arising high on the posterior digital nerve that travel with the ligament of the ergot. If these branches are left following posterior digital neurectomy, sensation is still present in the area of the navicular bursa. This undoubtedly accounts for some of the failures of this operation. Other variations are found, such as the anterior digital branch bifurcating and sending a branch posteriorly that will substitute for the posterior digital nerve (Fig. 2-7). These variations are so common that no definite anatomical description can be given.

STAY APPARATUS

A great deal of confusion seems to exist regarding classification of the stay, check, and reciprocal systems. These have not been classified in older literature, and thus there is no standard. Sisson's (1953) anatomy text mentions the stay system, but discrepancy exists between the description and the drawings. In consulting several anatomists, I found that the use of these terms is far from standardized. Therefore, I have changed the classification that I used in the first edition of this book and have made suggested changes in an attempt to standardize use of these terms. I realize there will be disagreement, but the descriptions used seem to be the most logical, and they reflect the thoughts of many authorities.

The stay apparatus of the limbs as interpreted from Sisson includes the suspensory apparatus of the fetlock joint as well as those structures aiding in supporting the horse while he stands. The stay apparatus supports the limb and fetlock, diminishes concussion, and prevents excessive extension of the fetlock, pastern, and coffin joints.

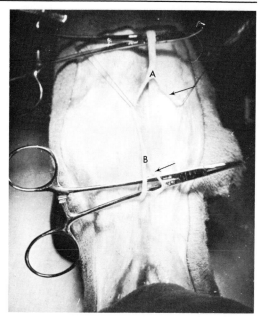

FIG. 2-7. Example of variation of nerve supply to foot. *A,* Normal bifurcation of medial volar nerve into anterior and posterior (upper arrow) digital nerves. *B,* The anterior digital nerve further bifurcates into anterior and posterior (lower arrow) branches. This posterior branch innervates the navicular area and can cause difficulty in diagnosis of navicular disease. This type of branching will cause poor results in posterior digital neurectomy.

Stay Apparatus of the Forelimb
(Figs. 2-8 and 2-9)

Distally

1. *The Intersesamoidean Ligament.* This ligament fills the space between the two sesamoid bones, forms a groove for the flexor tendons, and is more or less molded to their shape.

2. *The Collateral Sesamoidean Ligaments.* These ligaments, lateral and medial, arise on the abaxial surface of each sesamoid bone and pass forward, attaching to the distal end of the third metacarpal bone and to the proximal end of the first phalanx.

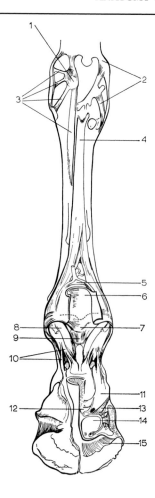

FIG. 2–8. Diagrammatic illustration of some structures in the stay apparatus. Some accessory structures are also shown. *1*, Accessory carpal bone; *2*, medial collateral ligaments of the carpus; *3*, ligaments of the accessory carpal bone; *4*, suspensory ligament; *5*, diverticulum of metacarpophalangeal (fetlock) joint; *6*, volar annular ligament of the fetlock (cut and reflected); *7*, intersesamoidean ligament; *8*, middle or oblique distal sesamoidean ligament; *9*, superficial or straight sesamoidean ligament; *10*, volar ligaments of proximal interphalangeal (pastern) joint; *11*, medial collateral ligament of the pastern joint; *12*, diverticulum of the distal interphalangeal (coffin) joint; *13*, suspensory ligament of the navicular bone; *14*, flexor surface of navicular bone; *15*, insertion of deep digital flexor tendon.

3. *Suspensory Ligament or Interosseous Ligament.* This ligament attaches proximally to the posterior surface of the third metacarpal/metatarsal bone and to the distal row of carpal/tarsal bones. It lies on the posterior surface of the third metacarpal or third metatarsal bone, and divides in the distal one-third of the metacarpus or metatarsus into two branches. These attach to the abaxial surface of the corresponding sesamoid bone, and a portion passes obliquely downward and forward from each sesamoid bone to the dorsal surface of the first phalanx, where they join the common or long digital extensor tendon.

4. *The Distal Sesamoidean Ligaments.* (A) *The superficial sesamoidean ligament* (straight or "Y" sesamoidean ligament) attaches above to the bases of the sesamoid bones and to the intersesamoidean ligament and below to the overhanging lip of the proximal end of the palmar (volar) or plantar surface of the second phalanx. (B) *The middle sesamoidean ligament* (oblique or "V" sesamoidean ligament) attaches to the base of the sesamoid bones and intersesamoidean ligament above and distally on the palmar surface of the first phalanx. (C) *The deep sesamoidean ligament* (cruciate or "X" sesamoidean ligament) consists of two layers of fibers that arise from the base of the sesamoid bones, cross each other, and end on the opposite proximal eminence of the palmar (volar) or plantar aspect of the first phalanx.

5. *Short Sesamoidean Ligaments.* These are short bands that extend from the anterior part of the base of the sesamoid bones and attach to the posterior margin of the articular surface at the proximal end of the first phalanx.

6. *Collateral Ligaments of the Fetlock.* Although not mentioned by Sisson, the collateral ligaments of the fetlock are included because of their common attachment with the collateral sesamoidean ligaments.

Proximally

7. *The Serratus Ventralis Muscle.* This muscle originates on the ribs and attaches to the costal area of the scapula on the facies serrata. The dorso scapular ligament attaches above from the third to the fifth thoracic spines; its lower fibers intersect the scapular fibers of the serratus ventralis muscle and attach to the scapula.

Anteriorly (Cranial)

8. The *biceps brachii* tendon and the extensor carpi radialis tendon (including the lacertus fibrosis tendon from the biceps to the extensor carpi radialis). The *biceps brachii* originates on the tuber scapulii and inserts on (1) the radial tuberosity; (2) the medial ligament of the elbow joint; (3) the fascia of the forearm and the tendon of the extensor carpi radialis. The *extensor carpi radialis* originates on (1) the lateral condyloid crest of the humerus; (2) the coronoid fascia; (3) the deep fascia of the arm and forearm and the intermuscular septum between this muscle and the common extensor. It inserts on the metacarpal tuberosity. It receives a tendon (lacertus fibrosis) from the biceps brachii toward the proximal end of the radius.

Posteriorly (Caudal)

9. *The Long Head of the Triceps Muscle.* This is the largest and longest of the three heads of the triceps. It originates on the posterior border of the scapula and inserts in the lateral and posterior part of the summit of the olecranon.

10. *The Superior or Radial Check Ligament.* This is often termed the radial head of the superficial flexor tendon. It originates on a ridge on the posterior surface of the radius below its center and near the medial border and fuses with the tendon of the superficial digital flexor near the carpal joint.

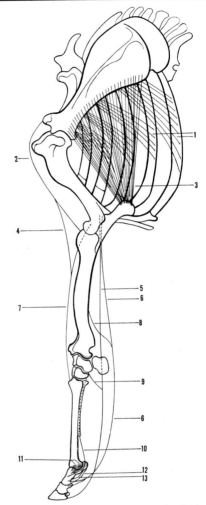

FIG. 2–9. Stay apparatus of forelimb (not all structures are shown). *1,* Fibrous sheet of serratus ventralis; *2,* tendon of biceps brachii; *3,* long head of triceps; *4,* lacertus fibrosus; *5,* deep digital flexor; *6,* superficial digital flexor; *7,* extensor carpi radialis; *8,* proximal (superior) check ligament; *9,* distal (carpal) check ligament; *10,* suspensory ligament; *11,* combined collateral sesamoidean ligament and collateral ligament of fetlock joint; *12,* superficial (straight) distal sesamoidean ligament; *13,* middle (oblique) distal sesamoidean ligament.

11. *The Superficial Flexor Tendon.* This muscle originates on (1) the medial epicondyle of the humerus, (2) a ridge on the posterior surface of the radius below its center and near the medial border. This latter origination is termed the radial head or the radial or superior check ligament. The muscle inserts on the eminences of the proximal extremity of the second phalanx behind the collateral ligaments of the proximal interphalangeal joint and on the distal extremity of the first phalanx also behind the collateral ligaments.

12. *The Inferior (Carpal) Check Ligament.* The carpal check ligament originates as a direct continuation of the posterior ligament of the carpus. It joins the deep flexor tendon at approximately the middle of the third metacarpal bone.

13. *Deep Digital Flexor.* This muscle originates on (1) the medial epicondyle of the humerus, (2) the medial surface of the olecranon, and (3) the middle of the posterior surface of the radius and a small adjacent area of the ulna. It inserts on the semilunar crest of the third phalanx and the adjacent surface of the collateral cartilages of the third phalanx.

Stay Apparatus of the Hind Limb
(Figs. 2–8 and 2–10)

In the hind limb, the stay apparatus comprises structures 1 through 6 listed for the stay system of the forelimb, as well as the following:

7. *Tensor Fascia Lata.* This muscle originates at the tuber coxae and inserts on the fascia lata and thus indirectly to the patella, the lateral patellar ligament, and the crest of the tibia.

8. *The Gastrocnemius Muscle.* This muscle originates by two heads: the lateral head from the lateral supracondyloid crest of the femur and the medial head from the medial supracondyloid crest of the femur. It inserts on the posterior part of the tuber calcis in conjunction with the

superficial digital flexor tendon. It is included here because of its close association with the superficial digital flexor.

9. *The Peroneus Tertius Muscle.* This muscle is primarily tendinous and originates in the extensor fossa of the femur. It divides before insertion into dorsal (cranial) and lateral branches. The dorsal branch inserts on the proximal extremity of the third metatarsal bone, and the lateral branch inserts on the fibular and third and fourth tarsal bones laterally.

10. *The Deep Digital Flexor.* The origin of this muscle actually has three heads, which unite into a common tendon. It originates on (1) the posterior edge of the lateral condyle of the tibia, (2) the border of the lateral condyle of the tibia just behind the facet for the fibula, and (3) the middle third of the posterior surface and upper part of the lateral border of the tibia, the posterior border of the fibula, and the interosseous ligament. It inserts on the semilunar crest of the third phalanx and the adjacent surface of the collateral cartilages.

11. *The Tarsal Check Ligament.* Tarsal check ligament originates from the posterior ligamentous tissue of the hock and joins the tendon of the deep digital flexor just below the hock joint.

12. *Superficial Digital Flexor.* This muscle originates in the supracondyloid fossa of the femur and inserts on (1) the tuber calcis and (2) the eminences on each side of the proximal extremity of the second phalanx and the distal extremity of the first phalanx behind the collateral ligaments of the pastern joint.

CHECK APPARATUS

The check apparatus will be defined in this text as that part of the stay apparatus involving the check (accessory) ligaments. This includes the superior (radial) and inferior (carpal) check ligaments and the superficial and deep flexor tendons in the forelimb. In the hind limb the check apparatus includes the tarsal (inferior) check ligament and the superficial and deep digital flexor tendons. These structures aid in supporting the palmar (volar) surface of the forelimb and the plantar surface of the hind limb. However, in the hind limb, only the tarsal (inferior) ligament is present.

SUSPENSORY APPARATUS OF THE FETLOCK (Fig. 2–8)

The suspensory apparatus of the fetlock joint is that portion of the stay apparatus that supports the fetlock (metacarpophalangeal) joint and prevents it from dropping to the ground. The support extends from the carpus distally in the forelimb and from the hock distally in the hind limb. The following structures are included in the suspensory apparatus:

The suspensory ligament (interosseous ligament)
Proximal sesamoid bones
The intersesamoidean ligament
The distal sesamoidean ligaments (superficial, middle, deep)
Short sesamoidean ligaments
The superficial and deep flexor tendons. These must be included because of their support to the fetlock joint.

RECIPROCAL APPARATUS OF THE HIND LIMB

The reciprocal apparatus is that portion of the stay apparatus in the hind limb that causes reciprocal movement of the hock and stifle joints. The reciprocal apparatus causes the hock to flex whenever the stifle joint flexes and the stifle to extend when the hock extends, provided all structures are normal. The action is strictly mechanical and can be changed only if one of the reciprocal structures is ruptured. This apparatus also aids in preventing fatigue in the standing position. Structures that compose the reciprocal apparatus of the hind limb are as follows:

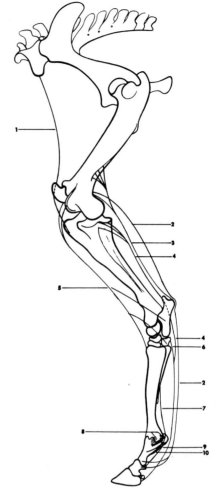

Fig. 2–10. Stay apparatus of hind limb (not all structures are shown). *1,* Tensor fascia lata; *2,* superficial digital flexor; *3,* gastrocnemius; *4,* deep digital flexor; *5,* peroneus tertius; *6,* tarsal (inferior) check ligament; *7,* suspensory ligament; *8,* combined collateral sesamoidean ligament and collateral ligament of fetlock joint; *9,* superficial (straight) distal sesamoidean ligament; *10,* middle (oblique) distal sesamoidean ligament.

Anteriorly

Peroneus Tertius Muscle. This muscle is entirely tendinous in structure. It originates in the extensor fossa of the femur, and inserts on the anterior surface of the proximal extremity of the third metatarsal bone, the third tarsal bone, and on the fibular and fourth tarsal bones. Occasionally this muscle is ruptured after exertion. This results in inability of the hock to flex normally when the stifle joint is flexed (see Rupture of the Peroneus Tertius, Chap. 6, p. 317).

Posteriorly

1. *Superficial Digital Flexor Tendon.* This muscle lies between and under cover of the two heads of the gastrocnemius in its proximal part. It consists almost entirely of a strong tendon. It inserts on the tuber calcis as well as the distal extremity of the first phalanx and proximal extremity of the second phalanx. The fact that it inserts at the tuber calcis causes a reciprocal action with the peroneus tertius muscle. At its origin, and again near its tarsal insertion, the muscle is intimately associated with the gastrocnemius muscle.

2. *Gastrocnemius Tendon.* Although this muscle is not ordinarily classified as a portion of the reciprocal apparatus, it must be considered because of its close attachment to the superficial flexor. Rup-

ture of the gastrocnemius causes the hock to drop. If both are cut, the hock joint will drop to the ground. The combined tendons above the hock are known as the Achilles tendon.

PHYSIOLOGY OF MOTION

Concussion

In a fast gait there is tremendous concussion exerted upon the limbs of the horse. The forelimbs of the horse bear 60 to 65 percent of the body weight and thus are subjected to greater concussion and to a greater incidence of lameness. In the Standardbred, using the trotting and pacing gaits, there is a more balanced concussion to the fore and hind limbs which nearly equalize the incidence of lamenesses. Concussion to the foot and limb is produced by the weight of the horse and the counterpressure of the earth. A second strain occurs when the limbs leave the ground. This is the compression of propulsion.

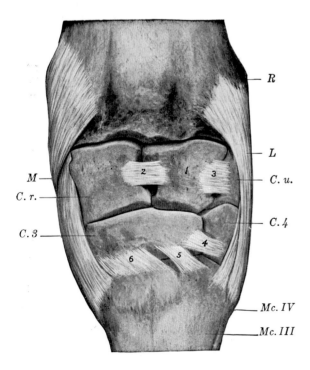

FIG. 2-11. Left carpal joints of horse; dorsal view. The joint capsule is removed. R, Lateral distal tuberosity of radius; M, medial ligament; L, lateral ligament; C.r., radial carpal bone; C.u., ulnar carpal bone; C.3., third carpal bone; C.4., fourth carpal bone; McIII, McIV, metacarpal bones; 1, intermediate carpal bone; 2–6, dorsal ligaments. (Sisson and Grossman, *Anatomy of Domestic Animals*, courtesy of W. B. Saunders Company.)

The construction of the limbs and feet are such that concussion is countered in numerous ways.

The Carpal Joint (Fig. 2-11)

The carpal joint is composed of three main joints and numerous ligaments. The radiocarpal and intercarpal joints have the greatest range of movement, while the carpometacarpal joint has very little motion. There is more movement of the seven or eight carpal bones during motion than there is in the tarsal bones. The carpal bones can move in three planes, which greatly diminishes concussion. The carpal

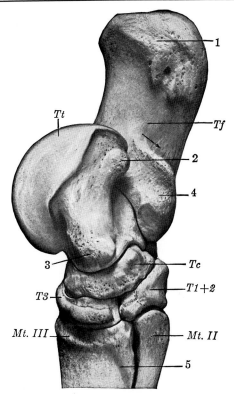

FIG. 2-13. Right tarsus and proximal part of metatarsus of horse; medial view. *Tt*, Tibial tarsal (trochlea); *Tf*, fibular tarsal; *Tc*, central tarsal; *T1 + 2*, fused first and second tarsals (dotted line indicates division between two elements); *T3*, third tarsal; *1*, tuber calcis; *2,3*, proximal and distal tuberosities of tibial tarsal; *4*, sustentaculum; *5*, groove for great metatarsal vein; *Mt. II, Mt. III*, metatarsal bones. Arrow indicates course of the deep flexor tendon in tarsal groove. (Sisson and Grossman, *Anatomy of Domestic Animals*, courtesy of W. B. Saunders Company.)

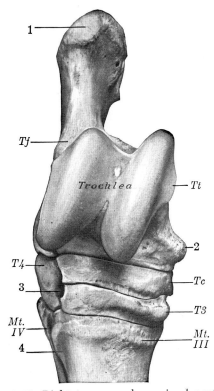

FIG. 2-12. Right tarsus and proximal part of metatarsus of horse; anterior or dorsal view. *Tt*, tibial tarsal bone; *Tf*, fibular tarsal; *Tc*, central tarsal; *T3*, third tarsal; *T4*, fourth tarsal; *1*, tuber calcis; *2*, distal tuberosity of tibial tarsal; *3*, vascular canal; *4*, groove for great metatarsal artery; *Mt. III, Mt. IV*, metatarsal bones. (Sisson and Grossman, *Anatomy of Domestic Animals*, courtesy of W. B. Saunders Company.)

bones themselves are bound together by a complex series of ligaments. Injury to this ligamentous structure is common and occurs predominantly over the radial, intermediate, and third carpal bones.

The Tarsal (Hock) Joint
(Figs. 2-12, 2-13, and 2-14)

The hock joint, as the carpus, is composed of numerous bones; however, there is not the degree of motion in these six

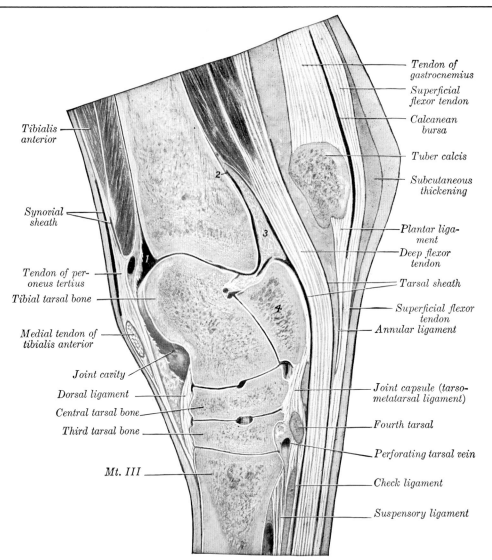

Tibialis anterior

Synovial sheath

Tendon of per- oneus tertius

Tibial tarsal bone

Medial tendon of tibialis anterior

Joint cavity

Dorsal ligament

Central tarsal bone

Third tarsal bone

Mt. III

Tendon of gastrocnemius

Superficial flexor tendon

Calcanean bursa

Tuber calcis

Subcutaneous thickening

Plantar liga- ment

Deep flexor tendon

Tarsal sheath

Superficial flexor tendon

Annular ligament

Joint capsule (tarso- metatarsal ligament)

Fourth tarsal

Perforating tarsal vein

Check ligament

Suspensory ligament

FIG. 2–14. Sagittal section of right hock of horse. The section passes through the middle of the groove of the trochlea of the tibial tarsal bone. *1,2,* Proximal ends of cavity of hock joint; *3,* thick part of joint capsule over which deep flexor tendon plays; *4,* fibular tarsal bone (sustentacu- lum). A large vein crosses the upper part of the joint capsule (in front of 1). (Sisson and Grossman, *Anatomy of Domestic Animals,* courtesy of W. B. Saunders Company.)

bones that there is in the carpal bones. The partial flexion of the hock joint at all times aids in diminishing concussion.

The oblique ridges in the tibial tarsal bone of the horse cause some differences in the action of the hock when compared with other animals in which the ridges are usually straight. As the body weight

passes over the hind limb, it is not un- common to observe a considerable out- ward twist of the hock joint in some horses. At the same time, the stifle joint and the toe turn in. This effect is due to the ascent of the lower end of the tibia on the oblique ridges of the tibial tarsal bone. During flexion, the oblique setting of the ridges on the tibial tarsal bone apparently aids in turning the stifle joint outward, which allows clearance past the posterior ribs.

The Femorotibial (Stifle) Joint
(Figs. 2-15 and 2-16)

The stifle joint is the largest in the body. One function of this joint is to cause the limb to become rigid when the foot is on the ground. This is done by the contraction of the muscles inserted into the patella. The first joints flexed in advancing the hind limb are the coffin, pastern, and fetlock joints. In upward fixation of the patella where no flexion of the stifle and hock can occur, these lower joints can still be flexed (Fig. 6-120). The semiflexed position of the stifle joint aids in decreasing concussion.

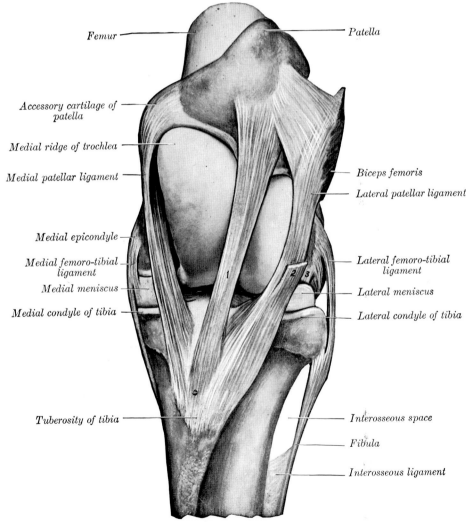

Femur

Patella

Accessory cartilage of patella

Medial ridge of trochlea

Medial patellar ligament

Biceps femoris

Lateral patellar ligament

Medial epicondyle

Medial femoro-tibial ligament

Medial meniscus

Medial condyle of tibia

Lateral femoro-tibial ligament

Lateral meniscus

Lateral condyle of tibia

Tuberosity of tibia

Interosseous space

Fibula

Interosseous ligament

FIG. 2-15. Left stifle joint of horse; front view. The capsules are removed. *1*, Middle patellar ligament; *2*, stump of fascia lata; *3*, stump of common tendon of extensor longus and peroneus tertius. (Sisson and Grossman, *Anatomy of Domestic Animals*, courtesy of W. B. Saunders Company.)

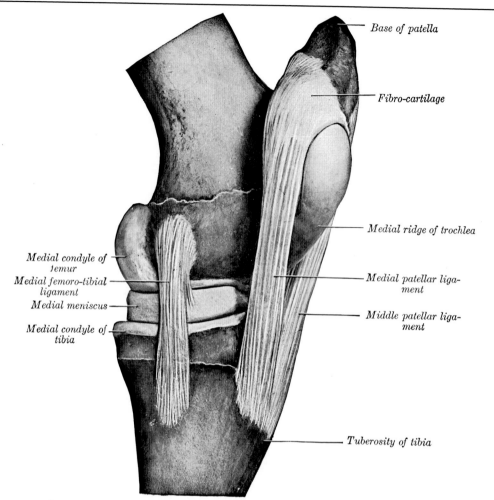

Base of patella

Fibro-cartilage

Medial ridge of trochlea

Medial condyle of femur

Medial femoro-tibial ligament

Medial meniscus

Medial condyle of tibia

Medial patellar ligament

Middle patellar ligament

Tuberosity of tibia

FIG. 2–16. Left stifle joint of horse; medial view. The capsules are removed. (Sisson and Grossman, *Anatomy of Domestic Animals,* courtesy of W. B. Saunders Company.)

The Metacarpophalangeal (Fetlock) Joint (Figs. 2–3 and 2–17)

The fetlock joint has a great degree of anticoncussive action. The stay apparatus changes the direction of concussion and weight distribution. In other words, weight is partially directed anteriorly from the distal end of the cannon bone instead of entirely straight down. The joint is supported by the suspensory apparatus of the fetlock.

The posterior cul-de-sac of the fetlock joint capsule is so constructed as to allow a great degree of motion. Of all joints, the fetlock is subjected to the greatest stress, and at times the entire body weight may be pressed upon one fetlock joint.

The suspensory ligament has slight elastic properties. Histologically, it contains some muscular fibers, and some regard it as a modified muscle (Rooney, 1969). The suspensory ligament, sesamoid bones, and the posterior half of the metacarpal phalangeal articulation carry most of the weight of the horse. That portion of the suspensory ligament that joins the common extensor tendon has very little stress on it and is rarely, if ever, injured. If the suspensory ligament is divided, the

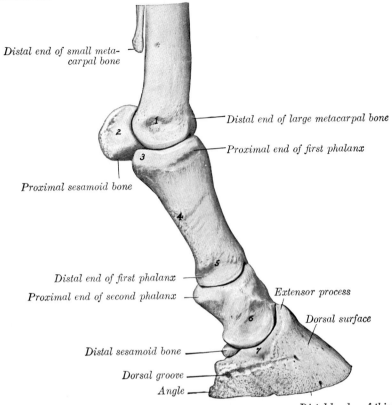

Distal end of small meta-
carpal bone

Distal end of large metacarpal bone

Proximal end of first phalanx

Proximal sesamoid bone

Distal end of first phalanx
Proximal end of second phalanx

Extensor process

Dorsal surface

Distal sesamoid bone

Dorsal groove
Angle

Distal border of third phalanx

Fig. 2-17. Skeleton of digit and distal part of metacarpus of horse; lateral view. *1-7*, Eminences and depressions for attachment of ligaments. Cartilage of third phalanx is removed. (Sisson and Grossman, *Anatomy of Domestic Animals,* courtesy of W. B. Saunders Company.)

fetlock sinks but does not come to the ground. If the superficial flexor tendon is cut, a slight sinking of the fetlock occurs. To bring the fetlock completely to the ground, both flexors must be divided, as well as the suspensory ligament. This shows that all three structures support the fetlock joint.

The suspensory ligament is subjected to a great deal of the initial shock when the foot lands (Figs. 2-18 and 1-22). It is commonly injured at the same time the superficial or deep flexor tendons are damaged. In some cases, it is injured in only one branch, and this may occur during the initial shock of landing (Rooney, 1969). The suspensory ligament is also capable of contraction resulting from disuse. New-

born foals with contracted deep and superficial flexor tendons also often have contraction of the suspensory ligament. Before tenotomy is done to the superficial or deep digital flexor tendons, the foal should be closely checked for contraction of the suspensory ligament. In some cases, this contraction is so severe that the limb cannot be pulled into normal position even after tenotomy of the superficial and deep flexor tendons.

The Proximal Interphalangeal (Pastern) Joint (Figs. 2-3 and 2-17)

This is the least movable of the phalangeal joints. There is a minimal amount of anticoncussion activity at this joint, and

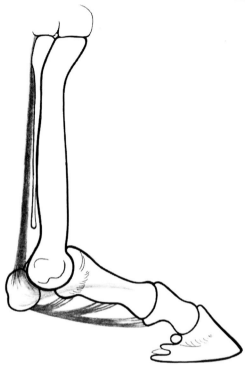

FIG. 2–18. Schematic example of fetlock joint in overflexed position. At this point, chip fracture of the proximal end of the first phalanx, injury to the suspensory ligament, sesamoid bones, and the distal sesamoidean ligaments is possible. Tendosynovitis of the superficial and deep flexor tendons (not shown) may also occur. (Courtesy of Dr. W. Berkley.)

it is possible that this renders it more subject to pathological conditions such as ringbone. Because the foot exerts upward and forward propulsion to the body when the foot is leaving the ground, much of the resulting shock is distributed to the pastern joint.

The Distal Interphalangeal (Coffin) Joint (Figs. 2–3 and 2–17)

The coffin joint is composed of the second and third phalanges and the navicular bone (distal sesamoid bone). This joint has a great degree of elasticity and motion, because of the placement of the navicular bone, and considerable anticon-

cussive action. Direct concussion to the coffin joint is averted by the partial distribution of weight from the second phalanx to the navicular bone. From the navicular bone, the weight is then transferred to the third phalanx, which descends slightly because of a yielding of the sensitive and insensitive laminae. The sole also descends slightly from pressure by the third phalanx.

The navicular bone could not withstand great pressures but for the deep flexor tendon supporting it from behind and below. The navicular bursa has a smooth lubricating surface that reduces friction, and the surface of the deep flexor tendon is closely fitted to the surface of the navicular bone.

There is no "pulley" action at the coffin joint because no leverage is gained; there is merely a change in direction of the weight distribution. The greatest pressure between the navicular bone and the deep flexor tendon does not occur when the foot hits the ground, but rather as the body weight passes over the foot. The central ridge of the navicular bone is subjected to greater pressure than any other portion of the bone.

The Laminae (Figs. 2–2 and 2–3)

The laminae help absorb shock, as does blood in the vessels of the foot, which in normal horses is retained as a hydraulic cushion by the outward movement of the cartilages compressing the venous plexus lateral to the cartilages.

The Digital Cushion (Fig. 2–3)

This structure decreases concussion in the foot proper as described below.

The Frog (Figs. 1–38 and 2–2)

The normal resilient qualities of the frog aid in diminishing concussion; in addition, the frog distributes concussion to the digital cushion.

PHYSIOLOGY OF THE FOOT

In the process of evolution, the horse has developed from a multiple-digit to a single-digit animal. This subjects the single digit to great stress. The frog is the foot pad of the horse and is the most elastic structure of the foot. When the foot strikes the ground, the heels expand, aiding in distribution of concussion. The heel normally lands slightly before the toe, and this results in immediate heel expansion due to the action of the frog. As the frog is forced upward, the frog stay (Fig. 2–2) acts as a wedge in the digital cushion. This forces the digital cushion to expand, primarily in an outward direction, because it is confined by structures of the foot in the dorsal, volar, and proximal directions. The frog stay coming up from below naturally limits distal expansion of the digital cushion. Descent of the second phalanx from above may also aid in the expansion of the digital cushion (Rooney, 1969).

The digital cushion expands outward and exerts pressure against the lateral cartilages of the third phalanx. These cartilages are normally elastic and expand outward and backward, thus compressing the veins of the coronary plexus; at the same time, the cartilages act as a pump to force venous blood up the limb. The compression against the veins of the coronary plexus serves the purpose of valves, which are absent in this area. As the foot hits the ground, the blood in the vascular bed of the foot is partially held by the pressure of the lateral cartilages against the coronary plexus. This forms an efficient hydraulic cushion of blood for the third phalanx, which further aids in reduction of concussion.

When the lateral cartilages are affected by disease, i.e., sidebones, and lose elasticity, this function is lost. As a result, a foot affected with sidebones is subjected to greater concussion and to inefficient venous return of blood, which may account for a chronic swelling of the lower limb (stocking) with edema.

If no frog pressure is present, the movement of the digital cushion is downward and outward. Because it can move in a distal direction, it does not expand sufficiently in an outward direction to compress the lateral cartilages and aid in expansion of the foot. This usually causes foot contraction and atrophy of the digital cushion.

GLOSSARY OF TERMS

When reading old texts, one encounters many names for anatomical structures that differ from those cited in modern anatomy books such as Sisson's *Anatomy of Domestic Animals*. Some of these terms are offered below as an aid to the reader.

Modern Name	*Old Name*
BONES OF THE HIND LIMB:	
Hock	
Tibial tarsal bone	Astragalus, talus
Fibular tarsal bone	Calcaneus, os calcis
Central tarsal bone	Cuneiform magnum, scaphoid, navicular
First tarsal bone	Internal cuneiform
Second tarsal bone	Cuneiform parvum, middle cuneiform
Third tarsal bone	Cuneiform medium, external cuneiform
Fourth tarsal bone	Cuboid
Third metatarsal	Great metatarsal, cannon bone
MUSCLES OF THE HIND LIMB:	
Long digital extensor	Extensor pedis, anterior digital extensor
Peroneus tertius	Tendinous part of flexor metatarsi
Tibialis anterior	Tibialis anticus, flexor metatarsi
Deep digital flexor	Flexor perforans
Superficial digital flexor	Flexor perforatus

Modern Name	Old Name
BONES OF THE CARPUS:	
Radial carpal	Scaphoid
Intermediate carpal	Semilunar, lunar
Ulnar carpal	Cuneiform
First carpal	Trapezium
Second carpal	Trapezoid
Third carpal	Os magnum
Fourth carpal	Unciform
Accessory carpal	Pisiform
Splint bones or second and fourth metacarpals	Inner and outer small metacarpal bones

MUSCLES OF THE FORELIMB:	
Biceps brachii	Flexor brachii
Extensor carpi radialis	Extensor carpi magnus
Deep digital flexor	Flexor perforans
Superficial digital flexor	Flexor perforatus

FOOT:	
First phalanx	Os saffragenous, long pastern bone
Second phalanx	Os coronae, short pastern bone
Third phalanx	Os pedis, pedal bone, coffin bone
Navicular bone	Shuttle bone

REFERENCES

AXE, J. W. 1906. The Horse in Health and Disease. Vols. I and II. London: Gresham Publishing Co.

CAMP, C. L., and SMITH, N. 1942. Phylogeny and Functions of the Digital Ligaments of the Horse. Berkeley: University of California Press.

FRANK, E. R. 1959. *Veterinary Surgery*. 6th ed. Minneapolis: Burgess Publishing Co.

KOCH, T. 1940. Termination of the volar nerve in the horse. Vet. Reco. 52(2): 26.

KOVAK, G. 1963. The Equine Tarsus—Topographic and Radiographic Anatomy. Budapest: Publication House of the Hungarian Academy of Sciences.

LAMBERT, F. 1966. Role of moisture in hoof function. Vet Med. Small Anim. Clin. 61(4): 342–347.

ROONEY, J. R. 1969. Biomechanics of Lameness in Horses. Baltimore: Williams and Wilkins Co.

RUSSELL, W. 1907. Scientific Horseshoeing. 10th ed. Cincinnati: C. J. Krehbiel and Co.

SISSON, S. 1953. *Anatomy of Domestic Animals*. 4th ed. Grossman, J. D., ed. Philadelphia: W. B. Saunders Co.

SMITH, F. 1921. A Manual of Veterinary Physiology. 5th ed. Chicago: Alex Eger and Co., Inc.

SMITHCORS, J. F. 1961. The equine leg, Pt. I. Mod. Vet. Pract. 42: Pt. II, 42: 31; Pt. III. 42: 33.

STILLMAN, A. M. 1882. The Horse in Motion. Boston: J. R. Osgood and Co.

STUMP, J. E. 1967. Anatomy of the normal equine foot, including microscopic features of the laminar region. JAVMA 151(12): 1588–1598

TRAUTMAN, A., and FEBIGER, J. 1962. Histology of Domestic Animals. Ithaca, N.Y.: Comstock Publishing Assoc.

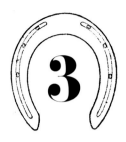

Examination for Soundness

The object of a soundness examination is to determine by examination of the horse his relative commercial value for the service in which he is to be employed. Soundness of the horse might be defined as that state in which there are no deviations from the normal that have resulted in, or that will predispose the animal to, pathological changes that interfere with intended use. This definition is deliberately vague since it must encompass all the purposes for which a horse may be used. Soundness might be subclassified as working soundness and breeding soundness, since a horse that is sound for breeding purposes is not necessarily sound for working, and vice versa. For this reason, all abnormal findings must be recorded during the original examination. Then, if the horse is resold, the veterinarian who made the soundness examination cannot be blamed for not identifying abnormalities that might interfere with a new use of the horse. For example, some minor unsoundnesses would not disqualify a horse for a child's use but would disqualify him for more strenuous work.

To certify a horse as sound implies that he passed both working and breeding soundness examinations. A statement as to soundness of the animal should be preceded by: "At the time of my examination," so that subsequent unsoundness cannot be construed as being present at the original examination.

A working horse must be checked closely for working soundness, and special emphasis must be placed on those qualities needed for the particular use to which the animal will be put. In addition, if there is a possibility that a stallion or mare may be used for breeding purposes, a breeding soundness examination must also be done. However, a stallion or mare may be purchased for breeding purposes and be unsound for work. In such a case, the weaknesses should not be inheritable, result from a conformation that might be inheritable, or be incapacitating.

One should also consider qualities that do not necessarily bear directly on the examination: e.g., the temperament of a horse being purchased for a child should be well suited to that purpose. A bad-tempered horse, even though sound in all other ways, might not pass such an examination. The size of the horse relative to the size of the rider should also be considered.

The American Association of Equine Practitioners is developing a standardized soundness examination form that will be helpful in performing soundness examinations (Flynn, 1969; Reid, 1969).

Insurance examinations should be complete and should follow the company's regulations. Stallions insured as such should always be checked for descent of both testes and for semen quality. The internal genital health of a mare should be checked if she is insured as a

53

brood animal. The external genitalia of both sexes are routinely examined if the animals are insured as breeding stock. Routine insurance examination includes a check of the locomotor, circulatory, respiratory, digestive, and nervous systems. The circulatory and respiratory systems should be examined before, during, and after exercise, and a stethoscope should be used as indicated in these examinations. Vision of the horse must be checked routinely, and conformational abnormalities predisposing to lameness should be noted on the insurance papers.

In some cases the soundness examination is limited by age. For example, the examination of yearlings will usually be confined to determining if infectious diseases are present and whether the horse has congenital or inheritable weaknesses. However, the heart should always be closely checked for abnormalities by a stethoscopic examination. Regardless of the type of horse being examined, careful and thorough examination is essential.

The increased incidence of equine infectious anemia (swamp fever), with the various syndromes that it may assume, plus the introduction of equine piroplasmosis into the United States, make it important to examine the horse closely for signs of icterus, anemia, edematous swellings of the limbs and abdomen, and temperature rise. The history of the horse should be checked to see if it could have originated in an area where these diseases are prevalent. At present, most states have potential equine infectious anemia sources, and piroplasmosis is known to exist in Florida.

Whenever there is reason to suspect the presence of equine infectious anemia, consideration should be given to testing the suspected horse, as well as others on the premises, by immunodiffusion test or other appropriate methods as they are developed. In addition, CBC, hemoglobin, sedimentation rate and packed cell volume determinations may be done. If piro-

plasmosis is suspected, peripheral blood from the ear vein may be drawn for staining purposes. However, in the carrier state, piroplasmosis is difficult to diagnose, and a carrier of equine infectious anemia may not show illness. Whenever possible, injection of blood from a suspected infectious-anemia horse should be inoculated intravenously into a nonexposed horse. If the disease is reproduced, a positive diagnosis can be made.

With the increased frequency of use of corticosteroids and phenylbutazone, there is always a possibility that a horse being sold is under the influence of one or both of these drugs to mask a lameness. In addition, a local nerve block or a neurectomy may have been employed to produce temporary soundness to promote sale of the horse. Atropine is sometimes used to mask the symptoms of pulmonary interstitial emphysema (heaves). Careful digital examination and needle prick check for neurectomy, alcohol block, and local anesthesia should be used. When in doubt, one should obtain a written guarantee stating that no masking drugs have been used and granting a week on the new owner's premises for the effects of any such drugs to disappear.

DISCUSSION OF UNSOUNDNESS

In some states the registration of stallions is required by law. In those states that do require an examination, certain unsoundnesses will exclude a stallion from a breeding license. The conditions listed below are considered to be unsoundnesses in some states and will disqualify the stallion for breeding license.

1. Splints (when accompanied by lameness)
2. Ringbone
3. Sidebone
4. Hernias (scrotal or umbilical)
5. Curb (when accompanied by curby conformation)
6. Bone spavin

7. Bog spavin
8. Thoroughpin
9. Stringhalt
10. Cryptorchid
11. Contagious disease
12. Blindness
13. Heaves
14. Periodic ophthalmia
15. Cataract
16. Roaring (laryngeal hemiplegia)
17. Parrot mouth
18. Shivering
19. Any form of venereal disease

In addition to this list many people regard the following as unsoundnesses. These must be understood to be only partial lists, as they do not include wounds or other conditions that might make the horse unsound. The combined lists should be used.

1. Hoof crack
2. Thrush
3. Corns
4. Quittor
5. Bowed tendon
6. Knee sprung
7. Dropped sole
8. Navicular disease
9. Laminitis
10. Leg interference of any type, e.g. scalping, forging, over-reaching, cross-firing, interfering, speedy cutting
11. Malignant neoplasms
12. Sweeny
13. Wind puffs (when due to arthritis)
14. Broken and decayed teeth
15. Poor apposition of teeth
16. Conformation predisposing to lameness

Some of these conditions may be either congenital or acquired. If congenital, the horse is not suited for breeding, but if acquired, the horse may in some cases be considered sound for breeding purposes.

The following conditions are considered blemishes and sometimes unsoundnesses:

1. Capped hock
2. Capped elbow (also known as olecranon bursitis, hygroma of the elbow, or shoe boil).
3. Windgalls (wind puffs) with no arthritis
4. Thoroughpin
5. Scars (especially when accompanied by extensive fibrous tissue)
6. Corneal scars associated with previous trauma
7. Firing marks
8. Saddle sores
9. Sit fast
10. Crooked tail
11. New bone growth (especially of large size in the lower leg).
12. Splints (when not accompanied by lameness).
13. Hygroma of the carpus

A blemish is a defect, pathological or otherwise, that is localized in a tissue such as skin or bone and that more or less diminishes the value of the horse by its appearance but does not diminish function.

Good judgment must be used in determining the importance of some of the above conditions. For example, a splint is a minor condition when not accompanied by poor conformation or lameness and when it does not involve any adjacent structure. It will be noted that there are some repeats here from the unsoundness list, such as thoroughpin and wind puffs. One must be able to decide whether these have been produced by sprains and are healed or whether they are due to poor conformation and consequently the result of secondary trauma. If they are due to trauma but the animal has good conformation, they are considered a blemish, provided there is no lameness. If they are due to poor conformation, they are considered unsoundness. It is obvious that no hard and fast rule can be made to apply to all cases.

When acting as an advisor in the purchase of a horse, one should note conformational defects not listed above and advise prospective buyer of their seriousness (see Chap. 1). Minor abnormalities should be noted when there is a possibility that they might cause pathological changes. The veterinarian must decide for himself when very minor blemishes are to be reported.

Conditions considered vices that might render some horses unsound for certain purposes are listed below:

1. Biting
2. Bucking
3. Cribbing, wind sucking, stump sucking, swallowing air
4. Kicking (either in the stall or at handlers)
5. Running away
6. Shying
7. Viciousness
8. Weaving
9. Stall-walking
10. Tail-wringing
11. Tail-rubbing

PROCEDURE FOR A SOUNDNESS EXAMINATION

A soundness examination should always be done in routine fashion so that the same qualities are checked and the possibility of overlooking defects is minimized.

The horse should always be observed in the box stall before being removed because at this time some conditions are obvious that will not be noticeable after the horse has warmed up. Careful observation of how the horse supports his weight on the limbs is important. Stringhalt or upward fixation of the patella may be evident.

General Appearance

A definite system of visual examination should be developed as a consistent routine. One should visualize the horse from the front, from each side, and from behind to determine any gross defects. If this is done in a routine fashion for every area of the horse, embarrassing mistakes can be avoided. Facial fractures, scars, torn ears, crooked tails, knocked-down hip (Fig. 3-1), and other defects that might otherwise be overlooked will be detected.

Locomotor System

Signs of lameness can best be detected while the horse is in motion. The way of going should also be observed to determine whether or not interference occurs or is likely to occur. Any conformational defects should be detected. The horse should be turned several times in a tight circle to check for the wobbler syndrome, or other causes of incoordination.

Close-up Examination

Forelimbs. The foot is observed carefully for any signs of laminitis, reshaping of the wall with a rasp, contraction or abnormal conformation. A hoof tester is applied for signs of sensitivity in any area. The lateral cartilages are examined and the feet observed for any cracks in the hoof. The pastern and fetlock areas are palpated for abnormal swellings, and the tendons and suspensory ligament are checked for damage. The carpal area is palpated for signs of joint capsule distention or swellings indicating chip fractures. The splint bone areas are palpated for signs of fractured splints or splint damage. The sites for neurectomies are closely checked for any signs of scarring, and needle-puncture tests are made as indicated. Any abnormal swellings are examined closely to determine their importance. Any atrophy of musculature or bony swelling should be noted and its importance determined. The shoulder area is carefully examined for any atrophy. The bicipital bursa can be examined by applying finger pressure to see if there is sensitivity in this area.

Hind Limbs. The hind limbs are examined like the forelimbs up to the hock. The foot is examined for any type of pathology and the pastern area palpated for ringbone. The tendons and suspensory ligament are closely examined, as is the sesamoid area. The hocks are examined closely for symmetry, and a spavin test is administered to each limb. The stifles are examined for signs of distention or thickening of the femoropatellar pouch. The patella of each hind limb is forced upward and outward to see if there is any sign of locking. The area of the greater trochanter of the femur is checked by pressure for pain of bursitis and for symmetry. Any sign of atrophy over the quadriceps or the gluteal muscles is noted. The tubera sacrala are examined for symmetry and for prominence at their junction with the sacrum. Abnormal prominence of one or both tubera sacrala would indicate a previous sacroiliac ligamentous separation. The tubera coxae are examined for any sign of asymmetry and fracture (Fig. 3–1). The back over the lumbar area is palpated for signs of pain indicating possible sensitivity over the dorsal spines of the lumbar vertebrae or from sacroiliac subluxation. The horse should also be observed in gaits at whatever work is planned for him.

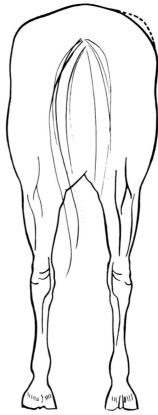

FIG. 3–1. Appearance of knocked-down hip (solid line) on right side. Dotted line shows where normal outline should be.

General Considerations

At the time of the close-up examination, any sign of infectious disease should be recorded. The lymph glands should be checked for enlargement that might indicate a developing respiratory disease complex. Any lacrimal discharge should be examined to see if it accompanies a disease of the eye, tearduct, or a systemic disease. The mucous membranes should be examined for normal color. If icteric or anemic membranes are present, diseases such as leptospirosis, piroplasmosis or equine infectious anemia may be involved, so laboratory tests should be made. The temperature should be taken routinely and should be within normal limits.

Respiratory System

The lungs should be checked at rest and after exercise by stethoscopic examination. Any signs of alveolar emphysema, indicating the presence of heaves, or any other lung pathology should be noted.

Dilation of the pupils and dryness of the mouth may indicate that atropine or belladonna has been administered to mask the symptoms of heaves.

After exercise, an examination for roaring should be made. This is done by placing the stethoscope over the larynx and palpating the larynx for muscular atrophy. If there is a suspicion that roaring is present, a rhinolaryngoscope* can be used to observe the laryngeal cartilages.

The trachea and larynx should be palpated to determine if previous tracheotomy or roaring operations have been done. The trachea should be examined for broken rings. While horse is working one can determine if normal wind is present. The nostrils should be observed closely to determine if there is a nasal discharge, which might indicate chronic guttural pouch infection, sinusitis, or other such conditions.

Circulatory System

The heart should be checked with a stethoscope from both the right and left sides. This examination should be conducted both at rest and after exercise, and any abnormalities noted. Auscultation should also be done immediately after startling the horse by slapping its abdomen with the open hand. Many cardiac abnormalities will become evident after this procedure. Common defects found in such an examination are valvular leaks, pericardial friction rub, tachycardia, and partial heart block. If there is any doubt concerning a cardiac ailment, an EKG can be used.

Both jugular veins should be checked for excessive jugular pulse, which usually indicates a right atrioventricular valvular leak. The jugular veins should also be checked for thrombosis resulting from subcutaneous injection of an irritant drug. The characteristics of the pulse should be noted in either the femoral artery or in the maxillary artery at the angle of the jaw.

**Genital System and
Inheritable Defects**

Under this system the second classification of soundness examination, or the

*Borescope, American Cystoscope Co.

breeding soundness examination, is given. In addition to unsoundnesses listed below, any inheritable abnormalities in the mare or stallion should classify the breeding animal as unsound. Any limb unsoundness present in the mare may become worse with the increased body weight caused by pregnancy.

*Conditions Considered To Be
Breeding Unsoundnesses in Mares*

1. Tipped vulva—this may cause sucking of air into the vaginal vault during movement. A mare with this condition, that makes an audible sound when air is sucked into the vagina, is often called a "gilflirt." A person should also check to see if the vulva has been previously sutured to prevent this condition, because special breeding precautions are necessary in such a case.

2. Rectovaginal fistula or perineal lacerations—the usual problem is a third-degree perineal laceration, where the entire shelf between the rectum and the vagina has been torn out to varying depths in the vagina. Occasionally, a single perforating fistula will be found. Mares rarely settle when afflicted with either condition and often abort if they do. Chronic vaginitis will be present with endometritis in some.

3. Abnormalities considered to be unsoundnesses when found on rectal examination—

a. Ovaries that are hard, fibrous, or excessively large, or that show evidence of adhesions in the fallopian tubes, should be considered abnormal. A single hard ovary is not usually abnormal if the other is normal. The hard ovary may be inactive, and subsequent examination will usually show it to be normal. If both ovaries are hard, small, and fibrous, the mare may be a nymphomaniac. A breeding history and heat cycle chart is helpful in determining the seriousness of this condition, since ovaries of the mare show many normal variations. In some cases, no ovaries are found, due to some congenital defect or because the mare has been spayed.

b. Abnormal uterus and/or cervix—Enlargement of the uterus due to pyometra or to thickened walls resulting from previous infection are unfavorable findings. A uterus that lacks proper tone and is flabby to palpation should be considered indicative of reduced breeding efficiency. Adhesions of the uterus to pelvic structures, and hematomas present on the wall of the uterus or in the region of the fallopian tubes due to rupture of uterine vessels during foaling reduce breeding efficiency. Occasionally, one will find an abnormally small uterus or complete absence of the uterus. This is due to a heritable factor, and the mare is obviously permanently infertile. A thickened cervix resulting from foaling lacerations or infection reduces breeding efficiency.

4. Abnormalities found on vaginal examination and considered unsoundnesses—

a. Adhesions of the vaginal wall or cervix, indicating previous tears.

b. Vaginal or cervical inflammation indicating infection and/or windsucking, which reduces breeding efficiency.

c. Abnormal exudate, indicating presence of infection.

5. Umbilical hernia—this condition is inheritable. The navel should be palpated to detect whether or not repair has been made.

6. The mammary gland should be checked for scar tissue from previous mastitis.

Some of the above unsoundnesses can be corrected, but all should be regarded as potential causes of unsoundness, and the purchaser should understand that the mare may not conceive or may not carry to term or that congenital conditions may be passed on to the offspring.

Conditions Considered To Be Breeding Unsoundnesses in Stallions

1. Undescended testicles—Testicles should be descended at birth, and any deviation from this is abnormal. Undescended testes may be unilateral or bilateral and are an inheritable characteristic.

2. Epididymitis—This is a comparatively rare finding in a stallion.

3. Penile pathology—The penis should be examined closely for any signs of pathological changes. Edema of the prepuce may indicate carcinoma, screwworm infestation, or other pathology in the penis and prepuce. A tranquilizer such as promazine* may be given intravenously to facilitate this examination.

4. Lack of libido—This may be accompanied by underdeveloped testes, or testes of poor consistency. In young stallions it can be due to shyness and may be overcome as the horse matures. Masturbation is a common cause of decreased libido, and use of a stallion ring should result in improved libido.

5. Umbilical and scrotal hernia—If there is any suspicion of scrotal hernia, a rectal examination should be done. If there is an enlargement of the internal inguinal rings, a hernia may occur, so this condition can be considered to be the same as a scrotal hernia. The umbilical area should be palpated for the presence of a hernia and for signs of previous repair.

6. Any unsoundness of the fore or hind limbs that will prevent the stallion from performing natural breeding service.

7. Poor semen quality—A semen evaluation should be done whenever possible, to determine the quality of semen and the

*Ft. Dodge Laboratories, Ft. Dodge, Iowa.

reproductive potential of the stallion (see below).

[Because of the lack of published information on accurate evaluation of stallion semen, I include here a section on this very important aspect of soundness examination in stallions. Although this discussion is perhaps more detailed than one would expect in a text of this nature, I feel that this information is important enough that it should be provided.]

Evaluation of Stallion Semen—

B. W. PICKETT, *B.S., M.S., PhD. Director, Animal Reproduction Laboratory, College of Veterinary Medicine and Biomedical Sciences, Colorado State University*

Introduction

Reproductive efficiency is lower in the equine than in any other species of farm animal. The primary causes of this low reproductive rate, as far as the stallion is concerned, are:

1. Lack of selection for fertility. Only a few stallions are booked to a sufficient number of mares each year to truly determine their reproductive capabilities.

2. Failure of the stallion owner to recognize that the stallion is a major factor in infertility and sterility. Too often, if a stallion will mount quickly and copulate vigorously, he is not suspected of being the primary cause of infertility until late in the breeding season.

3. Reluctance of stallion owners to present their stallions for semen evaluation prior to the breeding season. In most cases, no semen evaluation is made until the breeding season is almost over and many of the mares have returned several times. This is poor management and results in costly delays in the breeding program, and an excessive breeding schedule in an attempt to "catch up" frequently contributes to the stallion's breeding problem. The mares are either "held over"

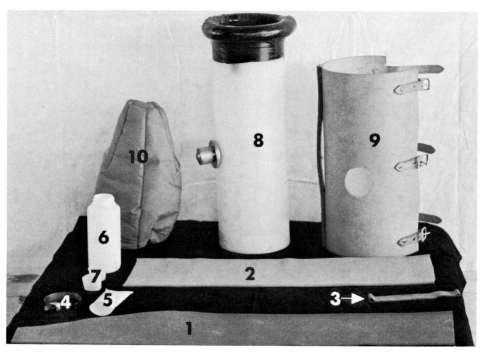

FIG. 3–2. The Colorado Model artificial vagina: *1*, Combination liner and cone; *2*, inner liner; *3*, large, heavy rubber band; *4*, hose clamp; *5*, filter; *6*, Nalgene collection bottle (500 ml); *7*, Nalgene laboratory stoppers, size 8 and 9; *8*, outer casing fitted with rubber vaccum hose and water plug; *9*, leather jacket; *10*, protector jacket for collection bottle.

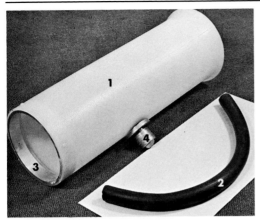

FIG. 3-3. The outer casing (1) is made from a Nalgene pipet jar, size E, $6\frac{1}{2}''$ by 27". The length is cut to $21\frac{1}{2}''$. The flared end of the pipet jar is fitted with a $\frac{3}{4}''$ vacuum hose (2) that has been split longitudinally and taped into place. The opposite end of the casing is fitted with an aluminum ring (3) $1\frac{1}{4}''$ wide by $\frac{1}{5}''$ thick and held in place with four plastic screws. The water plug (4) is stainless steel with an opening of 0.84".

until the next season or bred to a second-choice stallion late in the season. Semen should be evaluated enough in advance of the breeding season to permit other arrangements in the event the stallion is impotent or the semen is of poor quality.

4. Lack of sound, basic information on reproductive problems in the stallion. The horse has not enjoyed many of the benefits of modern scientific methods that have been applied to other species of livestock. For example, few if any controlled studies have been conducted on the transmission, cause of infection, or treatment of reproductive diseases such as that caused by *Klebsiella pneumoniae* var. *genitalium*.

5. The influence of season on fertility. Efforts to breed early in the season, when sperm production is low and mares are not cycling or ovulating normally, results in poor conception rates.

6. Failure of buyers to insist that each stallion undergo a thorough breeding soundness examination, including semen evaluation, prior to purchase. This proce-

dure could aid in establishing the frequency of infertility and sterility and serve as an incentive for owners to identify and correct breeding problems.

7. Difficulties in conducting a proper semen evaluation.

Proper Semen Evaluation

The following materials are necessary to a proper semen evaluation:

1. Mare in heat, natural or induced.
2. Hobbles and twitch.
3. Microscope, ideally a binocular, phase-contrast instrument.
4. Water bath or incubator to warm

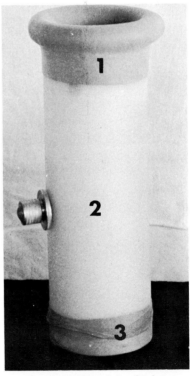

FIG. 3-4. The inner liner (1), which is approximately 29 inches in length, is manufactured of Gray Band Tubing by B. F. Goodrich, 7" by 0.063 G.A. This liner is placed through the outer casing (2) and turned back over each end of the casing, and the posterior end (toward the collection bottle) is held in place by a heavy rubber band (3), thus forming a water jacket.

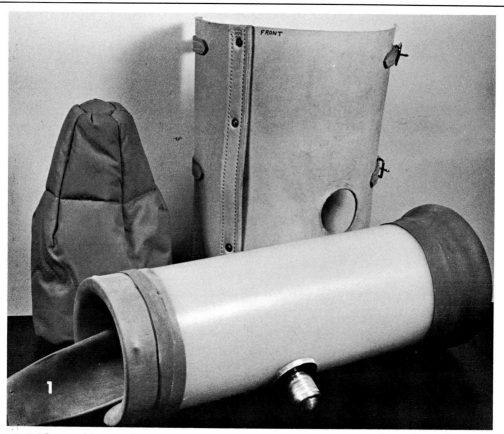

FIG. 3–5. The combination liner and cone (1), also made of Gray Band Tubing, is 30–32″ long. The last 12″ are cut to taper and vulcanized. This piece of tubing is placed through the casing and inner liner and turned back over the end where the stallion's penis is inserted. This forms a barrel for the stallion's penis and a funnel to direct the semen into the collection bottle.

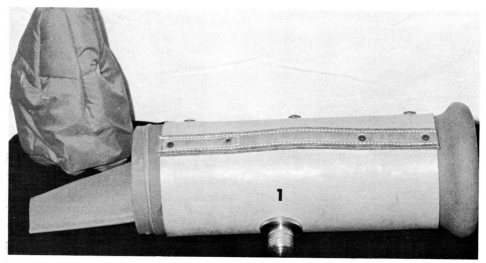

FIG. 3–6. The leather jacket (1), approximately 16″ long, is fitted over the outer casing and buckled into place.

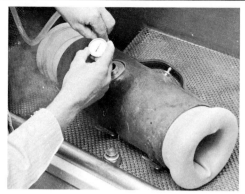

FIG. 3-7. The AV is then filled with 14 lb of water at a temperature of 57°C (134.6°F).

extender and keep the semen warm while it is being evaluated.

5. pH meter.

6. Apparatus for counting the spermatozoa. The simplest and least expensive is a hemocytometer. The method used for counting red blood cells can be employed for most samples; however, dilute samples must be diluted with a white blood cell pipette.

7. Artificial vagina (AV).* Although there are several available, we prefer the one developed at Colorado State University (Fig. 3-2). The material for construction and method of assembly of the AV is shown in Figures 3-2 through 3-11.

Gelatinous Secretion and Its Removal

The gelatinous material (gel) in the stallion's ejaculate is produced by the seminal vesicles. The secretion of this seminal fraction is highly seasonal and is reported to be greatly increased by intense sexual excitement. The precise function of this fraction of the ejaculate is unknown, but it is reported to inhibit bacterial growth

*Manufactured by Lane Manufacturing Inc., 2057 South Hudson, Denver, Colo. 802222.

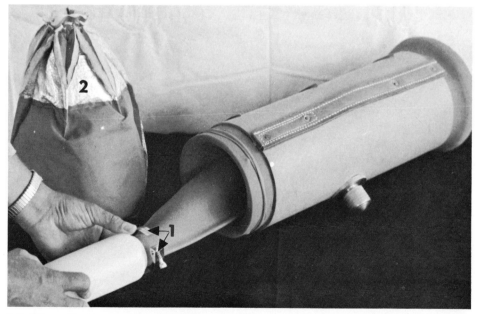

FIG. 3-8. The collection bottle, with filter in place, is removed from an incubator maintained at 38°C (100.4°F), fitted inside the tapered end of the combination liner and cone, and held in place with a hose clamp (1). Also shown is the inside of the protector jacket (2). The jacket is composed of an outer layer of nylon duck, a middle layer of insulation-type Dacron and an inner layer of Space Blanket.

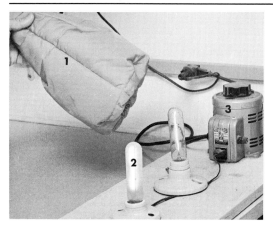

Fig. 3–9. The protector jacket (1) is placed over an electric bulb (2) maintained at slightly above body temperature by a rheostat (3). It requires about 10 minutes for the bulb to warm the inside of the jacket. Once the jacket is warmed and placed over a prewarmed collection bottle, the temperature inside will be maintained at about body temperature for 15 minutes even on cold days.

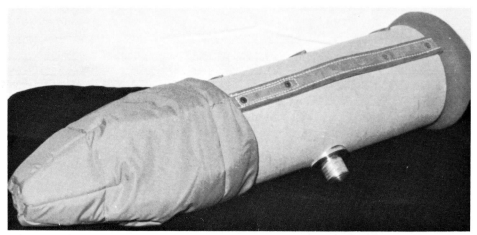

Fig. 3–10. Artificial vagina completely assembled.

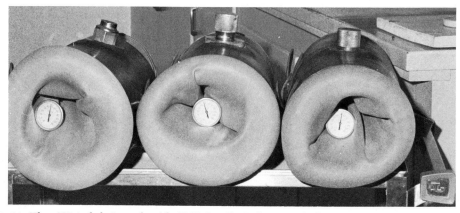

Fig. 3–11. The AV is lubricated with K-Y Sterile Lubricant (Johnson and Johnson), and a dial thermometer is placed inside. When the internal temperature is 44° to 48°C (111.2° to 118.4°F), the vagina is ready to use. Although some stallions may work better if the temperature is about 50°C, caution must be used to prevent damaging the spermatozoa with excessive heat.

and aid in spermatozoan survival. Although the appearance of gel in the ejaculate is seasonal, semen from some stallions rarely, if ever, contains gel. Consequently, the presence or absence of gel in an ejaculate may not reflect the potential fertility of that ejaculate.

To measure accurately the chemical and some of the physical characteristics of stallion semen, the gel must be removed from the ejaculate before it becomes mixed with the sperm-bearing fraction. Further, semen to be used for artificial insemination is easier to handle when the gel has been removed. Thus, a filtration system is used to remove the gel before it becomes mixed with the remainder of the ejaculate. The equipment for gel separation and method of assembly is presented in Figures 3–12 through 3–17.

Collection of Semen

In preparation for semen collection, the mare is hobbled, and her tail wrapped (Fig. 3–18). The stallion and mare are placed on opposite sides of a padded tease bar and teased until the stallion has an erection. His penis is washed with mild soap and warm water and thoroughly rinsed with clean water maintained at body temperature (Fig. 3–19). Care should be taken to remove the smegma from the preputial folds. Unless this is done, the skin in this area may dry, crack, and become infected. The mare is stationed in an area relatively free of obstacles, and the stallion is permitted to mount. As he mounts, the penis is deflected into the AV (Fig. 3–20) at an angle that does not cause bending of the penis.

As the stallion dismounts, the penis is "stripped" to collect the maximum volume of semen and number of spermatozoa (Fig. 3–21). Immediately after collection, the water-plug cap is removed, and the water is drained to reduce the internal pressure, permitting all the semen in the combination liner and cone to drain

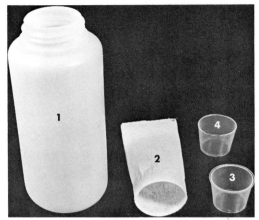

FIG. 3–12. The equipment used for gel separation is shown. The collection bottle (1) has a capacity of 500 ml and an opening of 1.6″. The filter (2) is a Surge Pipeline Milk Filter (Babson Bros. Co, 2100 S. York Rd., Oak Brook, Ill. 60521) cut to a length of 5½″ and doubly sewn at one end. The filter holders are Nalgene hollow stoppers, size 8 (3) and 9 (4). The bottoms of both stoppers and the rim from the size 9 have been removed.

into the bottle (Fig. 3–22). Unless this is done quickly, the spermatozoa may be damaged by excessive heat and drying.

In the laboratory, the protector jacket for the collection bottle and the hose clamp are quickly removed, the filter assembly removed and placed upside-down in a beaker. Although this filter system is quite effective, the gel will eventually pass

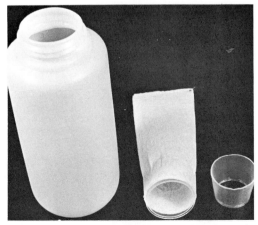

FIG. 3–13. The No. 8 stopper is placed inside the open end of the milk filter.

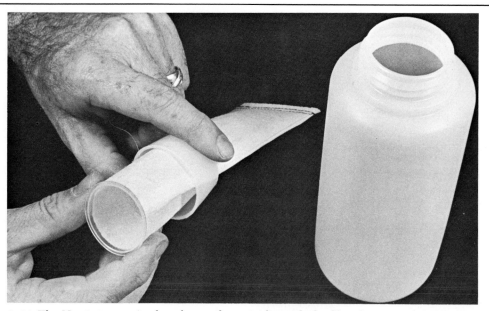

FIG. 3-14. The No. 9 stopper is placed over the outside, with the filter between the two stoppers.

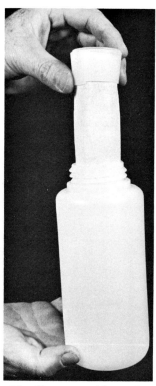

FIG. 3-15. The filter assembly is placed inside the collection bottle.

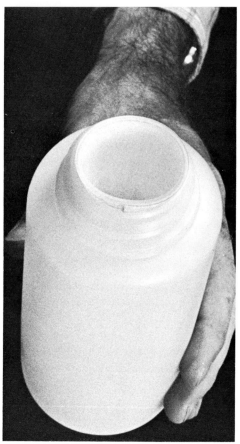

FIG. 3-16. The rim on the No. 8 stopper prevents the filter from falling into the bottle.

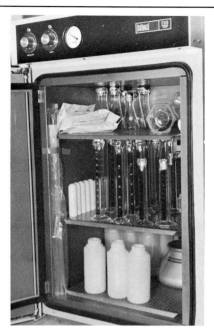

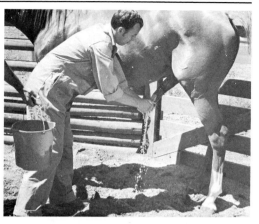

FIG. 3-19. Wash the stallion's penis with mild soap, and rinse well before collection.

FIG. 3-17. The collection bottles, with filters in place, are stored in an incubator maintained at 38°C (100.4°F).

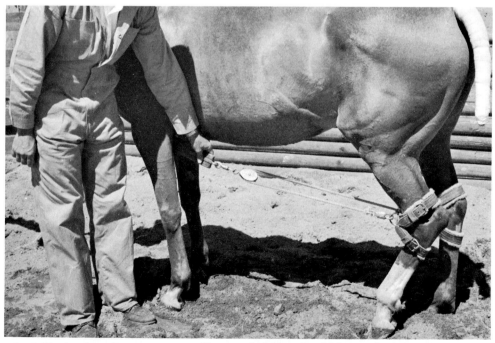

FIG. 3-18. During breeding or semen collection, hobbles should be used on the mare to protect the stallion. The hobbles consist of a neck strap and two hock straps connected by a $\frac{1}{4}''$ nylon rope. The rope passes through a pulley, which permits the mare to walk. The rope is attached to the neck strap and hock straps with "panic snaps" to permit rapid release.

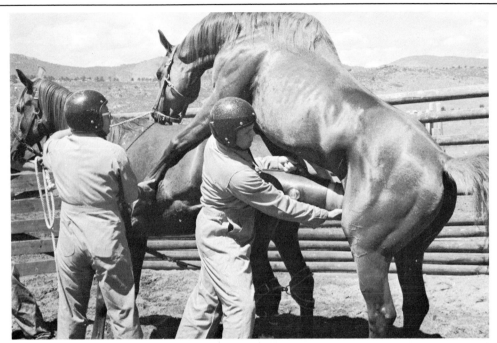

FIG. 3-20. The angle of the AV should approximate the position of the reproductive tract of the mare relative to the position of the stallion. The stallion handler should have his right hand behind the left foreleg of the stallion to protect the collector.

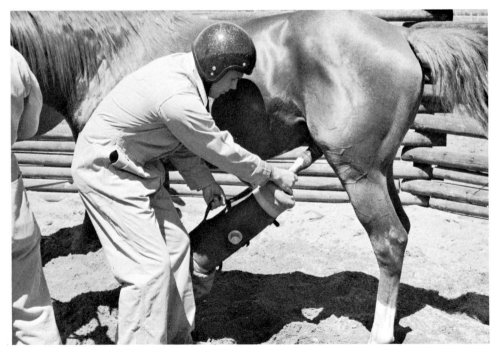

FIG. 3-21. "Strip" the stallion's penis to collect the maximum volume of semen and number of spermatozoa.

are to be truly representative of the ejaculate, semen evaluation must be completed immediately after collection. Further, the glassware and extender (this extender is used only for motility examination) that come into contact with the semen should be maintained at 37°C (98.6°F).

Evaluation of Semen

Semen from stallions to be used for breeding purposes should be evaluated prior to the breeding season. Seminal characteristics of the stallion and the sexual behavior and fertility of both sexes are influenced by season. To determine the influence of season and to develop recommendations for evaluation of semen, first and second ejaculates were collected approximately 1 hour apart, at weekly intervals, for 12 months, from each of three young Quarter Horse and two Thoroughbred stallions (Figs. 3–23 through 3–31).

Semen Volume. About half as much gel-free semen can be expected in the fall as at the height of the breeding season. Further, the volumes of second ejaculates, exclusive of gel, should be approximately the same as found in first ejaculates. The volumes (Fig. 3–25) are somewhat lower than those previously reported, probably because the earlier studies were done on collections made only during the breeding season, and gel was included in the seminal volume measurements; older stallions were also included in many previous studies. Regardless of these factors, the seasonal relationship is valid.

Sperm Concentration. Combined with semen volume, the concentration of spermatozoa can be used to calculate the total spermatozoa per ejaculate. Motility and total spermatozoa per ejaculate are the two most important measurements. For example, a stallion that produced only 20 ml of semen with 600 million spermatozoa per ml would be more desirable than a stallion that produced 200 ml of semen

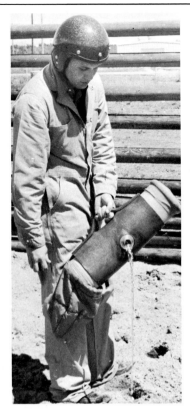

FIG. 3–22. Release the pressure in the AV immediately after collection to permit semen to drain into the collection bottle.

through into the gel-free semen unless the filter is quickly removed from the collection bottle.

The gel is discarded, and the following measurements are made on the gel-free semen:

1. Volume (ml)
2. Percent progressively motile spermatozoa
3. Spermatozoan concentration (millions per ml)
4. pH
5. Morphology

In addition to these measurements, a sample is also taken for culture.

Spermatozoa from the horse are generally less resistant to stress and less viable than spermatozoa from other species of farm animals. Thus, if the measurements

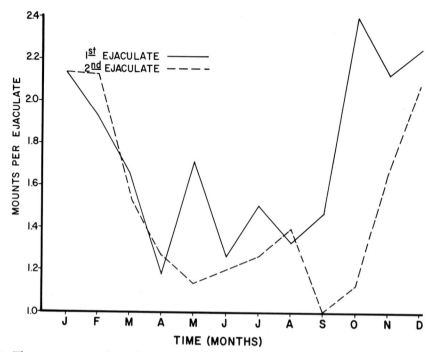

FIG. 3-23. The average number of mounts per first ejaculate over a 12-month period in experimental stallions was 1.8. The range was from 1.2 in April to 2.4 in October. The mean number of mounts per second ejaculate was 1.5; the low was 1.0 in September and the high was 2.1 in January.

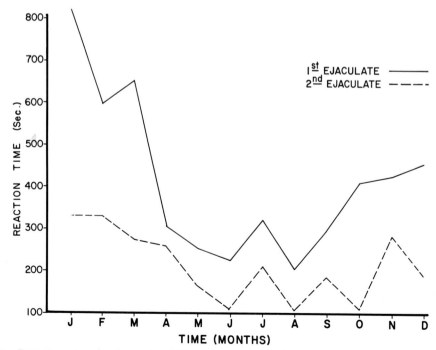

FIG. 3-24. Reaction time for first ejaculates was 414 seconds (6.9 minutes), ranging from a low of 206 seconds (3.4 minutes) in August to a high of 819 seconds (13.5 minutes) in January.

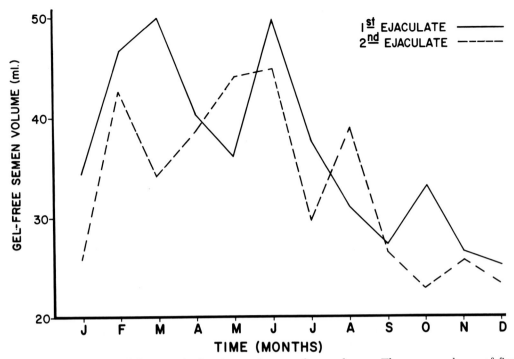

FIG. 3-25. The mean gel-free seminal volumes by month are shown. The mean volume of first ejaculates was 37 ml, ranging from 25 ml in December to 50 ml in March. Second ejaculates averaged 33 ml, ranging from 23 ml in October to 45 ml in June.

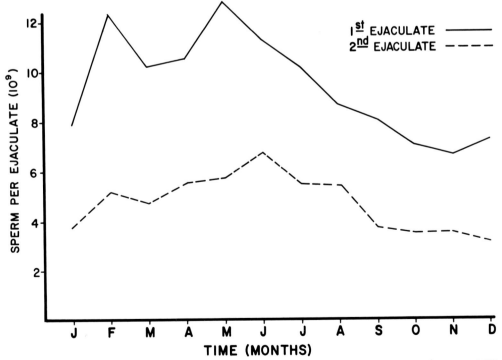

FIG. 3-26. There was an average of 9.4 billion sperm per first ejaculate, ranging from 6.6 billion in November to 12.7 billion in May. Second ejaculates averaged 4.7 billion, with a range of 3.1 billion in December to 6.7 billion in June.

71

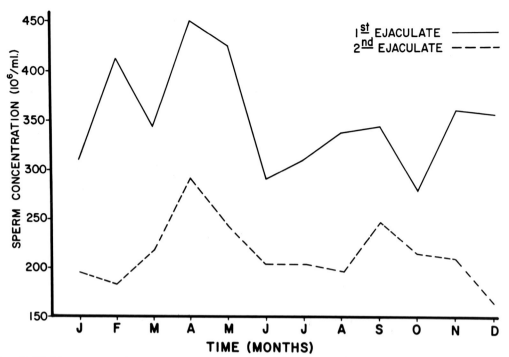

FIG. 3-27. Mean spermatozoan concentrations in millions per ml. First ejaculates averaged 348 million sperm per ml, compared to 212 million in second ejaculates. The range for first ejaculates was from 279 million sperm per ml in October to 451 million sperm per ml in April. Second ejaculates ranged from 164 million sperm per ml in December to 291 million in April.

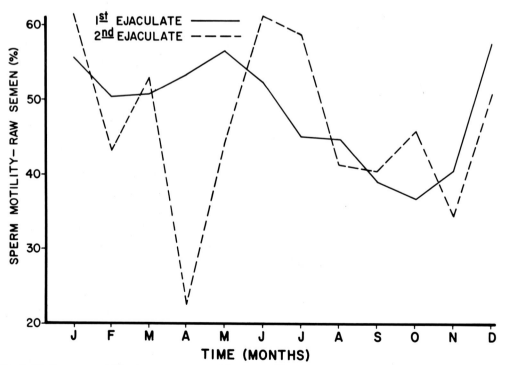

FIG. 3-28. Sperm motility in raw semen. Mean motility of spermatozoa in first ejaculates was 48%, with a low in October of 37% and a high in December of 58%. Second ejaculates averaged 47% motile cells and ranged from 23% in April to 61% in January.

72

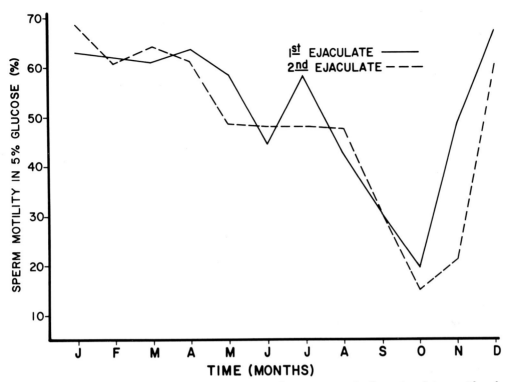

FIG. 3-29. Sperm motility in 5% glucose. Mean motility was 50% in first ejaculates, with a low of 19% in October and a high of 67% in December. Motility in second ejaculates was quite similar: mean motility was 47%, with a range of 15% in October to 69% in January.

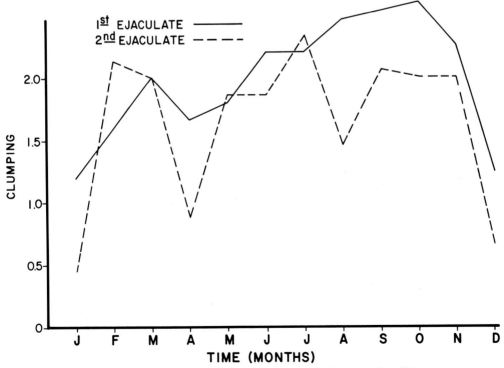

FIG. 3-30. Monthly variation in degree of clumping or agglutination of stallion spermatozoa in raw semen.

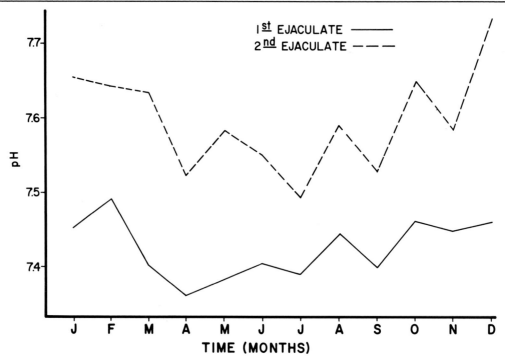

Fig. 3–31. First-ejaculate pH averaged 7.43; April was the lowest month with a mean of 7.36, and February was highest with 7.49. Second ejaculates averaged 7.60 and ranged from 7.49 in July to 7.73 in December.

with only 20 million spermatozoa per ml, because sperm output from the first horse was 12.0 billion cells per ejaculate, while sperm output of the second was only 4.0 billion.

Considerable variation in concentration of spermatozoa can be expected even from the same stallion, and only about half as many spermatozoa can be expected in the second ejaculate as in the first if approximately an hour is permitted to elapse between collections.

There are several procedures that can be used to estimate the number of spermatozoa per ml. The hemocytometer is the simplest and least expensive. However, if many samples have to be counted, a more rapid method is desirable. Spermatozoan concentrations in the semen samples in this study were estimated in the Bausch & Lomb "Spectronic 20" spectrophotometer shown in Figure 3–32. The original calibration was done with a

hemocytometer. After the instrument is calibrated, a portion of the ejaculate is diluted in a 10% formalin/0.9% NaCl solution, and the percent transmittance is measured. Then a chart of the calibration is consulted to determine the number of spermatozoa per ml. For example, in Figure 3–32 the indicator is on 59% transmittance; this corresponds to 469,961,328 spermatozoa per ml, as indicated from the table in Figure 3–33.

The data in Figures 3–25 and 3–27 were used to calculate total spermatozoa per ejaculate, which is presented in Figure 3–26. The dramatic change in spermatozoa output due to season may reflect a quantitative change in spermatogenesis. The difference between first and second ejaculates was about the same, regardless of season, which is evidence for altered spermatogenesis or ejaculatory function due to season. For example, in the fall, only 59% as many spermatozoa were

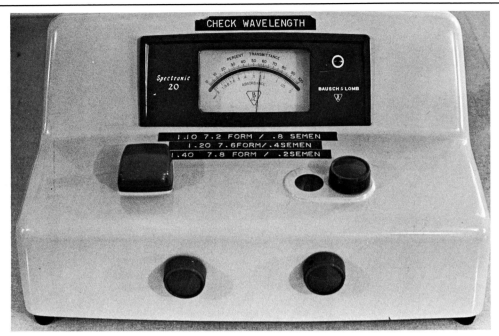

FIG. 3–32. Bausch & Lomb "Spectronic 20" spectrophotometer used to measure sperm concentration.

present in first ejaculates as in the spring, while the comparable value for second ejaculates was 57%. The difference between first and second ejaculates was quite similar throughout the year. There were approximately one-half as many sperm in the second ejaculate as there were in the first ejaculate.

Since there is a significant change in spermatozoan output due to season, this factor must be taken into account when stallions are evaluated for breeding soundness, particularly during the non-breeding season. Second ejaculates should also be collected and evaluated, because second ejaculates from stallions that have been sexually rested for one week should contain approximately half the number of spermatozoa found in first ejaculates in approximately the same volume of semen. When the number of spermatozoa in first and second ejaculates differs by some figure other than 50%, one or more of the following situations can be expected: one of the ejaculates was in-

complete; the stallion has low spermatozoan reserves, either naturally or due to depletion; or spermatozoa have accumulated in the reproductive tract (raising the number of spermatozoa in first and second ejaculates to be similar). When second ejaculates contain approximately the same number of spermatozoa as the first, a third or fourth ejaculate should be collected, and, if possible, the stallion should be scheduled for another evaluation a week later. In cases where a previous illness or injury is suspected as the primary factor in poor seminal quality, the stallion should be evaluated again in 60–90 days.

Sperm Motility. Spermatozoan motility was estimated in raw semen at 200 magnifications with a phase-contrast microscope, and the results are presented in Figure 3-28. Samples of raw semen were diluted 1:20 with 5% glucose to aid in microscopic evaluation (Fig. 3-29). Since stallion spermatozoa tend to agglutinate or clump, which interferes with the estimation of motility, a highly subjective

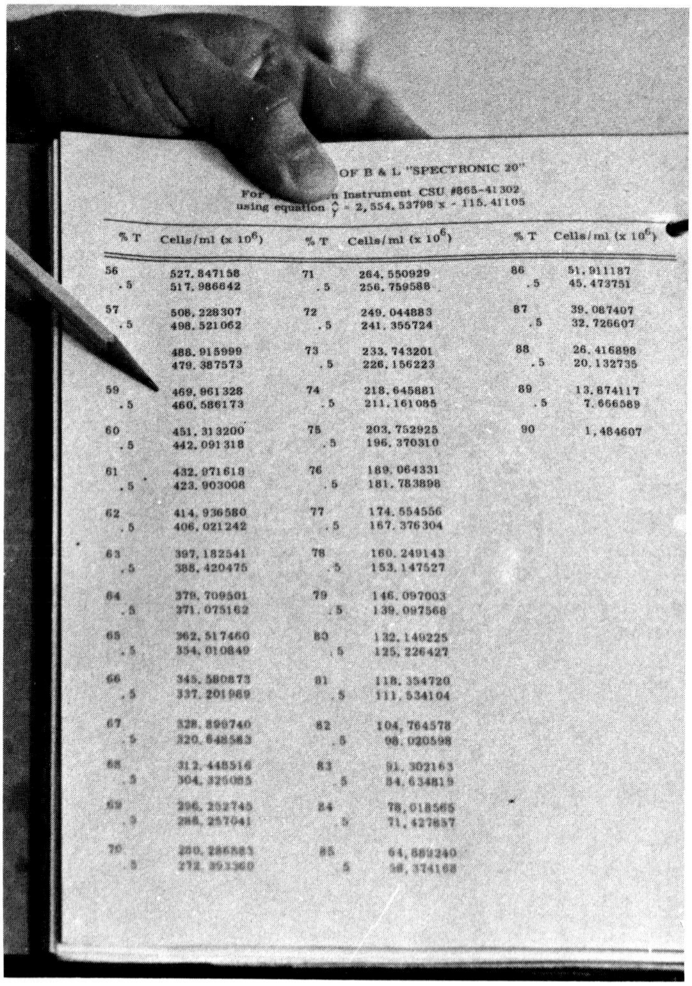

OF B & L "SPECTRONIC 20"
For … Instrument CSU #865-41302
using equation $\hat{y}$ = 2,554.53798 x - 115.41105

% T	Cells/ml (x 10^6)	% T	Cells/ml (x 10^6)	% T	Cells/ml (x 10^6)
56	527.847158	71	264.550929	86	51.911187
.5	517.986642	.5	256.759588	.5	45.473751
57	508.228307	72	249.044883	87	39.087407
.5	498.521062	.5	241.355724	.5	32.726607
	488.915999	73	233.743201	88	26.416898
	479.387573	.5	226.156223	.5	20.132735
59	469.961328	74	218.645881	89	13.874117
.5	460.586173	.5	211.161085	.5	7.666589
60	451.313200	75	203.752925	90	1.484607
.5	442.091318	.5	196.370310		
61	432.971618	76	189.064331		
.5	423.903008	.5	181.783898		
62	414.936580	77	174.554556		
.5	406.021242	.5	167.376304		
63	397.182541	78	160.249143		
.5	388.420475	.5	153.147527		
64	379.709501	79	146.097003		
.5	371.075162	.5	139.097568		
65	362.517460	80	132.149225		
.5	354.010849	.5	125.226427		
66	345.580873	81	118.354720		
.5	337.201989	.5	111.534104		
67	328.899740	82	104.764578		
.5	320.648583	.5	98.020598		
68	312.448516	83	91.302163		
.5	304.325085	.5	84.634819		
69	296.252745	84	78.018565		
.5	288.257041	.5	71.427857		
70	280.286883	85	64.889240		
.5	272.393360	.5	58.374168		

FIG. 3–33. Calibration table used to determine the number of spermatozoa per ml of semen.

estimate of degree of clumping was made when motility in raw semen was estimated (Fig. 3–28). From possible scores of 0, 1, 2, or 3, representing no clumping, slight, moderate, and severe clumping, respectively, first ejaculates averaged 2.0 and ranged from 1.2 in January to 2.6 in October. Second ejaculates averaged 1.7, with a low of 0.5 in January and a high of 2.3 in July (Fig. 3–30).

From the data in Figures 3–28, 3–29, and 3–30, it appears that there was an inverse relationship between motility and clumping. For example, there was more clumping in first ejaculates during October than during the other months, and with the exception of April for second ejaculates, October was also the month of lowest motility. Therefore, in all probability, clumping of spermatozoa is seasonal and interferes with an accurate evaluation of motility. From more recent data, it has been found that clumping can be prevented by extending the semen 1:20 in an aqueous extender containing 0.24% Tris buffer, 20% egg yolk, 5% glucose, and 5% glycerol. It is essential that an extender that prevents clumping of spermatozoa be used for reliable motility estimations. *Under no circumstances should this extender be used in a breeding program.*

pH Measurements. The pH varies with

season, and pH of second ejaculates was always higher than that of first ejaculates (Fig. 3–31). These observations are so consistent that any time the pH of the first ejaculate is higher than the corresponding second ejaculate, the first ejaculate should be considered incomplete or abnormal. When pH is consistently high, the possibility of infection should be considered. Under these circumstances, pH becomes a useful diagnostic tool in evaluation of stallion semen. There are numerous methods for measuring pH; because of the importance of the test, pH paper is not recommended. An accurate instrument used to measure pH is shown in Figure 3–34. It is a single-electrode digital pH meter.* The sample being measured has a pH of 7.47, which is in the normal range for first ejaculates.

Morphological Examination. Another measurement that is essential for a thorough seminal evaluation is a morphological examination of 100 individual spermatozoa from each of two slides per ejaculate. The staining procedure and slide preparation technique were adapted for stallion semen from the method outlined by Casarett (1953).

A. The following solutions are prepared:
   1. A 5% solution of aniline blue (200 ml)
   2. A 5% solution of eosin B (100 ml)
   3. A 1% solution of phenol (100 ml)
B. Mix the three solutions, filter and store the stain in a stoppered bottle
C. The slide preparation and staining procedure is as follows:
   1. Prepare a thin, uniform smear of fresh semen on a clean, dry microscope slide
   2. Fast-dry the smear over an open flame
   3. Fix in ethanol:ethyl ether (1:1) solution for three minutes

*Sargent-Welch, Model S-30000; 4040 Dahlia St., P.O. Box 7196, Denver, Colo. 80207.

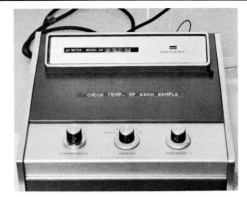

FIG. 3–34. Single-electrode digital pH meter.

4. Dry in air
5. Stain for 6 minutes over a steam bath (95°C)
6. Wash the residual staining fluid from slides with distilled water
7. Dry in air
8. Mount and examine under oil immersion

Shown in Figure 3–35 is a sheet used to record the spermatozoan abnormalities. Too few stallions with known breeding histories have been evaluated to predict a precise relationship of percent and type of abnormality with fertility. However, any stallion that consistently has more than 40% abnormal spermatozoa, excluding abaxial midpieces, should be considered potentially infertile. Abaxial midpieces are probably not abnormal in the stallion since as many as 90% of the spermatozoa have exhibited this characteristic and are still within normal ranges of fertility. Photomicrographs of normal and abnormal forms of stallion spermatozoa are shown in Figures 3–36, and 3–37. It has been reported that the appearance of leukocytes and erythrocytes is a relatively common occurrence in stallion semen. This has been observed only rarely in our laboratory and was generally associated with cases of urethral bleeding.

Bacteriological Examination. No stallion seminal evaluation is complete without a bacteriological examination of the

STALLION SPERMATOZOA MORPHOLOGY

Colorado State University Animal Reproduction Laboratory

Stall ion _____   Date _____

Owner _____   Address _____

Morphology	(Types of abnormalities per 100 cells counted)					
	Ejaculate 1		Ejaculate 2		Ejaculate 3	
	Slide 1	Slide 2	Slide 1	Slide 2	Slide 1	Slide 2
Normal						
Head						
Midpiece (Coils, irregular, etc.)						
Abaxial midpiece*						
Separated head & neck						
Reversed & coiled tails						
Proximal droplets						
Distal droplets						
Total Cells Counted						

* Abaxial midpieces in stallions are considered normal at this laboratory.

Remarks _____

_____

_____

FIG. 3–35. Data sheet used to record the results of morphological examination of stallion spermatozoa.

semen. Immediately following removal of the filter assembly, 0.25 ml of semen is pipetted from the collection bottle into a culture tube of thioglycolate medium. Although this sampling procedure may permit contamination from other sources, it is a valuable procedure. *Klebsiella pneumoniae* var. *genitalium* and β-hemolytic streptococci are of primary concern. Although the number of ejaculates from which these organisms have been cultured is limited, the spermatozoa in these ejaculates generally exhibit lowered motility and a higher percentage of abnormal forms. Considering the limitations of the sampling method, a stallion cannot be considered free of the organisms even if they are not cultured from the semen. However, their presence is indicative that the semen was contaminated.

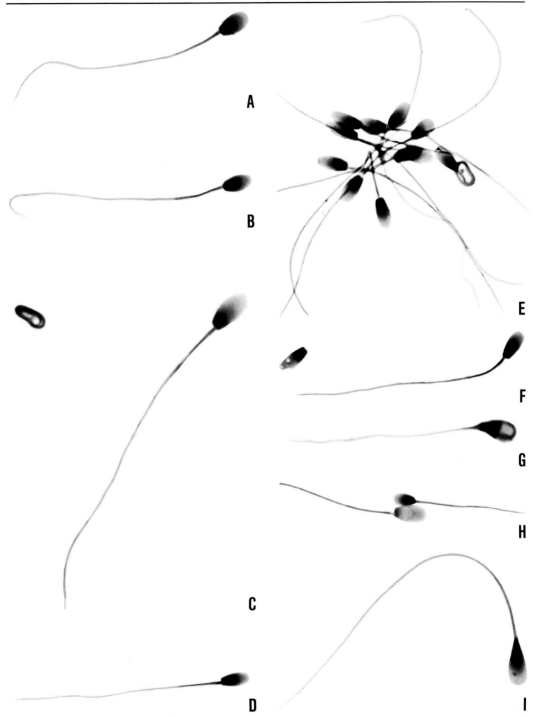

FIG. 3-36. *A*, Normal stallion spermatozoon with abaxial midpiece. *B*, Normal. *C*, Normal (right) and a misshapen, microcephalic head with tail tightly coiled around the head. *D*, Normal. *E*, Clumping or agglutination of normal and abnormal spermatozoa. *F*, Normal and a detached, vacuolated head. *G*, Pyriform head; midpiece is either very short or absent. *H*, Bovine (bottom) and stallion spermatozoa with abaxial midpiece. *I*, Pyriform head.

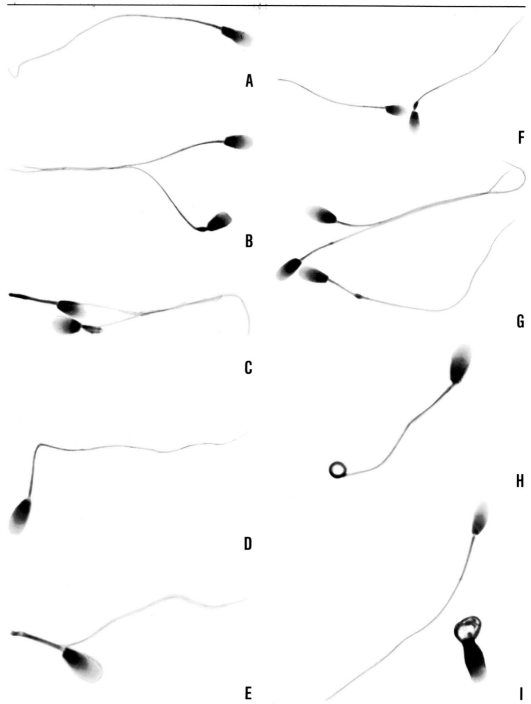

FIG. 3–37. *A*, Constricted, asymmetrical head. *B*, Normal sperm and sperm with asymmetrical head and proximal protoplasmic droplet. *C*, Reversed tail and coiled midpiece. *D*, Bent tail; this may be an artifact or a deviation from the reversed-tail defect. *E*, Reversed tail. *F*, Normal sperm and sperm with proximal protoplasmic droplet. *G*, Normal (top), vestige (center) of distal droplet, and distal droplet (bottom). *H*, Coiled tail. *I*, Normal and macrocephalic head with tightly coiled midpiece and tail.

Variation in Seminal Characteristics

An indication of the extreme variation in seminal characteristics that can be expected from a group of Thoroughbred and Quarter Horse stallions under almost identical husbandry is shown in Tables 3–1, 3–2, and 3–3. Semen from a random sample of stallions presented for routine evaluation can be expected to exhibit even greater variation. It must be concluded that the random fluctuations in seminal characteristics, particularly in seminal volume and spermatozoan number are so great that the error of a single sampling can be very large. Thus, a single ejaculate can provide only a general estimate of the precise value. Ideally, a second and perhaps a third ejaculate should be collected followed by daily collection for at least seven days.

The data presented in Table 3–1 do not include information on gel. However, 112 first ejaculates and 55 second ejaculates of those presented in Table 3–1 contained gel. The characteristics of those ejaculates with gel and results of the gel measurements are presented in Table 3–2. Since the production of gel is highly seasonal in both number of ejaculates containing gel and in gel volume per ejaculate, comparison with the data in Table 3–1 is not valid. The data in Table 3–2 is much more characteristic of what would be expected during the breeding season. It appeared that ejaculates containing gel required fewer mounts per ejaculate, a shorter reaction time and contained a higher volume of gel-free semen than those ejaculates that did not contain gel. Perhaps stallions producing gel have a more satisfactory endocrine pattern, favorably influencing libido and secondary-sex-gland secretions than those not producing gel.

The 112 first ejaculates that contained gel represented 30.9% of the first ejaculates collected, while only 16.7% of the second ejaculates contained gel. Further, gel volumes of second ejaculates were much lower than those of first ejaculates; yet there was little difference in gel-free

Table 3–1 First and Second Ejaculates of Stallion Semen Collected over a 12-Month Period

Characteristic	First ejaculate			Second ejaculate		
	N^a	Mean	SD	N^a	Mean	SD
Semen, gel-free						
Volume (ml)	363	36.4	91.0	329	34.0	18.0
Sperm conc./ml (10^6)	362	337.2	120.1	323	207.8	89.9
Sperm conc./ejaculate (10^6)	362	9,383.5	3,771.2	323	4,933.7	1,986.9
Clumping	340	2.0	0.97	321	1.68	0.94
pH	359	7.42	0.28	329	7.55	0.42
Motility (%)						
Raw semen	329	46.6	16.2	318	47.3	16.7
Diluted semen	358	52.5	22.2	322	45.9	23.8
Extended semen	316	71.9	8.9	291	72.8	8.0
Sexual behavior						
Mounts/ejaculate	363	1.6	0.75	328	1.4	0.70
Reaction time (sec)	355	349.5	369.9	325	167.6	179.0

[a] Number of ejaculates.

From Pickett, B. W.: Paper presented at the 3rd NAAB Technical Conference on Artificial Insemination and Reproduction, National Association of Animal Breeders, Chicago, Ill., Feb. 19–20, 1970.

Table 3–2 Stallion Seminal Characteristics of Ejaculates Containing Gel

Characteristic	First ejaculate			Second ejaculate		
	N^a	Mean	95% Confidence interval	N^a	Mean	95% Confidence interval
Gel						
Volume (ml)	112	31.6	23.4 – 39.8	55	19.3	11.7 – 26.9
Sperm conc./ml (10^6)	96	69.5	50.0 – 88.9	36	38.5	19.9 – 57.0
Sperm conc./ejaculate (10^6)	96	1,234.6	970.1 – 1,499.1	36	706.2	389.2 – 1,023.1
pH	106	7.53	7.50 – 7.56	54	7.60	7.55 – 7.66
Semen, gel-free						
Volume (ml)	112	48.6	42.7 – 54.4	55	48.3	40.5 – 56.1
Sperm conc./ml (10^6)	111	245.5	215.5 – 275.5	54	117.1	96.0 – 138.2
Sperm conc./ejaculate (10^6)	111	9,009.6	8,120.2 – 9,899.0	54	4,490.0	3,728.4 – 5,251.6
Clumping	110	1.98	1.78 – 2.18	54	1.74	1.49 – 1.99
pH	111	7.43	7.40 – 7.46	55	7.54	7.51 – 7.56
Total semen volume (ml)	112	80.2	70.2 – 90.1	55	67.6	56.1 – 79.1
Total sperm/ejaculate (10^6)	96	10,098.1	9,161.2 – 11,035.0	35	4,871.0	3,958.0 – 5,784.1
Motility (%)						
Raw semen	108	43.3	39.9 – 46.7	53	44.7	40.0 – 49.4
Diluted semen	109	45.7	40.3 – 51.1	55	35.6	27.9 – 43.4
Extended semen	110	71.3	69.3 – 73.2	54	71.6	69.2 – 73.9
Sexual behavior						
Mounts/ejaculate	112	1.3	1.20 – 1.48	54	1.1	1.01 – 1.28
Reaction time (sec)	107	115.3	87.4 – 143.2	51	82.2	51.3 – 113.1

^{a} Number of ejaculates.

From Pickett, B. W.: Paper presented at the 3rd NAAB Technical Conference on Artificial Insemination and Reproduction, National Association of Animal Breeders, Chicago, Ill., Feb. 19–20, 1970.

seminal volume between first and second ejaculates. Apparently, gel is not replenished as rapidly as secretions of the other accessory sex glands. The relationship between month and gel volume is presented in Table 3–3. It is important that these relationships be taken into account during stallion seminal evaluation.

During these studies, spermatozoa were counted in 96 gel samples. Approximately 12.2% of the total number of spermatozoa in the ejaculate was found in this fraction. It is customary at some horse-breeding establishments to collect the "dismount" sample and inseminate the mare. Considering that this is the very "tail end" of the ejaculate it is of doubtful value, since in all probability it contains less than 5% of the total sperm and is heavily contaminated with bacteria and debris.

Sexual Behavior

During the course of collecting semen from stallions throughout the year, an attempt was made to study the influence of season on sexual behavior. This type of information should be of value in treating stallions with abnormal sexual behavior and in developing recommendations for breeding management of stallions. It can be seen from the data in Figure 3–23 that the number of mounts per ejaculate were greatly affected by season. The results for the spring months are in agreement with the number of mounts required per ejaculation in natural service. This is further evidence that the artificial vagina shown in Figure 3–2 is a very effective device for collection of stallion semen.

Reaction time is defined as the number

Table 3–3   Effect of Month on Characteristics of Stallion Gel

Month	Ejaculate	N^a	Semen volume (ml)	Gel volume (ml)	Percent of total ejaculates
Jan.	1	2	95.0	21.0	8.0
	2	1	50.0	2.0	4.3
Feb.	1	4	94.0	11.5	16.7
	2	0	—	—	0.0
Mar.	1	5	88.4	23.4	21.7
	2	0	—	—	0.0
Apr.	1	10	60.2	22.3	33.3
	2	1	55.0	31.0	5.0
May	1	10	67.8	27.7	27.0
	2	3	76.0	11.3	9.4
June	1	19	45.3	73.5	57.6
	2	10	59.3	45.0	32.3
July	1	15	41.6	42.9	39.5
	2	14	54.4	18.1	41.2
Aug.	1	15	45.4	24.7	41.7
	2	5	54.0	11.0	13.9
Sept.	1	14	29.8	14.6	43.8
	2	3	34.0	6.3	10.3
Oct.	1	14	30.2	13.4	39.9
	2	9	31.1	15.7	25.7
Nov.	1	4	36.0	8.5	14.3
	2	9	35.2	8.6	32.1
Dec.	1	0	—	—	0.0
	2	0	—	—	0.0
Mean	1	112	48.6	31.6	30.9
	2	55	48.3	19.3	16.7

^{a} Number of ejaculates.

From Pickett, B. W.: Paper presented at the 3rd NAAB Technical Conference on Artificial Insemination and Reproduction, National Association of Animal Breeders, Chicago, Ill., Feb. 19–20, 1970.

of seconds between the moment when the male is near enough to the female for stimulation and the beginning of copulation (Fig. 3–24). The reaction time for second ejaculates followed essentially the same pattern that was exhibited for first ejaculates, but less reaction time was required for second ejaculates. It generally requires more time to prepare an animal to collect the second ejaculate than to collect the first; however, in this study the opposite was true. It is believed that this unexpected reaction was due to the use

of young stallions. Apparently, the first ejaculate served as a stimulus for the second ejaculate.

The sexual behavior of stallions that have been collected throughout the year changes during the fall and early winter; this change is evident in the number of mounts per ejaculation, reaction time, and other less definable aspects. For example, there was a greater tendency for the stallion to "savage" the mare by excessive biting and striking, both before mounting and during copulation. This problem became so severe that it was necessary to muzzle some stallions (Fig. 3-38). The stallions that exhibited this type of behavior were those in which the effect of season, as measured by increased reaction time and number of mounts, was most pronounced. Perhaps stallions in this category have an altered secretion of hormones that control sexual behavior, or they may be more quickly conditioned to a particular stimulus and therefore require more stimulus pressure to maintain a satisfactory level of libido conducive to normal sexual behavior. It is not difficult to imagine certain of these conditions as endocrine-mediated, but pharmacologic treatment cannot be recommended until physiological levels have been determined. There is little or no experimental evidence of a beneficial effect of hormone therapy in cases where libido is excellent but seminal quality is "poor" as evidenced by low motility and number of spermatozoa, accompanied by an elevated number of abnormal spermatozoa.

In addition to the possibility of abnormal sexual behavior being mediated through the endocrine system, there is the fact of psychologically abnormal sexual behavior induced by faulty management. Stallions with abnormal sexual behavior that have been presented to the Animal Reproduction Laboratory at Colorado State University have been classified into the following categories:

1. Failure to attain or maintain an erection.
2. Incomplete intromission and lack of pelvic thrusts after intromission.
3. Dismounting at onset of ejaculation.
4. Failure to ejaculate in spite of a complete prolonged erection and repeated intromissions. In the past, this condition has often been diagnosed as aspermatogenesis or blockage of the reproductive tract.

Most of these cases are suspected of being due primarily, if not entirely, to psychological causes. These stallions responded well to retraining, and recoveries were essentially complete without pharmacologic treatment. Retraining consisted of presenting the stallion to a mare or series of mares, observing his behavior, classifying him in one of the categories, then letting him act independently until a given situation elicited a sexual response. In most cases, this required extreme patience until the desired sexual response was obtained and the first few ejaculates were collected. Generally, after the stallion has had several complete ejaculations, he will response to limited correction. Many times it requires several days and occasionally weeks to obtain the first ejaculate. However, after this has been accomplished, all but the most severely maladjusted stallions will respond.

For example, an 11-year-old Thoroughbred stallion was presented for treatment with a case history of having been

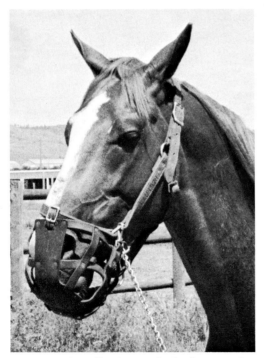

FIG. 3-38. An effective method of preventing the stallion from biting.

severely injured by a mare during the act of copulation. Prior to the incident, the stallion had completed three highly successful breeding seasons. No concerted effort was made to use the stallion after the injury until the following breeding season, at which time he appeared to have recovered physically. However, he refused to cover a mare and continued this attitude for three successive breeding seasons.

At initiation of treatment, his reaction toward mares was favorable as long as a tease rail was between him and the mare. If placed in close proximity to the mare, he would lose the erection and exhibit complete indifference. Attempts to force him to mount a mare in heat resulted in extremely active resistance.

Therapy consisted of using the patient to tease mares each day, but only as long as he showed an active interest. If he showed more than usual interest in a particular mare, she was placed in an adjacent paddock for several hours, or as long as interest was evident. During this period, semen was collected from other stallions where the patient could observe. Any time he showed considerable interest in the sexual act, an attempt was made to collect semen with an artificial vagina.

After 15 days, during which the patient became more aggressive, an ejaculation was collected. For several weeks thereafter, semen was collected from this stallion every third or fourth day. At first, the stallion would dismount at onset of ejaculation, but after several weeks of retraining, he had recovered sufficiently to settle 22 of 26 mares the following breeding season.

Shy, young stallions are also treated in this fashion. It must be remembered that each case is different, and successful treatment requires close observation of the behavior of the individual patient. Conditions necessary for treating such cases are (1) a variety of mares in heat,

(2) other stallions, and (3) extreme patience.

Although only a limited number have been observed, stallions that were severely injured during copulation are the most difficult horses in which to obtain complete recoveries. Racing and show stallions, regardless of breed, appear more frequently for treatment than any other group. It is suspected that, in many cases, the training methods and discipline necessary for racing and showing are not consistent with good breeding management.

These observations indicate that other conditions of abnormal behavior resulting in a "poor" response to mares probably should be treated as psychological problems. If this is true, most endocrine therapy would not be beneficial. Drugs such as psychic energizers, stimulants or even certain tranquilizers, in low doses, might be more effective than hormones.

Masturbation is a vice in breeding stallions, and the most commonly recommended treatment is to use a stallion ring. Masturbation should be classified as abnormal sexual behavior and treated as such. A stallion ring may eliminate the problem but will not correct the condition. Breeding stallions that are well adjusted with regard to the sexual act will not masturbate with sufficient frequency to reduce libido. Further, it is questionable whether a stallion can reduce his normal extragonadal sperm reserves by masturbation.

Some management practices that alter sexual behavior are:

1. Overuse of stallions at 2 to 3 years of age.
2. Unnecessary roughness while handling a stallion during breeding, particularly a young stallion. A stallion should not be allowed to endanger personnel or the mare, but he should be permitted to be aggressive.
3. Maintenance of a stallion in com-

plete isolation from other horses during the nonbreeding season.

4. Frequent use or semen collection during the fall and winter.
5. Forcing a stallion to breed certain mares to which he has considerable objection.
6. Excessive use of a stallion as a teaser, although judicious use as a teaser may serve as a stimulant.

Other Management Factors

A common cause of infertility in popular stallions is overuse. Some stallions can be used daily and occasionally twice a day without reducing sperm reserves below the number required for maximum reproductive efficiency. However, many stallions cannot maintain sperm reserves at a frequency of one ejaculate per day. Sperm production in bulls and boars is directly related to testicular size, and sperm output can be predicted. To date, however, not enough information is available to make such predictions with the stallion. However, it is suspected that this relationship will also be true for stallions, and it should be considered when a stallion is examined for breeding soundness.

Much has been written about the proper nutrition for maximum reproductive efficiency, and numerous recommendations are available. However, there is no experimental evidence to prove definitely what is needed. Thus, in all probability, if a stallion is receiving a sufficient quantity of a well-balanced ration, nothing can be added to increase libido or improve semen quality.

It is commonly believed that a breeding stallion needs a relatively large amount of exercise. Stallions have been maintained in 50' by 16' paddocks at Colorado State University for up to three years, rarely being taken out for anything other than breeding purposes. To date, there have been no detectable detrimental effects on seminal quality. However, no experiments have been designed specifically to study the effects of exercise on seminal quality.

Conclusions and Recommendations

Conclusions

1. The volume of gel-free semen in second ejaculates should be approximately equal to the volume of first ejaculates.
2. The volume of first and second ejaculates is half as large in the late fall and early winter months as during the spring and early summer.
3. Total spermatozoan output per ejaculate of normal stallions will vary from 3 to 40 billion spermatozoa, depending upon testicular size, frequency of ejaculation and season.
4. Total spermatozoan output in the fall and winter months of both first and second ejaculates will be approximately half the number at the peak of the breeding season. Second ejaculates follow the same pattern and normally contain about half the number found in first ejaculates.
5. The pH of normal first ejaculates is always lower than the pH of corresponding second ejaculates.

Recommendations

1. Semen from each stallion should be evaluated before the breeding season and before sale for breeding purposes.
2. The stallion should have at least one week of sexual rest prior to semen evaluation.
3. At least two ejaculates should be collected at approximately hourly intervals for the evaluation.

4. For reliable estimations of motility, equine semen should be extended (1:20) in an extender that will prevent clumping of the spermatozoa.

5. The morphology of 100 spermatozoa from each of two slides per ejaculate should be determined.

6. Each sample of stallion semen should be cultured.

7. The variation due to season in stallion seminal characteristics is extremely large, and this must be taken into consideration during semen evaluation.

8. The most common cause of abnormal sexual behavior is mismanagement.

9. Collect semen from the stallion with an artificial vagina every other day, and inseminate all mares that have been in heat two days or longer with 500 million sperm from undiluted semen.

Digestive System

The teeth should be checked for dental caries. The age, as indicated by the teeth, should be determined to see if it coincides with that given by the seller. The incisors should also be checked for presence of parrot mouth, which is considered an inheritable unsoundness (Fig. 3–39). A wearing of the outside edges of the incisors indicates that the horse is a cribber (Fig. 3–40). The molars should be checked for irregularities and missing teeth. Any sign of a split tooth or receding of the gum indicates a defective molar. Caps on the premolars in young horses should also be noted. Both upper and lower jaws should be checked for bony swelling that indicates previous fractures or dental caries.

The tongue should be examined for bit lacerations that may limit its action. The breath should be checked for odors indicating dental problems or necrosis of tis-

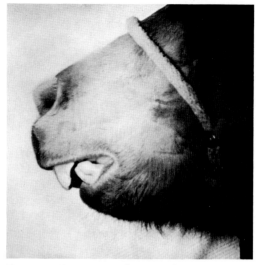

FIG. 3–39. Parrot mouth. Note that upper incisors overlap the lower incisors.

sue. It is desirable to examine the feces for parasite eggs; a rectal examination to determine the existence and extent of aneurysms at the anterior mesenteric artery or in the iliacs is also advisable.

Nervous System

The horse should be appraised to determine if his mental attitude is normal. Examination of the locomotor system should

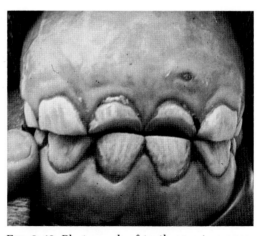

FIG. 3–40. Photograph of teeth on a two-year-old horse that cribs. Note that the outside portion of the upper central incisors is worn off. This change indicates an unsound horse.

have been done previously, and incoordination detected, if present. Incoordination problems include wobbling and shivering syndromes, after-effects of encephalomyelitis, and injury to the head or back.

The head should be raised reasonably high with the hand and then released quickly to determine the horse's balance. If he has pathological changes in the area of the semicircular canals, vertigo will be induced by this test.

The eyes should be examined, along with the nervous system, for the following conditions:

1. Corneal opacities and laceration. Ulcers can be detected by the use of fluorescein.
2. Blindness—this examination should include the use of an ophthalmoscope.
3. Hypopyon—this is the presence of a purulent exudate or blood in the anterior chamber of the eye.
4. Adhesions of the iris—these may be detected when determining the reaction of the pupil to light. An anterior synechia is an adhesion of the iris to the cornea. A posterior synechia is an adhesion of the iris to the lens.
5. Cataracts—which may be due to senility, injury or periodic ophthalmia.
6. Reaction of the pupil to light.
7. Evidence of carcinoma, especially on unpigmented eyelids and on the third eyelid.
8. Follicular lymphoma, a blemish on the sclera, is not an unsoundness. Corneal scars in the line of vision are an unsoundness because they interfere with light transmission and cause astigmatism, which is especially troublesome for jumpers. Congenital cysts may occur in the iris and be nonpigmented, but this is not unsoundness unless vision is impaired.

Hearing should be tested by observing the reaction of the horse to various sounds.

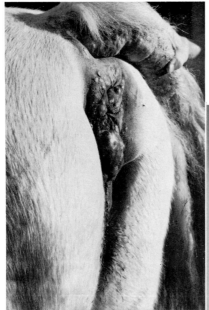
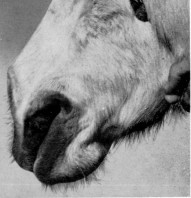

FIG. 3–41. Melanoma formation on the tail, anal sphincter, vulva and mouth of a mare. When these are in an early stage they can be overlooked in a superficial examination.

Common Integument

The skin should be checked for evidence of external parasites and fungus infection. The bursae at the withers, poll, tendon of the biceps brachii, point of the hock, and point of the elbow should be examined for abnormalities. Examination also should be made for melanoma and squamous-cell carcinoma or other tumors. The area of the anus, vulva, penis, and eye are the most common sites for squamous-cell carcinoma. Melanomas are most commonly found around the anus (Fig. 3–41). The back should be checked for scar tissue and other lesions that would interfere with a saddle. These lesions are often due to subcutaneous larvae similar to *Hypoderma bovis*. The tail should be elevated to test its muscular strength and checked visually for proper carriage. Lack of strength in the tail may indicate a tendency to the wobbles syndrome.

Excessive white (unpigmented) areas, although not an unsoundness, should be considered undesirable when found on the feet, eye, eyelids, vulva, anus, or penis, which are more subject to squamous-cell carcinoma under such circumstances. Also, white feet tend to wear faster and crack more easily than pigmented feet. Nonpigmented eyes (glass eyes) are considered undesirable and seem to be more subject to internal eye disease.

Not all types of unsoundnesses have been discussed in the above examinations; therefore, other conditions that occur should be evaluated for their seriousness after careful consideration by the veterinarian.

REFERENCES

Axe, J. W. 1906. *The Horse in Health and Disease. Vol. III.* London: Gresham Publishing Co.

Boddie, G. F. 1969. *Diagnostic Methods in Veterinary Medicine.* 6th ed. Philadelphia: J. B. Lippincott Co.

Casarett, G. W. 1953. A one-solution stain for spermatozoa. Stain Technol. 28: 125.

Coggins, L., and Norcross, N. L. 1970. Immunodiffusion reaction in equine infectious anemia. Cornell Vet. LX(2): 330–335.

Cook, W. R. 1964. The diagnosis of respiratory unsoundness in the horse. Proc. Brit. Equine Vet. Assoc., 18–37.

Cook, W. R. 1965. The diagnosis of respiratory unsoundness in the horse. Vet. Rec. 76: 516.

Equine Medicine and Surgery. (68 Authors.) Santa Barbara, Calif.: American Veterinary Publishers (1963).

Evans, L. H., and Reid, C. F. 1968. The soundness examination and soundness examination form. Proc. AAEP, 57–63.

Evans, L. H., and Panel 1968. Soundness examination form. Proc. AAEP, 65–79.

Flynn, D. V. 1969. The issuance of a soundness certificate—Ethical and medico-legal considerations—Scope, wording and distribution. Proc. AAEP, 175–191.

Frank, E. R. 1964. *Veterinary Surgery.* 7th ed. Minneapolis: Burgess Publishing Co.

Frank, E. R. 1964. Examining for soundness. Haver Lockhart Messenger 44(2): 4–5.

Gendreau, L. A. 1947. Warranty, soundness, unsoundness, vice and blemish. Can. J. Comp. Med. 11: 17.

Hafez, E. S. E., Williams, M., and Wierzobowski, S. 1969. The behavior of horses, Chap. 12. In E. S. E. Hafez (ed.), The Behavior of Domestic Animals. Baltimore: Williams & Wilkins Co.

Jones, W. A. 1936. Soundness in horses. Aust. Vet J. 12: 115.

Malkmus, B., and Opperman, T. 1944. *Clinical Diagnostics.* 11th ed. Chicago: Alex Eger, Inc.

Nishikawa, Y. 1959. Studies on Reproduction in Horses. Japan Racing Association. Tokyo: Shiba Tamuracho Minatoku.

O'Rourke, M. J. 1943. Examination of thoroughbreds. Vet. Med. 38: 404.

Peters, J. E. 1961. Physical examination of the horse for soundness. Proc. AAEP 109.

Pickett, B. W. 1968. Collection and evaluation of stallion semen, p. 80. Proceeding of the Second Technical Conference on Artificial Insemination Reproduction, National Association of Animal Breeders.

Pickett, B. W., Faulkner, L. C., and Sutherland, T M. 1970. Effect of month and stallion on seminal characteristics and sexual behavior. J. Anim. Sci. 31: 713.

Proctor, D. L. 1961. What is a sound horse? Western Livestock J. 39(51): 59.

Reid C. F. 1969. A field form for soundness examination. Proc. AAEP, 169–173.

Roberts, S. F., and Haynes, W. B. 1970. Laboratory Diagnosis of Equine Infectious Anemia. Report

New York State Veterinary College. Ithaca, N.Y.: Cornell University.

RUBIN, L. F. 1963. Some aspects of soundness examination relative to the eye. Proc. AAEP, 121.

RUSSELL, W. 1907. *Scientific Horseshoeing*. 10th ed. Cincinnati: C. J. Krehbiel and Co.

SMYTHE, R. H. 1959. *The Examination of Animals for Soundness*. Springfield, Ill.: Charles C Thomas.

U.S. Department of Agriculture. 1925. USDA Farmers Bulletin. No. 779, Revised. Washington, D.C.

WAYLAND, F. W. 1964. Breeding soundness examination in stallions. Proc. AAEP, 305–310.

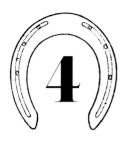

Diagnosis of Lameness

DEFINITION OF LAMENESS

Lameness is an indication of a structural or functional disorder in one or more limbs that is manifested in progression or in the standing position; it is sometimes called claudication. Lameness can be caused by trauma, congenital or acquired anomalies, infection, metabolic disturbances (rickets), circulatory and nervous disorders, or any combination of these. The diagnosis of lameness requires a detailed knowledge of the anatomy and physiology of the limbs, and there are cases of lameness where even the most experienced veterinarians differ in opinion. To the young veterinarian, this fact is apt to cause uneasy moments, since a mistake in diagnosis may interfere materially with a successful start in practice. To him it should be said: Never express a decision until you are thoroughly satisfied that it is correct.

Whenever possible, the horse should first be observed in a box stall. At this time some conditions are obvious that will not be noticeable after the horse has warmed up. Careful observation of how the horse supports his weight on the limbs is important. Stringhalt or upward fixation of the patella may be evident at this time and not after the horse has been moved.

Lameness has been classified by Dollar (O'Connor, 1952) as follows:

1. *Supporting-Leg Lameness.* This is evidenced when the horse is supporting weight on the foot or when he lands on it. Injury to bones, joints, collateral ligaments or motor nerves and to the foot itself are considered causes of this type of lameness.

2. *Swinging-Leg Lameness.* This lameness is evident when the limb is in motion. Pathological changes involving joint capsules, muscles, or tendons are considered to be the cause.

3. *Mixed Lameness.* This is evident both when the leg is moving and when it is supporting weight. Mixed lameness can involve any combination of the structures affected in swinging- or in supporting-leg lameness.

By observing the gait from a distance, one can determine whether it is supporting-leg, swinging-leg, or mixed lameness. A veterinarian may use this classification as an aid to diagnosis, but he cannot rely on it completely. Some conditions that cause supporting-leg lameness may cause the horse to alter the movement of the limb to protect the foot when it lands. This could lead to a mistaken diagnosis of swinging-leg lameness.

Complementary Lameness. Pain in a limb will cause uneven distribution of weight on another limb or limbs, which can produce lameness in a previously sound limb. A relatively minor condition in one foot, for example, can produce a more severe lesion in either the same limb or in an opposite limb. Rooney (1969) gives examples of lameness in one foreleg leading to lameness of the other foreleg and of lameness of one hind leg leading to lameness of the foreleg on the same side;

however, he states that lameness of one foreleg does not lead to lameness of a hind leg, and lameness of one hind leg does not lead to lameness of the other hind leg. In my experience, it is most common to have a complementary lameness produced in a forelimb as a result of a lameness in the opposite forelimb. For example, a lameness in the left forelimb causes enough stress on the right forelimb to produce lameness, often expressed as bowed tendon. Even minor changes in weight-bearing can produce complementary lameness at high speeds, especially over long distances. The suspensory ligament, sesamoid bones, and flexor tendons seem to be the structures that suffer most. However, horses that are slightly calf-kneed often fracture both carpi in identical places, possibly shifting weight unevenly after one carpal bone is fractured. When lameness is in a forelimb, the horse often assumes a lead in the opposite forelimb to protect the unsound limb. The resulting stress on the lead forelimb may cause injury because normal change of leads does not occur. Moreover, one must always be alert to the possibility of an additional lameness occurring in the same limb that already has a minor ailment. The cause of complementary lameness is increased stress on a sound limb resulting from an attempt to protect an unsound limb or, in the case of new injury in an unsound limb, stress to otherwise healthy structures trying to protect a painful area in that limb. This situation can lead to a confusion in diagnosis. For example, a horse with navicular disease usually lands toe first. This constant landing on the toe can cause a bruised sole in the area of the toe, and in extreme cases this soreness of the toe will be so painful that the horse will land excessively on the heel, because the toe bruise hurts more than the navicular area. In other cases, the horse may land on the toe to protect a sensitive area in the heel and cause additional stress on the suspensory ligament.

The character of the stride of a limb is also important to diagnosis of lameness. When observing the stride, the following characteristics are noted:

1. *The Phases of the Stride* (Fig. 4–1). The stride consists of an anterior phase and a posterior phase. The anterior phase of the stride is in front of the footprint of the opposite limb, and the posterior phase is behind it. In lameness, the anterior or posterior phases may be shortened, although the length of the stride must be the same as that of the opposite limb if the horse is to travel in a straight line. If the anterior phase is shortened, there must be a compensatory lengthening of the posterior phase, and vice versa. If there is no compensatory lengthening of the anterior or posterior portion of the stride, the horse will travel sideways with the body at an angle instead of in a straight line.

2. *The Arc of Foot Flight* (Fig. 4–2). The arc of foot flight is changed when there is pain anywhere in the limb. The arc of one foot is compared to that of the opposite member. In some cases the arc is changed in both forefeet (bilateral navicular disease, laminitis) or in both hind feet (bilateral bone spavin). In the hind limb, the arc may be changed enough to cause the toe to drag when the limb is advanced (bone spavin or gonitis) because of reduced flexion of the hock or stifle joints. Navicular disease, laminitis, nail punctures, and other such conditions cause a lowering of arc because of an effort to reduce pain when the foot lands. Painful conditions of the carpus cause a lowering of arc because of reduced flexion of the carpus.

3. *The Path of the Foot in Flight*. If the foot travels inward, there may be an interference problem causing medial fracture of a splint bone or painful lesions of the carpus. When the foot travels in an outward path (paddling) no special problem usually results.

4. *How the Foot Lands*. When a painful lesion is present in the foot, the horse will

usually indicate the pain by placing his weight opposite to the pain. For example, in navicular disease the greatest pain is near the heel, so the foot is placed down toe-first. In a nail puncture of the toe, the weight is placed on the heel. If the lesion is on the lateral portion of the sole, the weight is carried on the medial side of the foot, and vice versa.

Close observation of the above stride characteristics will aid in diagnosis of the lameness.

The majority of lamenesses are found in the forelimb, and of those in this region, 95 percent are in the carpus or below. Approximately three lamenesses will be seen in the forelimb to every lameness in the hind limb. However, in the Standardbred, hind-limb lameness is involved in approximately 40 percent of the lameness diagnoses, a result of his balanced gait. The greatest number of lamenesses occur in the forelimb because they carry 60 to 65 percent of the weight of the horse and are thus subject to much greater concussion than the hindlimbs. The hind limbs act as propelling limbs, while the forelimbs receive the shock of landing. In the hind limb, most lamenesses occur in the hock and stifle. One must remember that the horse may be lame in more than one limb or may have more than one pathological condition in the limb showing lameness. The veterinarian must also realize that *lameness in one area of the limb may cause the horse to injure a second area in the same limb or to injure the opposite limb in an effort to protect the original injury.* (See Complementary Lameness, p. 91.)

Lamenesses in horses will also vary according to the type of work performed. Although there is considerable overlapping, the common lamenesses associated with the type of work should be suspected first: The Thoroughbred is commonly afflicted with carpitis, carpal fracture, injury to the metacarpophalangeal joint (traumatic arthritis), tendon and suspen-

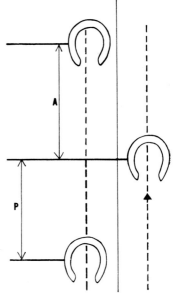

FIG. 4-1. Phases of a stride. *A*, Anterior phase of stride, which is that half of the stride in front of the print of the opposite foot. *P*, Posterior phase of the stride, which is that half of the stride in back of the print of the opposite foot.

sory ligament injury, and sesamoid injury. The Quarter Horse used for barrel racing, calf roping, reining, and cutting is more commonly afflicted with ringbone, fractures of the phalanges (first, second, and third), sidebone, and bone spavin. Navicular disease is common in both groups. A veterinarian should keep these facts in mind in diagnosis of lameness and should

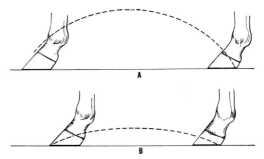

FIG. 4-2. Normal and abnormal arc of foot flight. *A*, Normal arc of foot flight. *B*, Low foot flight caused by lack of flexion in either the fore or hind limbs.

be sure to eliminate the common sites of lameness and the common lamenesses first. In all cases the foot should be suspected and eliminated as a cause of lameness.

In examining a horse for lameness, one should always consider the common things first. From experience we know that at least 95 percent of the lamenesses in the forelimb will occur from the carpus distally. Therefore, if the lameness is in the forelimb, all the common lamenesses from the carpus down should be eliminated before considering other lamenesses, unless some other condition is obvious. In the hind limb, approximately 80 percent of the lamenesses will be in the hock or stifle, so that after preliminary examination of the foot and lower limb, including examination with hoof testers, the hock and stifle are given primary consideration until conditions of those two joints can be eliminated. In difficult cases, nerve blocks are very helpful.

There are other factors to consider as the cause of lameness (Churchill, 1968). Horses that are improperly shod may become lame. Shoeing should be considered only a complementary aid to the way the horse goes; if not properly done, shoeing can produce lameness, especially at high speeds. The surface on which the horse runs on is frequently a contributing factor in lameness. Surfaces that are too soft, too hard, slippery, or rocky may aggravate conformational imperfections or may be the outright cause of lameness. Fatigue is one of the most important predisposing causes of lameness. Even in horses that have good conformation, fatigue will allow relaxation of tendons and ligaments and perhaps predispose to bone fracture, joint injury, or sprain (Figs. 1–15, 1–22). Improper conditioning of horses is a common thing, and many trainers do not fully understand the problems involved in proper conditioning of a horse. The age of a horse is often a factor in predisposition to lameness. With the emphasis on

racing 2-year-olds, many lamenesses are produced that would not occur in older, more mature horses. An immature skeletal system is not ready to accept the burdens of continual high speed. This problem will be with us as long as there is emphasis on 2-year-old racing.

ANAMNESIS

One should attempt to obtain an accurate history of every lameness case. In some instances, the anamnesis is invalid because the owner has recently purchased the animal, because he deliberately attempts to falsify the history (especially as to duration of the lameness), or because he actually believes that the animal is lame in one of the other limbs. In most cases falsification of the history is not malicious; the owner is often merely hesitant to admit that he has not called for professional services more quickly. The successful veterinarian soon acquires the ability of obtaining information in a manner suited to the particular client. This may be done by direct questions or by subtle suggestion to obtain facts essential to the diagnosis.

It is important that the following questions be answered in the anamnesis:

1. *How Long Has the Horse Been Lame?* If lameness has been present for a month or more, it can be considered a chronic condition, since permanent structural changes may have taken place that render complete recovery impossible. The prognosis should always be guarded in this case. A veterinarian should keep in mind that a young horse has a better chance for recovery from a chronic condition than does a mature one.

2. *Does the Owner Know What Caused the Lameness?* The owner may be able to say that he removed a nail from the foot or actually saw the injury occur. This description should include the character of the lameness at the time first noticed. If the lameness was acute initially, this

might indicate a condition such as a fractured third phalanx; if it developed insidiously, an arthritic type of disease might be present.

3. *Does the Horse Warm Out of the Lameness?* If so, muscular structures or arthritic joints (such as bone spavin) may be involved.

4. *Does He Stumble?* Stumbling may be the result of some interference with the synergistic action of the flexor and extensor muscles. It also may indicate that the animal has pain on heel pressure, as in navicular disease or heel puncture wounds, and thereby attempts to land on the toe, which causes stumbling. Painful conditions of the carpus and rupture of the extensor carpi radialis may interfere with flexion enough to cause stumbling and should be ruled out.

5. *What Treatment Has Been Done, and Was It Helpful?* This type of history may influence the prognosis of the case. If the owner has attempted to pass a needle into a synovial structure, suppurative arthritis or tenosynovitis may result. If the horse has received certain types of recommended therapy with no results, the prognosis is guarded, because results from further treatment may be unsatisfactory. It is very important to find out if the horse has been on parenteral corticoids or phenylbutazone derivatives. These will mask symptoms of lameness and give a false impression of recovery. Joint injection with corticoids may have been done, and in some cases, it may lead to infectious arthritis when improperly done. If a joint is painful and swollen, careful inquiry must be made about this possible complication.

6. *When Was the Horse Shod?* Sometimes a nail may be driven into sensitive tissue and then pulled out. In this case, evidence of infection may not manifest itself for several days. In other cases the nail remains in the sensitive tissue, and the shoe must always be removed to discover these potential causes of lameness.

If the nails do not enter sensitive tissue, but are close to it, they may cause lameness from pressure on the sensitive tissue. This is commonly called "nail bound" and it will not be relieved until the nails are pulled.

PROCEDURE FOR EXAMINATION

Visual Examination

The horse should first be observed after confinement. At this time one may observe any swellings, enlargements, or defects in conformation that would be helpful in diagnosis. The horse is more apt to show lameness following confinement than if he has had exercise. Allow the horse to stand for a short time and observe the efforts he may make to compensate for pain in supporting-leg lameness. These compensating efforts will often be a clue to the location of the lameness and to the structures involved. For example, if the horse stands with the carpus forward and the heel raised, the carpal, posterior fetlock and heel areas should be examined closely. If the horse points with the affected foot, navicular disease or fracture of the extensor process of the third phalanx may be present. If a forelimb is held posteriorly and the carpus flexed with the toe resting on the ground, the shoulder on that side should be considered in the diagnosis. Elbow joint lameness will often result in the forearm being extended, the knee being flexed and the foot being on a level with or posterior to its opposite member. In addition, the elbow may have a "dropped" appearance. When the limb is carried, fractures, nail punctures, severe sprains, and septic phlegmon are considered.

A veterinarian can compare the above findings with the normal attitude of the limbs. In the normal attitude, the forelimbs bear an equal amount of weight and are exactly opposite each other. In bilateral involvement of the forelimbs, the weight may be shifted frequently from one foot to the other, or both limbs may be placed too far out in front, called "camped in front" (Fig. 1–20B). In the hind limbs it is normal for the horse frequently to shift the weight from one limb to the other. If the horse consistently rests one hind limb and refuses to bear weight on it for a length of time, or cannot be forced to bear weight on it at all, a veterinarian should consider the possibility of lameness in that hind limb.

Next, the characteristics of the gait of all limbs should be observed from a distance. In most cases it is advantageous to observe the forelimbs first and follow this with observation of the hind limbs. Once a person is able to accommodate his eye to observing all limbs at once, diagnosis of lameness is simplified. Coordination of all limbs can be checked at this time to rule out diseases such as "wobbler" syndrome. The horse also should be backed to determine any lameness in this motion. The shoe, if present, should be removed before examination.

Proper examination includes watching the horse coming toward the examiner, from the side view, and going away from the examiner. In general, forelimb lamenesses are best observed from the front and side views, while hind limb lameness is best diagnosed by watching the horse from the rear and side views.

It is very helpful to examine the horse at the trotting gait on a hard surface where the feet can be seen and heard. There is usually an obvious difference in noise on landing between sound and unsound feet. The unsound foot makes less noise because less weight is put on it and it doesn't land as hard. There is a louder noise when the sound foot hits because most of the weight is taken on that foot. This is true when examining either front or hind limbs.

The Forelimbs

As a result of lameness in a forelimb, the head will drop when the sound foot lands. When weight is placed on the unsound foot or limb the head will rise. If acute lameness is not present, the trot should be used for diagnostic purposes, because any lameness evident in the walk will be increased in the trot because there is only one other supporting foot on the ground. One must be cautious not to confuse a left hind lameness with a right fore lameness, or a right hind lameness with a left fore lameness, in the trotting gait. This could happen, because when a hind limb is lame in the trotting gait, the horse will land more solidly on the sound diagonal limbs, sometimes causing confusion in cases where there is little or no nodding of the head. For example, if a left hind limb is lame in the trotting gait, the horse will land more solidly on the right hind and left fore diagonals. On a hard surface, this could give the impression that the horse was yielding on the right fore and landing solidly on the left fore. The most confusion would occur in watching the horse from the side view. Watching him from behind would reveal the hip elevation typical of hind limb lameness. No head movement is present in bilateral involvement of the limbs or in mild lameness.

In the normal gait the heel is lifted first when the limb is advanced. When the foot lands, the heel should hit just before the toe. If there is pain on concussion to the heel, the horse will attempt to land on the toe, as in navicular disease, or a nail puncture in the heel area. If there is diffuse pain in the foot, such as with laminitis, the horse will make an exaggerated effort to land on the heel and thereby avoid concussion to the bottom of the foot. This is also the case when pain is present in the area of the toe. If pain is present in the lateral portion of the foot, the weight will be carried medially. In general, involvement in the toe of the foot will cause a shortened posterior phase of the stride, and involvement of the heel area of the foot will cause a short anterior phase of the stride. The arc that the foot makes in flight should be observed (Fig. 4–2). If it is too low in the forelimb, there is interference with flexion of the shoulder or carpal joints due to pain or mechanical injury. Fixation of these joints will reduce the arc of the foot flight, limit the anterior phase of the stride, and lengthen the posterior phase. In shoulder involvement, the scapulohumeral joint usually remains semifixed during progression, and the head shows marked lifting and may be pulled toward the unaffected side. When involvement of both forefeet is present, the limbs show a stilted action that causes a false impression of shoulder involvement.

If interference of the limbs is suspected but cannot be seen, the hoof walls can be coated with chalk; the contact will leave a mark of chalk on the limb. The can be done for both the fore and hind limbs.

Various forms of limb contact are defined as follows:

1. Brushing: This is a general term for light striking, especially as in forging or interfering.

2. Cross-firing: This is generally confined to pacers and consists of contact on the inside of the diagonal fore and hind feet. It usually consists of the inside of the hind foot hitting the inside quarter of the diagonal forefoot (Fig. 4–3B).

3. Elbow hitting: This is when the horse hits the elbow with the shoe of the same limb. It rarely occurs except in those horses with weighted shoes.

4. Forging: The toe of the hind foot hits the sole area of the forefoot on the same side (Fig. 4–3C).

5. Knee hitting: This is a case of high interference, generally seen in Standardbreds.

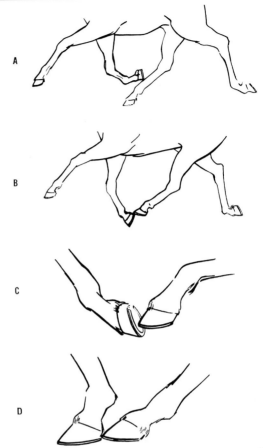

FIG. 4–3. A, Example of scalping. The toe of the forefoot hits the dorsal surface of the pastern or metatarsal area of the hindlimb on the same side. B, Example of cross-firing. The inside of the toe of the hind foot and the inside of the forefoot on the opposite side make contact. This occurs in pacers. C, Example of forging. The toe of the hindfoot hits the bottom of the forefoot on the same side. D, Example of how overreaching can cause pulling of the front shoe.

6. Interfering: This occurs both in the front and hind feet. It is a striking, anywhere between the coronary band and the cannon, by the opposite foot which is in motion (Fig. 1–9, page 7).

7. Overreaching: The toe of the hind foot catches the forefoot on the same side, usually on the heel. The hind foot ad-

vances more quickly than in forging, stepping on the heels of the forefoot. The toe of the hind foot may step on the heel of the shoe of the forefoot on the same side and cause shoe pulling (Fig. 4–3D).

8. Scalping: Here the toe of the front foot hits the hairline at the coronary band or above on the hind foot of the same side. It may hit the anterior face of the pastern or cannon bone. This is generally a fault of the trotting horse (Fig. 4–3A).

9. Speedy cutting: Speedy cutting is difficult to determine since it apparently has no positive definition. It may be the same as cross-firing, or it may mean that the outside wall of the hind foot comes up and strikes the medial aspect of the front leg on the same side. Since there is no positive definition, it can literally be defined as any type of limb interference in the fast gait.

Contact problems can occur in horses with good conformation as a result of the type of work—for instance, barrel racing, cutting, pole bending, and reining, where the weight is suddenly shifted and the horse may be off balance.

The Hind Limbs

In observing the movement of the hind limbs, the arc of the foot flight should be determined (Fig. 4–2). Involvements of the hock and stifle joints reduce the arc of the foot flight and thereby shorten the anterior phase of the stride with a compensating lengthening of the posterior phase. Because of the reciprocal apparatus, incomplete flexion is characteristic of involvement of both the hock and stifle joints. The hock joint is the most common site of lameness and should be inspected first. The toe is worn excessively (dubbed off) in involvement of the hock or stifle, and the horse may kick up dirt or small stones when advancing the limb due to reduced arc of foot flight.

When the sound hind limb strikes the ground, the hip drops on the sound side, and the head rises at the same time. The hip on the affected side rises and the head drops when weight is put on the unsound limb. It is best to observe the horse from behind in checking for hip movement.

In lameness of the hind limbs, as the horse pushes off of the sound hind limb, he raises both hips and thrusts the unsound hip higher than the sound one in an effort to advance the limb with a minimum of flexion. Because of the muscle tension over the gluteal region, one may get the impression that the sound hip is higher because of the tenseness of the muscles. However, if one will observe this action carefully, it can be seen that the affected hip is thrust into the air to aid its advance, while the apparent raising of the hip on the sound side is actually due to tensing of the muscles. This examination, when combined with observing the feet on a hard surface to listen for the differences in sound when the foot of the affected and unaffected limb hits the ground, will usually give accurate determination of which hind limb is involved. Watching the horse from behind and watching the action of the hips will usually differentiate between front and hind limb lameness. When a hind limb is involved, there will be a "hiking" or elevation of the affected hip as the sound limb pushes off the ground.

In involvements of either the fore or hind limb, the horse should be checked on both rough and smooth surfaces to determine the effect of concussion and of uneven pressures on the sole.

Examination by Palpation

Following observation of the animal from a distance, close examination of the limbs by palpation and, of course, by sight, is in order. A systematic method of palpation should be used so nothing will be overlooked. In palpating, start at the bottom of the foot and make a complete examination of the entire limb.

The Forelimbs

1. Examination of the bottom of the foot. Determine whether there is contraction of the heels. Observe the condition of the frog and determine if the sole appears normal. At this time the sole and frog should be examined with a hoof tester to determine any areas of sensitivity. If the entire sole shows pain upon pressure of a hoof tester, you should consider laminitis, fracture of the third phalanx, and a diffuse pododermatitis from a puncture wound. If the area of sensitivity is localized, you should check for sole bruising, puncture wounds, and separation of the white line (gravel) causing infection. Any separation at the white line, or discoloration of the sole, should be thoroughly explored with a hoof knife until the discoloration disappears or the bottom of the discoloration is found. If a sensitive area is localized in the center third of the frog, navicular disease should be considered, after puncture wounds of the frog have been ruled out. Pain in other areas of the frog may be caused by puncture wounds.

2. Examination of the hoof wall. The hoof wall should be checked for excessive dryness, contraction, cracks, and evenness of wear. Cracks may lead to the sensitive laminae, thereby causing lameness. These are most common in the toe and quarter areas of the wall. The shape of the wall should be examined to determine if the hoof is wearing abnormally.

3. Examination of the coronary band. The coronary band should be palpated for increase in heat. This is done by using the back of the hand to compare the coronary region on the affected limb with a sound limb. Increased heat, and a roughening of the hair at the anterior portion of the coronary band, might indicate a developing low ringbone. Drainage at the heel area of the coronary band would indicate a puncture wound in the foot. Drainage near the quarters might indicate quittor.

4. Examination of the lateral cartilages. The cartilages should be examined both with the foot on the ground and with the foot off the ground to determine if calcification has occurred (sidebones).

5. Examination of the pastern area. This area should be examined for change in temperature and swellings that might indicate ringbone. The posterior digital arteries should be palpated to determine if increased pulsation is present.

6. Examination of the fetlock joint. This joint should be examined for areas of pain on pressure, especially over the sesamoid bones and the dorsal part of the joint capsule. Distention of the posterior cul-de-sac of the fetlock joint capsule may indicate the presence of a joint disease. This distention occurs between the posterior aspect of the distal end of the cannon bone and the suspensory ligament and is termed swelling of the volar pouch. This swelling may or may not be indicative of pathology. The joints should be moved with the weight off the limb to check for crepitation and pain on movement. Swelling on the anterior surface of the fetlock joint may indicate osselets or chip fracture of the first phalanx.

7. Examination of the cannon bone area. This area should be checked on the lateral and medial side for the presence of splints; these are most commonly found on the medial side. The anterior surface of the cannon bone should be examined for the presence of periostitis (bucked shins). Other abnormalities easily found are usually in the form of traumatic exostoses.

8. Examination of the suspensory ligament. This ligament should be carefully examined by palpation both in the standing position and with the limb flexed. This ligament lies just posterior to the cannon bone. Damage to this structure is most often in the distal third of the cannon bone in the branches of the ligament. Pain on pressure or scar tissue in this structure indicates pathology.

9. Examination of the inferior check ligament. This joins the tendon of the deep flexor tendon at about the middle of the cannon bone. Damage to this structure can be determined by evidence of pain on pressure over the deep flexor tendon about halfway between the carpal and fetlock joints.

10. Examination of the flexor tendons, both superficial and deep. These tendons should be closely examined for tendosynovitis, pain on pressure, and fibrosis. Swelling of the tendon sheath and fibrosis indicate bowed tendon, fibrosis from external trauma, or an infectious tenosynovitis. Swelling of the tendon sheath is most common just above the fetlock joint. This swelling lies between the suspensory ligament and the deep flexor tendon, which differentiates it from swelling of the volar pouch of the fetlock joint capsule (wind puffs).

11. Examination of the carpus. The carpus should be carefully examined for swellings on the posterior or anterior aspect. Posterior swelling medial to the accessory carpal bone indicates distention of the carpal sheath carrying the flexor tendons and may be associated with fracture of the accessory carpal bone. Synovial swellings on the anterior face of the carpus include distention of the joint capsules; swelling of the tendon sheath of the extensor carpi radialis, the common or lateral extensor tendon sheath; and swelling of the carpal bursa. Swellings of the tendon sheaths, joint capsules, and bursa in this area commonly are called hygroma. Firm swellings over the anterior face of the carpus indicates fibrosis and/or exostosis that might be caused by carpitis (popped knee) and/or fracture of one of the carpal bones. The carpal joint should be flexed to determine if movement causes pain or if there is any mechanical limitation to movement. The radial, intermediate, and third carpal bones should be palpated while the carpal joint is flexed to determine if swelling indicating fracture is present. The cavities of the radiocarpal and intercarpal joints are usually separated, and careful palpation will determine in which one excess synovial fluid is present (Fig. 4-4).

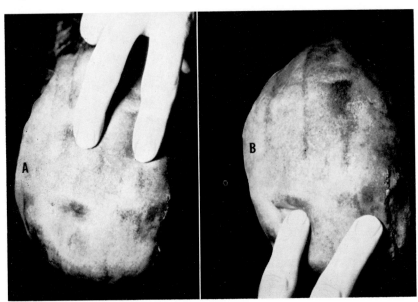

FIG. 4-4. Palpation of the carpal joints. A, Palpation of flexed carpal joint with the fingers in the radiocarpal joint space. B, Palpation of flexed carpus with fingers in the intercarpal joint space.

12. Examination of the soft tissues between the carpus and the elbow. These tissues should be examined carefully for swelling, pain, and puncture wounds.

13. Examination of the elbow and shoulder joints. These joints should be carefully palpated for the presence of pain and crepitation on movement. The bursa at the point of the shoulder should be checked for bicipital bursitis.

14. The forearm and shoulder and scapular areas should be examined for muscular atrophy indicating a long-standing lameness or sweeny.

The Hind Limbs

The hind limbs are checked in the same manner as are the forelimbs up to the hock joint.

1. The hock joint should be examined carefully for the presence of bog spavin, bone spavin, occult spavin, curb, thoroughpin, and capped hock. Bog spavin swelling is found at the antero-medial aspect of the tarsal joint, or occasionally at the posterior aspect of the joint where the capsule is not limited by surrounding tissues on the medial and lateral side. Thoroughpin is found anterior to the proximal end of the os calcis and is a bilateral distention of the tarsal sheath enclosing the deep flexor tendon of that limb. Bone spavin occurs at the medial aspect of the hock joint and involves the medial aspect of the proximal end of the third metatarsal and the medial side of the third and central tarsal bones. A routine spavin test should be done in hind-limb lameness by holding the hind limb in flexion for one or two minutes (Fig. 4–5). Immediately following this flexion the animal should be moved; if the lameness has worsened, the test is considered to be indicative of occult or bone spavin.

2. The stifle joint should be examined carefully for the presence of upward fixation of the patella and for gonitis. Examine the femoropatellar pouch between the

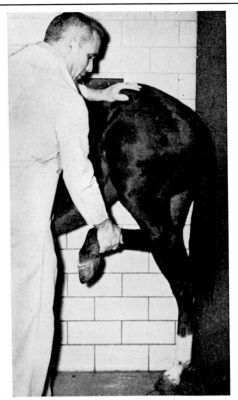

FIG. 4–5. Spavin test. The hind limb should be held in this position for one to two minutes and the horse observed for increased lameness in the first few steps he takes. Increased lameness is considered to be a positive reaction to the spavin test.

middle and lateral patellar ligaments and between the middle and medial patellar ligaments. This examination will disclose distention of this pouch or thickening of the capsule. Distention or thickening of the pouch means that an inflammatory change is present either between the patella and femur or in the femorotibial joint. Both stifle joints are examined carefully for comparison. If there is slight distention of the femoropatellar pouch on both hind limbs, the finding may or may not be serious. Prominent bilateral distention usually means that important changes have occurred in both stifles.

The next step is to force the patella upward and outward so that the medial patellar ligament will lock over the medial trochlea of the femur (Fig. 4–6). This test will reveal whether or not the patella can be locked on the medial trochlea of the femur; it may also reveal crepitation as the patella is forced over the upper part of the trochlea. If crepitation is present as the patella is moved back and forth over the upper part of the trochlea, chondromalacia of the patella is probably present and could be the source of irritation. If the patella can be locked, chondromalacia of the patella could be present, and the medial patellar ligament should be cut. Horses three years of age and under should have radiographs of the stifle to eliminate the possibility of concurrent osteochondritis dissecans (Fig. 6–129).

The stifle is then examined for looseness or tearing of the medial collateral or anterior cruciate ligaments. Facing cranially, the hand next to the horse is placed on the medial aspect of the hock joint, and the lower part of the limb is pulled outward while the stifle is forced inward with the shoulder. The other hand is held over the medial aspect of the stifle joint to detect opening of the joint (Fig. 4–7B, C). If one can detect opening of the medial aspect of the joint with this test, the medial collateral ligament is loosened or torn (Fig. 6–124). Next, the proximal aspect of the tibia is grasped between the hands as in Figure 4–7A and given a quick backward pull. If the anterior cruciate ligament is ruptured, crepitation can be felt between the tibia and femur. The prognosis in stretching or rupture of either of these ligaments is very unfavorable, and chronic lameness will result. If either collateral or the anterior cruciate ligaments are ruptured or stretched, there will be damage to the medial meniscus of the femorotibial joint. If both chondromalacia and ligamentous rupture can be ruled out, but there is distention of the femoropatellar pouch and a pronounced lameness, medial meniscus damage should be suspected. This diagnosis can be arrived at only through a process of elimination.

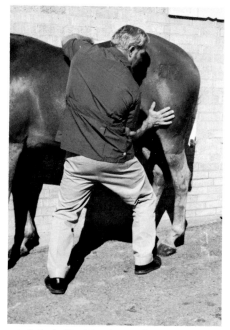 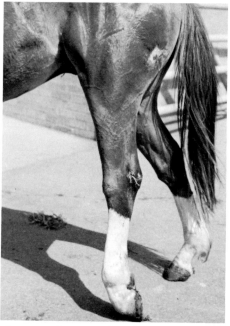

FIG. 4–6. *Left*, Positioning to force patella upward and outward as an aid in diagnosis of upward fixation of the patella. *Right*, Typical attitude of upward fixation of the patella: Extension of the stifle and hock joints and flexion of the fetlock joint are evident.

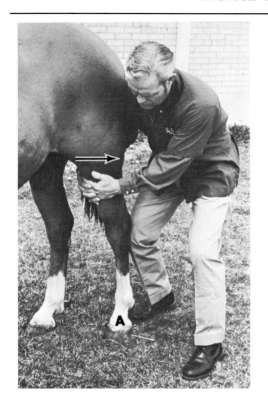

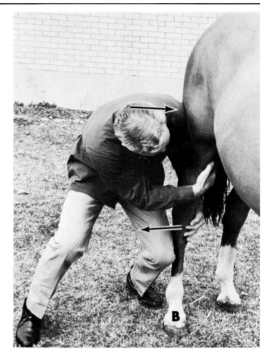

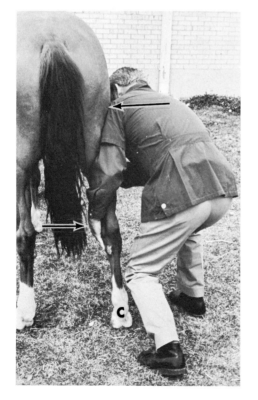

FIG. 4-7. A, Testing for rupture of anterior cruciate ligament. With knee behind the point of the hock, the proximal part of the tibia is jerked posteriorly (arrow). Any looseness or crepitation felt when the tibia moves posteriorly, or when it slides forward, indicates rupture of the anterior and possibly the posterior cruciate ligament(s). No movement between the tibia and femur can be produced in the normal horse. B and C, Testing for rupture of the medial collateral ligament of the stifle: B, The arm next to the limb is placed with the hand on the inside of the hock. The other hand is placed on the medial aspect of the femorotibial joint to check for opening of the joint. With the shoulder pushing in against the stifle joint, the hock is pulled out with the hand (arrows). Any opening felt by the hand on the medial aspect of the stifle joint indicates rupture of the medial collateral ligament of the stifle. C, Same test as B, from a different angle.

In the mature horse, the most common changes in the stifle joint are between the patella and femur in the form of intermittent upward fixation or chondromalacia resulting from the patella riding too high. If this finding is negative, ligamentous rupture is differentiated as described. Medial meniscal damage is cause for an unfavorable prognosis, because at the present time there is no satisfactory surgical procedure for removal of the meniscus and the continuous irritation in the joint causes osteoarthritis (Figs. 6–126 and 6–127). Most changes in the femorotibial joint are limited to the medial side, taking the form of ligament injury or damage to the medial meniscus. The lateral aspect of the joint is not commonly involved.

When examining a foal or a young horse (3 years and under), an additional change in the stifle joint that must be considered is osteochondritis dissecans of the joint. This is also known as aseptic necrosis and may involve either the femur or tibia. These changes involve the articulation and can be diagnosed only on radiographic examination. This change may be present in very young foals or in horses up to three years of age. However, in most cases the changes will be evident before the horse is a year old (Fig. 6–129).

If a suppurative or infectious arthritis is present in the joint, obvious heat, pain, swelling, and temperature rise will be present, and one can aspirate abnormal synovial fluid. This type of arthritis usually occurs in the young foal and is one of the changes in navel ill.

3. All soft tissue over the stifle and hip areas should be examined for pathological changes, including atrophy. Atrophy of the gluteal and quadriceps musculature will be present in chronic lameness of the hip and chronic painful stifle lameness.

4. The hip joint should be examined by palpation and by observation of the gait. Involvements of this joint produce a supporting-leg lameness and often an accompanying swinging-leg lameness. When the round ligament of the hip joint has ruptured, the stifle joint and toe will point outward, while the hock goes inward. This same appearance will be present in complete luxation of the joint. This typical attitude cannot be assumed unless the round ligament is ruptured. The femoral head may still be in the acetabulum, but the increased range of motion will produce severe osteoarthritis.

5. The pelvis should be examined by rectal examination for the presence of fractures. Manipulate the tuber coxae and tuber ischii, while one hand is in the rectum, to determine if any movement is produced at the symphysis pubis or at other potential fracture sites (Fig. 4–8). The sacroiliac and lumbosacral junctions should also be examined rectally at this time. Pain produced by rectal pressure over these areas or the iliopsoas muscles may indicate damage in these areas. If necessary, the horse should be walked a few steps while the hand is in the rectum to see if motion indicates a possible fracture or other pathological changes. Fractures are often accompanied by hematomas that are palpable. Separation of the symphysis pubis may not be accompanied by hematoma. If there is separation of the sacroiliac junction, only crepitation, with no hematoma, will be present; discrepancy of the ilium at the junction with the sacrum will be seen. One or both tubera sacrala will be elevated (see Chap. 6, p. 292).

Special Considerations

Hyperthermia is best checked by testing the area with the back of the hand and comparing this with the opposite limb. One should bear in mind that an area that has been clipped will feel warmer than an unclipped area, and the sun's rays on one limb will make it feel warmer.

Crepitation may be produced in normal joints, and there is more movement in the

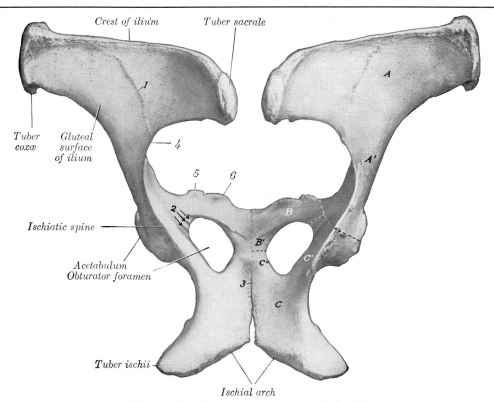

FIG. 4–8. Ossa coxarum of horse, dorsal view. *A*, Wing; *A'*, shaft of ilium; *B*, acetabular branch of pubis; *B'*, symphyseal branch of pubis; *C*, body of ischium; *C'*, acetabular branch (or shaft) of ischium; *C"*, symphyseal branch of ischium; *1*, gluteal line; *2*, grooves for obturator nerve and vessels; *3*, symphysis pelvis; *4*, greater sciatic notch; *5*, iliopectineal eminence; *6*, pubic tubercle. Dotted lines indicate primitive separation of three bones, which are potential fracture sites. (Sisson, *Anatomy of Domestic Animals*, courtesy of W. B. Saunders Company.)

pastern and coffin joints of some horses than in others. One should always compare the lame limb with the opposite limb to determine if abnormalities are present.

Areas of both limbs may appear to show pain on pressure, so it must be determined whether the animal is actually exhibiting pain or, through nervousness, is pulling away. Young animals are more difficult to examine than horses that are well disciplined. Some mature horses, though, have nervous temperaments that hamper examination procedures, so some allowances should be made for nervousness or fear. Tranquilization may be necessary, or at least helpful, in conducting a thorough examination.

One cannot judge the seriousness of enlargements in the limbs by palpation alone, but one must be able to evaluate carefully the importance of these swellings and their proximity to articular or other structures.

Special Methods of Examination

Hoof Tester

The use of the hoof tester has been discussed in the section on the examination of the sole. This is not necessarily a special method of examination, but is certainly one that always should be used.

One cannot begin to diagnose lameness without using a good hoof tester of sufficient size and construction that considerable force can be exerted (Fig. 4–9).

Local Nerve Blocks

These are of considerable aid in determining the site of some types of lamenesses. They are also valuable in proving a diagnosis to an owner who is not convinced. There are times when a positive diagnosis of a lameness cannot otherwise be made. In these cases, local anesthesia can be used in a systematic manner to pinpoint the site of lameness. Once the site is located, a detailed examination of the suspected area can be made clinically and radiographically. It is helpful to know the area of pathologic change in order to avoid excessive expenditure for radiographs. In the long run, there is a considerable saving of time to the practitioner when local anesthesia is used because the lameness can be pinpointed more quickly.

In all cases, the amount of local anes-

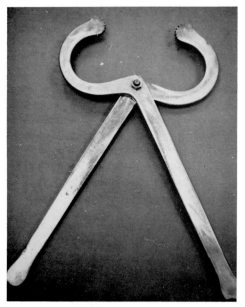

FIG. 4–9. Hoof tester made from plow steel. A hoof tester must be well constructed and large enough to conduct on adequate examination.

thetic used should be minimal because of residual tissue irritation. Adding a steroid such as Predef 2X* at the rate of 1:10 cc will decrease the irritant effect of the local anesthetic. In addition, local anesthesia should always be done as an aseptic procedure. To prevent infection resulting from injection, the area should be clipped closely, shaved when practical, and scrubbed with soap and water; skin antiseptics should be applied. When joints are injected, the skin should be shaved.

Recommended Anesthetic Solutions. In most cases the best agents for local anesthesia are 2 percent Lidocaine HCl,† 1 percent Hexylcaine HCl,‡ or 2 percent Mepivacaine HCl.§ These solutions are very potent and have rapid effect. They are also quite irritating, and minimal amounts should be used. Two percent procaine hydrochloride can be used but is not as effective as the above drugs. Procaine has no topical effect and is of no value in intra-articular injection for diagnosis of lameness.

Sterile needles, sterile syringes, and sterile anesthetic solutions should always be used. In no case should the same needle be used on more than one horse without sterilization between usages.

Diagnostic Local Anesthesia Techniques in the Forelimb. Once the veterinarian has satisfied himself that he has not been able to determine the lameness in the limb either by clinical examination or by hoof tester examination, the following methods of local anesthesia can be used to aid in localizing the lameness.

Local anesthetics containing epinephrine should not be used in ring block anesthesia below the carpus and the hock. The use of epinephrine may cause necrosis of the skin on the dorsal surface of the third metacarpal or metatarsal bones.

1. The medial and lateral posterior digi-

*Upjohn Co., Kalamazoo, Michigan.
†Xylocaine, Astra Laboratories.
‡Cyclaine, Sharpe & Dohme Laboratories.
§Carbocaine, Winthrop Laboratories.

tal nerves are anesthetized (Fig. 4–10) with 1.5 to 2 cc of anesthetic solution and a 25-gauge, $\frac{5}{8}''$ needle. These nerves are located just anterior to the superficial flexor tendon. The anesthesia is done about halfway between the fetlock and the coronary band. The needle is inserted just in front of the superficial flexor tendon. This block desensitizes the posterior third of the foot. Too much local anesthetic will cause the effect to spread to the anterior digital nerve, leading to a false interpretation of the block. If the horse is sound after anesthesia of the two nerves, such conditions as navicular disease, fracture of a wing of the third phalanx, puncture wounds of the heel, corns, and other involvements of the posterior third of the foot can be considered.

When doing a posterior digital nerve block for diagnostic purposes, one can expect approximately the same relief from a posterior digital neurectomy as obtained from using a small amount (1 to 1.5 cc) of a local anesthetic over the posterior digital nerve. If there is only a partial response to this block, one can expect that whatever lameness is evident after the posterior digital nerve block will still be present after a posterior digital neurectomy. There are several reasons a horse with navicular disease may not respond completely to a posterior digital nerve block:

a. Fibrous adhesions between the navicular bone and the deep flexor tendon. When adhesions are present between the deep flexor tendon and the navicular bone, it is nearly impossible for the horse to modify his gait. The gait will improve slightly after posterior digital nerve block because of some pain relief, but the foot will still hit toe first with a short anterior stride. This is a mechanical interference with the gait and cannot be modified by nerve block.

b. Possible arthritis of the coffin joint. In severe cases of navicular disease, the changes in the navicular bone may extend

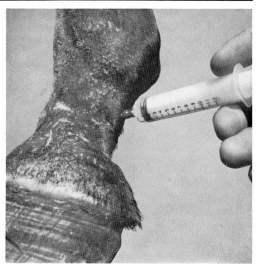

FIG. 4–10. Blocking the lateral posterior digital nerve. The needle (25-gauge, $\frac{5}{8}''$) is placed just anterior to the tendon of the superficial digital flexor tendon. The medial nerve is blocked in an identical way. (Courtesy Norden Laboratories.)

into the coffin joint. In this case, there is a coffin-joint arthritis present, and posterior digital neurectomy will only partially relieve the lameness. One can then inject local anesthetic into the coffin joint, as described on page 451, to desensitize the coffin joint. If complete relief of the lameness is obtained, it is reasonably certain that there is arthritis in the coffin joint. This means that a posterior digital neurectomy would be only partially successful, since the coffin joint would still be painful.

c. Accessory nerve supply from the anterior digital nerve or from the posterior digital nerve (Fig. 2–7). Sometimes the accessory branches from the posterior digital nerve will be separate enough from the main posterior digital nerve to escape blocking in a differential diagnostic block. In other cases, the anterior digital nerve will bifurcate and send a posterior branch back to the navicular area. In either case, this accessory nerve supply will be responsible for only a partial response to the posterior digital nerve block. Unless

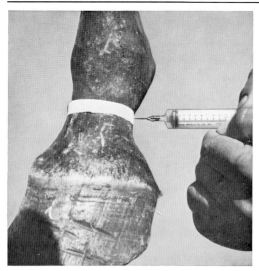

FIG. 4–11. Needle in position where the posterior digital nerve is blocked. The line of white tape indicates the area injected to complete the ring block above the pastern joint. (Courtesy Norden Laboratories.)

all nerve supply is severed to the navicular area, there will be poor response to the posterior digital neurectomy. Accessory branches of the posterior digital nerve can usually be found during surgery, but a posterior branch from a bifurcation of the anterior digital nerve must be searched out (Fig. 2–7). In racing horses, the anterior digital nerve should not be cut.

d. In severe cases of navicular disease, the horse bruises the soles in the toe areas from landing on the toe. In this case, the hoof tester examination should reveal pain over the toe area of the sole; this finding should be taken into consideration when doing posterior digital neurectomy. The lameness caused by the sole bruising at the toe will still be present after the posterior nerve block.

e. Concurrent traumatic arthritis of the fetlock. Pasterns that are too straight also predispose to traumatic arthritis (osselets) of the metacarpophalangeal (fetlock) joint. Navicular disease and traumatic arthritis of the metacarpophalangeal joint may be present at the same time. Injection of the volar pouch of the metacarpopha-

langeal joint with local anesthetic after blocking the posterior digital nerves will reveal how much lameness is due to each condition.

f. Improper or incomplete anesthesia. Skin sensation can be checked medially and laterally on the same foot, and one foot can be compared to the other. A hoof tester may also be used, and if sensation is still evident over the center one-third of the frog, the anesthesia is inadequate. In this case, the block should be repeated after reviewing the landmarks.

2. If, after the posterior digital nerve blocks, the horse is still unsound, a ring block can be done just above the proximal interphalangeal (pastern) joint, as shown in Figure 4–11. In this case, following anesthesia of the medial and lateral posterior digital nerves, additional anesthetic solution is injected subcutaneously around the anterior surface of the first phalanx above the proximal interphalangeal joint and over the flexor tendon area posteriorly. This ring block desensitizes the foot below this line. This desensitization will include the distal interphalangeal (coffin) joint and proximal interphalangeal (pastern) joint, provided the block is done above the latter joint. If the horse is sound following this procedure, the lameness has been localized to a point below the ring block. Attention can then be given to defining the type of lameness using radiography if necessary.

3. The next step in localizing a lameness that has not responded either to blocking the posterior digital nerves or to a ring block in the pastern area is anesthesia of the medial and lateral palmar nerves 2″ to 3″ above the metacarpophalangeal joint (Fig. 4–12). Two to three cc of anesthetic solution is deposited over each of the medial and lateral palmar nerves. These nerves lie between the suspensory ligament and deep digital flexor tendon, just anterior to the deep digital flexor tendon. The nerves are relatively deep but can be reached by a 25-gauge $\frac{1}{2}″$

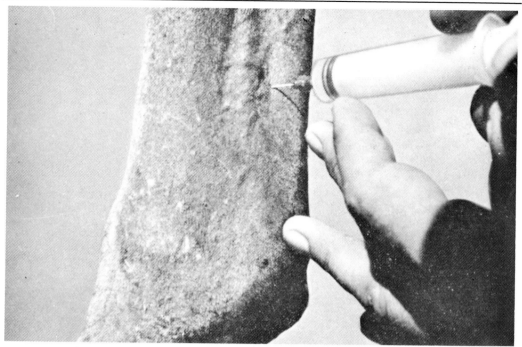

FIG. 4–12. Needle in position to block the lateral palmar nerve just in front of the tendon of the deep digital flexor. The medial nerve is blocked in the same fashion on the medial side of the leg. (Courtesy Norden Laboratories.)

needle. If the horse is sound after this block, but not sound after the ring block in the pastern area as described above, the area of the fetlock joint can be examined for lameness. However, it is a common experience to find that intra-articular lesions of the metacarpophalangeal joint do not respond to a simple palmar nerve block (Adams, 1966a).

4. If the horse is unsound after block of the two palmar nerves, a ring block is done as shown in Figure 4–13. Approximately 10 cc of a local anesthetic is necessary to complete the ring block. The area between the two blocked palmar nerves and over the flexor tendons is injected subcutaneously. Special attention is given to blocking the area where the second and fourth metacarpal bones join the third metacarpal bone. At this point, there is often a small nerve present that must be anesthetized to obtain a complete ring block. If, following this ring block, the

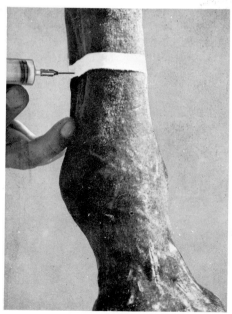

FIG. 4–13. Needle in position over the medial palmar nerve. The white tape indicates the line blocked to complete a ring block above the fetlock joint. (Courtesy Norden Laboratories.)

horse is sound but did not respond to the pastern ring block, a detailed examination for articular lesions of the metacarpophalangeal joint should be done. These lesions include small chip fractures of the first phalanx (Fig. 4–14) and osselets. Other lesions include longitudinal fractures of the third metacarpal bone and first phalanx (Fig. 4–15). These fractures can be present with minimal swelling and very little lameness. Lesions of the sesamoid bones are also considered. Further proof of an intra-articular lesion can be obtained by injecting the distended volar pouch of the metacarpophalangeal joint capsule. Injection of this pouch is done on the lateral side of the joint between the suspensory ligament and the third metacarpal bone at the level of the sesamoid bones (Fig. 11–12). A mixture of 5 cc of local anesthetic solution and 2 cc of a corticoid solution is used.

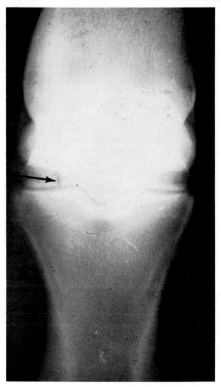

FIG. 4–15. An example of a fracture of the third metacarpal bone into the articulation of the metacarpophalangeal joint. This type of lesion may show minimal swelling, and the pain may not disappear following an ordinary palmar nerve block. A ring block above the fetlock joint or an intra-articular block may be required to localize the pain to this area.

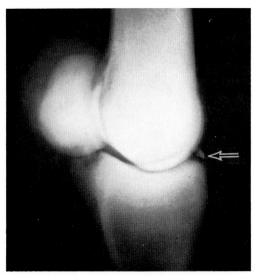

FIG. 4–14. Radiograph of a small chip fracture from the first phalanx (arrow) This type of lesion is not usually desensitized by an ordinary medial and lateral palmar block. A ring block above the fetlock joint must be completed to desensitize this lesion effectively. It can also be desensitized by an intra-articular injection of the metacarpophalangeal joint (Fig. 11–12). (Courtesy JAVMA 148: 360, 1966.)

5. If, after the ring block above the fetlock joint, the horse is still unsound, the carpal joints can be anesthetized. There are three joints in the carpus: the radiocarpal joint, the intercarpal joint, and the carpometacarpal joint. In most cases, the joint fluid that is present in the radiocarpal joint is separate from that enclosed by the intercarpal and carpometacarpal joints (Van Pelt, 1962). This means that to block the carpal joints effectively a local anesthetic must be injected into both the radiocarpal and intercarpal joints, as shown in Figures 4–16 and 4–17. Detailed examination will quite often reveal distention of a joint capsule or thickening of

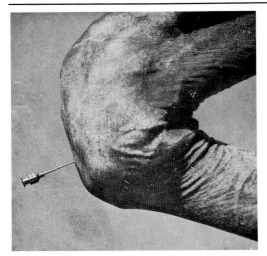

FIG. 4–16. Flexed left carpus showing 18-gauge 2″ needle in position in the intercarpal joint. (Courtesy of Norden Laboratories.)

soft tissues over these joints when pathological changes are present.

After proper preparation of the skin area, the carpal joint is flexed and a small skin bleb is made with a local anesthetic using a 25-gauge $\frac{1}{2}$″ needle. An 18- or 20-gauge 2″ needle is then placed into the intercarpal joint (Fig. 4–16). Five cc of 2 percent Xylocaine or other suitable topical anesthetic is placed in the joint. The author includes a corticoid solution in the injection. If there is no response to blocking the intercarpal joint, the radiocarpal joint is blocked in a similar manner (Fig. 4–17). Flexing the carpus greatly aids passage of the needle directly into the joint.

One should allow fifteen minutes for the local anesthetic to have a topical effect in the joint, whereas in blocking a nerve locally, the effect should be noticed within five to ten minutes. One of the local anesthetics mentioned above is recommended for use in a joint, since procaine has no topical anesthetic qualities. Some inflammatory effects may be noted after injection of a joint, but they are minimal and, if the injection has been done under aseptic conditions, no problems will result. A corticoid included in

the injection will minimize inflammatory effects. The steroid produces no adverse effects in most horses, and some may even show improvement in the lameness, provided the site of lameness is localized to this area.

If soundness results following one or both of these injections, osteoarthritis and carpal bone fractures are considered as possibilities and radiographs of the carpus are taken.

6. The entire carpal area and lower leg can be anesthetized by blocking the median, ulnar, and musculocutaneous nerves (Figs. 4–18 and 4–19). This procedure can be used to localize the lameness to the shoulder and elbow when other blocks have failed. These blocks eliminate the lower limb as the site of lameness, leaving the elbow and shoulder areas as the cause of lameness. In most cases, one should be able to localize the site of lameness without the use of these blocks.

The median nerve is blocked on the caudal aspect of the radius and cranially to the muscular portion of the flexor carpi radialis muscle. The needle is inserted through the skin about 2″ below the elbow joint or where the pectoral muscles

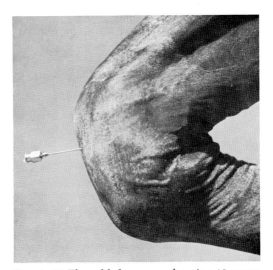

FIG. 4–17. Flexed left carpus showing 18-gauge 2″ needle in position in the radiocarpal joint. (Courtesy of Norden Laboratories.)

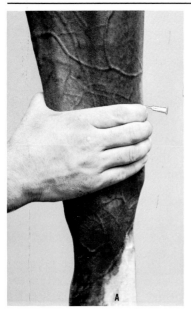
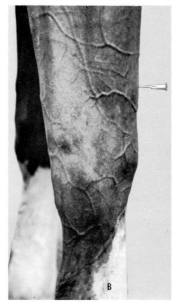
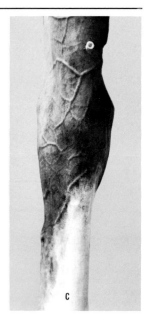

FIG. 4-18. Blocking the ulnar nerve. A, Needle between the ulnaris lateralis and flexor carpi ulnaris, a handbreadth (4″) above the accessory carpal bone, on caudal aspect of the left forelimb. B, Same view as A, with hand removed. C, Caudal aspect of left forelimb showing needle in place between ulnaris lateralis and flexor carpi ulnaris muscles, 4″ above the accessory carpal bone.

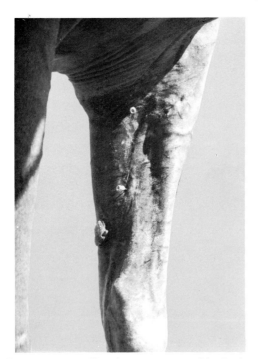

FIG. 4-19. Needles in position to block the median nerve (upper needle) and the musculocutaneous nerve (lower needle).

flatten to join the forelimb. The needle penetrates through the skin and fascia, and the local anesthetic should be deposited superficially and as deep as 1″ to $1\frac{1}{2}$″. The median nerve is large and not always definitely situated, making it advisable to use 10–20 cc of a local anesthetic solution (Fig. 4-19).

The musculocutaneous nerve is blocked on the medial surface of the radius halfway between the elbow and carpus and just in front of the cephalic vein. The nerve is usually just below the skin; its location can vary somewhat. It is best to block the subcutaneous tissues both in front of and behind the cephalic vein (Fig. 4-19).

The ulnar nerve is blocked approximately 4″ above the accessory carpal bone on the caudal aspect of the forearm. Careful palpation will reveal the groove between the flexor carpi ulnaris and the ulnaris lateralis muscles. The needle is inserted through the skin and fascia to the nerve. The depth of the nerve will vary somewhat but is usually about $\frac{1}{2}''$ below the surface. Using at least 10 cc of local anesthetic, one can block both superficially and deep in the area and usually ensure success (Fig. 4–18).

7. For other lesions that may be causing lameness, such as bony enlargements on the metacarpal bones (splints) or swellings that are suspected of causing lameness, an infusion of local anesthetic around the lesion down to the periosteum will produce soundness if the lesion is the cause of lameness. In this way, a specific lesion such as a possible fractured splint or metacarpal bone lesions can be anesthetized, and if the lesion is causing lameness, the horse will be sound, provided the local anesthetic is carried down to the periosteum.

8. The humeroradial (elbow) joint is somewhat difficult to palpate for injection. The joint is flexed repeatedly until the articulation can be distinguished. The needle can be passed from either the cranial or caudal aspects into the joint (Fig. 11–17).

9. The scapulohumeral (shoulder) joint is injected in a notch between the two parts of the lateral tuberosity of the humerus (Fig. 11–18). In most cases the tuberosity can be palpated, and the needle is carefully passed into the joint (*see* Chapter 11).

Diagnostic Local Anesthesia Techniques in the Hind Limb. In the hind limb, the posterior digital block, pastern ring block, plantar nerve block and the fetlock ring block are the same as in the forelimb. When the tarsal (hock) joint is reached, other techniques are employed.

1. If a bone spavin is suspected, local injection of the spavin area and bursa of the cunean tendon with a local anesthetic and a 2″ 20-gauge needle will sometimes alleviate the signs. The needle is pushed directly into the spavin area until it reaches bone, and approximately 8 cc of anesthetic solution are used to block this area. If a bone spavin is obviously present and if the block relieves it, one can assume that the cunean tendon is involved in the lameness. A more effective block that may anesthetize the hock joint sufficiently to be of diagnostic value in bone spavin is anesthesia of the tibial and deep peroneal nerves or of the tarsometatarsal and distal intertarsal joints.

a. Local anesthesia of the tibial nerve. This nerve is blocked in conjunction with the deep and superficial peroneal nerves in the diagnosis of bone spavin. The site of injection is approximately 4″ above the point of the hock on the medial aspect of the limb, between the Achilles tendon and the deep flexor tendon (Fig. 4–20). When the horse is bearing weight on the limb, the nerve lies close to the caudal edge of the deep flexor tendon. The nerve can be palpated by forcing weight off of the limb and grasping firmly in front of the Achilles tendon with the thumb and forefinger. The nerve can be felt as a structure approximately $\frac{1}{4}''$ in diameter just in back of the deep flexor tendon. Depending upon the temperament of the horse, tranquilization may or may not be necessary. A twitch should usually be used as a routine procedure for protection to the operator. The nerve may be blocked from two positions: (1) Stand on the lateral side of the limb to be blocked; and (2) stand on the lateral aspect of the limb opposite the one to be blocked and reach across to insert the needle. The method used depends a good deal on the horse and the operator. An area approximately 4″ above the point of the hock is clipped and shaved and prepared for injection. At this time, a 25-gauge needle is forced through the skin over the nerve, and a small amount of local anesthetic injected intradermally and subcutaneously. This makes it easier for passage of the larger (18-gauge, $1\frac{1}{2}''$) needle. The larger needle is forced through the skin, and when it is obvious that the needle has penetrated the fascia enclosing the nerve, 15 to 25 cc of

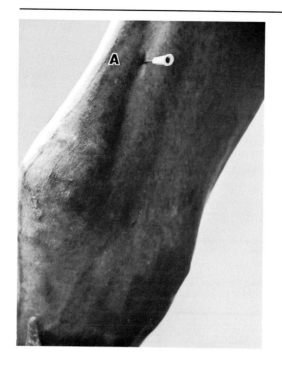

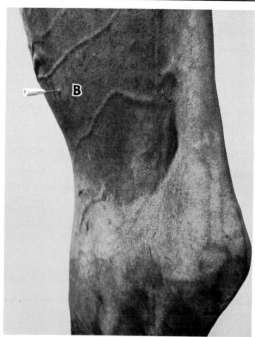

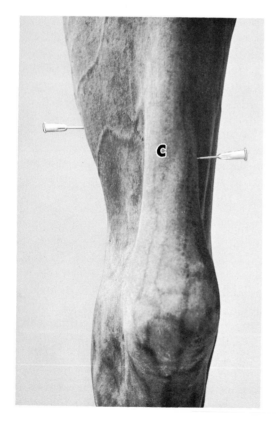

FIG. 4–20. Blocking the posterior (caudal) tibial and deep peroneal nerves. *A,* $1\frac{1}{2}''$ 18 gauge needle over posterior tibial nerve on medial aspect of left hind limb. *B,* $2''$ 18 gauge needle between long and lateral extensors on the left hind limb. This is the location to block the deep peroneal nerve. *C,* Caudal view showing needles for above blocks in position, approximately $4''$ above the point of the hock.

a local anesthetic agent is used, moving the needle superficially and deeply and caudally and cranially until the area is adequately infused. Care should always be used that the horse does not move quickly and break off the needle.

　b. Local anesthesia of the deep and superficial peroneal nerves. These nerves are usually blocked in conjunction with the tibial nerve for diagnosis of hock lameness, especially bone spavin. The location of injection is just distal to the most prominent portions of the lateral digital extensor and the long digital extensor in the groove formed between these two muscles. This is usually about 4″ above the point of the hock on the lateral aspect of the limb (Fig. 4–20B). The deep peroneal nerve lies near the lateral edge of anterior (cranial) tibial muscle and close to the bone. The superficial peroneal nerve lies slightly caudal to the septum of the two extensor muscles and more superficially. The groove between these two muscles is identified, and the area is clipped, shaved, and prepared for injection. Depending on the individual animal, tranquilization may or may not be necessary. A twitch should be used for protection of the operator. A 25-gauge needle is forced through the skin in the groove between the two muscles, and a small amount of local anesthetic is injected intradermally and subcutaneously to ease the passage of a larger needle. An 18-gauge 2″ needle is then passed through the intradermal bleb in a slightly caudal direction. It is passed deeply until the operator believes that the needle point is close to the lateral edge of the anterior (cranial) tibial muscle. To block the deep peroneal nerve, 10 to 15 cc of local anesthetic is injected on the deep edges of the two extensors and the lateral border of the anterior tibial muscle, close to the tibia. The needle is then retracted and 10 to 15 cc of local anesthetic is injected more superficially, with the needle moving cranially and caudally to be sure that the superficial peroneal nerve is blocked. The depth of the superficial peroneal nerve can vary, so the injection should include an area from $\frac{1}{4}$″ to at least 1″.

When the tibial and superficial and deep peroneal nerves have been blocked, some horses have difficulty with extension of the digit.

In many cases, satisfactory anesthesia of the individual joints of the hock can be obtained by inserting a 25-gauge $\frac{5}{8}$″ needle into the individual tarsal joints (Moyer, 1972) (Fig. 4–21). The technique is as follows: The anteromedial aspect of the hock is prepared for injection. A 25-gauge $\frac{5}{8}$″ needle is used to anesthetize the skin and subcutaneous tissues over the antero-medial surface of the hock. The injection site is more anterior than medial. The tarsometatarsal joint is blocked first, using the head of the second metatarsal bone as a landmark for approximate height of the joint space. A 25-gauge $\frac{5}{8}$″ needle is inserted through the skin and deep tissue to the bone. Probing along the bone with the needle point will usually allow the small needle to enter the joint space. The needle is inserted to the hub, and 3–5 cc of local anesthetic such as Xylocaine or Carbocaine is injected into the joint. The distal intertarsal joint is located approximately $\frac{1}{2}$″ above the tarsometatarsal joint, and the proximal intertarsal joint is located about $\frac{1}{2}$″ above the distal intertarsal joint. These blocks are very helpful in localizing the exact site of lameness in bone spavin, and are helpful in diagnosing the site of lameness in occult spavin.

The tibiotarsal joint cavity of the hock can also be anesthetized for suspected lesions such as chip fracture of the tibia or tibial tarsal bone. The injection site used is medial or lateral to the saphenous vein, directly over the joint capsule (Figs. 11–19 and 11–20). This is not a good block for diagnosis of bone spavin because the distal intertarsal and tarsometatarsal joints do not communicate with the tibiotarsal joint.

2. The stifle joint may be anesthetized by infusing a local anesthetic, but this is complicated somewhat by the separation of the capsule of the femorotibial joint and the femoropatellar pouch. The stifle joint of the horse is composed of two principal joints: the femoropatellar and femorotibial joints. The femorotibial joint is divided into medial and lateral joint cavities. The femoropatellar joint cavity communicates with the medial femorotibial joint cavity by a slit-like opening. A similar but smaller opening may exist between the femoropatellar pouch and the lateral femorotibial joint cavity (Van

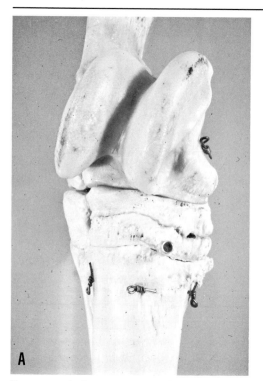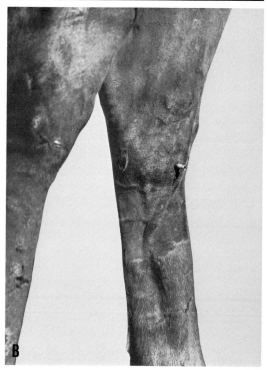

FIG. 4–21. *A,* ⅝″ 25 gauge needle in tarsometatarsal joint of right hock. *B,* ⅝″ 25 gauge needle in tarsometatarsal joint of left hock.

Pelt, 1966), but this is not a consistent finding. The femoropatellar pouch can be injected, and one can expect anesthesia of the medial femorotibial joint capsule but not the lateral femorotibial joint capsule.

The femoropatellar pouch is usually most easily infused between the middle and medial patellar ligaments (Fig. 4–22) but may be infused between the middle and lateral patellar ligaments at the distal margin of the patella. Thirty to fifty cc of 2 percent Xylocaine or other suitable local anesthetic is infused into the femoropatellar pouch for diagnostic purposes. A corticosteroid is included with the local anesthetic to minimize any inflammatory effects of the local anesthetic. If the lesion in the joint is subpatellar, this block will usually relieve signs of lameness. If the lesion is in the medial femorotibial articulation, the femoropatellar block will usually anesthetize this area. Since lesions

of this joint are most commonly located in the medial side, this is an important block. If desired, the medial femorotibial joint may be injected between the medial patellar ligament and the medial collateral ligament of the stifle joint.

The lateral femorotibial joint can be injected between the lateral patellar ligament and the lateral collateral ligament of the stifle joint. Since the femoropatellar joint cavity communicates with the lateral femorotibial joint cavity in only 18 to 25 percent of the stifle joints, it will be necessary to inject this joint cavity directly (Van Pelt, 1965). An 18 gauge 2″ needle is used to inject the cavities of the stifle joint after anesthetizing the skin with a 25 gauge ⅝″ needle.

3. The coxofemoral (hip) joint is injected through the notch that lies just cranial to the trochanter major of the femur. The trochanter major is followed down on the anterior edge, and the needle is passed

through the notch in front of it into the joint as shown in Figure 11-22.

4. The sacroiliac joint can sometimes be blocked successfully, but most often subluxation of this joint is diagnosed by clinical signs and differentiation of other similar lamenesses (see the section on subluxation of the sacroiliac joint, p. 292).

Radiography

Radiographs of suspected pathological areas are invaluable in diagnosis and prognosis. It is sometimes impossible to determine if some hard swellings are bony or fibrous in nature without the use of radiographs. Radiographs are also extremely helpful in determining the proximity of new bone growth to a joint surface. Some fractures of the carpus and the third phalanx are nearly impossible to detect without the use of radiographs. However, radiographs can never replace careful examination and palpation for disease of the soft tissues. See Chapter 12 for a complete discussion of radiological technique.

Thermography as a Diagnostic Aid

A thermograph has been described as a heat camera (Blakely, 1959) because it records an image—a thermogram of the skin temperature distribution pattern. The camera scans the area at which it is directed and collects infrared radiation and converts it into visible light that exposes a polaroid film. The relative darkness or lightness of a given region of film negative is proportional to temperature of the corresponding region of skin, so temperature distribution of an area of skin can easily be visualized. Delahanty (1965) described experiences with this machine in horses. His conclusions indicated that there are possible indications for use of thermography as a diagnostic aid for lameness. However, the cost of the unit, the difficul-

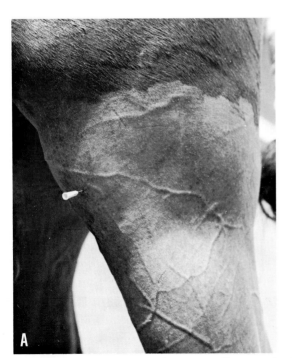 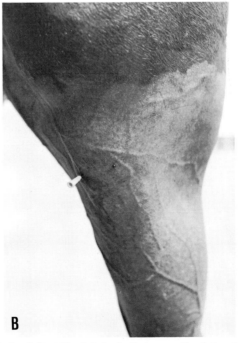

FIG. 4–22. Injection of the femoropatellar pouch of the left stifle joint. *A,* Between the lateral and middle patellar ligaments. *B,* Between the medial and middle patellar ligaments.

ties with restraint and the length of time (6 min.) required for examination make improvements necessary before it will receive wide acceptance. It is obvious that an aid of this nature could be very helpful in elucidating the causes of obscure lamenesses. The use of thermography would show inflamed areas in the limb that might go unnoticed in usual examination procedures. Thermography can also be used on other areas of the body besides the limbs. At present, it could probably be safely stated that it is generally impractical; but further improvements in the instrument, making possible a more rapid examination, plus possible cost reduction, might make its use more widespread.

REFERENCES

ADAMS, O. R. 1966a. Chip fractures of the first phalanx and the metacarpophalangeal (fetlock) joint. JAVMA. *148*(4): 360.

ADAMS, O. R. 1966b. Local anesthesia as an aid in equine lameness diagnosis. Norden News (Jan.).

BARNES, R. B. 1963. Thermography of the human body. Science, 140: 870.

BLAKELY, R. F. 1959. Radiographic diagnosis of injury to the foot of a horse. Ill. Vet. 2(3): 69.

BRENNAN, B. F. 1962. Symptoms of hind limb lameness in standardbreds. Proc. AAEP Convention, 194–96.

CARLSON, W. D. 1967. *Veterinary Radiology.* 2nd ed. Philadephia: Lea & Febiger.

CHENOT, A. 1904–05. Clinical study of lameness. Amer. Vet Rev., *28:* 806.

CHURCHILL, E. A. 1968. *Care and Training of the Trotter and Pacer.* Columbus, Ohio: U.S. Trotting Association.

DAUBIGNY, F. T. 1916. Halting or lameness in the horse. JAVMA 49: 648.

DELAHANTY, D. D. 1965. Thermography in equine medicine. JAVMA *147*(3): 235.

FOWLER, W. J. R. 1939. Diagnosis and treatment of lameness. Can. J. Comp. Med. *3:* 91.

FOWLER, W. J. R. 1940. Diagnosis and treatment of lameness. Can. J. Comp. Med. 4: 249.

FRANK, E. R. 1964. *Veterinary Surgery.* 7th ed. Minneapolis: Burgess Publishing Co.

GAUBAUX, A., and G. BARRIER. 1892. *The Exterior of the Horse.* 2nd ed. Philadelphia: J. B. Lippincott Co.

GERSHON-COHEN, J., *et al.* 1965. Medical thermography: A summary of current status. Radiol. Clin. N. Amer. 3(3): 403.

GIBBONS, W. J. 1966. Diagnosis of equine lameness. Mod. Vet. Pract. 47(9): 62.

GIBSON, S. J. 1945. Lameness in horses. Can. J. Comp. Med. *9:* 103.

HICKMAN, J. 1964. Veterinary Orthopaedics. Philadephia: J. B. Lippincott Co.

KIERNAN, J. 1894. Hints on Horseshoeing. Washington, D.C.: Office of Library of Congress.

LA CROIX, J. V. 1916. Lameness of the horse. Vet. Pract. Ser. No. 1, Amer. J. Vet. Med.

LIAUTARD, A. F. A. 1888. Lameness of Horses, New York: W. R. Jenkins.

McKILLIP, M. H. 1918. Lameness, some basic principles of diagnosis. Am. J. Vet. Med. *13:* 387.

MERCK & CO. 1973. Merck Veterinary Manual. 4th ed. Rahway, N.J.

MILNE, F. J. 1967. Examination and diagnosis of foot lameness. JAVMA 151(12): 1599–1608.

MOYER, W. 1972. Kennett Square, Pa. Personal communication.

O'CONNOR, J. J. 1952. Dollar's Veterinary Surgery. 4th ed. London: Bailliere, Tindall & Cox.

ROONEY, J. R. 1969. Biomechanics of Lameness in Horses. Baltimore: Williams & Wilkins.

SISSON, S. 1953. *Anatomy of Domestic Animals.* 4th ed. J. D. Grossman, ed. Philadelphia: W. B. Saunders Co.

SZBUNIEWCZ, M. 1969. Use of the hoof hammer in diagnosing lameness. VM/SAC 64(7): 618–627.

VAN PELT, R. W. 1962. Intra-articular injection of the equine carpus and fetlock. JAVMA 140: 1181.

VAN PELT, R. W. 1965. Intra-articular injection of the equine stifle for therapeutic and diagnostic purposes. JAVMA 147(5): 490.

VAN PELT, R. W. 1966. Arthrocentesis and injection of the equine tarsus. JAVMA 148(4): 367.

VAUGHN, J. T. 1965. Diagnosis of equine foot lameness. Mod. Vet. Pract. 46(4): 58–59.

WAY, C. 1935. Lameness and arthritis in horses. N. Amer. Vet. 16: 19.

WESTHUES, M., and R. FRITSCH. 1964. *Animal Anesthesia.* Philadelphia: J. B. Lippincott.

WHEAT, J. D. 1962. Detection of the site of lameness. Proc. 8th Annual A.A.E.P. Convention. 198–202.

WILLIAMS, W. 1891. *The Principles and Practices of Veterinary Surgery.* New York: W. R. Jenkins.

WYMAN, W. E. A. 1898. *Diagnosis of Lameness in the Horse.* New York: W. R. Jenkins.

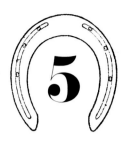

Diseases of Bones, Joints, and Related Structures

ARTHRITIS

Arthritis can be defined simply as inflammation of a joint. This inflammation may involve any or all of the components of a joint, which include the bones forming the joint, the articular cartilages, the joint capsule, and the associated ligaments. The ligaments of a joint consist of the periarticular or collateral ligaments, and, when present, the intra-articular ligaments. The shoulder joint of the horse is the only joint without collateral or intra-articular ligaments.

The joint capsule is composed of an outer fibrous layer and an inner, or synovial, layer, which secretes the synovial fluid. The volume of synovial fluid, which acts as a lubricant in the joint, increases in the presence of inflammation. The capsule's fibrous outer portion is strong, and when it is pulled from its bony attachment, periostitis and new bone growth may result.

Synovial fluid is a transparent, pale yellow, viscous protein containing dialysate of blood plasma. Hyaluronic acid (hyaluronate) secreted from the synovial cells imparts to the synovial fluid its lubricant character. Viscosity is highest during slow movement and increases as the rate of movement increases, reducing resistance to motion and ensuring adequate lubrication (Hollander, 1972).

Normal synovial fluid does not clot at room temperature. It contains relatively few cells, and these consist of lymphocytes, neutrophils, monocytes, eosinophils, macrophages, synovial cells, and undifferentiated cells. Most of the cells are phagocytic. Fluids, electrolytes, colloids, and protein will pass in both directions through the permeable synovial membrane between the blood vessels, lymphatics, and synovial fluid (Hollander, 1972). In injury to the joint, fibrinogen, normally absent, enters the synovial fluid imparting to it the ability to clot. The proportion of leukocytes increases, changing the color of synovial fluid to a turbid darker yellow. The viscosity of the fluid is increased by a lowered mucin production, and destruction of hyaluronate reduces the lubricant quality of the fluid.

According to Rooney (1969), synovial fluid has four important properties: constant load bearing; lubrication or wetting of surfaces; good heat conductivity; and elasticity and the ability to become semisolid instantly on impact, which prevents squeezing out from between the articular surfaces. If synovial fluid becomes less viscous for any reason, it may be squeezed from between the joint surfaces, allowing the surfaces to come into direct contact, causing increased friction. If the cartilage is damaged, there will be an increase in the shearing effect on the cartilage, and a decrease in the total area of contact. This concentrates the load on a smaller area of cartilage.

Rooney (1969) further states that the acute pathological response of a joint to an aseptic injury (such as trauma) is acute inflammation of the synovial membrane with increased production of synovial fluid that is deficient in hyaluronate. Leakage of serum and blood may occur, further disturbing the viscosity of the synovial fluid. When an inflamed joint is worked, the changes in synovial fluid result in increased damage.

Other things will change the ability of synovial fluid to lubricate a joint. Infection will almost always alter lubricant properties enough to cause destruction of cartilage, along with the destructive factors produced by the infection itself. Infection of the joint, especially with a suppurative-type organism, produces a rapid destruction of articular cartilage. Rarely does a joint recover after infection. Under these circumstances, cartilage can be destroyed in a matter of hours by the enzymatic substances produced by the organisms and white cells.

Articular cartilage consists of three layers: a narrow calcified base layer bound to the subchondral bone, a broad intermediate layer of great shock-absorbing capacity due to its high content of water, and a very narrow superficial layer of tangential collagen that resists shear and joint motion (Johnson, 1962).

Cartilage nutrition is by diffusion through and across the cartilage from two capillary beds, the capillary bed of the synovium and the capillary bed of the two bone ends. The rate of diffusion varies in a cycle controlled by use and rest. There is an associated variation in thickness of articular cartilage with activity.

Destruction of most of the articular cartilage in a joint usually results in ankylosis of that joint. Articular cartilage is usually described as being unable to regenerate. However, if the irritant causing degeneration is removed, the cartilage has remarkable healing qualities (Riddle, 1970). For example, a chip fracture in the carpal joint may cause considerable damage to the articular surface of the third or radial carpal bones. Removal of the chip fracture allows healing to occur, and, in many cases, the horse returns to complete soundness. Subsequent examination of the joint several years later reveals a well-healed articular surface.

In horses, the progression of pathological events leading to total destruction of the joint begins with microscopic changes in the cartilage of the bearing surface (MacKay-Smith, 1962). Race horses generate many millions of foot-pounds of force per mile, and the wear and tear produced in both support and propulsion contributes to the production of osteoarthritis.

According to Sippel (1942), in arthritis the cartilage loses its translucence, becomes more or less discolored, and with use is worn away in fragments ranging in size from microscopic to several millimeters. Scoring or grooving of the cartilage is often observable before the bone is exposed. As subchondral surfaces are laid bare, eburnation becomes marked. Periarticular proliferation of bone commonly accompanies this phase. As more bone is uncovered, the periarticular reaction accelerates. In joints that retain motion, the bare bone may become scored with wear. In an immobilized joint, peri- and intra-articular ankylosis progresses until the joint is solidified. Capsular changes vary directly with the speed of progression and with the stage of the disease. Fibrosis may be very extensive in the late stages.

Arthritis may be either primary or secondary. Examples of primary arthritis are trauma to a joint or direct penetration into a joint cavity by a foreign body. Examples of secondary arthritis are disease of the bone, such as rickets, or localization of a systemic infection in a joint. In other words, primary arthritis is a disease of the joint itself, while secondary arthritis results from localization of a metabolic disease or systemic infection in a joint; secondary arthritis may also be a result of poor conformation that causes trauma to a joint.

Enlargement of a joint can be the result of several causes. An effort should be made to ascertain which structures are involved in the swelling. This determination usually can be made by careful clinical and radiological examinations. The following are causes of joint enlargement, either singly or in any combination:

1. Enlargement of the bones forming the joint.
2. Thickening of the joint capsule.
3. Distention of the joint capsule with synovia or other fluid.
4. Swelling of the periarticular tissues.

Methods of Classifying Arthritis

Classification by Activity

Acute. Acute forms of arthritis cause severe inflammation of the joint and thus are self-evident. They may resolve, leaving a normal joint, or develop into a chronic arthritis.

Chronic. Chronic forms of arthritis consist of a low-grade joint inflammation that may exhibit acute flareups. Chronic arthritis almost always leaves a horse with permanent damage to the joint.

Classification by Type

In earlier editions of this work, I classified arthritis by type and by etiology. Now, in an effort to simplify this classification, I am combining these classifications into a single classification that will describe etiology under the type of arthritis. It should be remembered that one type or form of arthritis may progress into another type or form. For example, an infectious type of arthritis may lead to

ankylosis of the joint, at which time it is reclassified as ankylosing or adhesive arthritis.

1. *Serous Arthritis (Traumatic Arthritis).* In nearly all instances, serous arthritis is due to trauma. It may or may not be accompanied by sprain of the associated ligaments. It is characterized by an inflammation of the synovial membrane and increased synovia, which causes increased capsular pressure and swelling. Aspirated synovial fluid appears to be normal. If the inflammation persists, erosion of the joint cartilage and osteoarthritis may result. Serous arthritis can be caused by trauma due to poor conformation that causes constant stress on certain joints. As long as the stress on the joint is mild, the arthritis can remain a chronic serous arthritis that interferes little, if at all, with locomotion. Radiographically, the bony structures of the joint appear normal.

One cannot always determine the exact time that a serous arthritis will begin to develop the characteristics of osteoarthritis. Once the characteristics of osteoarthritis develop, the condition will not return to a simple serous arthritis. Serous arthritis should be considered a mild inflammatory change in the joint without any irreversible changes in the joint.

What begins as a serous arthritis can become complicated by infection. Infection can result from tapping the joint to inject corticoids or to aspirate fluid. Infection can also be the result of lowered resistance caused by the arthritis itself or by previous injection of corticoids. If infection occurs when the joint has not been recently injected, it is apparently the result of bacteria localizing in an area of injury. Bacteria reach the joint by way of the bloodstream (bacteremia). Since an injured or injected joint is an area of low resistance, an infectious type of arthritis may develop. Once serous arthritis has progressed either to an osteoarthritis or to infectious arthritis, the prognosis is much poorer.

2. *Osteoarthritis (Osteoarthrosis, Hypertrophic, or Degenerative Arthritis)* (Figs. 5–1 and 5–2). Osteoarthrosis and degenerative joint disease are the most accurate terms, since the disease is usually noninflammatory and is characterized by deterioration of articular cartilage and joint surfaces. The term osteoarthritis is used here because of its common use.

Osteoarthritis can apparently begin in either the bone or cartilage. In most cases it probably begins as a disease of cartilage, but in a few cases primary alteration of the bone may occur. It is recognized also that osteoarthritis can be primary or secondary. In primary osteoarthritis there is intrinsic degeneration of articular carti-

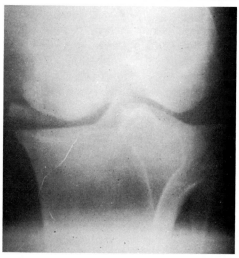

FIG. 5–2. An example of osteoarthritis of the stifle joint. Note the "lipping" on the articular edges of the tibia and the radiographic density of the damaged medial meniscus.

lage underlying the development of the disease (Hollander, 1972). In the secondary type there are predisposing causes, such as trauma, allowing osteoarthritis to supervene on other types of pre-existing damage to the joint, such as traumatic or serous arthritis. Osteoarthritis can occur in horses of any age but is most common in older horses. There is a distinct possibility that there are genetic factors that contribute greatly to osteoarthritis in horses.

Osteoarthritis commonly results from the continued trauma of use of a horse with serous arthritis. The use of corticoids to mask the pain of a serous arthritis will increase the possibility of development of osteoarthritis. The source of trauma may also be conformational. In some cases, the condition occurs as a result of age and results from "wearing" of the joint cartilages.

Osteoarthritis is characterized by degeneration of the cartilage and hypertrophy of bone. There is thickening of the synovial membrane; this membrane often develops numerous villi. Radiographically, osteoarthritis is characterized by

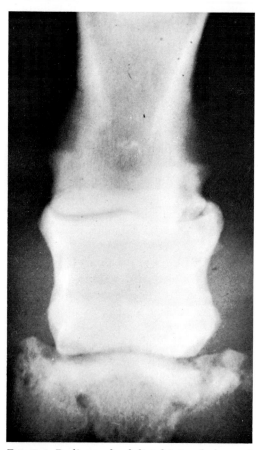

FIG. 5–1. Radiograph of distal interphalangeal (pastern) joint showing uneven joint space, an early radiographic sign of osteoarthritis.

uneven joint spaces (Fig. 5-1), variable amounts of "lipping" and hypertrophic new bone growth around the joint. Sclerosis of adjacent bone may be evident. Long-standing cases may develop a tendency to ankylose as a result of articular cartilage damage and hypertrophic bone. A joint space can always be identified in osteoarthritis even though there may be much new bone growth around the joint. Ringbone of the pastern joint and bone spavin of the hock begin as osteoarthritis and often end up as ankylosing arthritis. Osteoarthritis may become infectious arthritis as a result of repeated injection of corticoids (Fig. 5-3). The changes in osteoarthritis are usually irreversible, and treatment is directed at preventing further deterioration of the joint.

3. *Infectious Arthritis (Suppurative Arthritis, Pyogenic Arthritis)* (Figs. 5-3, 5-4, and 5-5). Infectious arthritis may be caused by several mechanisms: direct wound into the joint (including needle injection); blood-borne infection (metastatic); and extension from neighboring areas of infection. The metastatic form of infectious arthritis is most frequent, and the infecting organisms may spread by way of the bloodstream from any focus of infection or by bacteremia. This type of infection may also involve the joint if it has been injured, such as in sprain, and a bacteremia makes it possible for organisms to localize in an injured joint because of lowered resistance. The injection of corticoids into a joint also lowers its resistance and may allow bacteremic or injected organisms to cause infection of a joint. There may be a mild synovitis or a markedly destructive lesion of the joint.

Infectious arthritis may be suppurative or nonsuppurative, depending upon the organism involved. The infection of the

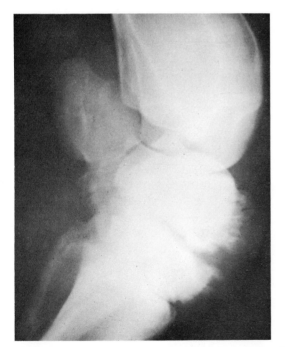

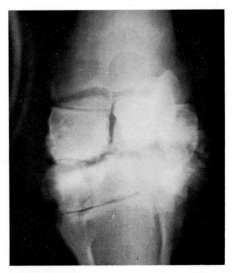

FIG. 5-3. Infectious arthritis of the intercarpal and carpometacarpal joints. The "sunburst" effect in the bone growth indicates infection. This is typical of the type of arthritis that can occur following injection of corticoids in the joint, or following surgery for carpal fracture, when corticoids have been used in the joint prior to surgery. Ankylosis of the affected joints is the usual end result.

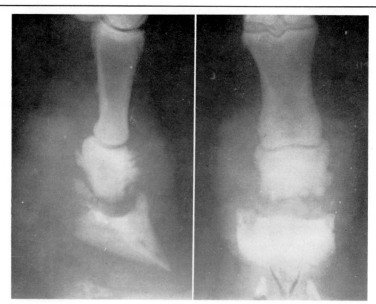

FIG. 5–4. Infectious arthritis and osteomyelitis in a horse. The animal was deeply cut by a barbed wire. It was treated with antibiotics, but infectious arthritis developed. There is extensive destruction of the cartilage and adjacent bone. The joint space appears much widened, which is typical of infectious arthritis and osteomyelitis. There is secondary new bone proliferation involving the second phalanx. (Carlson, *Veterinary Radiology*, Lea & Febiger.)

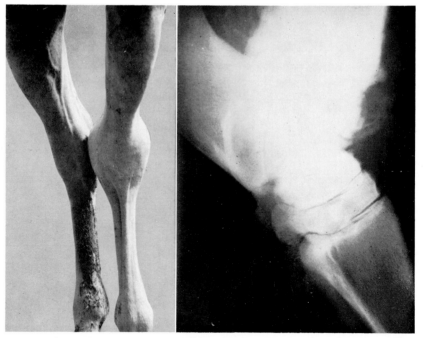

FIG. 5–5. Periarticular arthritis of infectious origin. The picture of the clinical case on the left shows involvement of the left hock. The disease starts with diffuse swelling of the periarticular structures and eventually works its way into the joint, leaving either a severe osteoarthritis or ankylosis of the joint. The radiograph on the right shows the same hock. Note the extensive bone changes on the distal end of the tibia and tibial tarsal bone. There are also periosteal changes on the cranial aspect of the central and third tarsal bones.

joint is characterized by distension of the joint capsule with pus or infected fluid, heat, pain, abnormal synovia on aspiration, temperature rise, and acute lameness. Temperature rise is variable, being elevated in acute streptococcal types but not in less acute forms. In newborn foals, navel ill (joint ill) is the most common example of infectious arthritis; here, the joints are often involved bilaterally, and numerous joints are usually involved. The joint involvement in this case is secondary to a septicemia that usually enters through the navel of the newborn foal. The joints may or may not develop suppurative exudate, depending on the organism involved. If the organism is *Streptococcus,* a purulent exudate is usually formed. Other organisms that are commonly involved are *Shigella equirulis* (*Actinobacillus equuli*) and *Escherichia coli.* In some cases, foals develop infectious arthritis after they have recovered from acute intestinal *Salmonella* infection (Rooney, 1962).

Organisms that cause suppuration cause rapid destruction of the joint cartilage and bone. Joint cartilage may be destroyed in a matter of hours, making early and effective treatment a necessity. Whether or not the organism is a pus-former, the cartilage is usually destroyed in time by the proteolytic enzymes produced by the organisms and white cells. Some organisms produce hyaluronadase, which destroys hyaluronic acid in the synovial fluid. This process destroys the lubricant properties of synovial fluid. If the infection is overcome, the joints are predisposed to osteoarthritis and/or recurrence of infection. If the infection is not controlled in a very short time, ankylosing arthritis is a common result.

In some cases, the joint presents all the appearances of infectious arthritis, but infection cannot be proved by culture. This is a common occurrence, and even though an organism cannot be cultured from the joint fluid, if clinical signs are those of infectious arthritis (heat, pain, swelling, rise in temperature, and acute lameness), it should be treated as such. Some types of infectious arthritis are identified by laboratory tests for agglutination as well as culture. Brucellosis and erysipelas have both been incriminated in arthritis of horses. In the experience of the author, some types of infectious arthritis cause no temperature rise. The joints involved with these more chronic types of infection often show periarticular swelling before the joint is actually involved. All other signs of infectious arthritis are present, and lameness is acute. These cases are chronic and have progressive degenerative changes, often ending in ankylosis of the joint.

Radiographic changes in infectious arthritis usually do not occur for two or three weeks after the onset of the infection and are not helpful in the early stages of the disease as a diagnostic aid. After radiographic changes appear, the new bone growth is characterized by a "sunburst" effect (Fig. 5-3).

Any infected joint that is untreated or treated inadequately or is unresponsive to treatment for one week or more can be considered a chronic infectious arthritis.

4. *Ankylosing or Adhesive Arthritis* (Figs. 5-6 and 5-7). Ankylosing arthritis is characterized by destruction of the articular cartilage, erosion of the joint surface, flattening of the underlying bone, and bridging of the joint by new bone growth. Ankylosing arthritis may be the end result of a severe osteoarthritis, infectious arthritis, or fracture and severe injury to the articulation. In fracture, ankylosis is a common consequence of fragmentation of the joint surfaces. Evidence of a joint space may be visible for some time even though the joint is immovable. In complete ankylosis, radiographic evidence of a joint space will eventually disappear.

5. *Metabolic Bone Disease (Rickets).* Signs of rickets occur in horses up to three years of age; however, foals between six months and one year are most commonly affected (Figs. 5-8 and 5-9). In older

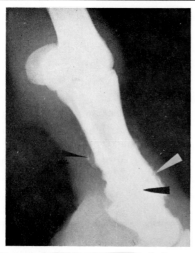

FIG. 5-6. Ankylosing arthritis of the pastern joint as the result of articular high ringbone. The upper dark arrow indicates new bone growth on the palmar aspect of the first phalanx. The light arrow indicates new bone growth at the joint space of the pastern on the dorsal surface of the first and second phalanges. The lower dark arrow indicates the area of the former joint space, now obliterated.

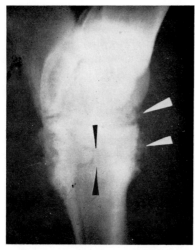

FIG. 5-7. Ankylosing arthritis of the hock joint resulting from infectious arthritis. The dark arrows indicate ankylosis of the intertarsal and tarsometatarsal joints. The upper light arrow indicates new bone growth on the tibial tarsal bone; the lower light arrow indicates new bone growth on the anterior surface of the central and third tarsal bones.

horses, osteoporosis can occur as a result of calcium or phosphorus deficiency. Prematurity predisposes to rickets. The skeleton is mineralized during the last three months of pregnancy, and premature foals are born without a full store of calcium.

Rickets of horses is primarily a disease of the epiphyses rather than of the joint itself. However, arthritis of the carpal, pastern, fetlock, and hock joints may occur. The arthritis of these joints is usually due to stresses caused by conformational changes resulting from epiphyseal changes in the bone. Rickets is a metabolic bone disease resulting from deficiency of calcium, phosphorus, vitamin D, vitamin C, or vitamin A. A deficiency of or imbalance between any one or combination of these elements can apparently cause the condition. Clinical study has led this author to believe that adequate levels of vitamin A and carotene are essential for proper metabolism of calcium and phosphorus. An adequate level of phosphorus is also essential for the proper absorption of vitamin A and carotene (Hickman, 1964). Many rations for horses that are high in protein and composed primarily of grain may contain practically no vitamin A. Vitamin A deficiency causes a rough and lusterless hair coat. It is not uncommon for both young and adult horses to exhibit pica—chewing on fences, gates, or other wood objects—when a deficiency of one or more of the above elements exists.

Some contend that this disease is primarily an epiphysitis and is not related to mineral deficiency (Rooney, 1963). However, although there is an epiphysitis present, it is the contention of this author that the disease is initiated by a mineral or vitamin imbalance. Compression of the epiphysis is given a primary consideration by one author (Rooney, 1963), and although this is undoubtedly a factor, it is not the cause of primary epiphysitis. The deviation of limbs must be initiated by some process and not merely by exercise.

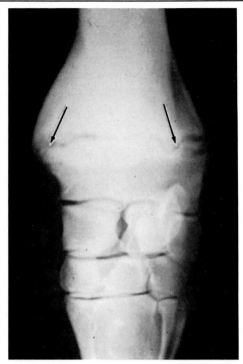

FIG. 5-8. Anterior-posterior radiograph of the carpus of a foal with rickets. The arrow indicates a ragged and widened epiphyseal line. Also note the enlarged metaphysis and epiphysis of the radius.

Radiographs reveal that the greatest area of epiphysitis in on the medial aspect of the epiphysis in medial deviation of the carpal joints. This is the area of least stress after deviation begins. The compression of the lateral portion of the epiphysis retards its growth. In many cases correction of the mineral or vitamin levels will stop the deviation and correct it before casts or stapling are necessary, if it is treated before severe deviation has occurred.

Deviation may be complicated by aseptic necrosis (see page 150). This complicates recovery, and it is important that deviations complicated with aseptic necrosis be corrected as soon as possible, or there is increased chance that the bones will be deformed, especially when the carpal and tarsal bones are involved (see Fig. 5-19).

In early phases, rickets causes a knuckling forward of the fetlocks of the front and/or hindlimbs, due to contraction of the flexor tendons (Figs. 5-10 and 11). Pain in the epiphyses may be a factor in the development of contracted tendons, because in some early cases of contraction, the signs can be relieved temporarily by local nerve blocks. It may be that the tendon contraction is an effort by these structures to "splint" or immobilize an area of pain; after a period of time the contraction is nearly irreversible. "Rachitic ringbone" (page 363) may develop in the pastern areas, and enlargement of the carpal, fetlock, and hock areas may occur. New bone growth, "lipping" of the joints, and destruction of cartilage, *do not* occur in early primary rachitic arthritis. Characteristic findings in joints affected with rickets are enlargement of

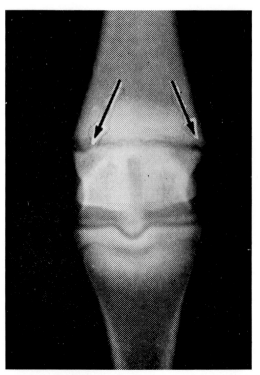

FIG. 5-9. Anterior-posterior view of the fetlock joint of a foal with rickets. Arrows point to a ragged and enlarged epiphyseal line at the distal end of the third metacarpal bone.

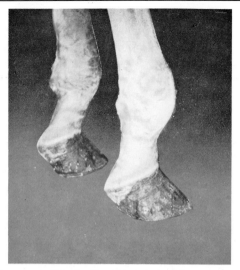

FIG. 5–10. "Cocked" ankles caused by contraction of the superficial flexor tendon. Note that the heel is still flat with the ground, which indicates that the deep flexor is not involved as much as the superficial flexor tendon.

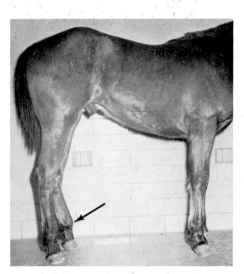

FIG. 5–11. An example of knuckling of the rear fetlocks due to mineral imbalance (rickets). Note that both rear fetlocks are displaced cranially. Also note a very upright positioning of front fetlocks. Contraction of the superficial digital flexor tendons is obvious.

the epiphyses of the bones forming the joint, irregular and widened epiphyseal lines (Figs. 5–8 and 5–9), and, in severe cases, demineralization of bone. The bones may become deformed by the epiphyseal damage or may fracture easily if demineralized (osteoporosis). Bog spavins may occur in rickets and, if so, are usually bilateral (see Chap. 6, p. 338). Windpuffs in the fetlock joint capsule, flexor tendon sheath, and in the carpal area may occur as a result of the rachitic syndrome. The deficient mineral(s) or vitamin(s) must be determined by a study of the diet and laboratory analysis of the blood.

Excessive feeding of grain can apparently cause the syndrome in horses under three years of age. In such a case, the disease may partly be due to increased growth rate stimulated by the concentrate diet. The high rate of concentrate intake must be reduced, and minerals and vitamins balanced before clinical improvement can be seen. Low calcium intake further increases the chance of the disease becoming evident. Phytic acid, found in oats and wheat, may interfere with the metabolism of calcium and contribute to rickets when horses are fed more grain than necessary for normal growth. Raising the levels of calcium and vitamin D intake will not help the horse offset the effects of high phosphorus and phytate intake. The grain ration must be reduced to the point where there is no danger of grain phytates tying up calcium ions in amounts great enough to prevent adequate absorption.

Krook and Lowe (1964) produced nutritional secondary hyperparathyroidism by decreasing the calcium intake and increasing the phosphorus intake. The horses so treated developed the typical osteoporosis seen in "Bran Disease" or "Miller's Head." Enlargement of the jaw bones and osteoporosis of the mandible were produced. Histologic examination of the bone showed generalized osteitis fibrosa. These authors maintain that osteomalacia, osteoporosis, and osteitis fibrosa are all the same disease. The horses showed progressive radiolucency in the mandibles and maxillae. The characteristic changes in the metacarpal bones were endosteal roughening and radiolucent linear striations of the cortex.

6. *Arthritis Due to Neoplasia of Joints.* This condition is seldom seen in horses, but synovial and other neoplastic growths may occur. Chondrosarcoma has been reported (Riddle and Wheat, 1971).

7. *Villous Arthritis.* This should not be considered a separate category since villi (finger-like growths from the synovial membrane of the joint capsule) are the result of chronic inflammation and not a cause or type of arthritis. They may occur in serous arthritis, osteoarthrosis, and infectious arthritis.

SPECIFIC REFERENCES

BARNETT, C. H., *et al.* 1961. *Synovial Joints.* London: Longmans.

CALLANDER, G. R., and R. A. KELSER. 1938. Degenerative arthritis—A comparison of the pathological changes in man and equines. Amer. J. Pathol. 14(3): 253–271.

COFFMAN, J. R. 1970. Joint ill in foals. VM/SAC 65(3): 274–279.

COLANDRUCCIO, R. A., and W. S. GILMER, Jr. 1962. Proliferation, regeneration, and repair of articular cartilage of immature animals. J. Bone Joint Surg. 44-A: 431–455.

DENNY, H. R. 1972. Brucellosis in the horse. Vet. Rec. 90(4): 86–91.

DINTENFASS, L. 1963. Lubrication in synovial joints: A theoretical analysis. Bone Joint Surg. 45–A(6): 1241–1256.

GIBBONS, R. W., and J. P. Manning. 1969. The prevalence of brucella agglutinins in the serum of horses. VM/SAC 64: 907–910.

HAAKENSTAD, L. H. 1969. Chronic bone and joint disease in relation to conformation in the horse. Equine Vet. J. 1(6): 248–260.

HICKMAN, J. 1964. *Veterinary Orthopaedics.* Philadelphia: J. B. Lippincott Co.

HOFFMAN-LAROCHE INC. 1965. *A Primer on Vitamin A for Farm Animals.* Nutley, N.J.: Agricultural Division.

HOLLANDER, J. L. (ed.) 1972. Parts 8, 9, 11, and 12. In Arthritis. 8th ed. Philadelphia: Lea & Febiger.

HOWELL, C. E., G. H. HART, and N. R. ITTNER. 1941. Vitamin A deficiency in horses. Am. J. Vet. Res. 2: 60.

HUTT, F. B. 1968. Genetic defects of bones and joints in domestic animals. Cornell Vet. 58 (Symposium on Equine Bone and Joint Diseases): 104–112.

JOHNSON, L. C. 1962. Joint remodelling as the basis for osteoarthritis. JAVMA 141(10): 1237.

LACK, C. H. 1959. Chondrolysis in arthritis. J. Bone Joint Surg. 41–B(2): 384–387.

LIVINGSTON, W. H. 1970. The C. L. Z. brucella complex of horses. Proc. AAEP, 155–160.

MACKAY-SMITH, M. P. 1962. Pathogenesis and pathology of equine osteoarthritis. JAVMA 141(10): 1246.

MENNEL, J. McM. 1969. Joint Pain. Boston: Little, Brown.

MORGAN, J. P. 1968. Radiographic diagnosis of bone and joint diseases. Cornell Vet. 58 (Symposium on Equine Bone and Joint Disease): 28–47.

RAKER, C. W., R. H. BAKER, and J. D. WHEAT. Pathophysiology of equine degenerative joint disease and lameness. Proc. 12th Ann. AAEP, 229–252.

RAKER, C. W. 1968. Clinical observations of bone and joint diseases in horses. Cornell Vet. 58 (Symposium on Equine Bone and Joint Diseases): 15–28.

RIDDLE, W. E., Jr. 1970. Healing of articular cartilage in the horse. JAVMA 157(11): 1471–1479.

RIDDLE, W. E., Jr, and J. D. WHEAT. 1971. Chondrosarcoma in a horse, JAVMA 158(10): 1674–1677.

RIDDLE, W. E. and J. D. WHEAT. 1969. Liquid silicone for intra-articular use in the horse. JAVMA 155(8): 1367–1369.

ROONEY, J. R. 1963. Epiphyseal compression in young horses. Cornell Vet. 53(4): 567.

ROONEY, J. R. 1967. Equine arthritis: Pt. I. Mod. Vet. Pract. 48: 49–53.

ROONEY, J. R. 1967. Equine arthritis: Pt. II. Mod. Vet. Pract. 48:(9) 44–49.

ROONEY, J. R. 1969. Biomechanics of Lameness in Horses. Baltimore: Williams & Wilkins.

SIPPEL, W. L. 1942. Equine Degenerative Arthritis. Master of Science Thesis, Cornell University, Ithaca, N.Y.

SIPPEL, W. L., *et al.* 1964. Nutrition consultation in horses by aid of feed, blood and hair analysis. Proc. 10th Ann. AAEP, p. 139.

VAN PELT, R. W. 1970. Intra-articular betamethasone in arthritis. JAVMA 156(1): 1589–1599.

VAN PELT, R. W. 1971. Monarticular idiopathic septic arthritis in horses. JAVMA 158(10): 1658–1673.

VAN PELT, R. W., and W. F. RILEY, Jr. 1969. Septic arthritis in foals. JAVMA 155(9): 1467–1480.

TREATMENT OF ARTHRITIS

Serous Arthritis

In the acute phase, local anesthesia and sedation can be used to reduce pain. The affected joint or joints should have absolute rest; in some cases it is necessary to use a plaster cast over the joint to enforce this rest, especially if the injury includes moderate or severe sprain (p. 147). If a cast is not used, the joint should be bandaged heavily so that it will receive support and counterpressure. The joint can be injected with a corticoid (p. 448) to relieve inflammation. These injections are valuable, even though theoretically they delay healing, but they *must* be accompanied by adequate rest. Following two weeks of complete immobilization or supportive wraps, hot Epsom salt packs and application of liniments should be used to aid mobility. If the joint has been severely injured, immobilization of the joint by wrapping should be continued for four to six weeks. Antiphlogistic packs such as Denver Mud* aid in relieving inflammation. Phenylbutazone and oxyphenylbutazone will give temporary relief of pain (p. 447). Corticoids, given intramuscularly, will also reduce pain and inflammation and may be continued one or two weeks as indicated. Giving full doses of both phenylbutazone and corticoids systemically is contraindicated.

In the chronic phase of serous arthritis, corticoids may be used intra-articularly to reduce inflammation (p. 448). Once inflammation is controlled, heat, liniments, and exercise should be used to promote motion. In some chronic cases, the joint may be blistered or fired, or radiation therapy may be used in the form of x or gamma radiation with cobalt or radium. When x-radiation therapy is used, about 750 to 1,000 roentgens is the usual dose; this dose is usually divided into two treat-

*Demco, Inc., Denver, Colorado.

ments of 350 to 500 roentgens each. Gamma radiation is applied with cobalt-60 needles or radium, and the material is strapped directly to the affected part. The dosage is calibrated so that it is distributed over several days. The usual total dosage is approximately 700 to 1,000 roentgens. Firing and radiation therapy promote an acute inflammation of the joint; when the acute inflammation subsides, the arthritis may heal and a sound joint result (see Chap. 11 for complete discussion of radiation therapy).

Ultrasonic therapy is of doubtful value for joint injury. Although it produces a deep heat, the effect is transitory. Such therapy can be dangerous, for if used to excess, it may cause bone necrosis. Ultrasound is of most value in relieving the pain of muscle spasms. Diathermy is helpful in producing deep heat in the joint, and by this means aids in mobility (see Chap. 11).

Adrenocorticotrophic hormone (ACTH) parenterally may be of some use in prolonged cases of arthritis if used to follow up corticoid therapy. The administration of ACTH stimulates the adrenal cortex to secrete hydrocortisone (p. 451).

An adequate rest period of one to six months, depending on severity of the disease, must be enforced if proper healing is to occur. Working a horse prematurely may cause the arthritis to fail to respond to treatment or a recurrence of the injury, or may lead to osteoarthritis, and ulceration of joint cartilage.

Prognosis. The prognosis is usually favorable if bone changes have not occurred. Bone changes and chronicity make the prognosis unfavorable.

Infectious Arthritis
(Suppurative Arthritis)

It is important to aspirate a joint and study the fluid when infectious arthritis is suspected. Before treatment, a sample of the joint contents should be cultured;

if growth is obtained, a sensitivity test should be done to determine the most effective antibiotic. With the many antibiotics to choose from, it is important to select an effective group in treatment of infectious arthritis. Since identification of any organism may take several days, it is helpful if a Gram stain can be done first. When the identity of organism is not known, and while waiting for results of culture, it is very important to inject the joint immediately with an antibiotic combination that will give a broad antibacterial coverage. Penicillin, streptomycin, neomycin, and choramphenicol are some of the commonly used antibiotics. Two effective drugs are crystalline penicillin (1,000,000 units) and crystalline chloramphenicol (0.5 gm) administered in the joint. One or both of these can be used until culture results are known. Before each injection of the joint with antibiotics, the joint fiuid should be aspirated as completely as possible to rid the joint of damaging enzymes and factors that inhibit the action of antibiotics. In addition to local joint injection, parenteral therapy with suitable antibiotics should also be begun. If culture and sensitivity tests indicate more effective antibiotics, a change is made in therapy. The joint should be immobilized as much as possible by bandaging during the treatment period.

Joint cultures are often negative in suspected cases of infectious arthritis, but other changes in the joint fluid, such as rise in neutrophils, may aid in the diagnosis. If the joint capsule is distended with infected synovia, it should be drained by needle and the joint flushed out with an antibiotic solution, saline, and if desired, an enzyme solution.

Two needles can be placed in an infected joint to allow thorough flushing with antibiotics and saline solution at each treatment or on a continuous basis for several hours. The drainage needle should be larger than the injection needle and, if possible, should be placed low in the joint. The solution is injected through the smaller and more proximal needle, and the joint is flushed thoroughly at least once daily, and preferably twice or more daily. This rinses out infected material that destroys the lubricating quality of the synovial fluid. After the infection has been controlled, heat therapy and exercise should be used to maintain mobility of the joint.

Treatment must be continued for a long period (at least 10 to 14 days) and for five days after signs of infection have ceased. Whenever an arthritis appears to be infectious, it should be treated as such, even if cultures are negative.

If the joint is open and draining, an effort should be made to establish drainage as low on the joint capsule as possible. The joint is flushed with the above mixture of antibiotics and saline daily until one is certain that the infection is overcome. The joint can then be immobilized in a plaster cast, when practical, to allow the joint capsule to heal. When the joint is open, it should be bandaged so that the opening will not be exposed to air.

Any infectious arthritis that is untreated, inadequately treated, or is resistant to therapy for one week or more may be considered to have developed the pathological changes of chronic infection. In chronic bacterial arthritis, the blood supply to the lesion is diminished by vascular thrombosis and may be shut off altogether by a wall of fibrous tissue. In such cases, it is useless to attempt to treat the central necrotic and suppurative portion solely by the administration of antibiotics that must reach the focus by way of the bloodstream. The same is true for the local injection of antibiotics that cannot reach the entire lesion since there are usually numerous localized areas of infection. Prolonged administration of an antibiotic prior to surgical treatment in chronic bacterial arthritis may only serve to produce sublethal concentrations of the agent in the localized foci, thereby fostering the development of antibiotic-resistant bacteria. Early surgery is recommended in chronic infections and should consist of open drainage and thorough excision of the infected bone, soft-tissue foci, and all sinuses.

Surgical therapy consists of incision of the joint and suturing a soft rubber drain of appropriate size to the capsule—not permitting this to intrude into the joint. Active motion is begun as soon as possible. This type of treatment is by necessity limited to those areas where the drains and joint can be protected by sterile bandaging (Hollander, 1972).

In some cases, when a joint capsule opens after routine orthopedic procedures, it is quite difficult to get it to heal, whether or not there has been an infection present. When healing of the joint opening is desired, it is best to immobilize the joint in a plaster cast whenever possible. If the joint is immobilized for seven to 10 days with a plaster cast, the joint capsule will usually heal closed. If, upon removal of the cast, it is found that it has not healed, another cast is applied for approximately seven days.

Prognosis. The prognosis of infectious arthritis is always guarded. Bone and cartilage changes within the joint capsule, especially on the articular surfaces usually occur in a matter of hours, and destruction of joint cartilage may be complete in as little as eight hours after the infection begins. Unless the infection is controlled early, osteoarthritis or ankylosing arthritis often results and causes chronic lameness. Ankylosis is the result of destruction of the cartilage and hypertrophic bone growth. In all cases of infectious arthritis, the owner of the horse should understand that, at best, the end result will be a lame horse. Only if the infection is overcome in the first few hours is there a chance for a sound joint.

Osteoarthritis (Hypertrophic or Degenerative Arthritis)

This type of arthritis usually is chronic and may result from arthritis of other types. This arthritis sometimes is treated by counterinflammation, such as firing, blistering, or radiation therapy. These forms of therapy cause acute inflammation of the joint, and the resulting healing process may cause enough remission of symptoms that the horse may be used.

Firing has sometimes been acclaimed for its ability to remove osseous growth. This is not true, and in some cases it actually promotes additional bone growth. The inflammation it produces rarely causes any demineralization, and reduction of swelling occurs only in the soft tissues that are involved. This is true also of radiation therapy. Healing of the inflammation causes a smoothing of bone, as in fractures, but not destruction of new bone growth.

The true effects of x-ray therapy, and other forms of radiation therapy, are not precisely known at present. Various claims have been made for the pain-relieving effect of radiation therapy, which may be due to destruction of sensory nerve endings. The effect of radiation therapy, as claimed by some, is the destruction of leukocytes that may later stimulate phagocytosis. It also has been claimed that decalcification of tissue can be accomplished through radiation therapy by increasing the blood supply to aid in demineralization. Radiation therapy is helpful in some cases of osteoarthritis, but it is not a cure-all by any means. It will not remove bony proliferations, and the smoothing of bone that occurs is through normal healing processes.

In some cases, arthrodesis (surgical fusion of the affected joints) is the only answer to relief of pain. This operation is most successful in the proximal interphalangeal (pastern) and distal tarsal joints (*see* Ringbone and Bone spavin, Chap. 6).

Intra-articular injections of corticoids are often of temporary value in treatment of osteoarthritis, since they reduce inflammation and pain (*see* p. 448). Parenteral use of corticoids or phenylbutazone also may cause temporary amelioration of lameness as long as the therapy is continued; signs usually appear once corticoid or phenylbutazone therapy is stopped. Too often, corticoid or phenylbutazone therapy allows the horse to be used, causing further injury before healing has taken place. Repeated injections of corticoids may lead to eventual infection in a joint (Fig. 5–3). The corticoids lower the local resistance of the joint, and infection may develop as a result of organisms injected through the needle if poor technique is used or from a bacteremia. In bacteremia, the organisms cause infection at the site of low resistance created by the repeated injection of corticoids. Corticoids are more detrimental than helpful unless used with good judgment. Asepsis should be maintained at all times when injecting joints.

Prognosis. The prognosis is guarded to unfavorable. If new bone growth occurs on the articular surfaces, mechanical factors result in chronic lameness. Under proper therapy, some cases become asymptomatic. In bone spavin or high ringbone, soundness may result after natural or surgical ankylosis of the affected joint(s).

Ankylosing or Adhesive Arthritis

In this type of arthritis, immobility and ankylosis usually result, so there is little chance that the horse will be useful for purposes other than breeding. In some joints, such as the proximal interphalangeal joint, afflicted with hypertrophic arthritis in the form of ringbone, ankylo-sis may occur, but the horse still may be functional. This is more often true when the hind limb is affected rather than the forelimb. A favorable result may also occur following ankylosis of the distal tarsal joints in bone spavin.

Ankylosis of the proximal interphalangeal joint should be stimulated surgically once ringbone has involved the articular surface. When the articulation of the proximal interphalangeal joint is involved, lameness will be present until ankylosis has occurred. As long as a joint space is visible on a radiograph, lameness persists, regardless of how much hypertrophic bone has built up around the joint. This joint must be stripped surgically of its articular cartilage and then immobilized in a cast for several weeks to enable the joint to ankylose (*see* Ringbone, Chap. 6). Once movement of this joint is suspended, pain usually disappears. Since this joint is only slightly movable in the

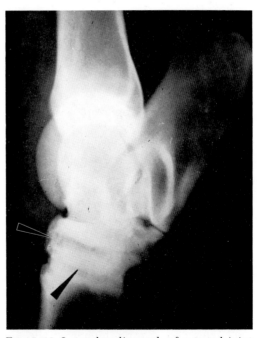

FIG. 5–12. Lateral radiograph of a tarsal joint affected by ankylosis of the distal intertarsal joint (top arrow) and the tarsometatarsal joint (lower arrow) as a result of bone spavin.

normal state anyway, the treated horse may be able to function normally.

Ankylosis also occurs in joints such as the distal intertarsal and tarsometatarsal joints in the hock of the hind limb (Fig. 5–12), resulting from bone spavin. Once ankylosis has occurred in these joints, the horse may be completely functional following tenectomy of the cunean tendon, which relieves the bursitis when it is present. Surgical ankylosis of the distal intertarsal and tarsometatarsal joints is often successful in chronic bone spavin (p. 333). Both articular ringbone and bone spavin usually begin as an osteoarthritis. The main articulation of the hock joint may ankylose as the result of trauma, suppurative arthritis, or periarticular involvement. This type of involvement makes the horse useless. Ankylosis may result from luxation of a joint if the articular cartilage is badly damaged (Fig. 6–172). Ankylosis of the joint may also follow an infectious arthritis, which rapidly destroys the joint cartilage even though the infection is brought under control very soon. The ankylosing process usually takes a long time and causes debilitation of the horse because of pain and disability of the limb.

Prognosis. The prognosis is unfavorable. In the case of ringbone and bone spavin, the prognosis is guarded to unfavorable until enough time has passed for final judgment.

Metabolic Bone Disease (Rickets)

The normal ratio of calcium to phosphorus in the horse is approximately 2:1 in the bloodstream. Although there is some variation, blood should contain about 10 mg percent of calcium and 5 mg percent of phosphorus. In foals, these levels may be slightly higher, while in adults the phosphorus level may be slightly lower. Blood levels of minerals are not always accurate indicators of mineral status because the blood uses minerals from the bone to maintain near-normal levels as long as possible. For the most accurate interpretation of calcium-phosphorus levels in the blood, samples should be taken from several horses on the premises. Establishing a definite trend in a calcium-phosphorus imbalance is very helpful in compounding a therapeutic diet. A reduced blood level of either calcium or phosphorus means that the deficiency has been present for some time. Sippel (1964) claims that hair analysis is a good method of determining mineral imbalance. It also represents the condition of the animal for the preceding six to eight weeks or whatever interval is required to grow out the full length of hair. Methods of handling the hair must be standardized to give accurate results. He used hair analysis to check for minerals other than calcium and phosphorus and found definite correlations between several of these ions. Others claim it is not an accurate means of determining mineral status (Wysocki and Klett, 1971). Further testing of this method may provide a more accurate method of determining the true state of mineral levels in the horse. Alkaline phosphatase levels are usually elevated in the active stages of the disease. The horse's daily ration should contain a ratio of 2:1 or 1.5:1 calcium to phosphorus. In areas deficient in phosphorus, this mineral must be artificially supplied to maintain the proper balance with calcium. Monosodium phosphate may be used for this purpose. Most authorities agree that horses require 25 to 45 gm daily of calcium and 15 to 28 gm daily of phosphorus. However, work done by Schryver *et al.* (1969, 1970) indicates that for a 1,000-lb horse, 25 gm of calcium and 12 gm of phosphorus daily are adequate for maintainance. Late-pregnant or lactating mares and working studs require the higher levels of calcium and phosphorus.

Show horses fed high-grain rations but little hay tend to lack in calcium; thus, this mineral must be supplied in the ration. If a horse is deficient in both minerals, it is possible to feed products, such as dicalcium phosphate, that balance both in the proper ratio. However, if a horse is deficient in only one of the minerals, then only that mineral, and not a combination, should be fed. If a combination is fed, the calcium-phosphorus ratio tends to become more unbalanced, if the supplement is a standard product containing more calcium than phosphorus.

Horses that are fed large amounts of grain to increase their growth rate also may show signs of rickets. In some cases this can be attributed to the increased demand for vitamins and minerals because of increased growth, but in other cases it appears that the excessive protein, or at least certain types of protein, in excess, interfere with mineral metabolism. High-protein diets also accelerate growth rate to the point that it is nearly impossible to furnish an adequate mineral intake. Protein supplements should not exceed 16 percent concentration, or problems may result. In addition, phytic acid, present in grains, tends to prevent absorption of calcium, causing further discrepancy in the Ca:P ratio. Such cases improve only upon withdrawal of the heavy ration and protein. The increase in demand for minerals and/or vitamins, under these circumstances, is apparently greater than the increase in growth rate. Four to six weeks is required after the diet is corrected for favorable changes in the rickets. Increased vitamin D should be fed whenever a horse is fed a high-grain ration. The increased vitamin D may aid absorption of calcium in the presence of phytates, but it cannot completely overcome their effect.

According to Knox (1970), availability of calcium and phosphorus is dependent on several factors:

1. *Solubility:* Calcium and phosphorus must be soluble at the point of absorption or they will be unavailable to the horse. An acid medium tends to promote the absorption of calcium, while alkaline intestinal contents tend to cause formation of insoluble and unabsorbable calcium salts such as tricalcium phosphate. Large intakes of iron, aluminum, and magnesium interfere with absorption of phosphorus by forming insoluble phosphates. High-fat diets form calcium salts with fatty acids and decrease absorption; however, small quantities of fat enhance absorption.

2. *Ca:P Ratio and Vitamin D:* A ratio of near 1.5:1 (normal limits are 1.5:1 to 2:1) encourages maximum absorption of both calcium and phosphorus. When the ratio varies from this, high intake of vitamin D becomes increasingly important.

3. *Forms of Ca and P:* The forms in which calcium and phosphorus are fed are very important. These minerals are available commercially in several forms:

   a. Phosphates—three basic types:
      · Metaphosphoric acid, which has low animal availability.
      · Pyrophosphoric acid, which has low animal availability.
      · Orthophosphoric acid, which has a reasonably high availability to animals.

   b. Calcium forms of orthophosphoric acid:
      · Monocalcium phosphate (superphosphate of lime), an excellent source of calcium and phosphorus.
      · Dicalcium phosphate (Dical); this is a good animal supplement.
      · Tricalcium phosphate, which occurs naturally in mineral deposits, is a primary form of (defluorinated) rock phosphate and a poor source of phosphorus.

c. Other forms of calcium and phosphorus:
- Defluorinated phosphates. The calcium and phosphorus are available to animals, but unless the fluorine is removed, they are toxic. The term "defluorinated" does not guarantee a safe product (if the ration contains 1 percent phosphorus, the phosphorus should not exceed 0.5 percent fluorine content).
- Colloidal phosphate (soft rock phosphate). This usually contains fluorine and is unsafe unless treated.
- Curacao phosphate. This special rock phosphate is naturally low in fluorine. It contains about 33 percent calcium and 14.5 percent phosphorus, both of which are available (60–70 percent).
- Phosphoric acid in available form.
- Phytic phosphorus: Half or more of the phosphorus in most mature plant seeds and their by-products is in this form. This cuts availability to the horse by at least one third. The utilization of phytin is lower than with organic phosphorus even when vitamin D levels are increased.

A number of substances may reduce absorption of calcium by forming insoluble compounds with it in the gut. Among these are phosphate, phytic acid, oxalic acid, and fatty acids. Citric acid and some other substances may increase the absorption of calcium. Phytic acid accounts for 40 to 90 percent of the total phosphorus content of cereals. There is more of it in oats than there is in wheat; it is present in the outer covering of the grain. Some phytate can be hydrolyzed by a phytase contained in the grain, but oats and maize contain no phytase.

Adequate calcium and phosphorus nutrition is dependent upon three factors: Sufficient supply of each element in an available form; suitable ratio between calcium and phosphorus (1.5:1 to 2:1); and presence of vitamin D.

There are three rules that should be followed: (1) Be sure horses are receiving enough available calcium and phosphorus. Young and growing horses should receive about 1 percent of the diet in calcium and 1 percent in phosphorus. Mature animals require slightly lower levels. The upper limit is 2 percent for either mineral. (2) The calcium:phosphorus ratio should not vary beyond the range of 1.5:1 to 2:1. Be aware of the form of calcium and phosphorus that the horse is consuming. (3) If horses are not consuming some cured hays, vitamin D should be supplied in the feed at a recommended level. Overuse of supplemental vitamin D can be harmful.

Under practical feeding conditions, it is particularly difficult to balance rations and ensure optimal levels and ratios of calcium and phosphorus. Most grass hays or legume hays are relatively abundant in calcium, and most grains (except corn) are low in calcium and relatively high in phosphorus. (See Table 5–1 for a listing of calcium and phosphorus content in various feeds.)

Apparently, more than the daily requirement of calcium can be fed as long as the daily requirement of phosphorus is not exceeded. If excessive amounts of calcium and phosphorus are fed in proper ratio (2:1–1.5:1) toxicity from excessive phosphorus may become evident if the total daily requirement of phosphorus is exceeded over a prolonged period (Krook, 1968; Schryver et al., 1970).

Animal bone meal, dicalcium phosphate, monocalcium phosphate, and animal bone charcoal supply both calcium and phosphorus, while calcium gluconate, ground limestone, and oyster shell flour supply only calcium. Monosodium phosphate and disodium phosphate supply only phosphorus. Mineralized salt blocks

Table 5–1 Calcium and Phosphorus Content in Feeds

Feed component	% Ca	% P
Forages		
Alfalfa	1.20	0.20
Bermuda grass	0.42	0.18
Biome grass	0.39	0.25
Clover	1.42	0.19
Fescue	0.44	0.32
Meadow	0.53	0.16
Prairie	0.46	0.07
Oat	0.23	0.21
Timothy	0.36	0.16
Vetch	1.20	0.30
Grains and other prepared feeds		
Dehydrated alfalfa	1.60	0.23
Barley	0.08	0.42
Beet molasses	0.16	0.03
Dried milk	0.87	0.79
Cottonseed meal	0.15	1.10
Linseed meal	0.44	0.89
Brewers grains	0.27	0.50
Corn	0.02	0.31
Oats	0.10	0.35
Rye	0.06	0.34
Milo	—	—
Soybean meal	0.32	0.67
Wheat bran	0.14	1.17
Wheat	0.09	0.30
Supplements		
Animal bone meal	29.0	13.6
Dicalcium phosphate (dical)	26.5	20.5
Defluorinated phosphate	26–36	12–18
Limestone	33.8	—
Animal-bone charcoal	22.0	13.1
Calcium phosphate	17.0	21.0
Sodium phosphate	—	22.4
Diammonium phosphate	—	20.0
Oyster shell	35.0	—

supplementing minerals is to combine the desired minerals with alfalfa meal and bind this with molasses. When supplementing minerals, one must recognize the fact that feeding one ounce of a particular mineral does not mean that the horse utilizes the whole amount. Depending on the product, absorption of the mineral in a supplement is usually 50 percent or less. A variation also exists in dietary sources of mineral: e.g., wheat bran is a poor supplement of phosphorus compared to monosodium phosphate (Hintz *et al.*, 1973; Krook, 1970). In all cases it is neces-

Table 5–2 Minimum Daily Requirements of the Weanling Foal* (4–12 Months)

Projected Mature Weight of 1,000–1,400 Pounds

4 months—Body weight = approximately
  300 pounds
    Total digestible nutrients (pounds). . 6.4
    Digestible protein (pounds) 1.16
    Carotene (milligrams). 22.5
    Calcium (grams) 30–40
    Phosphorus (grams) 18–24
6 months—Body weight = approximately
  400–500 pounds
    Total digestible nutrients (pounds). . 9.0–9.3
    Digestible protein (pounds) 1.17
    Carotene (milligrams). 30.7–37.5
    Calcium (grams) 33–45
    Phosphorus (grams) 21–28
8 months—Body weight = approximately
  450–600 pounds
    Total digestible nutrients (pounds). . 9.5–9.7
    Digestible protein (pounds) 1.19–1.30
    Carotene (milligrams). 33.8–45.0
    Calcium (grams) 33–45
    Phosphorus (grams) 21–28
12 months—Body weight = approximately
  550–800 pounds
    Total digestible nutrients (pounds). . 9.9–11.0
    Digestible protein (pounds) 1.22–1.30
    Carotene (milligrams). 41.3–60.0
    Calcium (grams) 33–45
    Phosphorus (grams) 21–28

The above table will give at least a foundation for supplementing the diet of the foal. These figures can be used as a basis for estimating a balanced ration.

*Tables 5-2, 5-3, and 5-4 from Nelson, A. W.: *Nutrient Requirements of the Light Horse*, Courtesy of American Quarter Horse Association.

do not provide an adequate supply of minerals for horses because not enough of the minerals can be obtained from licking a block. Minerals may be supplemented by mixing monosodium phosphate, for example, half and half with *crushed* salt (fine rock salt) and using this as the only source of salt. When minerals are supplemented in this way, the mixture should be weather-proofed, or the minerals will harden. One of the most effective ways of

Table 5-3 Minimum Daily Requirements of the Yearling (12-24 Months)

Projected Mature Weight of 1,000-1,400 Pounds

12 months—Body weight = approximately
700-800 pounds
    Total digestible nutrients (pounds). . 10-11.2
    Digestible protein (pounds) 1.30-1.35
    Carotene (milligrams). 52.5-60.0
    Calcium (grams) 16.9-45
    Phosphorus (grams) 16.3-28

24 months—Body weight = approximately
900-1,100 pounds
    Total digestible nutrients (pounds). . 11.4-11.9
    Digestible protein (pounds) 1.40-1.50
    Carotene (milligrams). 67.5-82.5
    Calcium (grams) 15-40
    Phosphorus (grams) 15-27

sary to analyze the diet on the basis of known mineral content of its ingredients. Only in this fashion can one arrive at an accurate interpretation of the total intake of minerals and vitamins. Mineral supplementation must be done in an intelligent manner and not haphazardly.

According to A. W. Nelson (1961) in his *Nutrient Requirements of the Light Horse:* "Vitamin A and Carotene have been explored as much, if not more than, other vitamins; however, no work was encountered that established the actual daily requirements for either vitamin A or carotene. The estimated daily requirements per 100 pounds of body weight for vitamin A ranges from 773 to 1,000 I.U. (Guilbert *et al.,* 1940) to 667 to 800 I.U. (Errington, 1937). The latest N.R.C. (1973) recommendations are 25-50 I.U. Vit A per kg body wt. per day. The estimated daily maintenance requirements per 100 pounds body weight for carotene ranges from 0.91 to 1.36 milligrams (Guilbert *et al.,* 1940), 0.9 to 1.4 milligrams (Errington, 1937), and 0.9 to 1.14 milligrams (Crasemann, 1945)." Hay is usually low in carotene and vitamin A in spite of the best efforts to preserve them. Unless horses are grazing on green grass, they nearly always need supplemental Vitamin A.

Vitamin A palmitate appears to be one of the better supplements of vitamin A, as this product is gelatin-coated to prevent oxidation. Natural sources of vitamin A, such as fish liver oils, oxidize rapidly, so their value is quickly diminished. Carotene can be supplemented by feeding fresh alfalfa meal or alfalfa leaf meal. Alfalfa pellets also are valuable as a source of carotene, provided they are fresh and have not lost the carotene content as a result of oxidation. These pellets should be fresh, or they may not contain sufficient carotene to prevent vitamin A deficiency. Whenever possible, the caro-

Table 5-4 Examples of Mineral Supplements

Mix No. 1
    1 lb Monosodium phosphate
    1 lb Monocalcium phosphate
    each ounce contains 2.25 grams of calcium* and
      6.6 grams phosphorus*
Mix No. 2
    1 lb Monocalcium phosphate
    2 lb Monosodium phosphate
    each ounce contains 1.5 grams calcium* and
      6.5 grams phosphorus*
Mix No. 3
    1 lb Monosodium phosphate
    each ounce contains 6.4 grams phosphorus*
Mix No. 4
    1 lb Dicalcium phosphate
    1 lb Ground limestone (calcium carbonate)
    2 lb Monosodium phosphate
    each ounce contains 6.1 grams calcium* and
      6.2 grams phosphorus*
Mix No. 5
    1 lb Dicalcium phosphate
    each ounce contains 7.5 grams of calcium* and
      5.8 grams phosphorus*
Mix No. 6
    1 lb Monocalcium phosphate
    1 lb Ground limestone (calcium carbonate)
    each ounce contains 7.7 grams calcium* and 3.4
      grams phosphorus*
Mix No. 7
    1 lb Dicalcium phosphate
    1 lb Ground limestone (calcium carbonate)
    each ounce contains 9.8 grams calcium* and 2.9
      grams phosphorus*

*Available mineral in each ounce
One ounce is equal to 30 grams

tene intake should be increased because carotene apparently is more efficient in raising the blood levels of vitamin A than any type of vitamin A supplement, including intramuscular injections. Parenteral injections of vitamin A often do not cause a demonstrable increase in the blood level of vitamin A. However, this should not discourage its use. The horse may convert carotene to vitamin A more efficiently than he can utilize a vitamin A supplement. Adequate phosphorus is necessary in the diet for optimal vitamin A and carotene utilization. Excessive nitrates in the diet may depress conversion of carotene to vitamin A. The role of the nitrate is not clear (Hickman, 1964).

When treating a vitamin A deficiency, vitamin A palmitate (30,000 units per gm) should be added to the grain at the rate of 50,000 to 100,000 units per day. Once signs of rickets have disappeared, 1 gm daily (30,000 units) of vitamin A palmitate should be adequate.

A. W. Nelson (1961) says: "Vitamin D requirements for the horse are not known. From information obtained in other species, 300 I.U. of vitamin D per 100 pounds of body weight is adequate to meet the daily needs of the adult horse (National Research Council, 1973). Way (1941) indicated that 700 to 1,000 USP units of vitamin D per 100 pounds body weight would be adequate for training and racing Thoroughbred horses. A pro-vitamin D or precursor of vitamin D has been found in the stomach wall and the wall of the first part of the small intestine of the horse and other species (*Nutritional Review*, 1958). Therefore, the horse may be able to produce at least small quantities of vitamin D." Show horses that are confined indoors most of the time to preserve coat luster will be deficient in vitamin D if this vitamin is not supplemented in the diet. Vitamin D can be supplemented by giving approximately 5,000 units of vitamin D in the form of irradiated yeast daily in the grain.

In cases that do not respond to treatment, injections of parathyroid extract are indicated for those with abnormal calcium metabolism. The feeding of iodinated casein to stimulate the thyroid gland and the subcutaneous implantation of thyroid pellets or oral administration of thyroid tablets (30–50 grains daily) are occasionally helpful in cases that may be the result of hypothyroidism.

Deviations of the tarsal joints, carpal joints, and the metacarpophalangeal joints are treated by means of casts and epiphyseal stapling. In general, casts are of the most value starting at about three weeks of age. If the foal is presented for treatment after it is approximately four months of age, epiphyseal stapling is more satisfactory because a cast cannot be left on long enough to correct the deviation (see Chap. 6).

SPECIFIC REFERENCES

American Quarter Horse Association. 1967. American Quarter Horse Research Report. J. Amer. Quarter Horse Assoc. 20(1): 78–84.

American Quarter Horse Association. 1970. American Quarter Horse Report: J. Amer. Quarter Horse Assoc. 23(1): 76–98.

BREUER, L. H. 1970. Horse feeding management and nutrition. Anim. Nutr. Health. 25(8): 4–8.

BURGESS, D. 1963. Leg abnormalities in foals, weanlings and yearlings. Proc. 2nd Ann. Cong., Brit. Equine Vet. Assoc., 11–17.

FORMESBECK, P. V., and L. D. SYMONS. 1967. Utilization of the carotene of hay by horses. J. Anim. Sci. 26(5): 1030–1038.

FOURMAN, P., et al. 1968. Calcium Metabolism and the Bone. 2nd Ed. Oxford and Edinburgh: Blackwell Scientific Publications.

HICKMAN, J. 1964. *Veterinary Orthopaedics*. Philadelphia: J. B. Lippincott Co.

HINTZ, H. F., et al. 1973. Availability of phosphorus in wheat bran when fed to ponies. J. Anim. Sci. 36(31): 522.

HOLLANDER, J. L. (ed.). 1972. Parts 8, 9, 11, and 12. In Arthritis. 8th Ed. Philadelphia: Lea & Febiger.

JOYCE, J. R., et al. 1971. Clinical study of nutritional secondary hypothyroidism in horses. JAVMA 158(12): 2033–2042.

KNOX, K. 1970. Calcium-phosphorus metabolism in horses. *In* 13th Annual Conference for Veterinarians, Colorado State University.

KROOK, L. 1968. Dietary calcium-phosphorus and lameness in the horse. Cornell Vet. 58(Suppl. Equine Bone Joint Dis.): 59–73.

National Research Council, Committee on Animal Nutrition. 1973. Nutrient Requirements of the Horse. Washington, D.C.: National Academy of Sciences.

O'MOORE, L. B. 1972. Nutritional factors in the rearing of the young thoroughbred horse. Brit. Eq. Vet. J 4(1): 9–16.

SCHRYVER, H. F., et al. 1969. Equine calcium metabolism. Proc. AAEP, 99–109.

SCHRYVER, H. F., et al. 1970. The calcium and phosphorus requirements of the horse. Proc. 16th Ann. AAEP., 117–126.

SCHRYVER, H. F., et al. 1971. Calcium and phosphorus: Inter-relationships in horse nutrition. Eq. Vet. J. 3(3): 102–109.

SIEGEL, E. T. 1968. Effect of hormones on bone. Cornell Vet. 58(Suppl. Equine Bone Joint Dis.): 95–103.

SIPPEL, W. L., et al. 1964. Nutrition consultation in horses by aid of feed, blood, and hair analysis. Proc. 10th Ann. AAEP, p. 139.

SPRATLING, F. R., et al. 1970. Osteodystrophy associated with apparent hypovitaminosis-D in yearling cattle. Br. Vet. J., 126(6): 316–323.

TEETER, S. M., M. C. STILLIONS, and W. E. NELSON. 1967. Recent observations on the nutrition of mature horses. Proc. AAEP, 39–49.

WHITTOCK, R. H., et al. 1970. The Effects of High Dietary Calcium in Horses. Proc. 16th Ann. AAEP, 127–134.

WYSOCKI, A. A., and R. H. KLETT. 1971. Hair as an indicator of the calcium and phosphorus status of ponies. J. Anim. Sci. 32(1): 74–78.

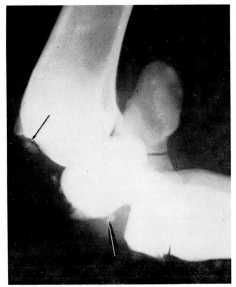

FIG. 5–14. Severe carpitis on a lateral flexed-joint radiograph. The upper arrow indicates the loose joint mouse in the radiocarpal joint, and the lower arrow indicates the joint mouse in the intercarpal joint.

JOINT MICE

Joint mice, or bodies within the joint cavity, may be formed by a splitting off of a piece of the joint cartilage, by a fracture of an arthritic osteophyte at the joint margin, or by a chip fracture of one of the bones forming the joint (Figs. 5–13 and 5–14).

When joint mice occur as free osseous bodies in a joint they may be surgically removed with success. Most of the common chip fractures remain attached to the joint capsule, facilitating their removal (see Chapter 6, Fracture of the Carpal Bones and Chip Fractures of the First Phalanx). Radiographic studies should be made of the joint to determine if erosion of the articular surfaces has occurred. If extensive erosion of these surfaces has occurred, little improvement will be obtained by removing the joint mouse. Lameness caused by joint mice often is characterized by a sudden onset and a sudden disappearance. Sometimes the

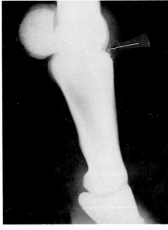

FIG. 5–13. Joint mouse (arrow) in the fetlock joint as viewed on a lateral radiograph.

horse will be sound until the joint mouse is caught between the articular surfaces; then he becomes acutely lame. The signs often disappear just as rapidly. Villi resulting from arthritis can cause similar symptoms if they become caught between the bones of the joint. Careful radiographic studies must be made prior to surgery since, in some instances, the calcified objects may be difficult to find.

Large bone chips have been removed from the femorotibial joint and from the scapulohumeral joint by the author. In general, removal of a bone chip is successful if it is removed soon after the injury occurs and if it does not involve much of the articular surface. The lateral tuberosity of the humerus and portions of the lateral aspect of the femoral condyles are subject to trauma from kicking and may chip off into the joint. These chips must be removed if soundness is to be regained.

INFLAMMATION OF SYNOVIAL STRUCTURES

Bursitis*

Bursitis may be defined as an inflammatory reaction within a bursa. This may vary from a very mild irritative synovitis to suppurative bursitis with abcess formation. A bursa is specifically designed to facilitate motion between contiguous layers of the body. Bursitis can be classified as true or acquired. An acquired bursitis results when a bursa develops as the result of trauma where a natural bursa is not normally present, e.g., carpal hygroma. A true bursitis results when a bursa that is normally present becomes inflamed; e.g., trochanteric bursitis.

Treatment. Treatment is directed toward prevention of repeated injury and

*Definitions for the conditions marked with an asterisk have been taken from O'Donoghue's text, *Treatment of Injuries to Athletes,* courtesy of W. B. Saunders Co.

reduction of the irritation within the bursa. Aspiration of fluid, local injection with corticoids, protection against direct trauma, and application of pressure bandage to oppose the walls of the sac are used. If the condition becomes chronic and the synovitis is persistent, surgical removal of the bursa may become necessary.

Cosgrove (1963) has suggested that *Brucella abortus* may be responsible for bursitis in the stifle, withers, and navicular bursa. He suggests the use of strain 19 vaccine when this etiology is suspected.

Bursitis of Specific Areas

Bursitis of the Points of the Elbow (Olecranon Bursitis, Shoe Boil, Capped Elbow)

Bursitis over the olecranon is caused by trauma at the point of the olecranon. It is usually an acquired bursitis and is due to trauma caused by the shoe on the foot of the affected limb hitting the point of the olecranon during motion or while the horse is lying down. A false subcutaneous bursa forms; the bursa under the triceps is not usually involved. Most trauma probably occurs while the horse is down with the foot under the point of the elbow. Gaited and Standardbred horses may hit the elbow with the foot while in motion. The disease is characterized by a prominent swelling over the point of the elbow, that may contain fluid or that, in the chronic stages, may be composed primarily of fibrous tissue. Lameness is usually mild, if present at all.

Treatment. In the acute stages, bursitis of the elbow can be treated with injection of corticoids (see Chap. 11). The swelling should be shaved and prepared for aseptic injection over its lateral aspect. After aspiration of the contents, part of the corticoid solution should be injected into the bursa and part into the surrounding connective tissue. (Do not use long-acting corticoids in soft tissues.) The corticoid injections can be repeated two or three times weekly, if necessary. If the cause is removed, and the case is treated before extensive fibrosis has occurred, results are often reasonably good. Most cases of this type will cause some blemish as the result of scar tissue formation.

Surgical removal is sometimes successful when the bursa is large and composed primarily of fibrous tissue. However, it is difficult to keep sutures in place because of stress, and an open wound may result that heals with extensive fibrous tissue. If surgical correction is used, the incision should be curved over the lateral portion of the bursa and should not be made on the posterior aspect of the elbow. This will reduce stress on the incision during flexion and extension of the elbow joint. Mattress sutures should be used in the skin, and a reinforcing quill suture is helpful. Berge and Westhues (1966) recommend that the center of the bursa be injected with 3 percent copper sulfate solution 4-5 days prior to surgery to aid dissection.

Cross-tying the horse for ten days postsurgically to prevent it from lying down will aid healing. Booting the foot or using donut padding below the elbow joint will protect this area from injury when the

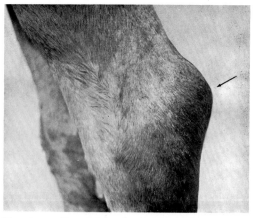

FIG. 5-15. Capped hock. Arrow indicates distention of the bursa over the point of the hock.

horse is getting up and down. This protection should be used during corticoid therapy or after surgical correction.

Capped elbow is sometimes treated by blistering or firing. These methods are usually ineffective, and the additional inflammation produced may result in even greater deposition of fibrous tissue.

Bursitis of the Hock (Capped Hock) (Fig. 5-15)

Bursitis of the hock is caused by trauma to the point of the hock. This is an acquired bursitis caused by trauma induced when the horse kicks a wall or trailer gate. Some horses develop the vice of wall kicking; they may only do it at night when they are not seen. The condition is characterized by a firm swelling at the point of the hock, and it may be accompanied by curb (Chapter 6, p. 342). Lameness is mild, if present, but the blemish is usually permanent. Swelling may be extensive and accompanied by edema when the injury has been severe.

Treatment. In the acute stage, bursitis of the hock can be treated with injection of corticoids. The area should be shaved and prepared for aseptic injection. After withdrawal of the synovial content of the bursa, part of the corticoid solution should be injected into the cavity and part into the surrounding tissue. (Do not use long-acting corticoids in soft tissue.) Corticoid injections can be repeated several times weekly, if necessary. Whenever possible, a pressure bandage should be used at the point of the hock. The hock is difficult to bandage and care must be used so that a skin slough over the Achilles tendon does not result. If the injury to the hock occurs only once, and the case is treated before extensive fibrosis has occurred, results are reasonably good. However, if the injury is repeated several times and extensive fibrous tissue results, little can be done to correct it. Surgical intervention may be used, but if the wound opens, a larger blemish than was present originally may result. When the blemish is very disfiguring, surgery may be done, dissecting out the fibrous-tissue portion of the mass. The incision should be made lateral to the bursa and not on the posterior aspect of the hock. This will ease the stress on the incision. Mattress sutures should be used in the skin, with a reinforcing quill suture to prevent tearing of the incision line. The horse should be kept tied following surgery to minimize motion. Counterpressure bandage should be used for ten to fourteen days.

SPECIFIC REFERENCES

BERGE, E., and M. WESTHUES. 1966. *Veterinary Operative Surgery.* Baltimore: Williams & Wilkins Co.

COSGROVE, J. S. M. 1963. Equine brucellosis. Proc. 9th AAEP. 161.

VAN PELT, R. W. 1962. Therapeutic management of capped hocks. Mich. State Univ. Vet. 23(1): 28.

VAN PELT, R. W.,and W. F. RILEY. 1968. Treatment of calcaneal bursitis. JAVMA 153(9): 1176–1180.

Trochanteric Bursitis (Trochanteric Lameness, Whorlbone Lameness)

This type of bursitis is apparently most common in Standardbred horses and can be classified as a true bursitis. Trochanteric bursitis is difficult to treat and usually requires repeated injections of corticoids. Results are inconsistent, and accurate diagnosis is necessary. Treatment is described in the discussion of this ailment in Chapter 6.

Hygroma

Hygroma is an acquired bursitis of the anterior surface of the carpus. It is the result of trauma that produces a bursa; the bursitis causes a diffuse swelling over the anterior surface of the carpus (Fig. 6-17) (see Chap. 6). An uneven swelling over the anterior surface of the carpus may be the result of a synovial hernia from either the radiocarpal joint or the intercarpal joint, or it may result from distention of the common or lateral digital extensor tendon sheath(s). Treatment of hygroma is discussed in Chapter 6, (p. 182).

Bicipital Bursitis

Bicipital bursitis is found between the biceps brachii tendon and the bicipital groove of the humerus. It is classified as a true bursitis. Description of the lameness and its treatment can be found in Chapter 6, p. 163.

Bursitis of the Cunean Tendon

Bursitis of the cunean tendon is described by Lutz and Gabel (1969) as a separate entity in the Standardbred. Signs of lameness are the same as those for bone spavin. In some cases of hock lameness, most of the signs are due to bursitis of the cunean tendon; these must be differentiated from those resulting from other disorders. Bursitis of the cunean tendon will usually exhibit swelling of the bursa over the cunean tendon. Injection of this area with a local anesthetic in and around the bursa of the cunean tendon will reveal how much of the lameness is due to bursitis and how much is due to bone spavin. If injection of the bursa of the cunean tendon causes the signs of lameness to disappear, cunean tenectomy is indicated (see p. 330). If little or no relief is obtained by injection of the bursa with local anesthetic, little relief of signs of lameness will result from cunean tenectomy.

SPECIFIC REFERENCE

LUTZ, W. H., and A. A. GABEL. 1969. Spavin in Standardbred horses. Mod. Vet Pract. 50: 38–42.

Synovitis

Inflammation of any synovial lining—joint, tendon sheath, or bursa.

Tendinitis

Tendinitis implies inflammation of the tendon only. This occurs where the tendons have no sheath.

Tenosynovitis (Tenovaginitis)

Tenosynovitis may be defined as inflammation of the synovium surrounding the tendons. This inflammation is usually due to strain from unaccustomed overuse or may be due to a direct blow or infection. The result is a reaction of the relatively avascular synovium characterized by increased blood supply, invasion by inflammatory cells, oversecretion of synovial fluid, and development of fibrin causing adhesions between the tendon and its surrounding synovium. The exact manifestations vary greatly, depending upon the tendon involved. Pain and distention of the sheath are the first signs of tenosynovitis. This is usually manifested during motion. As the condition progresses, the adherence between the tendon and synovium becomes firmer and finally results in complete inability of the tendon to glide within its sheath.

Treatment. Treatment is directed toward pathological changes and the principles of treatment are rest, local heat and local injection of corticoids. Specific treatment will vary according to the site of the condition.

Thoroughpin

Thoroughpin is tenosynovitis of the tarsal sheath that encloses the deep digital flexor tendon of the hind limb. The swelling occurs in the area of the hock at a level approximately the same as that of the point of the hock (Fig. 5–16). This swelling can be confused with bog spavin when bog spavin causes swellings on the medial and lateral sides of the hock joint. Thoroughpin swelling is located approximately 2″ higher than the swelling that occurs in bog spavin in the posterior part of the joint capsule. Thoroughpin swelling can vary from a small swelling to a large swelling involving most of the tarsal sheath. Thoroughpin is usually unilateral and due to trauma. Mild swellings of both tarsal sheaths may occur when the horse is worked hard. In this case, thoroughpin would be classified as wind puff. When treatment is indicated, the lateral aspect of the thoroughpin is shaved, and in aseptic conditions as much fluid as possible is drained. The cavity is then injected with a corticoid. It is usually best to infuse the skin with a small amount of local anesthetic, using a 25-gauge $\frac{1}{2}$″ needle. Then an 18-gauge 1″ or 2″ needle is inserted into the tendon sheath, the fluid withdrawn, and the corticoid injected. A tranquilizer and twitch can be used as

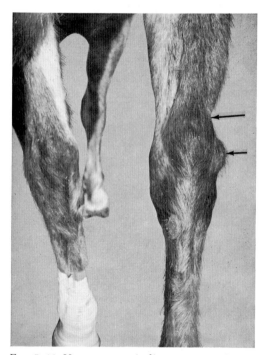

FIG. 5–16. Upper arrow indicates approximate position of thoroughpin. This example used because it shows the distention of the tarsal joint capsule (lower arrow) that can be confused with thoroughpin. This case shows no clinical evidence of thoroughpin, but a good comparison of their locations can be seen.

restraint if necessary. These injections may be repeated two or three times weekly until the swelling does not recur. Results are usually good. Firing and blistering of the area are contraindicated and will not achieve good results.

Tenosynovitis in Newborn Foals

Newborn foals occasionally show tenosynovitis of the extensors over the carpus (extensor carpi radialis, common digital extensor, and lateral digital extensor) and over the hocks (long digital extensor and lateral digital extensor). The etiology of this condition is unknown (Van Pelt, 1969b). The condition is noninfectious and is not associated with illness. The condition usually improves with age if the conformation of the foal is good. Some cases respond to treatment with injections of corticoids and antibiotics such as penicillin and streptomycin (Van Pelt, 1969b). Aseptic technique should be utilized when the tendon sheaths are injected in order to prevent the possibility of an infectious tenosynovitis. This type of tenosynovitis is differentiated from an infectious type in that there is no lameness, pain, heat, or rise of temperature associated with the condition.

Tenosynovitis of the Digital Flexor Tendons

The common tendon sheath of the deep and superficial flexor tendons of the forelimb is frequently injured in the fetlock area (this occurs occasionally in the hind limb). This injury produces a swelling that lies between the suspensory ligament and the deep digital flexor tendon. It must be differentiated from the swelling that occurs in the volar pouch of the metacarpophalangeal joint capsule between the suspensory ligament and the cannon bone. When treatment of these swellings is indicated, the lateral portion of the swelling at a distal point is shaved and prepared for aseptic injection. The horse is twitched, and a small amount of local anesthetic is infused in the skin with a 25-gauge $\frac{1}{2}''$ needle. A 18- or 20-gauge 1'' needle is then put into the tendon sheath, the contents withdrawn, and the corticoid infused into the cavity. These injections may be repeated two or three times weekly if necessary. Counterpressure should be applied. The horse must be rested until the injury has healed.

Open Tenosynovitis

Occasionally a tendon sheath is opened by a lacerated wound. These wounds are always slow to heal and can result in adhesions that will impair the action of the tendon and cause permanent unsoundness. Whenever possible, it is best to treat the wound soon after it occurs by irrigating the tendon sheath with antibiotics. Corticoids should not be used in treatment if there is any acute or chronic infection present. The wound should be sutured if it is believed that first-intention healing can be attained. It is then best to immobilize the area in a plaster cast. This cast is removed after approximately one week and the wound checked and treated locally and then recast. In approximately eight days the second cast is removed, and at this time the wound is usually healed; the limb should then be kept in supportive wrap for thirty days. Systemic antibiotics should be used for at least one week. If the wound does not heal by first intention, it must be treated locally by the infusion of antibiotics, enzymes and corticoids into the sheath. The wound is kept clean, and hair is shaved away from the site. The area is wrapped in pressure bandages, which are readjusted daily. Second-intention healing invariably results in a prolonged convalescence and the formation of some adhesions.

SPECIFIC REFERENCES

RAGLAND, L. 1968. Localized nodular tenosynovitis. Pathol. Vet. 5(5): 436–441.

ROBERTS, W. D. 1969. Treatment for shoe boil. Pract. Vet. 41(4): 126.

VAN PELT, R. W. 1969a. Tenosynovitis in the horse. JAVMA 154(9): 1022–1033.

VAN PELT, R. W. 1969b. Idiopathic tenosynovitis in foals. JAVMA 155(3): 510–517.

VAN PELT, R. W. 1969c. Inflammation of the tarsal synovial sheath. JAVMA 155(9): 1481–1488.

Tendosynovitis (Bowed Tendon, Tendovaginitis) (Figs. 6–40 and 6–41)

A tendosynovitis involves both tendon and sheath. The deep and superficial flexors are most commonly involved above the metacarpophalangeal (fetlock) joint (Chap. 6, p. 200). Actual pathology occurs within the tendon, and hemorrhage within the tendon fibers is present. In some cases, portions of the tendon fibers are torn, and the tendon may actually lengthen as a result of the tearing or stretching of these fibers. The tendon sheath is involved and usually there are adhesions between it and the tendon. Adhesions may also develop between the deep and superficial flexor tendons. Tearing of these adhesions causes recurrence of lameness.

Desmitis

Inflammation of a ligament, e.g., suspensory ligament injury or ligament injury from a sprain.

Windpuff (Windgall)

These are synovial swellings of joints or tendon sheaths that result from trauma, but they do not cause lameness. They are a form of synovitis and are classified as articular or tendinous windpuffs, depending on their location. The common sites are the metacarpophalangeal (fet-lock) joint, the flexor tendon sheath above the proximal sesamoid bones, the lateral and common digital extensor sheaths as they cross the carpus, the carpal sheath, and the tarsal sheath (thoroughpin) in the hock. When swellings such as these are present but are not accompanied by heat, pain, or lameness, they are called wind-puffs or windgalls. When these swellings are present and are accompanied by inflammation, they are considered signs of pathological change in the structure. Most hardworking horses have some windpuffs, especially in the metacarpophalangeal and tarsal sheath areas. Windpuffs tend to become smaller if work is decreased, and treatment is usually ineffectual.

Synovial swellings of the common digital and lateral digital extensor tendons in the forelimb and the lateral digital extensor tendon in the hind limb may also occur as congenital defects in newborn foals. Nutritional deficiencies may also produce windpuffs.

Ganglion*

Synovial hernia or ganglion is another condition involving a tendon sheath or sometimes a joint capsule. This condition usually results from a defect in the fibrous sheath of the joint capsule or tendon sheath that permits a segment of underlying synovium to herniate through it. The irritation accompanying this herniation results in continued secretion of fluid so that the sac gradually fills up and enlarges. As a rule, the synovial hernia will appear as a small, discrete, sometimes extremely hard nodule lying directly over or under the tendon. It may be impossible to tell whether the primary involvement is tendon sheath or joint capsule. It is uncommon in horses, but it does occur.

*Definitions for the conditions marked with an asterisk have been taken from O'Donoghue's text, Treatment of Injuries to Athletes, courtesy of W. B. Saunders Co.

I have observed ganglion underneath the long extensor tendon in the vicinity of the pastern joint in the hind limb. The same lesion has been observed under the common extensor tendon in the forelimb. These were diagnosed by the swelling that occurred when the horse was worked. When the horses were rested, swelling disappeared. The area was painful to the touch, and lameness was noted. When a local anesthetic was injected, the lameness disappeared.

Treatment. Treatment consists of incising directly into the area of swelling in the vicinity of the pastern joint on the anterior surface. The skin is prepared for aseptic surgery, and a ring block is used above the fetlock joint to produce anesthesia. The skin and tendon are both incised longitudinally before the ganglion is exposed when it lies beneath the tendon. Only the skin is incised when the ganglion is superficial to the tendon. The tissue and ganglion are dark blue and are obviously thickened synovium. The diseased tissue is completely excised. The tendon and skin are then sutured, and the wound kept under bandage for ten to fourteen days. If all tissue in the ganglion is not removed, it will recur.

SPRAIN AND STRAIN

The terms sprain and strain are often used loosely. O'Donoghue (1962) classifies these in a logical manner, and his classification is used here.

Sprain

Sprain can be defined as an injury to a ligament resulting from overstress. This causes some degree of damage to the ligamentous fibers or their attachment. Certain ligaments may bind two bones together firmly with relatively little motion, e.g., the ligamentous attachment between the second and third metacarpal bones or between the tibia and fibula. Other ligaments serve to reinforce the joint and permit a rather wide range of motion but prevent motion in an abnormal direction. Abnormal motion to a degree beyond the power of a ligament to hold it will cause a sprain. As abnormal force is applied, the ligament becomes tense and then gives way at one or another of its attachments or at some point in the substance of the ligament. If the attachment pulls loose with a fragment of bone, it is called a sprain fracture, but the mechanism is the same. The location of the damage will depend upon the weakest link in the chain of the ligament, which may be within the ligament itself or at one of its attachments, possibly at the site of an area of previous damage. The extent of the damage depends upon the amount and duration of the force. If the abnormal force is terminated promptly, there may be little actual functional loss to the ligament, and only a few of its fibers may be involved. In this instance there is localized hematoma formation with prompt deposit of fibrin in the hematoma. The fibrin is invaded by fibroblasts, and they repair the ligament. If the damage is so severe that there is disruption of numerous ligamentous fibers, there may be a considerable functional loss. When the ligament is completely torn, all function is lost. In this case, the findings will depend on the location of the tear. Ordinarily, there will be relatively extensive hematoma formation with swelling and edema. The process of repair will be much slower and much less complete and will result in scar formation rather than restoration of normal ligament.

Sprains are classified as follows:

Mild Sprain (Fig. 5–17A)

This is a sprain in which a few fibers of a ligament have been torn, with some resultant hemorrhage into the ligament but with no actual functional loss.

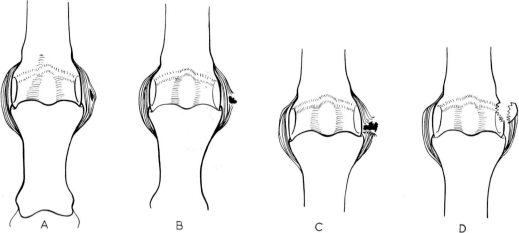

FIG. 5–17. Examples of sprain. A, Mild sprain—hemorrhage occurs in the fibers of the ligament. B, Moderate sprain—hemorrhage in the fibers of the ligaments and some of the fibers are torn. C, Severe sprain—complete tearing of the ligament and loss of function. D, Sprain fracture—the function of the ligament is lost in the same fashion as in C, but in this case the portion of bone to which the ligament was attached is fractured. (Redrawn from O'Donoghue, *Treatment of Injuries to Athletes,* courtesy of W. B. Saunders Co.)

Moderate Sprain (Fig. 5–17B)

A moderate sprain is one in which some portion of the ligament is torn and some degree of functional loss is sustained. The amount of damage may vary from a tear of a relatively small portion of the ligament to almost complete avulsion. One would not expect wide retraction of torn ligament ends in a moderate sprain. Union can, therefore, proceed in an orderly manner with replacement of fibrous scar by ligament during the process of repair. If the damage is relatively severe, however, there may be considerable permanent scar formation, with resultant weakness in this segment of the ligament.

Severe Sprain (Fig. 5–17C)

In severe sprain there is complete loss of function of the ligament. The stress tears it completely away from one of its attachments or pulls it apart along its length. There is usually a separation of the ends of the ligament. Efficient repair is dependent upon apposition of the torn ends of the ligament, and it is important to obtain apposition of the ends of the ligament. Ligaments that heal across a gap by scar formation never assume the characteristics of a normal ligament.

Sprain Fracture (Fig. 5–17D)

In this case, the portion of bone to which the ligament is attached becomes avulsed.

Treatment. In mild sprain, treatment is relatively unimportant and is aimed mostly at prevention of pain. In moderate sprain, the critical factor in treatment is protection in order to permit repair. In severe sprain and sprain fracture, where the ligament is ruptured or a portion of bone is avulsed, emphasis must be placed on reapposition of the ends of the ligament or bone in order to assure a ligament of normal length and strength. It is very important that accurate diagnosis is made in the management of ligament injuries. Adequate rest is mandatory to obtain healing of ligament damage. Immobilization in a cast for three to six weeks is essential for repair of the more severe sprains. Milder types can be supported by use of Gelocast* or Medicopaste†.

Strain

Strain may be defined as damage to a tendon or muscle caused by overuse or overstress. It is important to distinguish between strain and sprain, applying the former term to muscle and tendon and the latter to ligaments. Strain of the tendon could consist of anything from minor irritation to near complete avulsion of the tendon from its attachment or within its substance. Strain of the muscle includes those cases of overuse and overstretching short of actual muscular rupture. Strain can be classified as follows:

Simple Strain

In this type of strain there is no appreciable hemorrhage and the pathological changes are confined to a low-grade inflammatory reaction with swelling and edema and some disruption of adjacent fibers. Simple strain may completely incapacitate a horse for work until healing has occurred. To continue the work when the strain is present will lead to additional pathological changes.

Violent Strain, Musculotendinous Injury

Those injuries to the musculotendinous unit caused by a single violent injury may be of any degree. Tendinitis, tenosynovitis or tendosynovitis may occur. A tendon may be torn from the bone or pulled apart. The musculotendinous junction may be ruptured or the muscle itself may tear. These injuries result from either violent contraction of the muscle against resistance or from violent overstretching of the muscle while it is forcibly contracted.

*Gelocast, Duke Laboratories, South Norwalk, Conn.
†Medicopaste, Graham Field Laboratories, Woodside, N.J.

In the horse one of the most common locations for this type of injury is the attachment of the common digital extensor to the extensor process of the third phalanx. The extensor tendon may be torn from its attachment or avulsion of the extensor process may occur. The peroneus tertius is commonly ruptured in its length and not at its bony attachment.

Treatment. Treatment of simple strain consists of relieving the acute condition by injection of a local anesthetic and corticoids. Ultrasound therapy is often of value. Local heat and protection against movement that causes pain are additional methods of therapy. The amount of protection applied must vary with the degree of damage so that in some cases all that is necessary is to limit the patient's activity, while in others it may be sensible to prevent motion by immobilization of the part. The criterion for the amount of protection is pain. Function should be resumed as soon as pain is no longer felt. One must be careful that desire to rehabilitate the muscle by active use does not cause recurrence.

Treatment of violent strain should be preceded by accurate diagnosis. If at all possible, one should determine if there has been a complete disruption of the musculotendinous unit. If disruption has occurred and it is recognized early, immediate surgical repair is the best therapy when possible. Surgical repair may be impossible in horses because of an inability to immobilize the part. Immobilization by means of a plaster cast or other device must be used whether or not surgical apposition is accomplished. If the injury is less than a complete rupture, an attempt should be made to evaluate the degree of tearing and treat it accordingly. Immobilization of the part with plaster cast is one of the best methods of therapy. When tendons have been divided by lacerated wounds, a common lesion in the metatarsal/metacarpal area, a plaster cast with the foot in a flexed position is used. When the extensor tendon is cut, the foot is cast in an extended position. It is not uncommon to find that sutures will not hold in equine tendons, but good results may be accomplished with plaster immobilization. Changing a cast two or three times over a period of approximately eight weeks, followed by the use of corrective shoeing and fetlock support (see Chap. 6, p. 352), will often give gratifying results.

SPECIFIC REFERENCES

CRENSHAW, A. H. 1963. *Campbell's Operative Orthopaedics*. 4th ed. St. Louis: C. V. Mosby.
O'DONOGHUE, D. H. 1962. *Treatment of Injuries to Athletes*. Philadelphia: W. B. Saunders Co.

DISEASES OF BONE

Necrosis of Bone (Avascular Necrosis of Bone, Bone Cysts)

Definition

Necrosis of bone may be either septic or aseptic. Septic necrosis of bone is present in some sequestra and in some cases of osteomyelitis. To call either aseptic or septic necrosis "avascular necrosis" is redundant, since all necrosis of bone is avascular. Inflammation of bone with increased blood supply may be present around an area of necrosis, but the bone undergoing necrosis is avascular.

Aseptic necrosis may occur as a result of trauma, irradiation, infarcts, and numerous other causes. Idiopathic aseptic necrosis also occurs, and the most important example of idiopathic aseptic necrosis is osteochondritis dissecans.

Osteochondritis Dissecans

Definition

Osteochondritis dissecans usually affects only young horses in any weight-bearing joint. The lesion will involve the articulation, and the articular cartilage may or may not fracture. As long as the articular cartilage remains intact, there is a good chance the lesion will heal. Once the cartilage separates and allows the necrotic bone to be free, there is little chance that the joint will ever be sound. I have observed it in the carpal bones, tarsal bones, femur, distal end of the metacarpal bone and the third phalanx. Others (Pettersson and Sevelius, 1968) have reported the disease in other long bones.

Etiology

The process is one of degeneration and eventual replacement of the affected portion of bone. It is probable that this disease results from a change in vascularity and blood supply to the affected bone area. Ischemia results in death and demineralization of the affected portion of bone. It is assumed to be essentially an infarct within the bony epiphysis. Rare cases in man have yielded positive bacterial cultures, but in horses this has not been proven. However, a high white cell count (above 20,000) may be present (Morgan, 1962). In some cases, this disease has been attributed to hypothyroidism (Reid, 1970).

During the course of this disease, unless interrupted by surgery or other treatment, the necrotic bone and the cartilage overlying it may gradually separate from adjacent bone and cartilage and together become a loose body. Trauma may play a very prominent part in the cause of this disease.

Signs

The earliest radiographic changes consist of irregularity in the outline of the bone, followed by demineralization. Density of the bone in the early stages is irregular, with areas of lysis present. Joint capsule distention may be noted early in some cases. Fragmentation can occur in the tarsal or carpal bones, probably due to pressures that force the affected pieces in an anterior direction. Cartilage is not affected early in the disease, and the normal joint space remains preserved. However, complete destruction of the articular cartilage may occur later. Regeneration produces a bone of normal hardness, and irregularity varies with the degree of compression in the early stages. Later, bony ankylosis may bridge the intertarsal joints, and the tarsometatarsal joint may become fused. This is not the case when the metacarpophalangeal joint is affected. It is important that involvement of the tarsal bones does not later become confused with typical osteoarthritic (bone spavin) changes of the tarsal joints.

Signs of lameness are vague, but usually the swelling of the joint plus selective nerve blocking will localize the site. Pain in the joint is one of the most obvious clinical signs.

The lesion may be seen in one or more of many bones and has been described in the femur, tibia, tibial tarsal, central tarsal, third tarsal, fourth tarsal, third metatarsal, first, second, and third phalanx of the hind limb (Morgan, 1962).

In the forelimb, lesions have been seen in the humerus, radial, intermediate and ulnar carpal bones, third carpal bone, accessory carpal bone, third metacarpal, proximal sesamoids, first, second and third phalanges, and the navicular bone (Pettersson and Sevelius, 1968).

Diagnosis

Horses with osteochondritis dissecans seldom show a marked swelling of the joint area involved. Often the lameness has to be localized by use of nerve blocks (see Chap. 4). Radiography will reveal the avascular bone area as an area of decreased density on the articular surface (Fig. 5–18). Good-quality radiographs are necessary for diagnosis, and the quality

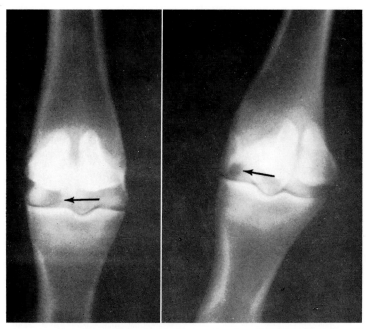

FIG. 5–18. An example of osteochondritis dissecans in the distal end of the third metacarpal bone. The figure on the left shows an AP radiograph with arrow pointing at the area of decreased density on the articular surface of the distal end of the third metacarpal bone. The figure on the right shows an oblique radiograph of the same area. Notice that the oblique radiograph confirms the findings on the AP radiograph. The lateral radiograph of this condition would not show the condition nearly so well.

must be uniform to allow accurate evaluation of healing. The area of decreased density may not be visible on one view but obvious on another. When osteochondritis dissecans is suspected, oblique views of the joint are helpful in outlining the defect (Fig. 5–18).

Treatment

A conservative attitude toward the treatment of osteochondritis dissecans seems best. Surgery is usually unnecessary, and if the cartilage overlying the avascular bone is well preserved and the joint is protected as much as possible from weight-bearing, the avascular bone will remain in place and become revascularized in three to seven months. Evans and Jenny (1970) on the other hand, have reported that forced exercise stimulated healing. Radiation therapy has been a successful treatment in the hands of the author in a few cases. However, it is difficult to say whether or not the condition

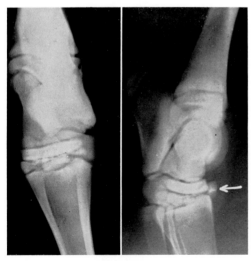

FIG. 5–19. Aseptic necrosis of the tarsal joint. Notice the crushing effect on the tarsal bones causing avulsion of a portion of the third tarsal bone. When aseptic necrosis involves the tarsal or carpal bones, the horse seldom recovers to full soundness (Carlson, *Veterinary Radiology*, Lea & Febiger).

would have healed without the therapy. When a portion of bone separates, the outlook for successful treatment is not favorable (Fig. 5–19). In this case the tarsal joint or carpal joint may become permanently deformed as a result of bone separation (Fig. 5–19). Surgical removal of a loose body would be indicated if the economic value of the horse warranted it. A large loose body could be fixed in place by use of a bone screw.

In those cases that are accessible by a surgical approach, surgical curettage and packing with cancellous bone from the tuber coxae has been said to be successful (Evans and Jenny, 1970).

SPECIFIC REFERENCES

American Jockey Club. 1965. Conference on Unsoundness of Thoroughbreds. Washington, D.C.: Armed Forces Institute of Pathology.

CARLSON, W. D. 1961. *Veterinary Radiology*. 2nd ed. Philadephia: Lea & Febiger.

CRENSHAW, A. H. 1963. *Campbell's Operative Orthopaedics*. 4th ed. St. Louis: C. V. Mosby, Vol. 1.

DeMOOR, A., *et al.* 1971. Osteochondritis dissecans of the tibiotarsal joint. 19th World Vet. Cong. 1: 378–381.

DeMOOR, A., *et al.* 1972. Osteochondritis dissecans of the tibiotarsal joint in the horse. EVJ 4(3): 39–143.

EVANS, L. H. and J. JENNY. 1970. Surgical and clinical management of subchondral "Bone Cysts." Proc. 16th Ann. AAEP, 195–197.

JENNY, J. 1970. A.S.I.F. Internal fixation of bone course. Davos, Switzerland.

MORGAN, J. P. 1967. Necrosis of the third tarsal bone. JAVMA 151(10): 1334–1342.

MORGAN, J. P. 1962. Personal communication.

PETTERSSON, H., and R. SEVELIUS. 1968. Subchondral bone cysts in the horse: A clinical study. BEVJ 1(2): 75–77.

PETTERSSON, H., and S. REILAND. 1969. Periarticular subchondral bone cysts. Proc. 14th Ann. AAEP, 245–264.

REID, C. F. 1970. Radiographic diagnosis and appearance of osseous cyst-like lesions in horses previously reported as periarticular subchondral "bone cysts." Proc. 16th Ann. AAEP, 185–193.

ROONEY, J. R. 1963. *Equine Medicine and Surgery*. Santa Barbara, Calif.: Veterinary Publications Inc.

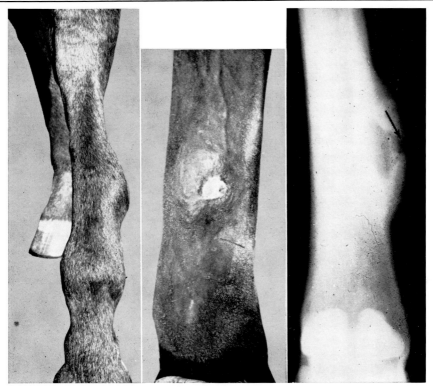

FIG. 5-20. Three views of a case of osteomyelitis on the lateral aspect of the left third metatarsal bone. *Left,* appearance of the clinical case with fibrous tissue and bony swelling. *Center,* close-up view of the draining tract after surgical preparation. *Right,* radiograph of the same limb with arrow pointing at "cloaca" typical of osteomyelitis in this area. A dead piece of bone was found inside the cloacal opening. The fibrous tissue and periosteal new bone growth were removed, and full clinical soundness resulted.

Osteomyelitis and Osteitis

Definition

By Dorland's definition (1965), osteo-myelitis is an inflammation of the bone caused by a pyogenic organism. Osteitis is an inflammation of bone involving the haversian spaces, canals, and their branches. In some cases it also includes inflammation of the medullary cavity. For the purposes of this discussion, the term osteomyelitis will be used and the inflam-matory reaction present presumed to be infectious in nature. These infections may occur with comminuted or compound fractures and can involve long bones, carpal or tarsal bones, and bones of the head and jaw.

Etiology

Osteomyelitis most commonly occurs following a compound fracture. In this case, the fractured ends of the bone have penetrated the skin and infection enters through the wound. This is always seri-ous, and it is rare for an adult horse to recover from this type of injury and in-fection. Young horses may recover after careful and diligent care.

Osteomyelitis may follow a commi-nuted fracture in which one of the bone fragments is separated from its blood sup-ply. In this case, a fragment of bone dies, and infection develops by hematogenous source.

Osteosis (necrosis) may occur in a small fracture fragment when a horse has been kicked on one of the metacarpal or meta-tarsal bones (Fig. 5-20). In this case, an abscess develops within the cortex of the bone and the infection does not break into the medullary cavity. This bone fragment acts as a sequestrum and must be removed before healing will occur. Osteo-myelitis may also occur in the carpal bones following carpal surgery. It is rare to encounter this difficulty following re-moval of chip fractures of the carpus, but when exostoses are removed from the carpal bones or when the joint has been injected with steroids prior to surgery, osteomyelitis will occasionally occur. The bone inflammation and infection usually appear two to three weeks after surgery, after the incision has healed by first in-tention. The source of infection is appar-ently hematogenous, acting on an area of low resistance. Why removal of bony periosteal new bone growth is more apt to result in osteomyelitis than is removal of chip fractures is not known.

Osteomyelitis is not uncommon when a second or fourth metacarpal or metatarsal bone has been fractured, leaving a portion separated from its blood supply (Fig. 6-45).

Signs

Osteomyelitis is characterized by chronic drainage from the wound. This has generally occurred as a result of a compound fracture; the wound shows persistent drainage and the bone does not heal at a normal rate. Many weeks are required for a bone callus to form, and union may never occur. This type of

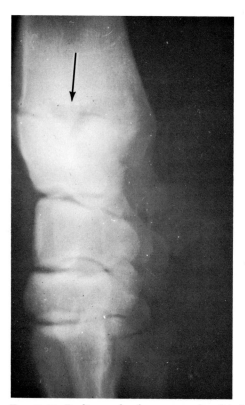
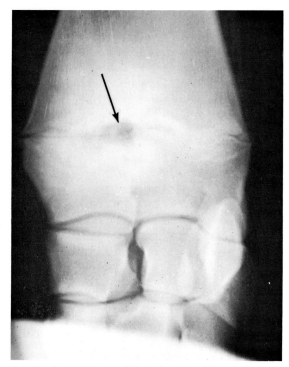

Fig. 5-21. Radiograph of an example of infection in the epiphyseal line (arrow). This is a form of osteomyelitis. It is characterized by heat, pain, swelling, and acute lameness. There is usually a rise in body temperature. Poulticing and parenteral administration of appropriate antibiotics for ten to fourteen days is required. Prognosis is guarded.

drainage will also eventually occur when a piece of bone has become necrotic in a comminuted fracture. Drainage will occur as long as the dead piece of bone is present in the fracture site.

In osteomyelitis where a portion of the cortex has fractured, the wound will apparently heal, only to break open repeatedly (Fig. 5-20). Drainage will be persistent until the bone fragment is removed. When a portion of a second or fourth metacarpal or metatarsal has been fractured and separated from its blood supply, it will also drain intermittently until the fragment is surgically removed (*see* Fractured Splint Bone, Chap. 6, p. 211).

Treatment

When a compound fracture is present, complete debridement of the wound must be done. The fracture is set and a cast put on over the fracture site. After eight to fourteen days the original cast is removed, and, if healing is not progressing normally by first intention, a new cast is put on and a window is cut into it over the wound site. The wound is then irrigated daily with antibiotics and enzymes until granulation has occurred. It is important to cover the bone with granulation tissue. Whenever possible, pull tissue over the bone by means of sutures. If osteomyelitis develops after a comminuted fracture and it is obvious that an abscess is developing, the fracture site should be opened and the piece of bone that is separated from its blood supply should be removed. A cast with a window cut into it can be used for local treatment of the wound. In all cases, parenteral antibiotics are used for a prolonged period (seven to fourteen days).

Whenever a window is used in a cast, it is extremely important that pressure be maintained against the wound to prevent bulging of the soft tissues through the window. When healing of the wound has occurred, a new cast without a window should be applied.

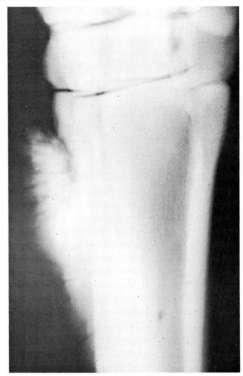

FIG. 5-22. An example of osteomyelitis of the second metacarpal bone. Infection in the active bone growth is indicated by the "sunburst" effect in the bone proliferation. In some cases, removal of this type of bone infection will result in a recurrence of the bone growth.

When a fractured piece of bone has become a sequestrum in a cortex (Fig. 5-20), simple surgical removal of the bone fragment will allow the lesion to heal. Bony proliferation and fibrous tissue over the bone fragment should be removed using aseptic surgical precautions. The bone should be trimmed to as nearly normal a shape as possible. The cavity where the bone fragment was removed should be curetted thoroughly and the subcutaneous tissues and skin sutured. A counterpressure bandage should be maintained for approximately two weeks over the incision. The use of bacterins in treatment of osteomyelitis has been described (Coffman, 1969).

SPECIFIC REFERENCES

COFFMAN, J. R. 1969. Autogenous bacterins in osteomyelitis therapy. VM/SAC 64(10): 899–902.

CRENSHAW, A. H. 1963. Campbell's Operative Orthopaedics. 4th ed. St. Louis: C. V. Mosby.

Dorland's Illustrated Medical Dictionary. 1965. 24th ed. Philadelphia: W. B. Saunders.

GUFFY, M. M. 1968. Bone sequestrums and nonhealing wounds in horses. JAVMA 152(11): 1638–1642.

GUSTAVESSON, P. O., and B. STROMBERG. 1966. Tibial osteomyelitis: Case report. J. Vet. Radiol. Soc. 7: 48–50.

JUBB, K. V. F., and P. C. KENNEDY. 1963. Pathology of Domestic Animals. New York: Academic Press. Vol. 1.

LEWIS, R. E., and C. D. HEINZE. 1970. Bone sequestration in the horse: Diagnosis, radiography and treatment, Proc. 16th Ann. AAEP, 161–169.

Hypertrophic Pulmonary Osteoarthropathy

Definition

In the horse, this disease is characterized by a marked change in the limbs with a distinct thickening and deformity by new bone growth. New bone growth is formed beneath the periosteum, which is pushed outward. The osteophytic growths are very irregular, and the bone becomes very rough. In conjunction with this, there is lung pathology in some form, e.g., lung tumor. In the horse it has been described with a granular-cell myoblastoma (Alexander et al., 1965). The bones usually affected are those of all four limbs from the femorotibial and scapulohumeral joints to the phalanges. The joint surfaces are not involved, although there may be periarticular proliferation and enlargement. Occasionally, a bone may attain twice its normal diameter. In later stages, there may be considerable pain on movement and palpation. The disease usually results in death, but the course is usually prolonged.

Signs

The disease has been described in man, dogs, sheep, deer, and lions (Jubb and Kennedy, 1963; Smith et al., 1972) as a primary respiratory disease. In these species, it is usually heralded by cough, dyspnea, or other pulmonary disturbances. In the horse, however, the most marked change is a noticeable thickening and deformity of the limbs by new bone growth (Fig. 5–23). Alexander et al. (1965) described a case in which the fetlock, carpal and tarsal joints were grossly enlarged and symmetrical. Passive movement revealed a decreased motion in the carpal and tarsal joints as a result of the bone growth. The horse was obviously lame when it walked. Auscultation of the lungs indicated areas of consolidation. Radiographs revealed extensive subperiosteal hypertrophic osteogenesis of the phalanges and the metacarpal and metatarsal bones. In the carpal and tarsal joints there was intracapsular involvement but in no case was the articular surface involved. None of the joints were actually fused. A lateral radiograph of the thorax revealed a discrete circular area of increased density approximately 6″ in diameter. Subsequent necropsy revealed this to be a granular-cell myoblastoma.

Etiology

The cause of hypertrophic pulmonary osteoarthropathy is unknown. Most believe that lung pathology is primary, with a possible toxin or chronic anoxia causing the bone reaction.

Diagnosis

A positive diagnosis is rather difficult without necropsy, since radiographs of the lung of a horse are difficult to obtain without powerful equipment. The best diagnostic feature is bilateral bony enlargement of the limbs as shown in Figure 5–23. It should not be confused with hereditary multiple exostosis, in which the lesions are more localized. Necropsy findings consisting of lung tumor plus the typical bone enlargements constitute

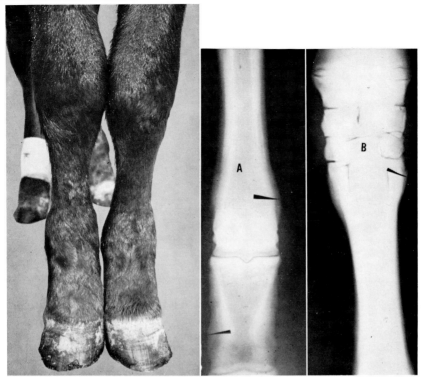

FIG. 5-23. Hypertrophic pulmonary osteoarthropathy. *Left,* appearance of the limbs of the clinical case. Note enlargement of the distal end of the radius, proximal end of the third metacarpal bone, distal end of metacarpal bones and pastern areas. The rear limbs showed similar enlargement. *Right,* radiographs of the same horse. *A* shows the thickening of the distal end of the third metacarpal bone and of the first phalanx. *B* shows the thickening of the proximal end of the second, third, and fourth metacarpal bones.

strong evidence of the disease. There is general agreement that the bone is not neoplastic. Metastatic neoplasms in the lung do not appear to be invariably associated with pulmonary osteoarthropathy.

Treatment

There is no known treatment.

SPECIFIC REFERENCES

ALEXANDER, J. E., G. H. KEOWN, and J. L. PALOTAY. 1965. Granular cell myoblastoma with hypertrophic pulmonary osteoarthropathy in a mare. JAVMA 146(7): 703.

CARLSON, W. D. 1967. *Veterinary Radiology.* 2nd ed. Philadelphia: Lea & Febiger.

HOLMES, J. R. 1961. A case of pulmonary osteoarthropathy in a mare. Vet. Rec. 73(114): 333-335.

JUBB, K. V. F., and P. C. KENNEDY. 1963. *Pathology of Domestic Animals.* New York: Academic Press.

SMITH, A. S., T. C. JONES, and D. H. HUNT. 1972. *Veterinary Pathology.* 4th ed. Philadelphia: Lea & Febiger.

Hereditary Multiple Exostosis

Definition

Hereditary multiple exostosis is a bone disease in which numerous abnormal projections of bone extend out from the normal contour of the affected bones. The new bone growths have a cortex and medulla that are continuous with that of the bones from which they arise. Such exostoses may occur on most of the long bones, as well as on the ribs and pelvis. This condition is a developmental anomaly of a proven hereditary nature.

Etiology

The disease has been reported in dogs, man, and horses (Aergester and Kirkpatrick, 1958; Morgan *et al.,* 1962). The disease is regarded as inherited in all these species. In man, the disease is presumed to be passed by the male. Two fillies from one affected stallion have been known to have the condition.

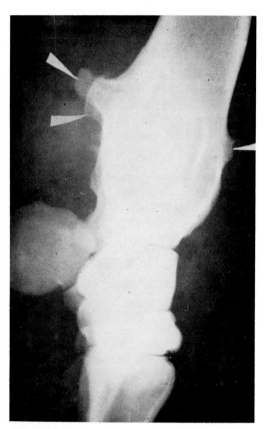

FIG. 5–24. Hereditary multiple exostosis. Pointers indicate the areas of exostosis on the distal end of the radius. Similar growths may occur at the distal end of the tibia; exostosis over the ribs also occurs.

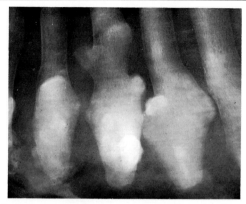

FIG. 5–25. Radiographic appearance of the costochondral rib articulations in inheritable multiple exostosis.

Signs

I have observed ten cases of this disease. In none of these were signs of lameness severe. A typical case showed enlargement of the carpal and/or hock joints; in one case the carpus had been drained of fluid several times and corticoids had been used intra-articularly. Clinical examination revealed the presence of firm swellings in the region of the distal ends of both radii (Fig. 5–24). Gross nodular swellings at the junction of the middle and ventral thirds of the ribs may be present. The lesions, which may occur on any rib, have been observed as far back as the twelfth rib (Fig. 5–25). They often are unilateral. In addition, lesions may affect the distal end of the tibia on one, or both, hind limbs. The tarsal joint capsule may be distended. The tuber calcis also may be involved.

Diagnosis

A horse that shows enlargements of the posterior aspect of the carpal joints, swelling of the hock joints, and bony swelling over the ribs should be suspected of having this condition. Radiographs should be taken of the joints mentioned to determine if these swellings are bone (Fig. 5-24).

Histopathological reports usually will show that there is no neoplasia present in the new bone growth. The medullary cavity of the bone will tend to follow the exostosis; the ends usually will be radiographically smooth on the surface.

Treatment

No known treatment is of value at present.

Prognosis

The prognosis is unfavorable because there is no known method of removing the exostoses. Some horses, however, may not show lameness and may be functional. The prognosis is unfavorable for a breeding animal.

SPECIFIC REFERENCES

AEGERTER, E., and J. A. KIRKPATRICK, JR. 1958. *Orthopedic Diseases.* Philadelphia: W. B. Saunders Co.

CARLSON, W. D. 1967. *Veterinary Radiology.* 2nd ed. Philadelphia: Lea & Febiger.

LUCK, J. V. 1950. *Bone and Joint Disease.* Springfield, Ill.: Charles C Thomas.

MORGAN, J. P., W. D. CARLSON, and O. R. ADAMS. 1962. Hereditary multiple exostosis in the horse. JAVMA 140: 1320.

SHUPE, J. L., *et al.* 1969. Hereditary multiple exostosis. Utah Sci. Agr. Exp. Sta. 30(40): 101–104.

REFERENCES

ADAMS, O. R. 1961. Nutritional deficiencies of foals. Amer. Quarter Horse J. 73(7): 142.

ANDREYEV, P. P. 1948. On the structure of the joints of horses. JAVMA 113: 483, (Trans. summary by R. E. Habel from the Veterinarya Feb. 25: 20, 1948.)

AXE, J. W. 1906. *The Horse in Health and Disease.* London: Gresham Publishing Co. Vol. II.

BAIN, A. M. and K. G. JOHNSTON. 1955. Bacteroid arthritis in a foal. Aust. Vet. J. 31: 210.

BORDEAUX, E. F. J. 1924. Bone disease in the horse: A clinical study. J. Comp. Path. Ther., 37: 27.

BUNN, C. E. E., and J. E. BURCH. 1955. Hydrocortisone in the treatment of traumatic arthritis in thoroughbreds. N. Amer. Vet. 36: 458.

CAMPBELL, D. M. 1934. Shifting lameness in the horse. Vet. Med. 29: 29.

CARLSON, W. D. 1967. *Veterinary Radiology.* 2nd ed. Philadelphia: Lea & Febiger.

CRAIGE, A. H., JR., and J. D. GADD. 1941. The determination and clinical correlation of variations in the calcium, inorganic phosphorus and serum proteins of horse blood. Am. J. Vet. Res. 2: 227.

CRASEMANN, E. 1945. Landwirtsch. Jahrb. Schweiz., 59: 504.

DILLON, R. 1956. Corticosteroids in the treatment of certain equine lamenesses. Vet. Med, 51: 191.

DIMOCK, W. W., and B. J. ERRINGTON. 1942. Nutritional diseases of the equine. N. Amer. Vet. 23: 152.

DODD, D. C., and D. W. RAKER. 1970. Tumoral calcinosis in the horse. JAVMA 157(7): 968–972.

EARLE, I. P. 1948. *Grassland crops as feed for horses,* p. 86–90. *In* Yearbook of Agriculture, Washington, D.C.: U.S. Department of Agriculture.

ERRINGTON, B. J. 1937. Variations in inorganic phosphorus and calcium content in blood of horses. Cornell Vet. 27: 1.

FERGUSON, A. B., JR., and J. BENDER. 1964. *The ABC's of Athletic Injuries and Conditioning.* Baltimore: Williams & Wilkins.

FRANK, E. R. 1964. *Veterinary Surgery.* Minneapolis: Burgess Publishing Co.

GARDNER, E. 1962. Structure and function of joints. JAVMA 141(10): 1234.

GREENLEE, C. W. 1939. Skeletal diseases of horses and their relation to nutrition. Cornell Vet. 29: 115.

GUILBERT, H. R., *et al.* 1940. Minimum vitamin A and carotene requirements of mammalian species. J. Nutr. 19: 91.

HAYES, I. E. 1954. Treatment of equine coxitis with intra-articular hydrocortisone. N. Amer. Vet. 35: 673.

HEINZE, C. D., and R. E. LEWIS. 1968. Bone growth in the horse determined by orthopedic markers. Proc. AAEP, 213–225.

HUTYRA, F., J. MAREK and R. MANNINGER. 1949. *Diseases of Domestic Animals.* 5th ed. Chicago: Alexander Eger. Vol. 3.

INGLE, H. 1907. The etiology and prophylaxis of equine osteoporosis. J. Comp. Path. Ther. 20: 35.

JAMIESON, R. A., and A. W. KAY. 1966. Surgical Physiology. Edinburgh and London: E. and S. Livingstone.

JENNY, J. 1962. Clinical diagnosis of osteoarthritis. JAVMA 141(10): 1253.

JOHNSON, L. E., M. A. THOM, J. B. CHASSELS, D. L. PROCTOR, and C. F. REID. 1960. *Equine radiology.* Proc. 6th Ann. AAEP.

JONES, V. B. 1946. Arthritis (a case of multiple arthritis in thoroughbreds). Vet. J. 102: 93.

JUBB, K. V. F., and P. C. KENNEDY. 1963. *Pathology of Domestic Animals.* New York: Academic Press. Vol. 1.

KATTMAN, J., and J. KRUL. 1960. Intra-articular injection of penicillin and streptomycin. Veterinarni Medicina 5: 55.

KELSER, R. A., and G. R. CALLENDER. 1938. Equine degenerative arthritis. Vet. Med. 33: 307.

KINTNER, J. H. 1940. The calcium phosphorus ratio in the ration of horses. Vet. Med. 35: 640.

KRIEGER, C. H., R. BUNKEFELDT, and H. STEENBOCK. 1940. Cereals and rickets. J. Nutr. 20: 7.

KROOK, L., and J. E. LOWE. 1964. *Nutritional Secondary Hyperparathyroidism in the Horse.* New York: S. Karger.

LA CROIX, J. V. 1916. Lameness of the horse. Veterinary Practice Series, No. 1. Amer. J. Vet. Med.

LIAUTARD, A. 1888. *Lameness of Horses.* New York: W. R. Jenkins.

MANNING, J. P. 1963. Equine hip dysplasia—osteoarthritis. Mod. Vet. Prac. 44(5): 44.

MANNING, J. P. 1962. Equine rickets. Proc. 8th Ann. AAEP, 78.

MELLANBY, E. 1949. The rickets producing and anticalcifying action of phytate (phytic acid). J. Physiol. 109: 488.

MERCK AND CO. 1973. *The Merck Veterinary Manual.* Rahway, N.J.: Merck & Co. 4th Ed.

M'FADYEAN, J., and J. F. EDWARDS. 1919. Observations with regards to the etiology of joint ill in foals. J. Comp. Path. Ther., 32: 42.

MILCH, R. A., G. J. BURKE, and I. W. FROCK. 1962. Surgical management of degenerative joint disease. JAVMA 141(10): 1276.

MILLER, W. C. 1961. Bone dystrophy. Irish Vet. J. 15(8): 156.

MILNE, F. J. 1962. Medical treatment of osteoarthritis and tenosynovitis. JAVMA 141(10): 1269.

MILNE, F. J. 1960. *Subcutaneously induced counterirritation.* Proc. 6th Ann. AAEP, 25.

MITCHELL, W. M. 1937. Rheumatic diseases in the horse (osteo-arthritis and allied conditions). J. Comp. Path. Ther. 50: 282.

National Research Council, Committee on Animal Nutrition. 1973. Nutrient Requirements of Horses. Washington, D.C.: National Academy of Sciences.

NELSON, A. W. 1961. *Nutrient Requirements for the Light Horse.* Amarillo, Texas: America Quarter Horse Association.

NICHOLAYSEN, R., *et al.* 1953. Physiology of calcium metabolism. Physiol. Rev. 33: 424.

Nutritional Review, 16: 16, 1958.

O'DONOGHUE, D. H. 1962. *Treatment of Injuries to Athletes.* Philadelphia: W. B. Saunders.

PROCTOR, D. L. 1956. *Meticorten in Equine Practice.* Abstracts of First Veterinary Symposium on Uses of Meticorten and Meticortelone. Bloomfield, N.J.: Schering Laboratories.

RAKER, C. W. 1962. Surgical treatment of osteoarthritis and tenosynovitis. JAVMA 141: 1273.

REID, R. L., M. C. FRANKLIN, and E. G. HALLSWORTH. 1947. The utilization of phytate phosphorus by sheep. Aust. Vet. J. 23:136.

RHODES, W. R. 1962. Radiographic manifestation of degenerative joint disease. JAVMA 141(10): 1256.

RILEY, W. F., JR. 1956. Corticosteroids in the treatment of certain equine lamenesses. Vet. Med. 51: 191.

ROONEY, J. R. 1963. *Equine Medicine and Surgery,* p. 414. Santa Barbara, Calif.: American Veterinary Publications Inc.

ROONEY, J. R. 1962. Joint ill. JAVMA 141(10): 1259.

ROONEY, J. R. 1969. Biomechanics of Lameness in Horses. Baltimore: Williams & Wilkins.

SCHMIDT, H. 1940. Calcium and phosphorus deficiencies in cattle and horses: Clinical picture, treatment and prevention. JAVMA 96: 441.

SHARPE AND DOHME. 1951. *Arthritis Pt. 1.* Seminar 13, No. 3 (Aug.), 3–19 *Pt. 2.* Seminar 13, No. 4 (Nov.), 3–17. Philadelphia.

SISSON, S. 1953. Anatomy of Domestic Animals. 4th ed. J. D. Crossman, ed. Philadelphia: W. B. Saunders.

SOKOLOFF, L. 1960. Comparative pathology of arthritis, p. 193–250. *In* Advances of Veterinary Science 6. C. A. Brandly and E. L. Jungher, ed. New York: Academic Press.

SOKOLOFF, L., O. MICKELSEN, E. SILVERSTEIN, G. E. JAY, JR., and R. S. YAMAMOTO. 1960. Experimental obesity in osteoarthritis. Amer. J. Physiol. 198: 765.

STECHER, R. M. 1962. Discussion of osteoarthritis. JAVMA 141(10): 1249.

SWENSON, M. J. 1962. Therapeutic nutrition of animals. JAVMA 141(11): 1353.

TEIGLAND, M. B., J. JENNY, J. D. WHEAT, and D. L. PROCTOR. 1960. *Panel on orthopedic surgery.* Proc. 6th Ann. AAEP.

TEMPLE, J. I. 1960. Fluoprednisolone in race horse practice. JAVMA 137: 136.

TRUM, B. F. 1959. Pathogenesis of osteoarthritis in the horse. Lab. Invest. 8.

VAN PELT, R. W. 1962. Anatomy and physiology of articular structures. Vet. Med. 57: 135.

VAN PELT, R. W. 1962a. Arthritides of the diarthrodial articulation. Mich. State Univ. Vet. 22(2): 71.

VAN PELT, R. W. 1962b. Therapeutic management of capped hocks. Mich. State Univ. Vet. 23(1): 28.

VIGUE, R. F. 1960. Clinical evaluation of prednisolone trimethylacetate in arthritis and general inflammatory conditions of horses. Southwestern Vet. 13: 103.

WHEAT, J. D. 1955. The use of hydrocortisone in the treatment of joint and tendon disorders in large animals. JAVMA 127: 64.

WILLIAMS, W. 1891. *The Principles and Practices of Veterinary Surgery.* New York: W. R. Jenkins.

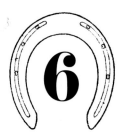

6

Lameness

LAMENESSES IN THE FORELIMB*

Atrophy of the Supraspinatus and Infraspinatus Muscles (Sweeny)

Definition

The term "sweeny" can apply to any group of atrophied muscles, regardless of location. In popular usage the term generally applies to atrophy of the supraspinatus and infraspinatus muscles caused by paralysis of the suprascapular nerve.

Etiology

Atrophy of muscles results from disuse or loss of nerve supply. In the case of injury to the suprascapular nerve, the etiology is usually trauma from a direct blow to the point of the shoulder, or from stretching of the nerve in a sudden backward thrust of the limb.

*For descriptive purposes, lamenesses have been divided into those affecting the forelimb, those affecting the hind limb, and those that are common to both fore and hind limbs. Lamenesses that occur in both fore and hind limbs, but are most common in front, appear in the discussion on lamenesses of the forelimb. Those lamenesses that can occur in both the fore and hind limbs, but are more common in the hind limbs, appear in the discussion of lamenesses of the hind limb. Where it was difficult to make a decision as to whether it was most common in the fore or hind limb, the discussion has been placed in the section dealing with lamenesses common to both fore and hind limbs.

Signs

Atrophy of the supraspinatus and infraspinatus muscles is obvious, for it causes the shoulder joint to appear more prominent (Fig. 6–1). The shoulder area appears flattened, and the spine of the scapula is prominent. Sometimes there is outward rotation of the affected shoulder during progression.

Diagnosis

Diagnosis of muscular atrophy is easy, but determining the etiology is another matter. A veterinarian should remember that atrophy may result from disuse of the limb as a result of lameness and is not necessarily due to paralysis of a nerve. The attitude of the limb during motion usually reveals whether lameness is present or whether the condition actually is due to paralysis. Muscular dystrophy can occur and must be differentiated from muscular atrophy (see p. 350).

Treatment

No known treatment is of any value for atrophy due to nerve injury. Antiphlogistic packs, ultrasound, and heat applications are probably beneficial to circulation, but they are of no value for nerve damage. Commonly, the areas are blistered or fired, but with poor results. Sometimes the atrophied area is injected with subcutaneous irritants to fill the area with scar tissue to create the appearance of a normal shoulder. This is of cosmetic value only. At the present time, I am trying a surgical approach, removing a piece of scapula 1½″ long and ½″ wide under the nerve to aid decompression of the nerve. Results are not yet known.

Prognosis

Prognosis is guarded to unfavorable. Judgment on the degree of nerve function return should not be made for at least six months, as a long period is required for regeneration of nerves.

Inflammation of the Bicipital Bursa (Bursa Intertubercularis, Bicipital Bursitis)

Definition

The bicipital bursa, which is quite extensive, is found between the biceps brachii tendon and bicipital groove of the humerus. Movement of the biceps brachii tendon over the groove in the humerus is cushioned by this bursa. The bursa, along with the biceps tendon, is sometimes affected by acute or chronic inflammation, which often is diagnosed as "shoulder lameness." The shoulder, though often blamed for the lameness, seldom is at fault. Race horse trainers often inject the skin over the shoulder with air because of a belief that it is "too tight." This is a ridiculous procedure, since the true cause of the lameness often is navicular disease.

Etiology

The most common cause of inflammation of this bursa is severe trauma at the point of the shoulder. Other structures also may be injured, and fractures involving the scapula or humerus may even be incurred. The same blow may cause sweeny as a result of damage to the suprascapular nerve. The bursa may become infected if it is opened or if an infection

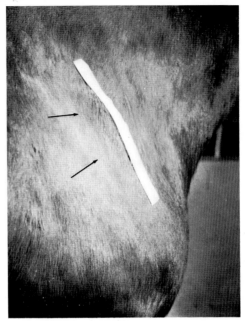

FIG. 6–1. Sweeny. Arrows indicate atrophy of the infraspinatus muscle. The tape is on the spine of the scapula.

causing a septicemia in a disease like navel ill, which results in a suppurative bursitis, localizes here. Bicipital bursitis sometimes occurs following influenza or other viral respiratory diseases.

Signs

Signs of shoulder lameness include:

1. Marked lifting of the head when the limb is being advanced. This results when the horse tries to advance the limb with a minimum of flexion of the shoulder joint.

2. Imperfect flexion of the limb causing the foot to be lifted only slightly off the ground.

3. Shortened anterior phase of the stride.

4. Stumbling due to insufficient foot clearance and to the short anterior phase of the stride, which causes the toe of the foot to land too soon.

5. Fixation of the scapulohumeral joint, evidenced by restricted movement of the

shoulder joint during progression. This is one of the more important signs of shoulder lameness.

6. Indifference to the hardness of the ground. Lameness signs will be approximately the same on hard or soft ground if it is level. Soft ground is more likely to impede movement because of the irregular surface.

7. Circumduction of the limb in an effort to overcome the difficulty of advancing it.

8. Dropped elbow if the inflammation is severe or if the radial nerve also is injured.

When the horse is in motion, he does not flex the limb properly because of the pain. In acute cases, the limb usually is carried while the horse makes a short jump on the sound limb; he usually will not make any attempt to lift the foot of the affected limb when going forward, but he may use the limb in backing. In less acute cases, observation of the horse during movement shows the fixation of the shoulder joint. When the horse is standing, the foot of the affected limb is back of normal position, and usually rests on the toe. In mild cases, signs similar to navicular disease may occur (p. 260).

Diagnosis

Diagnosis is based on the signs listed above. Swelling of the bursa at the point of the shoulder nearly always is present, but atrophy of the supraspinatus and other associated muscles should not be confused with bursitis; atrophy of these muscles causes the shoulder joint to appear to be more prominent. A fixation of the scapulohumeral joint is one of the most diagnostic signs of shoulder lameness. This is evident when the horse is in motion. Pain usually can be produced by pulling the limb upward and backward. If there is doubt about the presence of navicular disease, a diagnostic block of the posterior digital nerves can be done

to determine if it is present (p. 265). This lameness must be differentiated from fractures of the lateral tuberosity of the humerus, the deltoid process of the humerus, and the tuber scapulae and tuber spinae of the scapula.

Treatment

Injection of the bursa with corticoids, repeated at intervals of approximately one week for four to five injections, plus parenteral corticoid therapy, is one of the most effective methods of treatment for noninfectious bursitis. Counterirritation caused by blisters, injection of irritants, and firing commonly have been employed, but results have not been good. X-radiation might be helpful. The horse must be rested until signs of lameness disappear.

Prognosis

The prognosis is guarded to unfavorable. If the condition is chronic when the veterinarian is first called, the prognosis is unfavorable because permanent changes may already have occurred.

Arthritis of the Shoulder Joint (Omarthritis)

Definition

Arthritis of the shoulder joint can have multiple causes, most of which involve traumatic bone changes such as fractures. Fracture of the tuber scapulae of the scapula and fracture of the lateral tuberosity of the humerus are the most common of these. In these cases, the fractures do not involve large portions of the bone, so the stability of the joint is retained. The irritation caused by these fractures produces an arthritis that causes persistent lameness. In young horses, osteochondritis dissecans (aseptic necrosis) may cause damage that will remain as chronic osteoarthritis of the shoulder joint.

Etiology

Trauma is the etiology in most cases. Kicks, running into solid objects, and other forms of trauma are nearly always involved. The etiology of osteochondritis dissecans is not known.

Signs

The signs are highly variable. In some cases, they are severe in the early stages, becoming chronic at a later date. In general, the signs that are typical of shoulder lameness are present, i.e., holding the head to the affected side when advancing the limb, circumduction of the limb when advancing it to avoid flexion of the shoulder, and standing with the affected limb so that the foot is behind the opposite forefoot. In some cases, obvious swelling of the shoulder is present. However, in most cases it is difficult to distinguish any difference between the normal and abnormal side. During progression, the horse tends to fix the scapulohumeral joint. Careful observation of the shoulder area during movement will reveal the difference in movement in the normal and the affected shoulder.

Diagnosis

Because in many cases there is no obvious swelling of the affected side, differential nerve blocks are helpful. Blocking the median, musculocutaneous, and ulnar nerves will help to eliminate lamenesses of the lower portion of the limb. When unsoundness still exists after blocking these nerves, the shoulder and elbow joints should receive close scrutiny. Whenever possible, a radiograph should be taken of the shoulder. This requires a good x-ray machine. If the picture is taken obliquely through the shoulder joint, an adequate radiograph can be obtained. Arthritic changes visible on the radiograph are diagnostic of the condition. Injection of the scapulohumeral joint with 20 to 30 cc of Xylocaine and a corticoid are helpful in diagnosis (see Chap. 11).

Treatment

If osteoarthritis from trauma is in the joint, no treatment will be helpful. However, small chip fractures of the lateral tuberosity of the humerus can be removed successfully. Injection of the shoulder joint with a corticoid may give temporary relief.

Paralysis of the Radial Nerve

Definition

The radial nerve, often the largest branch of the brachial plexus, derives its origin chiefly from the first thoracic root of the plexus. The radial nerve innervates the extensors of the elbow, carpal, and digital joints and also supplies the lateral flexor of the carpus (ulnaris lateralis). Paralysis of the radial nerve inactivates these muscles.

Etiology

In most cases, paralysis of the radial nerve is due to trauma of the nerve as it crosses the musculospiral groove of the humerus; such trauma often accompanies fracture of the humerus. The nerve is traumatized by a fracture, and in some cases is completely severed by a bone fragment. A kick or a fall on the lateral surface of the humerus may produce enough trauma to cause paralysis of the nerve. Prolonged lateral recumbency on an operating table or on the ground may produce radial paralysis in the forelimb next to a hard surface. Whenever a horse is to be cast for a long period of time, it is wise to pad the shoulder if it is next to a hard surface. Rubber padding or a half-inflated tire inner-tube is helpful in preventing injury to the shoulder and radial nerve. Temporary paralysis of the radial nerve is sometimes seen following surgery even though the shoulder has been padded. It may or may not be accompanied by myositis of the triceps muscle. The condition is usually temporary, and the greatest danger is additional injury to the horse while the limb is not functioning.

Signs

The signs vary somewhat, depending upon the extent or degree of paralysis. When that portion of the radial nerve supplying the extensors of the digit is affected, the signs are characteristic. The horse cannot advance the limb to place weight on the foot. If the foot is placed under the horse, he can bear weight with no difficulty. In most cases the branch of the nerve to the triceps muscle also is involved, so the elbow is dropped and extended while the digits are flexed (Fig. 6–2). The muscles of the elbow are relaxed, as are the extensors of the digit, and the limb appears longer than normal. In severe paralysis, dragging of the limb may wear off the anterior surface of the fetlock joint. If the injury occurs at the point of the shoulder when the humerus fractures, the suprascapular nerve may be paralyzed, causing sweeny (p. 162).

Occasionally, radial-nerve paralysis is accompanied by paralysis of the entire brachial plexus. In this case, the limb shows paralysis of the flexor and extensor muscles and is unable to bear weight. The elbow is dropped, and the affected limb appears to be longer than the opposite limb. The humerus, radius and ulna must be carefully examined for fracture when radial paralysis is present, since many cases of radial paralysis are due to external trauma from kicks. Examination for crepitation is done by palpating the olecranon and humerus while moving the limb. These areas are also checked for abnormal motion.

Milder cases of radial-nerve paralysis may cause little lameness in a slow walk. Then, as the foot encounters an obstacle, the horse may stumble if the toe catches and the foot does not land flat. More difficulty is experienced on uneven ground.

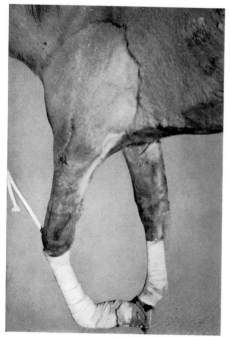

FIG. 6–2. Paralysis of the radial nerve. Note the "dropped" appearance of the elbow and the foal's inability to extend the leg and digits. This filly was later returned to a nearly normal condition by operation to free the nerve from adhesions and to correct trauma resulting from a fragment of the fractured humerus.

Treatment

Treatment in most cases is of no value, and the horse should be stalled to prevent further injury. The limb may be placed in a light plaster cast to prevent contraction of the flexors of the carpus and digits or protected with heavy bandages so that the skin will not wear off the anterior surface of the limb. Manual massage of the muscles of the limb is probably beneficial.

While waiting for recovery from the nerve paralysis, it is usually wise to place the forelimb in a light plaster cast or brace to prevent contraction of the flexor tendons. Then, if recovery does occur, contraction of the flexors is not advanced to the point that no correction can be made. This cast can be changed every two to three weeks.

Limited experience shows that in cases of humeral fracture, surgical correction may be beneficial in repairing the nerve as it crosses the fracture site. The nerve is freed from adhesions, and all prominent bone chips are removed so that the nerve is no longer traumatized. If the nerve has been completely severed, end-to-end anastamosis, if possible, is in order. In other cases, the nerve is stretched, torn, and traumatized by the bone fragments. Freeing the nerve, removing the bone fragments, and dissecting out scar tissue will produce a partial or complete recovery in some cases. This procedure should be done between eight and ten weeks following fracture of the humerus so that the nerve is given every possible opportunity to recover before surgical correction is undertaken. Unfortunately, most cases of radial-nerve paralysis accompanying fracture of the humerus are permanent, and operation is the only alternative for recovery.

Prognosis

The prognosis is guarded in mild cases and unfavorable in severe ones. Six months should be allowed for recovery after injury or corrective surgery before any final decision is made. If surgery is used in an attempt to correct the paralysis, it should be done no sooner than eight and no later than twelve weeks after injury, whenever possible.

SPECIFIC REFERENCE

ROONEY, J. R. 1963. Radial paralysis in a horse. Cornell Vet. 53:328.

Fracture of the Ulna (Olecranon)

Definition

The ulna is usually fractured in the olecranon process, but it can be fractured at a point distal to the humeroradial joint. Most cases of fractured ulna show signs similar to radial-nerve paralysis.

Etiology

Trauma is the etiology in all cases, and a direct kick by another horse over the elbow is the most common cause. Other cases result from being hit by a car or truck or from the horse hitting a solid object with the olecranon.

Signs

The signs are those of acute disability of the limb; some degree of radial-nerve paralysis is nearly always seen. The horse appears to be unable to flex the elbow joint and usually will not or cannot bear weight on the affected limb. The elbow joint appears to be "dropped." Manual manipulation of the limb will usually cause bone crepitation and pain. Those cases that have a fracture of the ulna through the articulation will show more pain than those that have fracture through the proximal end of the olecranon.

Diagnosis

Diagnosis is based on appearance of the limb, manual manipulation, and radiographic changes. Fracture of the ulna is to be differentiated from fracture of the distal end of the humerus and fracture of the proximal end of the radius, either of which may occur in conjunction with fracture of the olecranon.

Treatment

If there is no separation of the bone fragments, absolute stall rest for six weeks is usually the best treatment. A sling is helpful, providing the temperament of the horse is suitable. Surgical or mechanical interference when there is no separation of the fragments appears to be contraindicated. When the fracture fragments are separated, which is commonly the case, surgical reduction is indicated if restoration of function is desired. The great force exerted on the olecranon by the triceps muscle may bend most mechanical devices such as bone plates, pins, and bone screws. Compression plates using ASIF* equipment and the tension-band principle (Müller, 1970) with pins and wire appear to be the best method of treatment. Stall rest for six to ten weeks after surgical correction is necessary.

SPECIFIC REFERENCES

ARNJERG, J. 1969. Fracture of the ulna. Nord. Vet. Med. 21(7–8): 387–389.

JOHNSON, J. H., and H. C. BUTLER. 1971. Tension-band fixation of ulnar fracture, VM/SAC 66(6): 552–556.

MÜLLER, M. E., et al. 1970. Manual of Internal Fixation. New York: Springer-Verlag.

Rupture of the Medial Collateral Ligament of the Humeroradial Joint

Definition

Although this is not a common lameness, it does occur, especially when severe adduction is placed on a forelimb, as when a foot is caught in a rope or other restraint. The adduction can be severe enough to cause rupture of the medial ligament of the elbow joint.

Etiology

Severe abduction of the limb is the usual cause. A horse that is tethered by

a rope, either by one foot or from the neck, is the most subject to the condition. If the horse is frightened and starts to run with a forefoot caught in a rope or other restraint, the adduction stress may be sufficient to rupture the medial ligament of the joint.

Signs

Signs of lameness are rather obscure. Immediately after the rupture, the horse exhibits considerable pain in the limb, but usually the pain diminishes within twenty-four hours. Watching the affected forelimb from in front and behind during progression may reveal an outward movement of the limb from the elbow down. The sign that is pathognomonic for the condition is the "opening" of the joint on the medial side when the foot is adducted and the elbow joint is pushed in. This opening of the joint can be detected by palpation.

Treatment

Stall rest and confinement for four to six weeks are required. In some of the cases, the ligament will heal if the horse will cooperate. A sling is indicated for those horses whose temperaments are suitable.

Prognosis

Guarded to unfavorable.

Capped Elbow (see Chap. 5, p. 141)

Anterior Deviation of the Carpal Joints (Bucked Knees, Knee Sprung, Goat Knees)

Definition

Bucked knees is a deformity of the carpal joint, consisting of an anterior devia-

---

*Smith Kline Surgical Specialties, Philadelphia.

tion of the carpus, that causes an alteration in the articulations of the bones forming the joint and results in constant partial flexion of the carpus (Fig. 1–13B, p. 10).

Etiology

Several factors are involved in the etiology of bucked knees. Many horses exhibit a mild anterior deviation of both carpal joints, but this may not be serious, as it often is the result of a congenital condition. Congenital types may be the result of positioning of the limbs in the uterus or of a mineral or vitamin deficiency in the mare. The rickets syndrome of growing foals can produce the condition as a result of a calcium, phosphorus, vitamin A, or vitamin D imbalance or deficiency (Chap. 5).

Some cases of bucked knees are due to trauma, when certain lamenesses cause inactivity of the extensor group of muscles, allowing the flexors to contract. The muscles most involved are the ulnaris lateralis, flexor carpi ulnaris, and the deep and/or superficial flexor tendons. Injury to the suspensory ligament, to the deep and/or superficial flexor tendons, or to the heel of the foot, often causes a horse to rest the carpus in an anterior direction. If the pain persists, the tendons contract to such a degree that they cannot be straightened. In some cases carpal injury, such as carpitis, also may cause anterior deviation of the joint to relieve pain, which will cause contraction of the muscles and tendons. Bucked knee due to trauma is usually unilateral.

Signs

Severity of bucked knees varies considerably: in some cases the condition is very mild, while in others it is extreme. When the affected horse is in the normal standing position, one or both carpal joints will be flexed forward at varying degrees. This inhibits normal movement and gait, as there is a shortening of the anterior phase of the stride. The condition may be so pronounced that the horse falls to the carpal joints while standing or walking. The carpal joint, or joints, may be unable to support their share of weight, so damage may occur to other areas of the limb. Knuckling of the fetlock also may be present in this condition (Fig. 5–10, p. 128) as a result of digital flexor tendon contraction.

Treatment

Bucked Knees in the Foal. If the condition is not severe, meaning that the foal can put its feet flat on the ground without knuckling over to the carpus, and if nutrition has been corrected, treatment often is not necessary. Many foals straighten up remarkably well by the time they are six months old. However, if lateral or medial deviation of the carpal joints is present, in addition to bucked knees, corrective procedures may be necessary (see Knock knees, p. 171). If medial or lateral deviations are present, or if the condition is considered severe, the limbs may be put into plaster casts.

To correct bucked knees, the following method of casting should be used. The foal should be anesthetized and the limb padded with cotton or other suitable material. A light layer of 4″ plaster of paris bandage should be applied to the limb from hoof wall to elbow joint using three rolls of plaster. As the plaster dries, one or two pieces of moist yucca board or other suitable material (25″ long, $\frac{1}{8}$″ thick, $5\frac{3}{4}$″ wide) should be placed on the volar aspect of the limb, and two or three more rolls of 4″ plaster of paris bandage used to pull the carpus toward the rigid support. Considerable tension may be applied to this second layer over the yucca board if proper padding has been placed over the pressure points of the limb. The pressure points are the anterior surface of the carpal joint and two points on the volar aspect of the limb at the proximal and distal ends of the yucca board or other rigid support.

The foal should be left in the cast for approximately ten days to two weeks. In many cases it will not be necessary to reapply the cast, but if a new cast is necessary, it should not be applied until ten to fourteen days after the first cast is removed. This interval will allow the foal to partially overcome the effects of disuse atrophy in the musculature. A second cast should be applied in the same manner as the first and removed after ten to fourteen days. (Correction of medial deviation of the carpal joints is discussed on p. 171.)

A complete check of the horse's diet should be made, and the diet fortified, if necessary, with those elements considered deficient. Foals that develop bucked knees after birth should be considered rickets suspects and treated accordingly.

Bucked Knees Due to Injury. When a bucked-knee condition is due to injury to the carpus or other structures, it is necessary to direct treatment at correction of the original pathological changes. The bucked-knee condition will usually then take care of itself. Pathological changes in the flexor tendons, suspensory ligament, foot, or carpus are most often responsible for this type of bucked knee. If the condition is not of long duration and is corrected promptly, the tendons will gradually stretch, and the carpus will again assume a normal position.

Surgical Correction. When bucked knees are so severe in a foal that the condition cannot be properly corrected with plaster casts, or when the condition persists in a mature horse after injury to some structure, so that there is little hope of natural correction, a tenotomy of the ulnaris lateralis and the flexor carpi ulnaris tendons should be undertaken. This operation is most successful for bucked knees that result from trauma and is less successful for those that are congenital, as

the carpal bones are often deformed in congenital bucked knees, whereas in an acquired condition, the carpal bones are relatively normal. In addition, congenital bucked knees show contraction of the deep and superficial flexor tendons and the suspensory ligament, as well as the ulnaris lateralis and flexor carpi ulnaris tendons.

Surgical correction can be performed with the horse in standing position if he is tractable, but the horse should be anesthetized, thrown, and tied if unmanageable. Tranquilization with promazine,* $\frac{1}{2}$ mg per pound of body weight, intravenously, or some other suitable tranquilizer, may be necessary if the operation is to be done while the horse is standing. The operative area is 1″ to 1$\frac{1}{2}$″ above the accessory carpal bone on the volar aspect of the limb.

The area should be clipped, shaved, and prepared for aseptic operation. Anesthesia should be accomplished by injecting a local anesthetic, such as lidocaine hydrochloride.† If the horse is placed in recumbency, the tendons should be tensed by extending the carpus. The depression between the two tendons is located on the volar surface of the limb about 1″ above the accessory carpal bone. An incision 2″ long is made through the skin and subcutaneous tissue, and a blunt-pointed bistoury inserted through the wound at the side of the tendon of the ulnaris lateralis muscle. The tendon then should be severed by cutting outward with the bistoury until the knife edge can be felt beneath the skin. The length of the incision allows careful identification of the structure to be severed. The limb should be extended during the cutting procedure. The bistoury then should be turned and the tendon of the flexor carpi ulnaris severed. Care must be exercised not to cut too

*Sparine, Wyeth Laboratories; or Promazine, Fort Dodge Laboratories.
†Xylocaine, Astra Laboratories.

deeply, or structures underlying the muscles may be injured. Sutures are then placed in the incision and the area kept bandaged for at least ten days. The patient should not be worked for six to eight weeks. If the limb cannot be fully straightened following tenotomy, it is beneficial to place the limb in a cast from elbow to fetlock joint. This cast should be left in place ten to fourteen days.

Prognosis

The prognosis is guarded in all acquired cases of bucked knees, and it is to be expected that some horses will never be returned to full use. However, most such conditions can be improved so that the horse can serve as a useful brood animal. The prognosis is favorable in mild, congenital types if the nutrition of the foal has been good or is corrected. Severe congenital types result in an unfavorable prognosis.

Medial Deviation of the Carpal Joints in Foals (Knock Knees)

Definition

Knock knees in foals are usually a congenital condition (Figs. 6–3 and 6–4). The foal may be born with varying degrees of medial deviation of one or both carpal joints, and as he grows older the condition either improves or becomes so severe that permanent deformity results. Some foals born with reasonably straight limbs develop this deviation as they grow older. A condition similar to knock knees occurs in the hock joints of rear limbs. This will not be discussed as a separate condition because the etiology and treatment are similar to those for deviation of the carpal joints. Some cases of carpal or tarsal deviations may be due to an inheritable factor.

It is most important to correct a deviation in time to prevent damage to the small bones of the carpus or tarsus. It is also important to straighten the distal radial epiphyseal line and the distal tibial epiphyseal line.

Etiology

If the foal is born with medial deviation of the carpal joints, the condition may be inheritable or due to nutritional deficiency or it may be the result of intrauterine positioning. In cases that develop after birth, it is believed that nutrition, in the form of rickets, plays a role (Chap. 5). The importance of nutrition in those cases present at birth is not fully understood. All cases at birth should be closely checked for nutrition, and, if necessary, blood samples of several horses of the herd analyzed to determine if any deficiencies in calcium, phosphorus, vitamin A, carotene, or vitamin D are present.

Signs

The signs are obvious, but determination of the etiology can cause difficulty (Fig. 1–16B, p. 12, and Figs. 6–3 and 6–10). A blood analysis, as mentioned above, should be used if poor nutrition is suspected as a cause. Some mares repeatedly have foals of this type when bred to the same stallion. In this case, an inheritable characteristic should be suspected. Aseptic necrosis may also be present, requiring immediate casting of the carpus to prevent collapse of the affected bones.

Treatment

In most cases plaster casts are the most economical treatment for deviation of the carpal or hock joints (Fig. 6–5). Treatment should begin at an early age, preferably at about three weeks, or sooner if the deviation is severe or if aseptic necrosis is present. The sooner a correc-

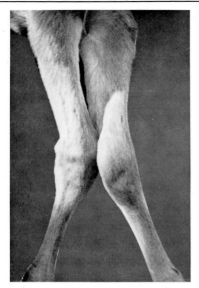

FIG. 6–3. Knock knees in a foal.

Orthoplast* may also be used for this purpose. The moist wood may be molded to conform to the shape of the limb. Strips of 2″ tape are used to hold these in position, and then an additional two rolls of blue label, Johnson & Johnson 4″ plaster of paris bandages should be placed on the limb, pinning the carpus as tightly as possible to the rigid support. Pressure should be especially heavy over the medial aspect of the carpus to straighten the limb. With larger foals, four rolls of 4″ plaster bandage may be necessary.

*Johnson & Johnson.

tive procedure is used, the sooner the deformity is corrected. The foal should be anesthetized, and the area to be in the cast covered with 2″ stockinette. The limb should be padded by placing cotton between the fetlock and coronary band and by covering the limb with combine pads of $\frac{1}{2}$″ thick cotton gauze. The combine pads should be covered with 3″ gauze, and a small amount of tape used to hold the padding in place. This type of padding should be used from coronary band to elbow joint. The pressure points should be given additional padding. These are the outside of the limb below the elbow joint, the outside of the coronary band, and the inside of the carpal joint. Following padding of these points with orthopedic felt, the limb should be wrapped with three rolls of blue label, Johnson & Johnson 4″ plaster of paris bandage. Just as the plaster starts to dry, two pieces of moistened yucca board or other suitable material such as bass wood or aspen wood* (25″ long, $\frac{1}{8}$″ thick, $5\frac{3}{4}$″ wide) should be placed over the outside of the limb.

*Berbert Surgical Supply, Denver, Colo.

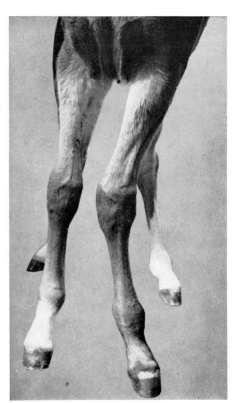

FIG. 6–4. An example of limb deviation due to uterine positioning. The right forelimb has slight lateral deviation of the carpus, and the left forelimb has severe medial deviation of the carpus. Both limbs are bowed toward the same direction. These would require opposite pressures in casts used to straighten the limbs.

The first two rolls of plaster of paris, plus the padding, greatly aid in preventing any complications of the plaster cast. The foot can be bandaged if the hoof wall is incorporated in the cast. The cast can end above the fetlock if there is no deviation in the fetlock. The foal and dam should be placed in a box stall so the foal gets little, if any, exercise. After ten to fourteen days, the cast should be removed and the foal left in the stall for another ten to fourteen days. At the time of removal of the cast, it will be noted that there has been considerable atrophy of the muscles of the forearm and that the flexor tendons have been weakened. These conditions will correct themselves. After ten to fourteen days, a new cast should be applied in the same fashion as the original, if it is deemed necessary. If the foal shows marked straightening of the limb, a second cast is not necessary because the limb will tend to continue to grow straight. In some cases the condition is bilateral, so casts should be placed on both limbs at the same time.

If the foal shows pain when using the limb, or limbs, while the cast is in place, the cast should be removed immediately. This may signify pressure necrosis. The first signs that the cast is causing trouble are disuse of the limb and an increase of temperature. Decreased use of the limb should be heeded immediately. Plaster casts provide a good method of correction, providing one is experienced in application of casts, and if the foal is left under experienced observation. Plaster casts can be disastrous if the foal is not confined to a box stall and if an experienced observer is not in charge of after-care.

Most affected foals can be almost perfectly straightened by the use of one or more casts. However, in some cases the epiphyseal growth centers are damaged so the bone grows more rapidly on the medial side, and permanent deformity re-

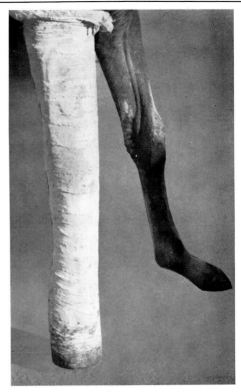

FIG. 6–5. Cast on forelimb of a foal suffering from medial deviation of the carpus. This cast was applied as described. Both forelegs may be cast at the same time, if necessary.

sults. This is especially true if the condition is unilateral. Epiphyseal staples are of value in this case. Epiphyseal staples are also of more value than casts when the foal has passed two months of age.

If the carpal joints have a lateral deviation (bowed knees), the casts should be applied in the same fashion, but the rigid support should be placed on the inside of the leg. The pressure points, under the top and bottom of the wood and over the outside of the carpal joint, should receive extra padding. The same type of therapy should be used when the hocks show a medial deviation. The cast should be applied in the same way, with the rigid support on the outside. However, a foal has difficulty moving if both hocks are cast at the same time.

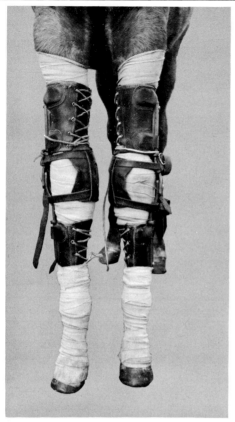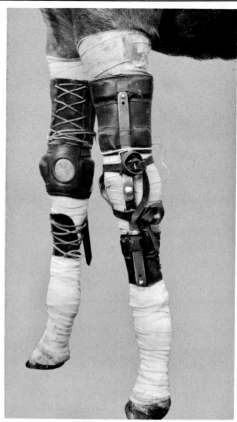

FIG. 6–6. Front and side views of hinged braces used to straighten mild medial deviation of the carpi. These braces can be reversed for lateral deviation. They must be adjusted daily to avoid pressure necrosis. Because the brace is hinged, there is very little muscle atrophy.

When the casts are removed, the flexor tendons will have weakened, and the fetlock will drop farther than normal. Until the flexor tendons have strengthened so that the fetlocks are raised to a normal position, the foal should be confined to a box stall. After the fetlock assumes a normal position, normal exercise can begin. Ordinarily, confinement should continue for ten' to fourteen days following cast removal.

Braces with hinge joints have been developed for knock knees and are successful if anterior rotation of the brace can be prevented (Fig. 6–6). Braces require daily attention and resetting. The advantage of braces is that muscular atrophy will not be as great (Fig. 6–6).

X-irradiation has been used on the distal radial epiphysis for correction of forelimb angulation in foals, but the disadvantages appear to outweigh the advantages (O'Brien and Meagher, 1971).

After the foal is approximately two months of age, epiphyseal stapling to limit growth of one side of the epiphysis is more effective than casts for straightening the limbs. Staples may be placed any time after two weeks of age, and if the deformity is severe, the limb can be placed in a brace or a cast while waiting for the surgical procedure. One must keep in mind that the staples must have several months in which to exert their effect. The various epiphyseal areas close at different times, making it mandatory that some areas be stapled sooner than others (e.g., the distal epiphysis of the third metacarpal or metatarsal bone closes between nine and twelve months). This means that any stapling of the fetlock joint must be done at least by four months of age and preferably sooner. In the case of the carpus and tibia, these epiphyses close at approximately 24 months of age. There is considerable variation, but 24 months is the standard age limit used. This means that whenever possible, the staples should be put in at least by 15 months of age, and preferably much sooner.

The fundamental of stapling an epiphysis is that the staples be put on the convex side of the curvature, thereby limiting growth on that side. This allows the concave side to grow and eventually straighten the bone. The concave side of the epiphysis carries more weight load as a result of the deformity; thus the growth rate on this side is slower than normal. Compression of an epiphysis limits growth, while reduction of weight load allows it to grow faster.

The stapling technique is relatively simple. The following description can be used for medial or lateral deviation of either the tarsus or carpus. In general, stapling the carpus is more successful than stapling the tarsus. The foal is anesthetized by a standard method. The convex side of the distal end of the tibia or distal end of the radius is clipped and shaved and prepared for aseptic surgery. A skin incision is made longitudinally over the convex surface of the bone. The epiphyseal line is located with a small needle prior to placement of the staple. In some cases, the epiphyseal line is quite wide; its limits can be determined with a needle so that the staple can be properly centered (Fig. 6–7). Heinze (1969) recommends removal of soft tissue longitudinally under the staple. An alternative is a single incision to the bone, which allows the staple to set firmly against the bone.

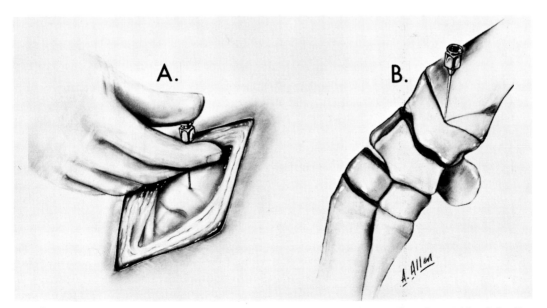

FIG. 6–7. Locating distal epiphyseal line of the radius by use of a needle. The width of the line can be delineated and the staple centered in this way. A, Through incision. B, Skeletal model. (From Heinze, 1969; courtesy of Dr. C. D. Heinze and American Association of Equine Practitioners.)

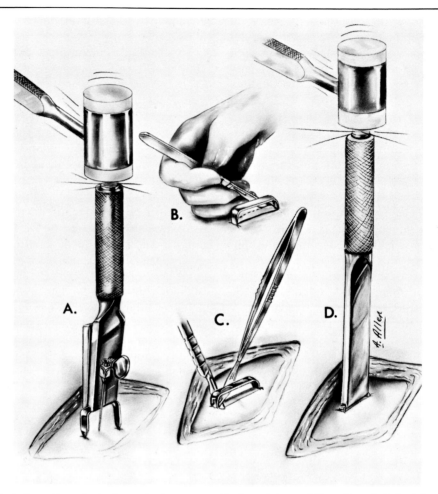

FIG. 6–8. *A*, Insertion of staple centering on needle in epiphyseal line. *B* and *C*, Incision of soft tissue under staple; if desired, the soft tissue can be removed as in *C*. *D*, Setting staple firmly next to bone. (From Heinze, 1969; courtesy of Dr. C. D. Heinze and American Association of Equine Practitioners.)

The staple should not be buried beneath the periosteum (Figs. 6–8 and 6–13, 14). Postsurgical radiographs are recommended, along with a sketch of the area showing the location of the staple(s) in relation to the skin incision to aid removal of the staples. In some cases staple removal is complicated by bone growth overlying the staple. This makes accurate knowledge of the placement of the staple very important. The staples are placed so that one leg of the staple is below the epiphyseal line and one above it (Fig. 6–13). One to three staples of cast vital-lium are placed in the distal radial epiphyseal line. The number and size depend on the size of the animal. Weanlings require at least two large staples in the distal radial epiphysis in most cases. Young foals may require only one staple if the deviation is not severe. Vitallium staples* with reinforced corners are far stronger than those made from Steinmann pins. The legs on the staples are approximately 1″ long, and the body of the staple is approximately 1″ long. They are driven into

---

*Howmedica, Inc., Medical Division.

the bone with a bone hammer. Special apparatus for holding the staples while driving them is available (Fig. 6–12). Ready-made staples are available and are preferred. The staples must be driven in firmly or they will loosen and come out. The subcutaneous tissue is closed over the pins with a 00 catgut suture. The skin is then closed with a noncapillary-type suture with simple interrupted pattern. A pressure bandage is kept in place over the incisions for approximately two weeks. Exercise should be limited for 60 days.

When stapling the tibia, the distal leg of the staple, which is inserted into the epiphysis, must be shortened or it will penetrate the tibiotarsal articulation. Stapling of the distal tibia requires very accurate placement of the staple because of the small area in which there is to place it. The epiphyseal line can be located with a needle, as in the distal radius (Fig. 6–7). One can check the preoperative radiographs with a staple to make sure that the staple will fit the bone. It is a good procedure to take postoperative radiographs, before incision closure, to make sure that the staple has been placed properly.

The foal should always be confined in a stall regardless of the method of angular correction. Confinement of about four weeks is usually necessary to prevent stress on the epiphyses.

When the carpus is deviated laterally, the same procedure is followed for surgery, except the surgery is done on the lateral aspect of the distal radial epiphysis.

One of the complications of epiphyseal stapling is the production of a large amount of fibrous tissue over the staples. Staple movement is probably the greatest single factor in development of fibrous tissue. Placing the staple firmly against the bone and bandaging properly will usually prevent this complication.

Removal of the staples often proves to be more difficult than placing them in the bone. They are difficult to find because

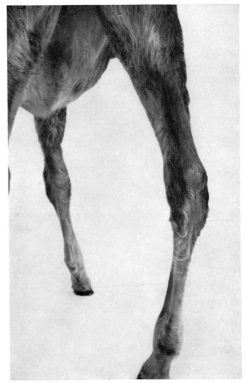

FIG. 6–9. An example of looseness of the lateral-collateral ligament of the tarsal joint. In this case the limb bows outward when weight is placed on it. At other times it can be pushed to a normal position by hand. This should not be confused with deviation of the limbs from nutritional causes. This type of condition is treated by placing the limb in a cast for approximately four weeks.

fibrous tissue covers them completely. One should have a special staple remover, or a screwdriver, to drive under the staples for removal. The staples are removed under the same type of anesthetic used to put them in place. The skin, subcutaneous tissue, and fibrous tissue over the staples are incised, and the staples located. Some fibrous tissue has to be removed before the staples can be found. A screwdriver-type blade is driven under the ends of the staple and they are lifted out with pliers. Once the staple is located they are usually quite easy to remove. Subcutaneous tissue is closed with 00 catgut, and the

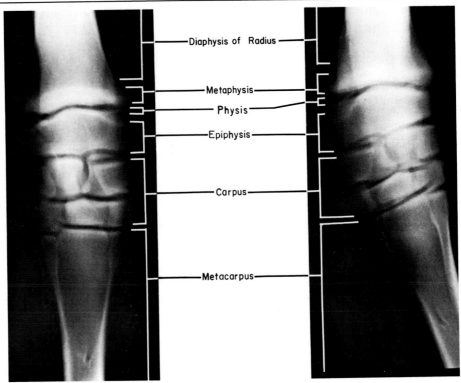

FIG. 6-10. Radiographs of a three-month-old colt. *Left*, right foreleg showing sclerosis and irregularity of the physis, although the limb is straight. *Right*, lateral deviation of the left foreleg, with sclerosis and irregularity of the physis. Anteroposterior views, radii parallel. The lesions may involve the epiphysis, epiphyseal plate, or metaphysis. Most often all three areas show evidence of altered growth. (From Heinze, 1969; courtesy of Dr. C. D. Heinze and American Association of Equine Practitioners.)

skin with a nonabsorbable skin suture. A pressure bandage should be kept in place for at least three weeks to aid in preventing excessive fibrous tissue formation.

The staples are not removed until the limb is completely straight. In a growing epiphysis, staples left too long can overcompensate and cause a deviation opposite to the one corrected. It is important to remove staples before overcorrection occurs. As soon as the limb is straight, the staples should be removed.

Corrective hoof trimming is indicated for all limb deviations. An attempt is made to keep the hoof wall level. When the carpal joints are bowed inward, excessive wear usually occurs on the inside wall, and when they are bowed outward, excessive wear is usually seen on the outside wall. In all cases check to see which wall the foal is landing on and trim the opposite wall. In deviation of the fetlock joints where the foot is deviated medially, excessive wear usually occurs on the outside wall. Corrective trimming must be done every two weeks to prevent the foot from wearing off-level.

Prognosis

The prognosis is guarded in all cases, but improvement can be expected. However, one must be exceedingly cautious in application of the cast to be sure that all areas are sufficiently padded to prevent complications.

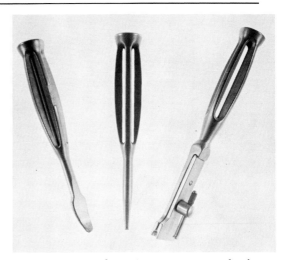

FIG. 6–12. Stapling instruments made by Howmedica Inc., Medical Division, Rutherford, N.J. *Left,* staple remover. *Center,* instrument for final imbedding of staple. *Right,* staple starter.

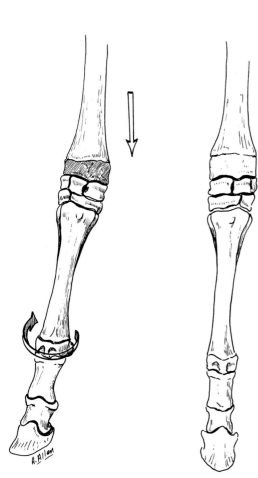

FIG. 6–11. Rotational effect that may accompany epiphysitis. (From Heinze, 1969; courtesy of Dr. C. D. Heinze and American Association of Equine Practitioners.)

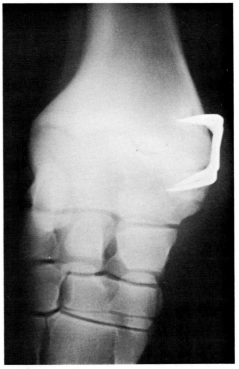

FIG. 6–13. Radiograph of epiphysitis case with two vitallium staples in the medial aspect of the distal radius. (Courtesy of Dr. J. Lebel.)

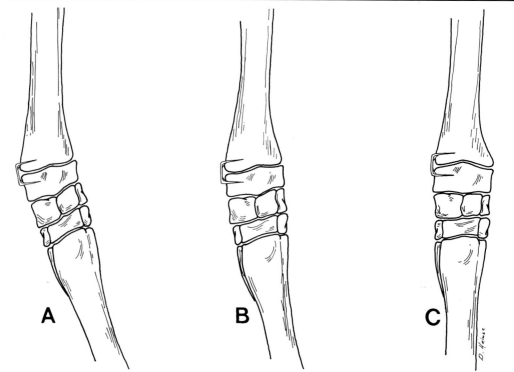

FIG. 6–14. Schematic drawing showing placement and effect of the staples in medial deviation of the carpal joints. (Courtesy of Dr. C. D. Heinze and American Association of Equine Practitioners.)

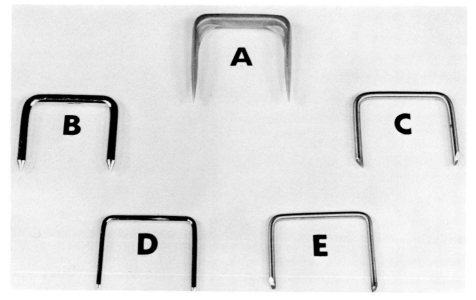

FIG. 6–15. Example of Steinmann pin (B, C, D, E) staples and ready-made human epiphyseal staple (A). The ready-made vitallium staple (A) is preferred. (From Heinze, 1969; courtesy of Dr. C. D. Heinze and American Association of Equine Practitioners.)

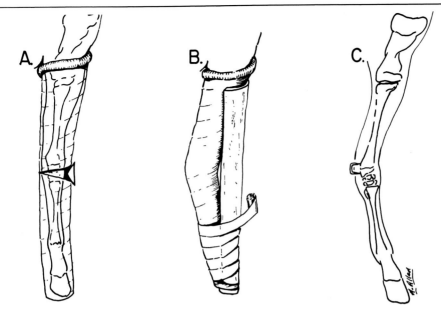

FIG. 6–16. Examples of various ways of correcting deviation of the forelimb. *A,* Wedging the dry cast. *B,* Yucca board applied over green cast. *C,* Stapling. (Courtesy of Dr. C. D. Heinze and American Association of Equine Practitioners.)

SPECIFIC REFERENCES

GUFFY, M. M., and J. R. COFFMAN. 1969. The variability of angular deformity in foals. Proc. AAEP., 47–57.

HEINZE, C. D. 1963. Proc. 9th Ann. AAEP, 203.

HEINZE, C. D. 1965. Proc. 11th Ann. AAEP.

HEINZE, C. D. 1966. General principles and surgical technique, p. 64–84. *In* Mod. Vet. Pract. Red Book.

HEINZE, C. D. 1966. Epiphyseal stapling in the horse. Mod. Vet. Pract. 47(10): 40–44.

HEINZE, C. D. 1969. Epiphyseal stapling—A surgical technique for correcting angular limb deformities. Proc. AAEP, 59–73.

HEINZE, C. D. 1971. Physeal stapling in the horse. Norden News, 24–30 (Summer).

MAY, V. R., and E. L. CLEMENTS. 1965. Epiphyseal stapling; with special reference to complications. Southern Med. J. 58: 1203.

O'BRIEN, T. R., and D. M. MEAGHER. 1971. X-irradiation of the distal radial epiphysis for the correction of forelimb angulation in the foal. Proc. 17th Ann. AAEP, 253–269.

Hygroma of the Carpus
(see Chap. 5, p. 143)

Definition

A hygroma is a synovial swelling over the anterior surface of the carpal joint. Most commonly, it is an acquired bursitis resulting from trauma. Normally there is no subcutaneous bursa in this area, but through trauma a bursa may form. The tendon sheath of the extensor carpi radialis or the common digital extensor, may also be involved. A synovial hernia of the radiocarpal or intercarpal joint capsule can occur. This causes a hygroma-like swelling that is almost indistinguishable from those caused by an acquired bursitis. However, careful examination will reveal that the swelling on the anterior surface of the carpus is irregular in outline and does not uniformly cover the carpus when a synovial hernia has occurred. Acquired bursitis shows an evenly distributed swelling over the anterior surface of the carpus.

Etiology

Trauma is the etiology in all cases. Horses that get up and down on hard ground most commonly are involved. Hygroma also can be produced as a result of a horse pawing and hitting the carpus on a hard surface such as a wall.

Signs

Signs are swellings of varying shapes over the anterior surface of the carpus. The swellings vary with the structure or structures involved (Fig. 6–17).

Treatment

Injection of corticoids, followed by counterpressure with elastic bandage, appears to be the most effective method of treatment. Injections should be repeated three to five times at intervals of a week (p. 447). Continued pressure of the elastic bandage is used to promote adhesions between the distended skin and underlying tissues. The distended skin will thicken, producing a permanent blemish. A second treatment is to open and drain the hy-

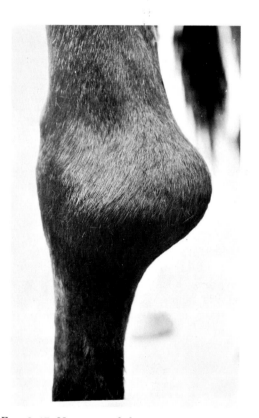

FIG. 6–17. Hygroma of the carpus. The distribution of the swelling indicates a primary involvement of the intercarpal joint capsule.

groma and swab the cavity daily with tincture of iodine. This causes a long continued drainage of the lesion. You must be absolutely certain that the carpal joint capsule is not opened, because it can enlarge in conjunction with a hygroma. Opening of the joint capsule can be disastrous. Injections of the bursal sac with Lugol's iodine also have been used, as have blistering and firing of the area, but these methods are less helpful. If the lesion responds to corticoid therapy, the healing time can be shortened.

A hygroma of long standing with a thickened synovial lining can be surgically removed under general anesthesia. The hygroma is carefully dissected out after preparing the area for aseptic surgery. An elliptical incision is made over the front of the swelling, and the mass is dissected out by using curved Mayo scissors to separate the tissues. In most cases the bursa can be dissected completely free without puncture. However, if the bursa is punctured, it can be dissected out by staying outside the thickened wall. If the joint capsule is involved, e.g., in a synovial hernia resembling a hygroma, the opening to it is closed with catgut. This opening is usually very small. Subcutaneous tissue is closed with 00 catgut, and the skin is sutured with a noncapillary suture using simple interrupted or vertical mattress suture pattern. The operative area is kept under pressure bandage for thirty days following surgery, and activity is limited to a box stall during this period.

Prognosis

Prognosis is guarded to favorable. Old cases will retain considerable swelling because of fibrous tissue that has been laid down in the inflamed area. Such cases usually are of unfavorable prognosis because adhesions may not form following corticoid therapy, and the lesion may require surgical drainage or removal.

Traumatic Arthritis of the Carpus (Popped Knee, Carpitis)

Definition

Carpitis is an acute or chronic inflammation of the carpal joint, often involving joint capsule, the associated ligaments of the carpus, and the bones of the carpus. In early stages, carpitis consists of a serous arthritis due to trauma. Later, the joint may become severely involved with osteoarthritis if the condition is not treated properly, if the original injury is severe, or if the joint is subjected to repeated trauma. New bone growth may occur on nonarticular surfaces from injury to ligamentous or joint capsule insertions.

Etiology

Concussion and trauma are primary causes of carpitis. The condition is especially common in race horses, as a result of hard training. Horses that are not in condition or are worked too hard are prone to develop carpitis. Also, poor conformation of the carpus may be an important factor in development of the condition. Bad conformation, such as calf knees or bench knees, shows poor bone alignment on radiographic examination, and poor bone alignment is probably a predisposing cause of the condition (Chap. 1). Infrequently, new bone growth occurs in these same areas after direct trauma to the anterior surface of the carpal joint as a result of the horse pawing and hitting a wall with the carpus.

Signs

Pathological changes occur predominantly on the anterior surface of the bones forming the carpus: the distal end of the radius, the proximal row of carpal bones, the distal row of carpal bones, and upon occasion, the proximal end of the third

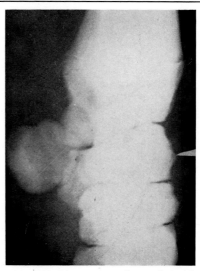

FIG. 6-18. Carpitis as viewed on a lateral radiograph of the carpal joint. The pointer indicates a healed area of new bone growth on the anterior surface of the intermediate carpal bone.

metacarpal bone. The radial and intermediate carpal bones in the proximal row and the third carpal bone in the distal row are the bones most commonly involved (Figs. 6-18, 19 and 6-20). The damage is usually in the form of new bone growth in these areas. If the injury is severe in the beginning or if the joint is injured repeatedly, new bone growth will result (Fig. 5-14, p. 140, and Fig. 6-19). In most cases, new bone growth is the result of periostitis, probably due to a pulling of the attachments of the joint capsule through the periosteum on the involved carpal bones. In some cases, it is possible that a pulling of the intercarpal ligaments between the carpal bones aids in production of new bone growth by disturbing the periosteum and causing a periostitis.

The degree of damage to articular cartilage is difficult to determine. One can assume that some changes occur in early traumatic arthritis, but these changes may be completely reversed if injury is not repeated. If osteoarthritis is present, irreversible changes in the cartilage are usually present.

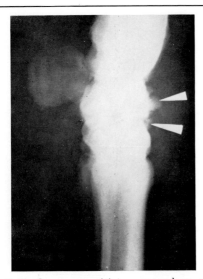

FIG. 6–19. Severe carpitis as viewed on a lateral radiograph of the carpus. Pointers indicate extensive new bone growth involving the radial, intermediate, and third carpal bones.

Osteoarthritis is present in those cases that show bone changes involving the articular surfaces (Fig. 5–14, p. 140, and Fig. 6–19). Mild cases that show no bone change are affected with a serous arthritis of the carpal joint.

In acute carpitis, lameness is very evident as a supporting- and swinging-leg lameness. A shortening of the anterior phase of the stride, due to decreased flexion of the carpus, is evident, and there is a tendency for the horse to hold the carpus slightly flexed in the standing position. Swelling is present, resulting from a distention of the joint capsule; associated periarticular structures also may be enlarged (Fig. 6–21).

In a chronic case, lameness may not be evident until the horse is used at a fast gait. Examination will reveal an enlargement on the anterior surface of the intermediate, radial, and third carpal bones and a fibrous inflammatory tissue over the area of the injury. It is sometimes difficult to tell if the fibrous tissue is bony enlargement or soft-tissue swelling unless a radiographic examination is made. Soft-tissue

crepitation will be evident under thumb pressure on the anterior surface of the carpal joint. Chronic cases may have well-developed exostosis present, the extent of which can be determined by radiographic examination.

Diagnosis

Carpitis, as such, usually is not difficult to diagnose on the basis of the symptoms described above. However, it is always important to bear in mind the possibility of a fracture of one of the carpal bones or other pathological changes (Fig. 6–22). The radial and third carpal bones are

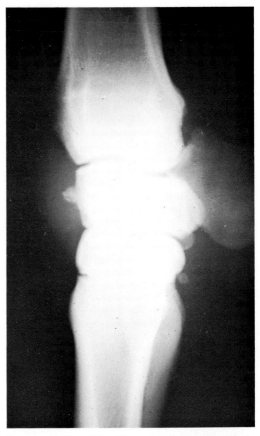

FIG. 6–20. Carpitis. The new bone growth is the result of injury to the attachment of the fibrous joint capsule. Surgical removal is not indicated, since no joint surface is involved.

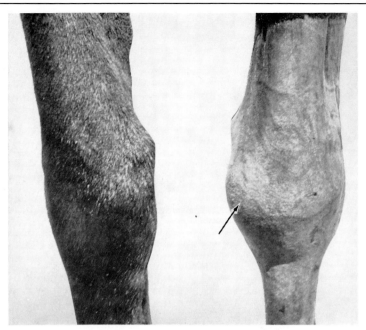

FIG. 6–21. The arrow indicates swelling commonly observed with carpitis. Without radiographs, this condition is difficult to distinguish from the swelling observed to result from fracture of the radial and third carpal bones.

most commonly fractured. Such a fracture can best be determined by taking radiographs of the lateral view, anterior-posterior view, oblique views, and lateral flexed joint view of the carpus. It is important that the carpus be flexed during palpation for diagnosis. Flexing the carpus aids in determining the exact location of the pathological changes (Fig. 4–4, p. 100).

Treatment

Cases for treatment should be selected on the basis of radiographic examination. If new bone growth is present on the articular surfaces of the radiocarpal joint, the intercarpal joint, or the carpometacarpal joint, treatment often is not successful. The owner should be advised of this fact and treatment undertaken only with proper understanding of the unfavorable prognosis.

If carpitis is in the acute stage, in the form of a serous arthritis, corticoids can be injected into the carpal joint (Chap. 11,

p. 453). Three injections of corticoids approximately one week apart are the most satisfactory. The carpus should then be bandaged and the horse rested for a minimum of four months. If new bone growth is present, corticoids will give temporary relief, but symptoms will recur as soon as the horse is put back in training, unless the proper healing time is allowed. The greatest difficulty in treating this condition with corticoids is that the relief afforded by the injections allows the owner to use the horse too soon; thus, reinjury occurs and more new bone growth can be expected. Bandaging the carpus for counterpressure and partial immobilization, following injection of corticoids, is also beneficial. The bandaging should be continued for approximately two weeks.

Blistering is common for this condition, but in general is not satisfactory treatment. If a person wishes to apply a counterirritant, it should be in the form of firing or radiation therapy. Carpitis is one

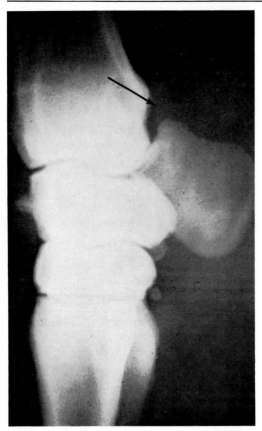

Fig. 6–22. Radiograph of a carpus showing carpitis with periosteal new bone growth on the radial carpal bone and rupture of the proximal ligament of the accessory carpal bone (arrow). Normally, the proximal portion of the accessory carpal bone lies close to the radius. Note how the accessory carpal bone is tilted downward. The prognosis would be unfavorable. Note the presence of the first carpal bone on the radiograph.

condition in which point firing appears to be beneficial. If the joint shows signs of new bone growth that is not encroaching on the articular surfaces, firing can be done after acute inflammation has disappeared. A leg paint should be applied for twenty-one days following the firing, and the horse should be rested approximately six months before being put back into training. Many horses treated in this fashion can be returned to racing.

Radiation therapy has proved satis-

factory in some cases of carpitis. Both x-radiation (approximately 1,000 roentgens) and cobalt-60 therapy, with gamma rays (750 to 1,000 roentgens), have been used. These are also methods of applying counterirritation (see Chap. 11, p. 445).

In summary, one might say that if carpitis is acute and in the form of a serous traumatic arthritis, intra-articular corticoid injections followed by prolonged rest are indicated. If new bone growth is present but is not encroaching on the articular surfaces, firing or radiation therapy is indicated and will aid recovery in most instances. In those severe cases where new bone growth is encroaching on the articular surfaces of the bones, firing or radiation therapy may be used, but with an unfavorable prognosis.

Most cases that show new bone growth encroaching on the articular surfaces can be made sound only by surgical removal of the bony growths. The surgical approach is very similar to that for fracture of the carpal bones. The new bone proliferations are removed by means of rongeurs and the surfaces curetted smooth. A cast is used for approximately eight days following surgery and then a pressure wrap for at least thirty days. The horse is confined to a box stall for thirty to forty-five days and no training begun for at least six months. Although the prognosis is less favorable than in chip fractures, this type of therapy sometimes yields a sound horse that could be cured in no other way.

Prognosis

The prognosis is guarded to favorable in early stages, if conformation is good. If new bone growth is present but is not encroaching on the articular surfaces, prognosis is guarded. If new bone growth is present and is encroaching on the articular surface, the prognosis is unfavorable. When poor conformation is a factor, the prognosis is always unfavorable, regardless of type, because of the likelihood of recurrence.

Fracture of the Carpal Bones

Definition

The radial and third carpal bones are the bones most commonly fractured in the carpal joint (Fig. 6-23). The intermediate carpal bone is fractured more rarely. The radial and intermediate carpal bones usually fracture with small chips from the proximal or distal portions of the bone on the anterior surface. The third carpal bone may fracture with a small chip or with a large slab fracture (Figs. 6-24 and 6-29). Chip fractures from the radius and

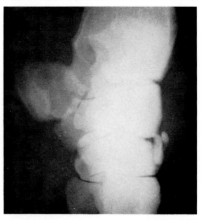

FIG. 6-24. Fracture of the third carpal bone. Note that two pieces of the third carpal bone have broken off. The large piece is a typical "slab" fracture.

from the third metacarpal bone can occur (Figs. 6-26 and 6-27). Fractures can occur from more than one carpal bone and can include any combination of those listed above.

Etiology

Trauma is the etiology of fracture of the carpal bones. From the appearance of the fractures it would seem that over-

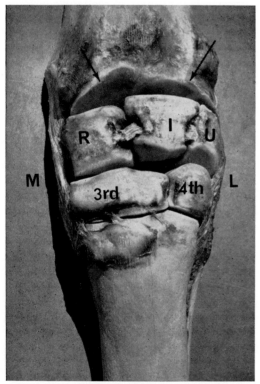

FIG. 6-23. Normal left bony carpus. *U,* Ulnar carpal bone. *I,* Intermediate carpal bone. *R,* Radial carpal bone. *3rd,* Third carpal bone. *4th,* Fourth carpal bone. Arrows indicate areas where chip fractures may occur on radius. *L,* Lateral side. *M,* Medial side.

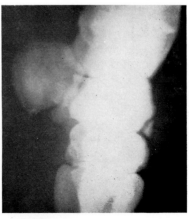

FIG. 6-25. Fracture of the radial carpal bone, viewed on lateral radiograph of the carpus. In this case, oblique views were necessary to determine whether the intermediate or the radial carpal bone was fractured.

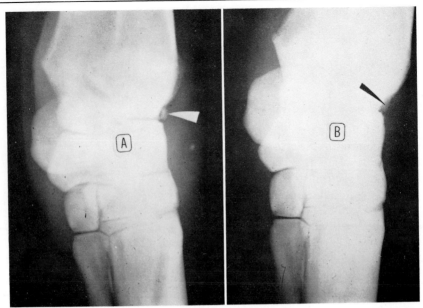

FIG. 6–26. Chip fracture of the radius. *A*, Pointer indicates chip fracture of the radius near the center of the anterior edge of the articular surface of the bone, as viewed on a lateral radiograph. *B*, Pointer indicates same area after chip fracture had been removed surgically.

extension of the limb is the probable cause in many cases (Fig. 6–28). This puts great stress on the anterior face of the carpal bones and radius, and portions may fracture off under these circumstances (Fig. 6–28). Fractures of the carpus are likely in calf-knee-type conformation (see Chap. 1).

Signs

Signs of fracture of the carpal bones are similar to those of carpitis: heat, pain and swelling of the carpal joint, and lameness. Often such fractures are fired for what is believed to be carpitis when radiographs have not been used for diagnosis. When no response is noted after firing of a carpitis, radiographs may reveal fracture of one of the above mentioned bones. In most cases, it is advisable to take radiographs of all cases of carpitis prior to treatment to eliminate the possibility of fracture; oblique views should be taken of the carpus to eliminate the possibility of overlooking a fracture (see Chap. 12). A

hard, prominent swelling is usually noted at the anteromedial surface of the carpal joint after the fracture has been present some time.

Diagnosis

The radial and third carpal bones are fractured most commonly, but chip fractures of the intermediate carpal bone and of the radius may occur (Figs. 6–23, 6–26). A positive diagnosis can be made only by means of radiographs. These radiographs should include an anteroposterior view, a lateral view, a flexed-joint lateral view, and medial and lateral oblique views of the carpus. Oblique views are necessary because these fractures are not evident unless the angle of the radiograph is such that the line of fracture will show up. Radiographs of the opposite carpus should be taken since fractures of identical nature may be present without showing clinical signs. Persistent lameness with hard swelling at the anteromedial aspect of the carpal joint should cause one

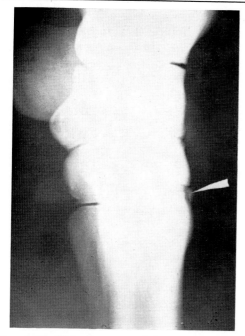

FIG. 6-27. Chip fracture of the proximal end of the third metacarpal bone. This type of fracture in the carpus is quite rare. It can be removed in a fashion similar to that described for other fractures by making an incision directly over the fractured portion, after determining by oblique radiographs on which side of the tendon it lies.

to suspect a fracture until this possibility is eliminated by complete radiographic examination. Careful palpation of the flexed carpal joint enables one to locate the fracture site with considerable accuracy once radiographs have shown that one is present.

If the synovial lining should form villi from a persistent traumatic arthritis in the joint, signs similar to those of fractured carpus may occur. If the villi become impinged in the joint as it closes, they cause persistent joint effusion and intermittent lameness. When lameness of this nature occurs, and no fracture is present, villi should be suspected. Villi are removed surgically when possible.

Treatment

The only effective treatment is surgical removal of the fragments or surgical fixation of the fragments by means of bone screws. Although carpal fractures will sometimes heal without surgical intervention, this is rare and takes many months, during which time considerable periosteal reaction may result, often involving the

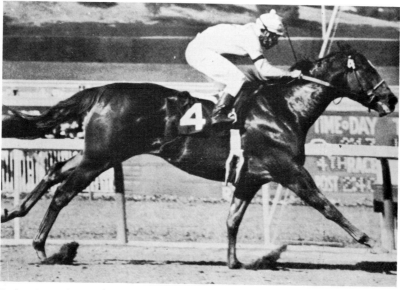

FIG. 6-28. Mechanism of carpal fractures. Notice severe overextension of left carpus. (Courtesy of Dr. W. Berkley.)

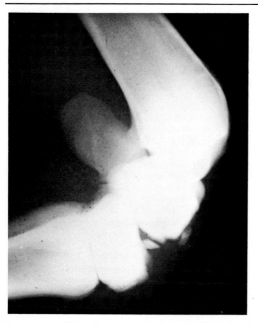

FIG. 6-29. Chip fracture of the distal end of the radial carpal bone and proximal end of the third carpal bone.

articular surfaces of the joints and causing permanent lameness. These same fragments may refracture when the horse is put back in training, making early surgical removal the best choice in most cases. The surgical approach to the fracture fragments should be carefully determined by radiographs and palpation. One must positively identify the radiocarpal and intercarpal joints so that the exact joint required may be exposed for fracture removal. Chip fractures of the radial and intermediate carpal bones may be removed either from the radiocarpal or intercarpal joints depending on whether they are located on the proximal or distal aspect of the bones. Fractures may come only from the top or bottom of these bones and the joint closest to the fracture should be selected. Fractures of the third carpal bone are removed by exposing the intercarpal joint. Fractures of the radius are removed by incision directly over the fracture site in the radiocarpal joint. Surgical removal of bone fragments is best

done as soon as possible after fracture has occurred (within ten to fourteen days after fracture). If the carpus has been injected with a corticoid, surgery is withheld at least 30 days, and the prognosis is much less favorable. The prognosis is also less favorable if a second operation is required on a carpus for refracture of a carpal bone.

The surgical procedure is as follows: The horse is anesthetized in a routine manner, preferably with halothane.* Clipping and shaving the leg before the horse is cast will shorten the time required in recumbency. If desired, the surgical area may be prepared and wrapped the day before surgery.

A tourniquet above the carpus is used to control hemorrhage. A pneumatic type that does not cause any arterial spasm is preferable, but broad rubber elastic bands over soft gauze rolls may be used.

The surgical site is prepared for aseptic surgery and protected with a sterile plastic drape† and muslin drapes. The joint is flexed so that the radiocarpal and intercarpal joints can be positively identified, and the incision is then made over the affected area. Most fractures will occur medial to the tendon of the extensor carpi radialis muscle on the radial carpal and third carpal bones. The incision is made so that the sheath protecting the tendon is not opened. The extensor carpi obliquus tendon usually lies far enough medially that it is easily avoided during surgery. Some fractures of the intermediate carpal bone require a more lateral incision, between the tendons of the extensor carpi radialis and the common digital extensor. This is also the approach to those chip fractures of the radius that occur in the center of its anterior surface.

The structures incised are the skin, subcutaneous tissue, dorsal annular ligament of the carpus, fibrous portion of the joint

---

*Fluothane, Ayerst Laboratories.

†Band-Aid Adhesive Drape, Johnson & Johnson.

capsule, and synovial layer of the joint capsule. The surgeon will find that after incision of the synovial lining of the joint capsule, joint fluid will run from the incision. Small bleeders encountered in the dorsal annular ligament and joint capsule can be controlled with cautery or by torsion and ligation. Visualization of the fracture is aided by flexing the joint so that the articular surfaces of the carpal bones can be observed. At this time, one can also appraise the amount of damage done to the joint surfaces, which will aid in prognosis (Fig. 6–30). Some irritation of the articular surfaces is always present as the result of the fracture, but this will often be repaired sufficiently to allow the horse to race again. Once the fracture is exposed, one is usually impressed with the proximity of the fragment to its normal position in spite of the wide separation that is apparently present on the radiographs. One will also find that there are often considerable fibrous adhesions present that make the fragment relatively immobile. Some fragments will have broken away completely and are attached to the joint capsule, making removal quite simple.

A periosteal elevator is used to gently work the fragment away from the adjoining carpal bone. The attachments of the joint capsule to the carpal bone on the anterior surface are freed by scalpel and the fragment removed (Fig. 6–34). The fracture area is then palpated for excessive roughness, and if present, the roughened areas are gently curetted till they feel smooth to palpation. The ragged edges of articular cartilage damage are also curetted smooth. Over a period of time the cartilage is replaced by fibrous tissue that eventually modifies and regenerates to articular cartilage. When villi have formed in the synovial layer of the capsule, they should be surgically removed. If they are not removed, they can be impinged in the joint during its closure, causing persistent joint effusion and pain.

They are dissected out using scissors and thumb forceps. This constitutes a partial synovectomy.

The joint cavity is then checked carefully to be sure that all fragments are removed and swabbed to remove hemorrhage. The cavity can be flushed with sterile saline solution if desired. The dorsal annular ligament and fibrous portion of the joint capsule are sutured with 00 medium chromic catgut or collagen* with swaged-on taper-point needle. One should be certain that the needle does not penetrate the synovial lining of the joint capsule, since this will sometimes cause rejection of the catgut at a later date. The sutures are placed close together; placing of corticoids and antibiotics into the joint

*Ethicon Inc., Somerville, N.J.

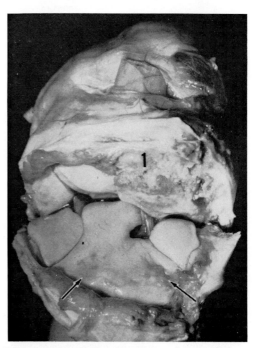

FIG. 6–30. Necropsy specimen of fractured radial carpal bone. The denuded area (1) shows where the fracture occurred on the radial carpal bone. Arrows indicate erosions in the articular surface of the third carpal bone. Areas such as this have some regeneration capability when the fracture is removed.

at this time is optional. The initial application of short-acting corticoids is apparently harmless, providing the joint was not injected with corticoids prior to surgery, and seems to aid in keeping inflammation minimal for a short time following the surgery. One million units of crystalline penicillin is also injected at the same time. The subcutaneous tissue is closed in the same fashion and the skin is sutured with a monofilament nylon or silk suture with swaged-on cutting-edge needle.

Occasionally it is found that the fractured piece of bone is so large that it would definitely harm the joint to remove it. This finding is most common in frac-

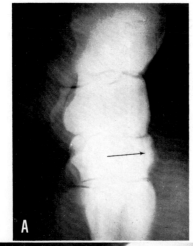

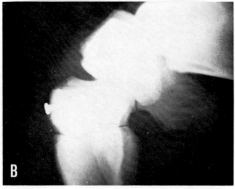

FIG. 6-31. Before and after insertion of bone screw for slab fracture of third carpal bone. A, Fracture prior to insertion of screw (arrow). B, Appearance of bone 60 days after bone screw was inserted.

ture of the third carpal bone. When this is the case, and the fracture is of a suitable type (one-piece), a bone screw is used to fix it into position (Figs. 6-31 and 6-32). This is done by making the incision described and drilling a hole in the anterior surface of the fragment and on into the affected carpal bone. Slab fractures are fixed into position using the "lag" principle. This consists of overdrilling the fragment to a size slightly larger than the threaded screw (Fig. 6-32). The solid portion of the bone is then drilled and tapped the proper size for the screw. When the screw is tightened, the fragment is then firmly fixed in place. The author prefers ASIF* cortical screws for this purpose. The drill hole in the fragment is countersunk so that the head will fit flush with the surface of the bone. If there are two large pieces in the slab fracture, each one is fixed into position with one screw as described. A slab fracture that requires a bone screw may slip upward (Fig. 6-24). This fragment is difficult to replace unless the carpus is flexed during surgery. Flexion of the joint causes the fragment to be pulled downwards because of the fibrous joint capsular attachment. This will greatly facilitate accurate positioning prior to placement of a bone screw. Cutting all attachments of the capsule to replace it has also been used (Dixon, 1969).

After suturing of the skin, sterile gauze sponges are placed over the wound, and the limb is bandaged from the hoof to above the middle of the forearm. The bandage may be of Gelocast,† which gives good support. Care should be taken to avoid ulcers on the accessory carpal bone and on the medial maleolus of the radius (Fig. 6-36). The limb should be padded with orthopedic felt over the prominence of the maleoli of the radius and the acces-

*Smith Kline Surgical Specialties, Philadelphia.
†Gelocast, Duke Laboratories, South Norwalk, Conn.; Medicopaste, Graham Field Labs, Woodside, N.Y.

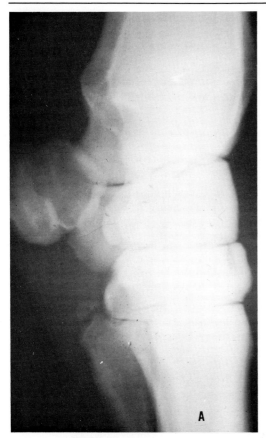 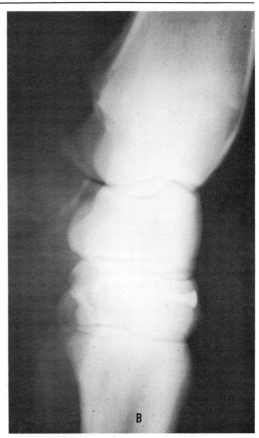

FIG. 6-32. Slab fracture of the third carpal bone repaired with an ASIF cortical screw using the compression technique. Radiographs were taken before (A) and after (B) surgery.

sory carpal bone. The bandage is intended to protect the joint while the animal recovers from anesthesia, and for the first five to seven days after the surgery, it will aid in keeping swelling to a minimum. The bandage is removed in five to seven days, and one often finds that the joint is the same size it was prior to surgery. At this time the joint is usually cared for by applying snug elastic bandages, and the horse is confined to a box stall for at least thirty days. Counterpressure is maintained by use of an elastic bandage and elastic tape for at least three weeks following surgery. A plaster cast is used when reoperating a joint or when corticosteroids have been previously administered. Parenteral antibiotics may be given for five to seven days after surgery.

Phenylbutazone derivatives to minimize pain and swelling after surgery should be covered by antibiotic therapy, and avoided when possible.

If any inflammation develops in the carpus after removal of the cast, use of an antiphlogistic poultice* is recommended till the inflammation disappears. Some authors recommend the use of radiation therapy following surgery. This is contraindicated in the experience of this author.

When exercise is first begun after surgery, the owner must be instructed to hand lead the horse, since the horse often feels so good that he wants to run and play, and he may reinjure the joint. For this reason, exercise following thirty days

*Denver Mud, Demco Corporation, Denver, Colo.

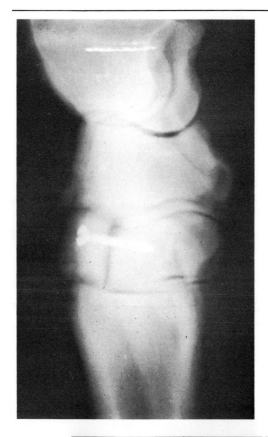

of confinement to a box stall is done at halter, and cantering is not permitted until the animal has been cared for in this way for at least an additional thirty days. The horse should not have any hard work for at least six months following surgery.

Prognosis

The prognosis for those cases that are carefully selected is good. About 75 percent of the selected cases will campaign successfully again. Large fractures, multiple fractures, and those cases that have excessive periosteal new bone growth, especially when near the articular surfaces, should be considered unfavorable surgical risks. Fractures that have had intra-articular injections of corticoids are bad risks, even though the last injection may have been several weeks before.

FIG. 6-33. Example of poor fixation of a slab fracture of the third carpal bone. Compression technique was not used.

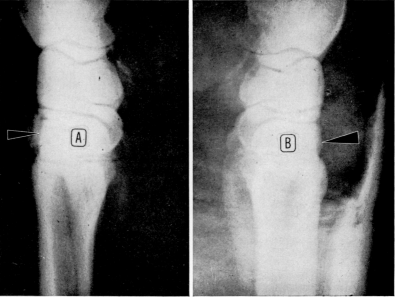

FIG. 6-34. Fracture of the third carpal bone. A, Dark pointer indicates line of slab fracture on third carpal bone. B, Dark pointer indicates the line of fracture after removal of the fragment from the same carpus. The areas of density around the limb are caused by the plaster of paris cast.

SPECIFIC REFERENCES

ADAMS, O. R. 1963. Surgical repair of equine carpal fractures. Norden News, 20 (June).

CHURCHILL, E. A., J. JENNY, J. D. WHEAT, C. W. RAKER, W. REED, and D. L. PROCTOR. 1959. Panel on orthopedic surgery. Proc. 5th Ann. AAEP.

DELAHANTY, D. D., J. JENNY, W. REED, and J. D. WHEAT. 1958. Panel on orthopedic surgery. Proc. 4th Ann. AAEP.

DIXON, R. T. 1969. Radiography of the equine carpus. Aust. Vet. J., 45: 171–174.

LARSEN, L. H., and R. T. DIXON. 1970. Management of carpal injuries in fast gaited horses. Aust. Vet. J. 46(2): 33–39.

MANNING, J. P., and L. E. ST. CLAIR. 1960. Surgical repair of the third carpal bone. Ill. Vet. 3: 106.

MANNING, J. P., and L. E. ST. CLAIR, 1972. Carpal hyperextension and arthrosis in the horse. AAEP 173–181, Dec.

MÜLLER, M. E. *et al.* 1970. Manual of Internal Fixation. New York: Springer-Verlag.

O'BRIEN, T. R., J. P. MORGAN, R. D. PARK, and J. L. LEBEL. 1971. Radiography in equine carpal lameness. Cornell Vet. 61(4): 646.

PARK, R. D. *et al.* Chip Fractures in the carpus of the horse: A radiographic study of their incidence and location. JAVMA 157, 1305–1312.

PROCTER, D. L. 1963. *Equine Medicine and Surgery.* Santa Barbara, Calif.: Veterinary Publications Inc. 725.

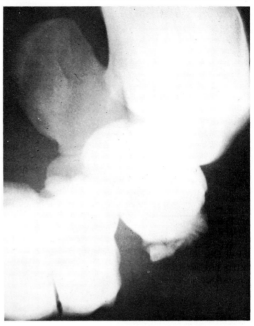

FIG. 6-35. Chip fracture of the distal end of the radial carpal bone and periosteal new bone growth on the cranial aspect of the radial carpal bone. The area of the fracture would require curetting, but the new bone growth need not be removed.

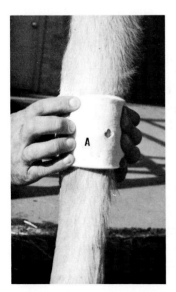
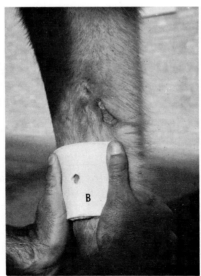
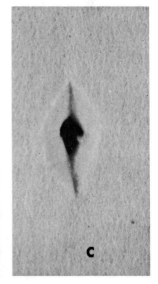

FIG. 6-36. A method of protecting the skin over the accessory carpal bone (A) and the medial malleolus of the radius (B) when bandaging or casting the carpus. An elliptical hole is cut in the orthopedic felt (C), and the felt is contoured over the prominence.

RIDDLE, W. E. 1970. Healing of articular cartilage. JAVMA 157(10): 1471–1479. December 1.

ROBERTS, E. J. 1964. Carpal lameness. Proc. 3rd Ann. Brit. Eq. Vet. Assoc., 18–28.

TEIGLAND, M. B., J. JENNY, J. D. WHEAT, D. L. PROCTOR, and W. REED. 1960. Panel on orthopedic surgery. Proc. 6th Ann. AAEP.

THRALL, D. E., et al. 1971. A Five year survey of the incidence and location of equine carpal fractures. JAVMA 158(8):1366–1368.

Fracture of the Accessory Carpal Bone

Definition

The accessory carpal bone is in a prominent position in the carpus and it may fracture from external trauma or from unknown causes. It often fractures in the groove that is formed for passage of the flexor tendons. The fragments usually separate because of the pull of the attachments of the flexor carpi ulnaris and ulnaris lateralis (Fig. 6–37). The articular portion of the bone is firmly attached by the accessory carpal ligaments.

Etiology

It is assumed that trauma is the etiology in most cases. However, most show no sign of external trauma on the skin and hair, and it may be that the bone can fracture as the result of stress from the tendinous attachments to it.

Signs

Signs of lameness are usually not acute. The horse may not put full weight on the limb soon after the injury, and if extensive swelling is not present, crepitation may be found in the early stages. Soon after the fracture, however, the ends are separated so that it is almost impossible to produce crepitation. The most prominent signs of the lameness are distention of the carpal sheath (Fig. 6–38) and pain on manual flexion of the carpus. Whenever the carpal sheath is distended, accompanied by pain on flexion, diagnostic radiographs should be taken to eliminate the possibility of accessory carpal bone fracture.

Diagnosis

Whenever a carpal sheath is distended and pain on flexion is evident, radiographs should be taken. The fracture will be evident on the lateral radiograph (Fig. 6–37).

Treatment

It is difficult to immobilize the fragments of accessory carpal bone because of the pull of the carpal flexors. Some-

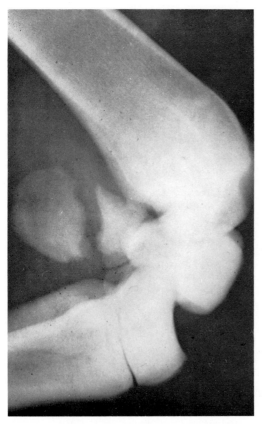

FIG. 6–37. Fracture of the accessory carpal bone. Notice the separation of the fragments caused by the pull of the carpal flexor tendons.

times, a bone screw fixation can be used. If a bone screw is to be used, a close study of the fracture must be made radiographically because of the curve in the bone. When using a bone screw, it is best to use the "lag" principle—overdrilling the first fragment to allow good apposition. It may be impossible to transfix the bone with a straight screw because of this curve. Surgical removal of fracture fragments of the accessory carpal bone can be done (Roberts, 1964), but cases should be selected carefully. Removal of small fragments may be beneficial, but large ones should be fixed in place with a bone screw or left alone. In many cases, the fracture is best left alone; eventually fibrous union of the fragments will take place. The horse may be able to return to light work after three to six months, and a few are successful at harder work. The carpal sheath may be injected with corticoids to alleviate the distention and relieve the inflammation.

Mackay-Smith (1972) has described a surgical method for relief of constriction of the carpal canal due to fracture of the accessory carpal bone or to other lesions in the carpal canal. The operation is described as follows:

An incision 15 cm long is made from 3 cm above to 5 cm below the accessory carpal bone, parallel to, and caudal to the common digital vein. Following dissection, a longitudinal elliptical strip of the volar annular ligament of the carpus is removed from between the veins that lie within the layers of the annular ligament. These veins run parallel to the long axis of the limb. The length of the strip removed should be somewhat longer than the zone of thickening, but rarely includes the entire length of the annular ligament. If intrathecal investigation is required, the synovial sheath is opened and any strictures are removed. If the intrathecal lesions can be localized to the tendon by palpation, the synovial sheath is not opened.

The subcutaneous fascia and skin are closed by layers and a firm adhesive bandage applied. The prominence of the ac-

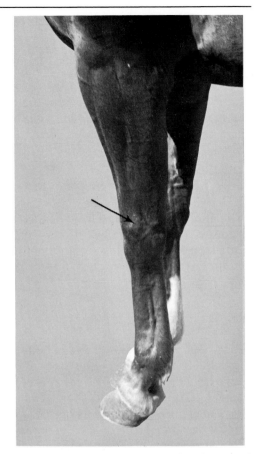

FIG. 6-38. Swelling of carpal sheath (arrow) caused by fracture of the accessory carpal bone.

cessory carpal bone is protected from excessive pressure (see Fig. 6-36).

A rest of three to six months should be enforced before attempting any work at all with the horse. Immobilization of the carpus by plaster cast may be helpful if the fracture is diagnosed soon after it occurs.

Prognosis

Guarded to unfavorable.

SPECIFIC REFERENCES

Mackay-Smith, M. P., et al. 1972. Carpal canal syndrome in horses. JAVMA 160(7): 993-997.
Roberts, E. J. 1964. Carpal lameness. Proc. 3rd Ann. Brit. Eq. Vet. Assoc., 18-28.

Rupture of the Extensor
Carpi Radialis

Definition

Rupture of the extensor carpi radialis tendon is comparatively rare. The signs of lameness are distinctive, making it easy to diagnose.

Etiology

The etiology is trauma. The logical conclusion is that overflexion of the limb would be most apt to cause rupture of this tendon. In most cases the actual etiology is not known.

Signs

With the resistance of the extensor carpi radialis tendon gone, the flexor tendons are able to overflex the limb. Careful observation of the gait will show that in the affected limb the carpus flexes considerably more than the carpus of the normal limb. Extension is accomplished by means of the common digital extensor and the lateral digital extensor. After the rupture has been present for a short time, atrophy of the muscular portion of the extensor carpi radialis begins. Palpation over the carpus will reveal the absence of the tendon on the anterior surface of the carpus.

Treatment

If the rupture is found soon after it occurs, it may be possible to bring the ends of the tendon together surgically. In this case, the limb would be kept in a cast for approximately six weeks. In cases of longer duration, it is impossible to bring the tendon ends together. One may be able to substitute the tendon of the extensor carpi obliquus by using tendon anastomosis.

Prognosis

Prognosis is unfavorable. In horses valuable enough to warrant surgery, either tendon anastomosis or substitution with extensor carpi obliquus may be used.

SPECIFIC REFERENCES

CATLIN, J. E. 1964. Rupture of the extensor carpi radialis tendon. VMSAC 59:1178.
WALLACE, C. E. 1972. Chronic tendosynovitis of the extensor carpi radialis tendon in the horse. Aust. Vet. (48): 585, 587.

Contraction of the Digital
Flexor Tendons

Definition

Contraction of the flexor tendons may be either congenital or acquired and may involve the deep and/or superficial digital flexor tendons. The degree of contraction is highly variable. The suspensory ligament is commonly contracted in foals affected with contraction of both the superficial and deep flexor tendons.

Etiology

Congenital types of flexor contraction result from inheritable characteristics, malposition of the fetus in the uterus, or nutritional deficiency of calcium, phosphorus, vitamin A, or vitamin D (see Chap. 5).

Acquired contraction of the flexor tendons may result from an injury that causes decreased use of the limb or from nutritional deficiency of the above-mentioned minerals after birth. Contraction of the flexor tendons due to injury is unilateral, while contractions resulting from nutrition, heredity, or malposition of the fetus in the uterus, are bilateral.

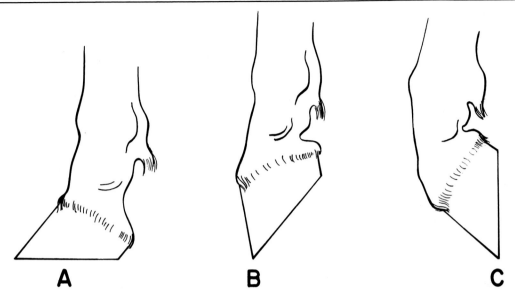

Fig. 6–39. Appearance of foot in contraction of the digital flexors. *A*, Primary contraction of the superficial flexor tendon characterized by dorsal rotation of the fetlock and pastern joints. "Cocked ankles" is the common term applied. *B*, Primary contraction of the deep flexor tendon, characterized by inability to place the heel of the foot on the ground. *C*, Contraction of both digital flexors and the suspensory ligament.

Signs

The signs vary with each case. If only the superficial digital flexor tendon contracts, the fetlock and pastern areas knuckle forward, causing "knuckling" of the fetlocks (Figs. 6–39A, 5–10, and 5–11). This may occur in either the fore or hind limbs. When the deep digital flexor contracts, the heel tends to lift from the ground. Contraction of the deep flexor alone seldom occurs; however, contraction of the superficial flexor can occur without the deep flexor showing comparable contraction. In some cases, the contraction of the deep digital flexor is so severe that the horse walks on the dorsal surface of the fetlock joint causing lesions that eventually open the joint capsule. These cases should be checked for contraction of the suspensory ligament.

Treatment

If contraction in the newborn foal is not too severe, the tendons may stretch as he grows, and treatment may not be required. If the foot can be placed flat on the ground, surgical correction usually is not advisable, provided progressive improvement is shown. If the fetlock and pastern areas knuckle over severely and the horse has difficulty keeping the foot flat on the ground, the affected limb should be placed in a plaster cast. Surgery can be performed later if there is insufficient response to the cast.

The foal should be anesthetized in a standard manner and the affected limbs covered with stockinette. The area between the fetlock and coronary band should be padded heavily with cotton. The limbs should be padded from just below the carpus or tarsus to the coronary band with heavy gauze and cotton pads. The limb then should be stretched under anesthesia to see if a normal position can be obtained. If the deformity still is severe, tenotomy of the deep and/or superficial flexor tendons may be advisable. If the heel of the foot remains on the ground when the horse is standing, only the superficial tendon should be cut. Two rolls of blue label, Johnson & Johnson 4″ plaster of paris bandage should be placed over the padding, and as it starts to dry, two pieces of yucca board, bass wood, or aspen wood (5$\frac{3}{4}$″ wide, $\frac{1}{8}$″ thick, and long enough to reach from the carpus to the hoof wall) should be placed on the back of the limb. Extra padding should be placed on the top and bottom areas of the wood and over the anterior surface of the fetlock and pastern joints. Two more rolls of blue label, 4″ plaster of paris bandage should be used to pull the fetlock and pastern area against the wood. The hoof wall should be incorporated in this cast. If moistened before application, the yucca board will conform fairly well to the shape of the limb. This cast should be left on for ten to fourteen days. The foal should be stalled during this procedure. After observation for ten to fourteen days of stall confinement after the cast has been removed, the decision to reapply the cast or to give no further treatment should be made. Flexor tendons tend to weaken when cast; this is helpful in the contraction syndrome.

If tenotomy is required, it should be done as follows: The foal should be anesthetized, and a small area over the lateral surface of the flexor tendons should be shaved and prepared for operation in the middle of the metacarpus or metatarsus. Using sterile gloves and instruments, a small Udall teat bistoury should be pushed between the two flexor tendons. A 2″ incision is used so the tendons can be adequately visualized. If only the superficial tendon is to be cut, the edge of the knife should be turned out, the tendon cut, and the skin sutured with monofilament nylon in a simple interrupted pattern. If both tendons are to be cut, the blade should be inserted under the deep flexor tendon through the incision, and, avoiding the large vessels in the area, both tendons then should be severed by turn-

ing the blade and cutting outward. The limb should be held in extension to tighten the flexor tendons while they are being severed. It is not necessary to cut both flexor tendons in the same spot. Some surgeons prefer to cut one of the tendons high and one low. This separates the tenotomies so that adhesions are less likely to occur. In addition, it is not necessary to cut the tendon through a small opening. The limb should then be cast in plaster with padding under the cast; a good supporting bandage may also be used.

If the cause of the condition has been found to be nutritional imbalance, the diet must be corrected to prevent recurrence.

Prognosis

The prognosis is favorable in cases that do not require tenotomy. It is guarded for those cases that do require tenotomy. It is unfavorable in those cases that cannot be pulled into a normal position after tenotomy is done. Such a condition indicates that the suspensory ligament also is contracted, but it should not be severed. If tenotomy of a flexor tendon is done, tetanus antitoxin should be administered; antibiotics usually are not necessary if aseptic procedures have been followed. Prognosis is unfavorable in cases where the fetlock joint capsule has been injured by trauma and suppurative arthritis is present.

SPECIFIC REFERENCE

Bedame, G. F. 1963. A corrective appliance for contracted tendons in foals. Proc. 9th Ann. AAEP. 91.

Tendosynovitis (Bowed Tendon, Tendinitis, Tendovaginitis)

Definition

The following definitions are taken from Bunnell (Boyes, 1964) to aid understanding pathogenesis of tendon damage.

Paratenon: This is a specialized loose tissue that fills space between a tendon and the immovable fascial compartment through which the tendon moves. It is elastic and pliable, with long fibers, allowing the tendon to move back and forth. Paratenon is not a true gliding mechanism; the tendon is not free, as in a sheath, but is intimately attached to the paratenon. The loose tissue is simply dragged with the tendon, its other end attached to fascia or some other fixed structure.

Tendon sheath: This is composed of two layers of synovia: a visceral layer covering the tendon and the parietal layer lining the fascial tunnel through which the tendon glides. Like enveloping peritoneum, the parietal joins the visceral layer in a double layer, the mesotenon. This mesentery-like structure is loose and filmy and does not limit motion of the tendon (normally).

As a tendon glides back and forth, the ends of the sheath form invaginating folds. The visceral layer enveloping the tendon is called the epitenon, and the outer layer is called the sheath. Fibrous septa running from the epitenon and dividing the tendon in bundles are called the endotenon. The mesotenon carries the blood vessels. The blood is supplied to a tendon from both origin and insertion, and the vessels enter the tendon in the mesotenon on the nonfriction side, run longitudinally in the epitenon, and send branches at right angles along the endotenon septa.

Annular ligaments are tough, fibrous, thickened parts of the fascial sheath lined with synovia. They act to prevent bowstringing of the tendon, which would destroy its mechanical efficiency. Tendons lying in firm tunnels or pulley mechanism (annular ligaments) suffer great damage when swelling from trauma or infection occur. Enclosed, they suffer ischemia, then necrosis. Sloughing tendon is replaced by scar tissue that involves the sheath, causing flexing and contracture.

When a tendon is partially severed or is crushed or bruised from a closed injury, it swells and softens, and it may rupture from ordinary pull several days to three weeks later.

Tendosynovitis results from an injury to the deep and/or superficial flexor tendons and their associated tendon sheath. The superficial digital flexor tendon is injured much more commonly than the deep digital flexor tendon. The injury is more common in the forelimb in running and working horses; in the Standardbred, the frequency of injury is nearly the same in front and hind limbs. The pathology has been described as a telescoping of the tendon sheath surrounding the deep and superficial digital flexors. The attachment of the mesotenon is torn from its position on the tendon, causing hemorrhage and inflammation. In the middle third of the metacarpal area, there is no sheath around the tendons. In this case, adhesions develop between the tendons, paratenon, and the surrounding subcutaneous tissues. Adhesions result that bind the tendons to the sheath, and, in addition, adhesions form between the deep and the superficial flexor tendons. Fibrous scar tissue also develops between the tendon sheath and surrounding connective tissue. Hemorrhage occurs within the tendon, and varying degrees of tearing of tendon fibers also occurs. Necrosis may occur within the tendon as a result of torn fibers. In some cases, many fibers are torn, causing lengthening of the tendon. The volar annular ligament of the fetlock often is involved, causing adhesions to form between this ligament and the superficial flexor tendon. When these adhesions contract, lameness may be caused by pressure on the tendon from the annular ligament (see the section on constriction of the volar annular ligament, p. 356). The "bowed" appearance, from which the disease gets its name, results from the fibrous adhesions on the volar aspect of the metacarpal area. Tendosynovitis is one of the more common causes of retirement of horses from racing.

Tendosynovitis occurs in the following areas:

1. High—just below the carpus
2. Middle—in the middle third of the cannon bone. In this area, the tendons lack a definite sheath, so the condition is essentially tendinitis.
3. Low—in the distal third of the cannon bone area, and may include the volar annular ligament. The deep flexor tendon may be injured below the fetlock, along with the insertions of the superficial flexor tendon and the distal sesamoidean ligaments.

Tendosynovitis may occur in the high or low areas alone, but usually not in the middle area alone. A severe case may involve all areas.

Etiology

Tendosynovitis occurs as a result of a severe strain to the flexor tendon area and is relatively common in the foreleg, but not so common in the hind leg. When it does occur in the hind leg, it usually involves only the low area. Predisposing causes include long, weak pasterns; forced training procedures; speed and exertion; muscular fatigue at the end of long races; improper shoeing; toes that are too long; muddy tracks; and horses that are too heavy for their tendon structure. The superficial flexor tendon is more commonly involved than is the deep flexor tendon. The time when tendosynovitis is most likely to occur is when the lead forefoot has all body weight on it while it is landing, and again just as it pushes off. Tight-fitting bandages or boots may predispose to injury to the tendons if a horse is worked in them.

Studies by Stromberg and Tufvesson (1969) indicate that degeneration of tendon cells begins before the acute lesion develops. They believe that this degeneration is evidenced by small swellings and heat in the tendon, which can be detected by careful palpation. It is their belief that these early lesions would heal if training were discontinued and the horse allowed to rest.

Signs

Signs of acute tendosynovitis lameness occur soon after injury, often toward the end of a long race, causing the horse to pull up lame, or to go lame shortly after the injury. In the acute phase, there is diffuse swelling over the involved area, and heat and pain are evident upon palpation. The condition, which is characterized by severe lameness, will cause the horse to stand with the heel elevated to ease pressure on the flexor tendon area. The carpus usually will be pushed forward while the horse is at rest, and in motion the animal will not allow the fetlock to drop because of the pain. Tendosynovitis also may occur in conjunction with suspensory ligament injury; a careful examination should be made to determine if this is true. The condition is considered more serious and the prognosis less favorable if the suspensory ligament is involved. In some cases the trauma is so severe that the fibers of the tendon actually are torn and stretched. This type of injury can be identified by an abnormal dropping of the fetlock. Stretching of the tendons occurs only in a small percentage of cases. Histological examination of the tendon will reveal various degrees of tendon tearing, necrosis, and hemorrhage in the tendon itself (Wheat, 1962). This means that there is injury within the tendon in all cases and that pathological changes are not limited to the peritenon or sheath. Signs of acute inflammation remain for several months, supporting the belief that at least a year's rest is necessary for healing. Regardless of cause of injury to a tendon, the tendon heals by fibrous scar tissue. Once scar tissue is present in the tendon, the tendon will never again have its normal strength. Although all collagenous tissue components are replaced, the elastin molecule is never replaced. Elastin was once thought to be part of the collagen molecule, but it has now been determined to be a separate molecule. Since elastin is never replaced, normal elasticity is never again present in the tendon.

A sign of chronic tendosynovitis is fibrosis in the area of the original injury (Figs. 6–40 and 6–41). Heat, pain, and lameness vary according to the degree of healing. A firm, prominent swelling usually is indicative of the condition. With chronic tendosynovitis, the patient often will be sound while walking or trotting, but will go lame under hard training.

If the volar annular ligament is involved, it will contract, causing a persistent lameness and chronic swelling of the tendon sheath above the sesamoid bones. Evidence of volar annular ligament involvement includes a "notching" or indentation visible on the posterior (caudal) aspect of the limb at the level of the volar annular ligament (Fig. 6–168, p. 357).

Careful palpation should be used to determine whether the inferior check ligament is also involved. The more structures involved, the more serious the condition. The structures should be palpated both with the foot on the ground and with the foot in a raised position when the structures are relaxed. There may be more lameness when the deep flexor and/or inferior check ligament are involved than when the superficial flexor tendon alone is involved.

The insertions of the superficial flexor tendon, the deep flexor tendon, and the distal sesamoidean ligaments may be injured individually or in any combination below the fetlock. Injured structures will be thickened.

Differential Diagnosis

Suspensory ligament injury and fracture of the proximal sesamoid bones can occur with bowed tendon; such a possi-bility should be considered. Tendosynovitis has a reasonably characteristic appearance, but only by careful palpation can suspensory ligament injury be determined. Radiographs can be used to determine if fracture of the proximal sesamoids has occurred. Below the fetlock, the insertion of the superficial flexor tendon may be injured, along with the deep flexor tendon and the distal sesamoidean ligaments. Careful palpation is required to identify these injuries (*see* p. 233).

Treatment

In early acute stages, the best treatment appears to be parenteral injection of a corticoid (Chap. 11, p. 447), combined

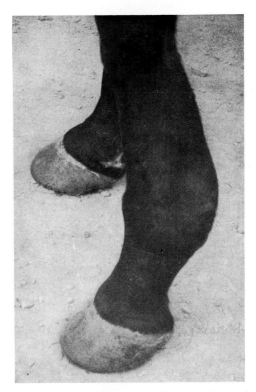

FIG. 6–40. Tendosynovitis (bowed tendon). Note the extensive swelling on the volar aspect of the limb above the sesamoid bones in the area of the flexors. This involvement includes all of the classification of high, middle, and low bowed tendon.

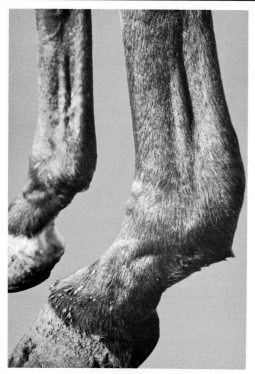

FIG. 6–41. Chronic low bowed tendon of left forelimb. Notice extent of swelling from the superficial flexor encompassing the deep flexor. This indicates tearing and adhesions of the common sheath. The left fetlock dropped lower than the right when the horse walked, indicating longitudinal tearing of the tendon(s) and an unfavorable prognosis. A tendon injury extending this low can involve the volar annular ligament (see the section on constriction of the volar annular ligament).

with the application of a plaster cast. The cast is applied from just below the carpus down to, and including, the hoof. Injection of parenteral corticoids is continued for ten days after application of the cast. At the end of two weeks, the cast should be removed, and, if necessary, another cast applied. If a marked improvement is evident after removal of the cast, the limb should be placed in supporting bandages for another 30 days. The horse should be rested for one year. Bowed tendon cases that are not severe may be exercised lightly in supportive bandage during the recovery period.

Formerly, the tendon was injected locally with corticoids, but calcification at the injection site occurs too frequently. Parenteral injection of corticoids is apparently just as effective as local injection.

This method of treatment gives most consistent results and is most apt to make it possible for the horse to return to racing. The use of parenteral corticoids plus a cast has given beneficial results, even when the case is not acute. Some cases of up to 30 days' duration that still have heat and swelling in the tendons respond favorably. This method of therapy is at least worth a try if signs of inflammation are still present. Antiphlogistic packs are sometimes used under bandages after the cast is removed.

If the case is no longer acute when the horse is examined, and he has developed fibrous tissue scarring in the tendon sheath area, little can be done except an attempt to correct the condition surgically or with radiation therapy to stimulate circulation. Firing and blistering are utilized, but usually these methods of therapy will not return the animal to soundness. Injection of the affected portion of tendon with irritants is sometimes used to promote increase in circulation. Various iodine preparations and mixtures of promazine and 50 percent dextrose have been used. It is doubtful that this type of therapy is of more value than radiation therapy for this purpose.

Shoeing with a raised heel will give some support to the damaged tendon. This should be used for no longer than ten weeks, in order to prevent contraction of the tendons.

Surgical correction has been used for tendosynovitis in recent years in an attempt to return a higher percentage of affected horses to racing. Such operations were successful in returning approximately one of five animals to racing; this percentage is probably no higher than would ordinarily return to soundness if other methods of treatment were used. If the volar annular ligament is constricted, it is necessary to cut it to relieve pressure on the tendon (see p. 356).

Asheim (1964) and others (Asheim and Knudsen, 1967; Maxwell, 1971) have described an operation for chronic bowed tendon and for suspensory ligament injuries. This operation was most successful when only the superficial digital flexor tendon was involved. Under general anesthesia and after surgical preparation of the skin, subcutaneous tissue and superficial flexor tendon are incised longitudinally in the center of the tendon on the volar or lateral aspect of the limb. The incision goes through the depth of the tendon, extending the full length of the damage and into normal tendon above and below. The tendon, subcutaneous tissue, and skin are sutured in separate layers. An alternative incision can be made over the lateral aspect of the tendon, splitting the tendon through its width over the length of the damage. The tendon can also be cut by the percutaneous method as described by Asheim and Knudsen (1967). After surgery, the limb is put in a plaster cast for two weeks. This cast is removed and replaced with another, which is allowed to disintegrate during a six-week box-stall convalescence. Gelocast* or Medicopaste† may be substituted for the second cast. The horse is rested for eight months; gentle exercise begun in two months.

Asheim claims that this operation increases the circulation to the tendon, thereby increasing its ability to heal. He supports this contention with histological studies. When the deep flexor tendon is involved, he recommends that the incision be made laterally into the tendon. Again, the incision extends the full length of the damaged tendon. Because there is evidence of necrosis in the tendon where it has been split by a long incision, it is possible that the stabbing technique will cause less damage to the tendon than a long splitting incision. This same technique is also used in a damaged suspensory ligament by using a longitudinal incision into the branch of the involved suspensory ligament. If the body of the ligament is damaged, the incision is made laterally into the ligament.

Sevelius (1964) reports that 28 of 40 horses operated on for injuries of the superficial flexor tendon and suspensory ligament returned to racing and Nilsson (1970) reports 65 percent success in the foreleg and 87 percent success in the hind leg.

In my experience, the surgery has not been this successful. I do differ on the method of suturing, since I do not believe the tendon sheath should be sutured with stainless steel. In my opinion, 00 catgut or collagen is preferable. Utilization of the lateral digital extensor tendon of the forelimb as a tendon graft into a damaged superficial digital flexor tendon has been described (Fackelman, 1972), but its value has not yet been determined.

Postoperative care is very important regardless of the treatment method. Swimming is an excellent exercise that does not overstress the tendon.

Prognosis

Prognosis is unfavorable in most cases because the lesion is easily reinjured. If treated in the early stages with a parenteral corticoid and a cast, the prognosis is better. In chronic stages when heavy scar tissue is present, the prognosis is strictly unfavorable. If tendosynovitis is accompanied by tearing of the suspensory ligament or fracture of a sesamoid bone, the prognosis also is unfavorable. Surgical splitting of the involved tendons may be more successful in Standardbreds because of their balanced gait. Only about 20 percent of horses suffering from tendosynovitis race successfully again. Not uncommonly, the horse may bow the tendons of the opposite leg, after apparent recovery from the original injury.

*Gelocast, Duke Laboratories. South Norwalk, Conn.
†Medicopaste, Graham Field Laboratories. Woodside, N.Y.

SPECIFIC REFERENCES

ASHEIM, A. 1964. Surgical treatment of tendon injuries in the horse. JAVMA 145: 447.

ASHEIM, A., and O. KNUDSEN. 1967. Percutaneous tendon splitting. Proc. AAEP, 255–259.

BOYES, J. H. 1964. Bunnell's Surgery of the Hand. Philadelphia: J. B. Lippincott.

FACKELMAN, G. E. 1972. The technique of tendon transplantation. Proc. 18th AAEP. 237–249.

FACKELMAN, G. E. 1973. The nature of tendon damage and its repair. Eq. Vet. J. 5(4): 141–149.

FISHER, W. F. 1961. Bowed tendons in the horse. Vet. Med. 56: 251.

FRANKS, P. W. 1970. Tendon and ligament injuries to race horses. Vet. Rec. 87(20): 637.

LACHOWICZ, S. 1966. Lesions of the flexor tendons in horses studied by means of radiography. Weterynaria Wroclaw 19: 47–68.

LINGARD, T. R. 1966. Strain of the superior check ligament. JAVMA 148(4): 364–366.

LUNDVALL, R. L. 1968: Tendon injuries of the lower leg. Norden News, 23–28 (Summer).

MAXWELL, J. A. L. 1971. Treatment of tendosynovitis in the horse by the tendon splitting operation. Aust. Vet. J. 47(5): 192–193.

NILSSON, G. 1970. A survey of the results of the tendon splitting operation for chronic tendinitis in the horse. Eq. Vet. J. 2(3): 111–114.

NORBERG, I. A. 1968. Tendons: Surgery. Proc. AAEP, 177–179.

Proceedings of the 4th Annual American Association of Equine Practitioners, 1958. Surgical Treatment of Tendinitis, a panel discussion.

PROCTOR, D. L. 1963. Tendinitis, p. 728. *Equine Medicine and Surgery,* Santa Barbara, Calif.: American Veterinary Publications Inc.

REED, W. O. 1962. Ligament and tendon injuries. JAVMA 141: 1258.

ROBINSON, R. C. 1968. The use of sclerosing agents in tendon repair of racehorses. Aust. Vet. J. 44(4): 200–202.

ROONEY, J. R. 1968. Tendons: Pathology. Proc. AAEP, 180–183.

SEVELIUS, F. 1964. Surgical treatment of bowed tendons and strained suspensory ligaments by Asheim's method. p. 28, *In* 3rd Ann. Cong. Brit. Vet. Med. Assoc.

SMITH, A. P. 1967. Corrective shoeing for bowed tendon. Mod. Vet. Pract. 48(2): 53.

STROMBERG, B., and G. TUFVESSON. 1969. Superficial flexor tendon lesions in race horses. Clin. Orthopaed. Rel. Res. 62: 113–123.

STROMBERG, G. 1973. Morphologic, thermographic and ^{133}Xc clearance studies on normal and diseased superficial digital flexor tendons in race horses. Eq. Vet. J. 5(4): 156–161.

STROMBERG, G., et al. 1974. Effect of surgical splitting on vascular reactions in the superficial flexor tendon of the horse. JAVMA 164(1): 57–60.

VAN PELT, R. W. 1969. Diagnosis and treatment of tendosynovitis. JAVMA 154(9): 1022–1033.

WHEAT, J. D. 1962. Pathology of tendon injuries. Proc. 8th Ann. AAEP, p. 27.

Metacarpal Periostitis (Bucked Shins, Sore Shins)

Definition

This is a periostitis of the dorsal surface of the third metacarpal or third metatarsal bone. It is frequent in young Thoroughbreds during the first few weeks of training. It is common in the forelimb but comparatively rare in the hind limb, although Churchill (1968) describes bruised metatarsal lameness in trotters as a result of gait compensation in hind leg lameness. Many cases are associated with fissure fractures and this possibility should always be considered.

Etiology

Concussion is probably the most important etiological factor, especially in young horses. In adult horses, the periosteal attachment to the bone is more mature, and periostitis is rarely evident after three years of age. The condition often occurs in both forelimbs at about the same time. The effect of the extensor tendon crossing the area and of the possible pulling of the peritenon tissues on the periosteum is not fully understood. Rooney (1969) stresses the importance of concussion and the probability of compression stress fractures. Injuries to the periosteum from direct trauma may also produce periostitis; this possibility should not be overlooked when the condition occurs in only one limb. Direct trauma to the metacarpal or metatarsal areas can produce periostitis in the mature horse. "Saucer" fractures of the third metacarpal bone may be present, as described by Wheat (1962). All cases should be radiographed to eliminate the possibility of such a fracture, since it is diagnosed with some frequency. The fracture may be seen on only one view, making a complete radiographic examination necessary.

Signs

A painful swelling on the anterior surface of the third metacarpal or, more rarely, the third metatarsal bone will be present. The condition is easily diagnosed, since this swelling is warm to palpation and painful when pressure is exerted. There will be a variable amount of edema in the subcutaneous tissues. Lameness will increase with exercise, and the stride will be characterized by a short anterior phase. If only one limb is involved, the horse will tend to rest the affected limb, but if both limbs are involved, he will shift his weight from one limb to the other.

Treatment

Rest is essential if complete recovery is to occur. Nearly all cases will heal if rest alone is used. Many practitioners apply antiphlogistic packs and cold applications during the first 24 or 48 hours the horse is affected, followed by firing in ten days after the limbs have cooled. The use of counterirritants, firing, x-ray therapy, and cobalt-60 therapy is controversial, especially if a fracture is present. All of these methods produce inflammation, but sufficient inflammation is already present in the condition. Subcutaneous injection of corticoids following proper skin preparation (Chap. 11) is a satisfactory treatment, but the rest period must be somewhat prolonged. The leg should be then wrapped and the horse rested for at least 30 days. The anti-inflammatory agent will reduce the swelling rapidly, and recovery will be complete if the rest period is suffi-cient. Unna's bandage may be helpful (see Chap. 11). The horse should be rested for at least one month or the condition may recur. Some trainers purposely work the horse heavily following appearance of the first symptoms of bucked shins in the hope that all pathological changes will occur at once. This could be very detrimental if a fracture is present, since prolonged rest and cast may be indicated. The very least one can do for a fracture is to apply supporting bandages and confine the horse for 45 days.

Prognosis

The prognosis is favorable in all cases if the trainer properly rests the horse. If the horse is not rested for a sufficient time, the condition recurs or persists, especially if a fracture is present. Permanent new bone growth may result if the periostitis is severe or recurs several times, or if a "saucer" fracture is present.

SPECIFIC REFERENCES

CHURCHILL, E. 1968. Care and Training of the Trotter and Pacer. Columbus, Ohio: U.S. Trotting Association.

GANNON, J. R. 1962. Treatment of sore shins with prednisolone. Aust. Vet. J. 38: 472.

LEWIS, R. D. 1968. Prevention of bucked shins in race horses. Mod. Vet. Pract. 49(8).

LINGARD, D. R. 1969. Fissure fractures of the equine metatarsus. VM/SAC 64: 895–898.

ROONEY J. R. 1969. Biomechanics of Lameness in Horses. Baltimore: Williams & Wilkins.

SLOCUM, D. B. 1967. The shin splint syndrome. Amer. J. Surg. 114(6): 875–881.

WHEAT, J. D. 1962. Bilateral fractures of the third metacarpal bone of a thoroughbred. JAVMA 140: 815.

Splints

Definition

. Splints, a disease of young horses, most often affect the forelimbs. Splints most commonly are found on the medial aspect of the limb between the second and third metacarpal bones. This is a disease associated with hard training, poor conformation, or malnutrition of a young horse.

Etiology

A disturbance of the fibrous interosseous ligament between the second and third metacarpal bones or between the third and fourth metacarpal bones causes splints. This irritation to the interosseous ligament causes periostitis and new bone growth. The condition may also occur, but is less common, between the second and third or between the third and fourth metatarsal bones. Splints also may be produced by trauma resulting from blows to the outside of the limb or from interference to the inside of the limb. Any trauma induced by slipping, running, jumping, or falling may be enough to disturb the interosseous ligament before it becomes ossified. Faulty conformation may produce splints due to malapposition of bones. Bench knees (Chap. 1, p. 13) commonly produces medial splints (Fig. 6–42). Deficiencies of calcium, phosphorus, or vitamin A or D also may predispose a horse to splints.

More splints occur on the medial side between the second and third metacarpal bones than on the lateral side between the third and fourth metacarpal bones because of the shape of the proximal ends of these bones. The proximal end of the second metacarpal bone is flat and articulates in a direct weight-bearing fashion with the carpal bones above. The proximal end of the fourth metacarpal bone is slightly oblique, thereby sliding the weight toward the inside. This puts the most direct weight-bearing on the second metacarpal bone, which explains why the interosseous ligament between the second and third metacarpal bones is more often disrupted than the one between the third and fourth metacarpal bones. When lateral deviation of the third metacarpal bone (bench knees) is present, there is even more concussion to the second metacarpal bone and less to the fourth metacarpal bone, thereby increasing the possibility of medial splint. Studies by Rooney and Prickett (1966) indicate that pressure by the second and third carpal bones forces the second metacarpal bone out of position during full extension. This displaces the interosseous ligament, thereby causing periostitis.

Signs

Lameness is most common in two-year-old horses undergoing heavy training, but cases occasionally occur among three- or four-year-olds. Splints most often are found on the medial aspect of

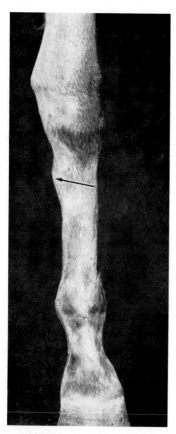

FIG. 6–42. Medial splint. This horse also was affected by bench knees.

the limb, because the second metacarpal bone normally bears more weight than does the fourth metacarpal bone; therefore, it is more subject to stress. Lameness is due primarily to concussion and is usually most obvious in the trot. Heat, pain, and swelling over the affected area may occur anywhere along the length of the splint bone. Splints most commonly occur about 3 inches below the carpal joint (Fig. 6-42). One large swelling or a number of smaller enlargements may occur along the length of the splint bone at its junction with the third metacarpal or third metatarsal bone.

If new bone growth occurs near the carpal joint, it may cause carpal arthritis. Extensive new bone formation on a splint may encroach on the suspensory ligament and cause chronic lameness unless it is removed. The existence of growths of this kind can be determined by palpation and radiographic examination. Splint lameness becomes more marked with exercise on hard ground. In mild cases no lameness may be evident in the walk, but lameness is exhibited during the trot. After the original inflammation subsides, the enlargements usually become smaller but firmer as a result of the ossification of the inflammatory process. The reduction in swelling is usually the result of resolution of fibrous tissue and not a decrease in size of the actual bone formation. In the early stages, the greatest bulk of the swelling is fibrous tissue, and this normally resolves to a much smaller size. This often misleads one into thinking that a method of treatment such as blistering or firing has reduced bony swelling. This is not true, and in many cases the actual new bone growth is larger than when originally treated. Some cases of splints may never cause lameness.

Diagnosis

Splints are a lameness of young horses. If the affected limb is examined carefully,

the obvious signs will lead to a diagnosis. Heat, pain, and swelling over the areas mentioned, plus lameness, are enough for diagnosis. Fracture of the splint bone is commonly confused with splints. In a fractured splint bone, the edema of the limb usually is distributed over a larger area and the animal remains chronically lame for a longer period. Whenever there is a suspicion that one of the splint bones is broken, radiographs should be taken (Figs. 6-43, 6-44, 6-45, and 6-46). An important part of diagnosis is to determine whether the carpal joint is involved or not and whether the new bone growth has extended posteriorly far enough that the suspensory ligament is involved. New bone growth resulting from trauma occurs on the third metacarpal or third metatarsal bones and may be mistaken for splints. Palpation and radiographs, though, will show that these swellings are anterior to the junction with the splint bones. This type of new bone growth is most often caused by interference. Radiographic examination reveals that the splint bone is not primarily involved and the bony growth is almost entirely on the third metacarpal bone. When doubt exists as to whether it is a splint or a growth due to interference, the medial aspect of the hoof wall should be marked with chalk, and the horse worked to see if chalk comes off in the area of the bony swelling.

Treatment

A number of treatments are used for splints. Some veterinarians prefer to treat the limb with hot and cold applications and then apply antiphlogistic packs* to reduce inflammation. Resting the horse for 30 days while continuing treatment often will permit the horse to be returned to training. Other veterinarians prefer to apply a blister or fire the splint area within two weeks of the occurrence of

*Denver Mud, Demco Corp., Denver, Colo.

pathological changes. Firing is probably more effective than the application of blisters because it produces more inflammation and, consequently, faster bone repair. In no case does firing or blistering ever reduce the amount of bone swelling. Healing of bone causes the swelling to lessen because it smooths the surface of the bone, but one should not be misled into believing that the inflammation produced by blistering or firing has done this. The swelling may lessen because of the reduction of swelling in the soft tissues surrounding the splint area. Radiographs taken before and after the application of blisters or firing of a splint will show that the bony exostosis actually may have become larger but that the swelling has been lessened because of the reduction in soft tissue swelling.

Another method of treatment is to inject the splint area with a corticoid (Chap. 11, p. 447). This treatment reduces inflammation and may help prevent excessive bone growth. Corticoid therapy should be accompanied by counterpressure bandage. In this case the horse must be rested longer than 30 days and should not be returned to training as rapidly as when counterirritation is used. However, the swelling may be considerably less. It is also true that a case of splints will heal without therapy, provided adequate rest is given. This rest should be a minimum of 30 days without training.

In some cases it is necessary to remove the bony exostosis that interferes with the action of the suspensory ligament or the carpal joint or is so large that it is being hit repeatedly by the opposite foot. In other cases, surgical removal of a splint is done because the horse is a halter-class horse and the owner feels that the blemish will lessen his chances of winning in the ring. Splints, though, should not be regarded by judges as a serious blemish, provided they are not accompanied by base-narrow, toe-out or bench-knee conformation. Successful removal of the bone

growth can be accomplished in about half of the cases; in the other half the bone growth will return to about the size it was before removal. The bone growth should be removed in the same manner that fractured splint bone is removed. If the bone growth has been caused by trauma from interference, the surgery will not be successful unless corrective shoeing will stop the interference.

In every case it is important to analyze the horse's diet and possibly his blood to determine if deficiencies exist that predispose the animal to the condition.

Prognosis

Prognosis is favorable in all cases except those in which the exostosis is large and encroaches on the suspensory ligament or the carpal joint or when it is due to interference.

SPECIFIC REFERENCES

O'CONNOR, J. P. 1962. Treatment of functional splints. Proc. 8th Ann. AAEP, 139.
ROONEY, J. R. and M. E. PRICKETT. 1966. Foreleg splints in horses. Cornell Vet. 56(2): 259–268.

Fracture of a Splint Bone

Definition

Fracture of a splint bone, commonly confused with splint lameness, may involve either the second or fourth metacarpal or metatarsal bones. Fracture, though, is most common on the second metacarpal (inside splint bone) as a result of the opposite foot hitting the bone. Fracture of the external splint bone (fourth metacarpal or fourth metatarsal bone) is less common.

Etiology

Trauma is the etiology in all cases. The bone may be broken anywhere along its

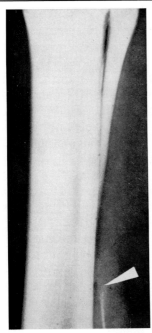

FIG. 6-43. Fracture of the distal end of the second metacarpal bone, as indicated by the pointer.

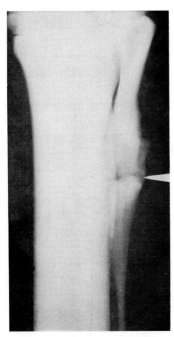

FIG. 6-44. Fracture of the fourth metatarsal bone, as indicated by the pointer.

length, but the break most commonly occurs in the distal third of the bone. Occasionally, a fracture may occur just under the carpal joint. When the second metacarpal or metatarsal bone is broken, it is usually because this bone has been hit by the opposite foot during turns or because of interference (Fig. 6-43). Rooney (1969) theorizes that the distal end of the second metacarpal bone may be fractured by pulling of the deep fascia as the carpus extends. Fracture of the outside splint bone (fourth metacarpal or fourth metatarsal bone) usually results from a kick or other external trauma (Figs. 6-44 and 6-45).

Signs

The horse often displays a typical splint lameness that becomes more marked upon exercise and is most noticeable at a trot. A swelling of the area is commonly present. This swelling is more diffuse than is the swelling with ordinary splints, and may extend the entire length of the splint bone. Chronic passive congestion may result in persistent swelling in the metacarpal area over the affected splint bone.

Diagnosis

A persistent swelling over the affected splint bone, exhibiting heat and pain when pressure is applied, should lead one to suspect fractured splint bone. Some fractured splint bones closely resemble the disease called splints. Some such fractures heal, but the bony swelling is confused with splints unless radiographs are taken. Radiographs are necessary to positive diagnosis of fractured splint bone and to differentiation of fracture of the splint bone from the disease called splints (Fig. 6-42). Rooney (1969) points out the necessity of differentiating between fracture and a distal epiphyseal line in the splint bone.

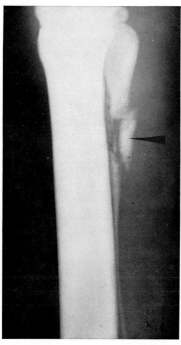

FIG. 6-45. Fracture of the fourth metatarsal bone with a chip broken from the bone as indicated by the pointer. Osteosis of the free portion was present.

Osteomyelitis may be present when a fragment of bone is separated (Chap. 5, p. 153; Fig. 5-20).

Treatment

If the splint bone is healed, as shown by radiographic examination, it is usually not advisable to disturb the condition, provided no lameness, swelling, heat, or pain are present and if the swelling is not so large it will be hit by the opposite foot. If the fracture has been present some time and shows no signs of healing, it should be removed, since healing often occurs more rapidly following surgical removal. In race horses, the fractured splint is sometimes removed soon after fracture rather than waiting for it to heal.

To remove the fractured bone, the operation should be performed with the horse in a recumbent position. The area over the fractured splint should be clipped, shaved, and prepared for operation. The horse is anesthetized in a routine manner and cast with the affected splint uppermost. An incision then should be made parallel with the anterior border of the affected splint bone, and the periosteum over the splint bone incised and reflected when easily identifiable. The distal fragment of the broken splint should be removed if it is short. Long distal pieces need not be removed if they appear to be normal. If removal is necessary, it should be done by teasing the bone away from its attachment to the third metacarpal bone with a chisel. The proximal end of the fracture should be left intact, but the distal end of this proximal segment should be tapered so that it will not cause irritation to the subcutaneous tissues. This also may be done by using a chisel. If the proximal fragment is short, it is fixed into position with a bone screw using the "lag" principle. The periosteum should be closed with No. 00 catgut or collagen followed by a layer of No. 00 catgut or collagen in the subcutaneous tissues. The skin then should be closed with simple interrupted sutures of a noncapillary, nonabsorbable suture. The line of incision should be covered with a sterile petrolatum gauze bandage; an elastic bandage should be applied to maintain compression on the area for at least two weeks. This bandage can be reapplied every two days to make sure that it maintains constant pressure. Sutures should be removed in two weeks. Recovery usually occurs. Training can begin in thirty days if sufficient recovery has occurred.

Prognosis

The prognosis usually is favorable, unless the new bone growth is large enough to involve the suspensory ligament behind or the carpal joint above.

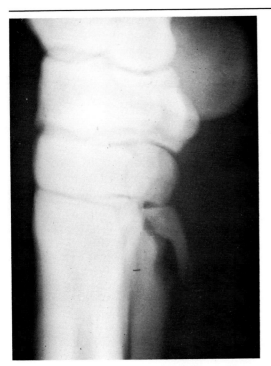

FIG. 6–46. Fracture of proximal end of second metacarpal bone. This type of fracture may require screw fixation to hold it in place.

SPECIFIC REFERENCES

METCALF, J. W. 1962. Removing fractured splint bones. Proc. AAEP, 142.

ROONEY, J. R. 1969. Biomechanics of Lameness in Horses. Baltimore: Williams & Wilkins.

WINTZER, H. J. 1960. Fractures of equine small metacarpal or metatarsal bones. Berl. Muench. Tieraerztl. Wochenschr., 73: 244.

Sprain (Desmitis) of the Suspensory Ligament

Definition

The suspensory ligament is the largest structure in the suspensory apparatus of the fetlock (see Chap. 2) and is commonly injured in race horses. It is a rare condition of the hind limb; most cases occur in the front limb. Standardbreds may be affected with suspensory ligament damage in both the fore and hind limbs (Rooney, 1969).

Etiology

Trauma is the etiology in all cases. At its point of bifurcation in the distal third of the metacarpal or metatarsal area, the suspensory ligament is subject to injury resulting from hyperextension of the fetlock joint. Injury most commonly occurs in one or both branches of the suspensory ligament where they attach to the sesamoid bones (Rooney, 1969). This type of injury, which tends to occur toward the end of a long race, is common in Thoroughbreds and Standardbreds, and causes periostitis and sesamoiditis (p. 228), with formation of new bone growth on the sesamoid bones (Fig. 6–61, p. 229). The ligament may tear longitudinally when injured at its bifurcation, but this is rare.

Signs

Injury to the suspensory ligament alone does occur, but the lameness often is due to injury to both the flexor tendons and the suspensory ligament. The lameness, which is similar to that evident in tendosynovitis (p. 200), is acute, causing swelling in early stages. The horse tends to hold his carpus forward and rest his heel lightly on the ground. The fetlock joint will be forward. When the horse walks, he will not allow the fetlock joint to descend to its proper level but will get off the affected limb as rapidly as possible. In the chronic form of the disease, there is considerable fibrosis and swelling of the suspensory ligament in one or both branches and at its attachment to the sesamoid bones.

Diagnosis

The diagnosis must be based on careful palpation and observation of the limb. The suspensory ligament should be palpated carefully at its bifurcation in the distal third of the metacarpus or metatarsus, at its branches, and at its attach-

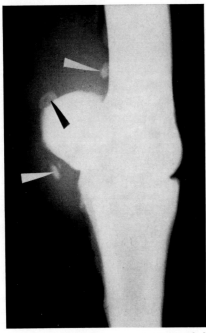

FIG. 6-47. Sprain of the suspensory and distal sesamoidean ligaments. The top arrow indicates calcification in the suspensory ligament. The middle arrow indicates new bone growth on the sesamoid bone or calcification in the attachment of the suspensory ligament; the lower arrow indicates calcification in the distal sesamoidean ligaments.

ment to the sesamoid bones. If scarring or thickening is present at any of these points, injury to the ligament has occurred. When the ligament is torn at its bifurcation, the horse will usually show considerable pain on pressure. Injury at this point must be differentiated from injury to the inferior check ligament, which joins the deep flexor in the middle of the metacarpus. Pain on pressure will identify which structure is damaged if careful palpation is done. In examining a horse with bowed tendon, one should carefully examine the suspensory ligament to be sure that this structure is not also injured. The prognosis of bowed tendon is even more grave if the suspensory ligament is injured. If the suspensory ligament is injured at its point of attachment to the proximal aspect of the sesamoid bones,

radiographic changes of these bones will be evident approximately 30 days after the injury, and these changes will be shown by new bone formation on the sesamoid bones (Fig. 6-61, p. 229), rarefaction of the sesamoid bones from inflammation, and calcification in the branches of the suspensory ligament above the sesamoid bones. Radiographs should be taken in the acute stage to be sure that no fracture of the sesamoid bones has occurred. In old injuries of the suspensory ligament at its attachment to the sesamoid bones, calcification of the ligament may show radiographically (Fig. 6-47). Desmitis and calcification of the distal sesamoidean ligaments are not uncommon.

Treatment

If the injury is seen in the acute stages, immobilization in a cast for two to four weeks and parenteral injections with a corticoid for ten days seems to be the best approach. After the cast is removed, the leg should be kept in supporting elastic bandages for a least a month. The horse should be rested for six to twelve months. The cast should include the hoof wall and extend proximally to just below the carpal joint. Some cases are treated with antiphlogistic packs on the limb to reduce swelling, and these packs are also valuable after the cast is removed.

In the chronic form of the disease, there is little treatment that is effective, since the scarred area is subject to reinjury because of decreased elasticity of the ligament and adhesions to surrounding tissues. Firing and blistering are often done but are of doubtful value. X- and gamma-ray therapy are said to be helpful in some cases, including those with calcification in the ligament. The horse should be rested for a year, and, if put back in training, he should be run in elastic or rubber supporting bandages.

A surgical method of correction for desmitis of the suspensory ligament has been described (Asheim, 1964; Sevelius, 1964). This method consists of a longitudinal incision into the affected branch or branches of the suspensory ligament. Under surgical anesthesia and proper preparation of the skin, the skin and subcutaneous tissues are incised, exposing the involved branch(es) over the medial and/or lateral aspect of the ligament. An incision is made into the ligament for the length of the involvement, going into normal tissue above and through the depth of the ligament. The incision in the ligament is then closed with simple interrupted sutures of catgut. The subcutaneous tissue is closed with 00 catgut, and the skin is closed with a 00 monofilament nylon. The orginator of this method (Asheim, 1964) uses stainless steel for suture, but it is unnecessary, and in many cases detrimental, to bury steel in an area such as this. The horse is then placed in a cast for two weeks, after which the cast is removed and a second cast put on and left for approximately six weeks. The horse then begins mild exercise but does no racing for eight months. A similar incision can be made into the body of the suspensory ligament if it is involved. After the same type of preparation, an incision on the medial or lateral side of the suspensory ligament is made and an incision extending the length of the involvement is made through the body of the ligament. This incision follows the same direction as the fibers of the ligament. The explanation given is that this increases the circulation to the ligament, allowing it to establish better healing. Injection of irritants into the damaged ligament have also been used. These methods of treatment are not highly successful.

Prognosis

Prognosis is unfavorable in nearly all cases. Some horses will return to racing if they are treated in the acute stages with corticoids and if the fetlock is immobil-ized in a plaster cast. Since tendosynovitis of the flexor tendons commonly occurs with injury to the suspensory ligament, only about 20 percent of the horses can be expected to race successfully again, although the success ratio may be higher in Standardbreds.

SPECIFIC REFERENCES

ASHEIM, A. 1964. Surgical treatment for tendon injuries in the horse. JAVMA 145: 447.

ROONEY, J. R. 1969. Biomechanics of Lameness in Horses. Baltimore: Williams & Wilkins.

SEVELIUS, F. 1964. Surgical treatment of bowed tendon and strained suspensory ligaments by Asheim's method, p. 28. In 3rd Ann. Cong. Brit. Equine Vet. Assoc.

Longitudinal Articular Fractures of the Third Metacarpal Bone into the Metacarpophalangeal Joint

Definition

Longitudinal fractures usually extend into the articulation and occur at the distal end of the third metacarpal bone. These fractures show little, if any, crepitation, and signs of lameness are often not severe. The diagnosis of the fracture may be missed entirely unless a radiograph is taken.

Etiology

Trauma is considered to be the etiology of this type of fracture. The great forces exerted on this bone during a full gallop plus possible unevenness of the terrain can produce uneven pressures in the joint. This probably forces a portion of the metacarpal bone to split away.

Signs

Signs of lameness are very similar to those caused by osselets and chip fracture of the first phalanx into the metacarpo-

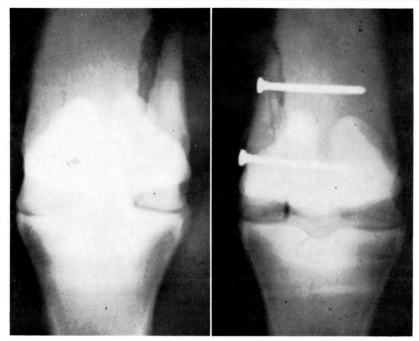

Fig. 6–48. Longitudinal fracture of the third metacarpal bone. On the left, appearance of the fracture prior to repair. The figure on the right shows the same fracture with two bone screws in place. Note that there is still some defect at the articulation. However, this horse went back into training for racing.

phalangeal joint. Lameness at the trot and swelling of the metacarpophalangeal joint and its capsule are present. Swelling of the joint capsule is best found between the suspensory ligament and the third metacarpal bone at the level of the sesamoid bones. Some pain may be exhibited on pressure over the area. Radiographically, varying types of fractures may be found. The type in Figure 6–48 is easily found radiographically, but the type shown in Figure 6–49 may be overlooked if careful examination of the radiograph is not made.

Diagnosis

Diagnosis can be established only by radiographic examination. A horse that shows considerable swelling of the fetlock and pain on pressure over the bony tissue should always be examined radiographically for the possibility of fracture.

Treatment

Treatment usually can be done in two ways. If there is no displacement of the fracture, the limb may be placed in a plaster cast for six weeks. This cast should be put on without padding and should enclose the hoof wall, extending to just below the carpal joint. When there is displacement, as in Figure 6–48, the fragment must be fixed. Bone screws may be used for this fixation; use of ASIF* cortical screws and the "lag" principle is preferred. The horse is anesthetized, the skin prepared for surgery, and a longitudinal incision made over the fracture site. The fragment is identified and forced into proper position. A radiograph may be taken at this point to see whether the fragment is properly fitted, but ordinarily this can be determined by digital palpation by dissecting the subcutaneous tis-

*Smith Kline Surgical Specialties, Philadelphia.

sues far enough to feel the fracture edges. A drill slightly larger than the bone screw is used to act as a guide hole for the screw in the outer fragment. If ASIF type equipment is not used, the hole in the inner fragment is drilled to a size only slightly smaller than the screw used. When the screw is tightened, it will force the fragments together. ASIF equipment provides a tap to thread the hole, permitting a better fit and better holding power. The subcutaneous tissue is sutured with an interrupted pattern of 00 catgut. The skin is closed with a monofilament noncapillary suture with a simple interrupted pattern. The limb is put in a cast for six weeks. This cast includes the hoof wall and extends to just below the carpus. This author does not remove the bone screws unless some complication occurs. Some surgeons prefer to put in a larger screw and remove it later.

Prognosis

The prognosis is guarded, but in many cases, the horse can be returned to normal function by the above procedures. The prognosis is better when there is practically no separation of the bone fragments. However, there is apparently good regeneration of tissue in this area, as evidenced by a return to soundness in cases with as much separation as shown in Figure 6–48.

Deviation of the Metacarpophalangeal (Fetlock) Joint

Deviation of this joint derives from nutritional causes as well as from uterine positioning and possible inheritable factors. It is very important that deviations of the fetlock in either the fore or hind limb be corrected as soon as noticed because of the early closure (6–12 months) of these epiphyses. While waiting to see if they will correct themselves, one may allow too much time to pass, making sta-

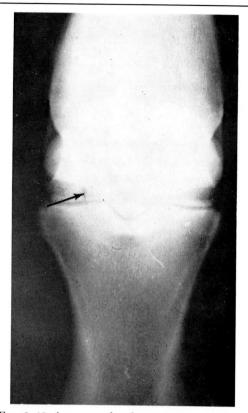

FIG. 6–49. An example of an articular fracture of the third metacarpal bone that can be repaired by using only a snug cast (arrow). The diagnosis of this fracture could be missed without careful examination of the radiograph.

pling unsuccessful. When the foal is two to three weeks old, the deviation can usually be corrected by means of a plaster cast. The foal is anesthetized in a routine manner, and the pastern area is padded with cotton so that it will blend with the prominence of the fetlock joint and coronary band. Stockinette is then placed over the limb and two rolls of 4″ plaster of paris bandage are applied to include the foot and extend to below the carpus or tarsus. A rigid support of bass wood or aspen wood is then placed on the concave side of the deviation. The proximal and distal portions of the wood are padded with cotton, as is the convex side of the metacarpophalangeal area. Two rolls of 4″

plaster of paris bandage are then wrapped around the wood and the limb so that pressure is exerted against the convex side of the fetlock joint, pulling it toward the rigid support. In most cases, it is not possible to produce complete straightening of the limb in the cast, but this is not necessary. It is apparently only necessary to get the limb started growing straight again. The cast is removed in ten to fourteen days and left off an additional ten to fourteen days before a decision is made whether to cast the limb in a similar fashion again. The mare and foal should be confined to a box stall for the entire period. Corrective trimming of the foot must be done every two weeks to keep the foot level. Ordinarily, one or two applications of a cast will produce a straight limb. Epiphyseal stapling may also be used.

If the foal is presented for treatment after it is three to four months of age, it is much more difficult to produce straightening with a cast. At this time, epiphyseal stapling is used (see p. 176). Under surgical anesthesia, the skin and subcutaneous tissues are incised over the convex side of the deviation. The epiphyses are more difficult to identify positively in these bones than in the radius or tibia. It may be best to take a radiograph prior to placing the staples to positively identify the proper positioning. Any metallic object can be used as a landmark to help identify the position of the epiphysis in the radiograph. Usually the epiphyseal line can be identified by probing the area with a sterile needle (25-20 gauge). The needle will sink into the epiphyseal line when pressure is applied. One or two staples are ordinarily sufficient to correct deviation of the metacarpophalangeal area (Fig. 6-50). One must keep in mind that staples must be placed in these bones much sooner than is required for the tibia

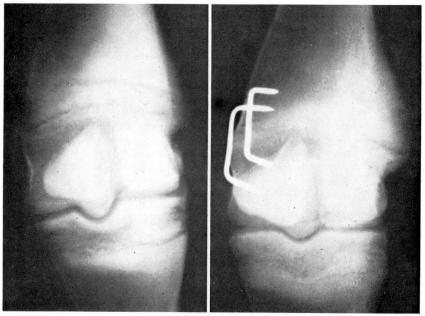

Fig. 6-50. Radiographs of the metacarpophalangeal (fetlock) joint before and after stapling. The radiograph on the left shows the deviation present in the distal epiphysis of the third metacarpal bone. The radiograph on the right shows the same limb a day after the staples were employed. This limb straightened adequately for normal use and appearance of the horse. The foal was four and one-half months of age when the staples were placed and not removed until after it was one year of age.

or radius. Ideally, the deviation will be corrected by means of a cast or stapling when the foal is just a few weeks old. If too much time has gone by to use a cast, staples are used. Preferably, staples are in place by four months of age so that when the epiphysis closes by nine to twelve months of age, the deviation is corrected.

Fracture of the Proximal Sesamoid Bone(s)

Definition

Fracture of the proximal sesamoid(s), most common in Thoroughbreds and Standardbreds, results from stress accompanied by fatigue as the result of a long race. Races of a mile to one and one-fourth miles so fatigue the limbs that the fetlock joints actually may touch ground (Fig. 6–28). It is at this point that injury is most likely to take place. Most fractured sesamoids occur in the front limb in the Thoroughbred and Quarter Horse, but in the Standardbred they are most common in the hind limb.

Etiology

Trauma is the etiology in all cases. The fatigue and strain of a long race are most likely to produce such injury, but cases have been recorded where a simple injury, such as stepping on a golf ball, produced the fracture. Interference may cause medial sesamoid fracture.

Some radiographs that I have seen showed signs of fractured sesamoids that appeared to be a congenital condition. In this case the proximal portion of the sesamoid bones showed fracture lines through both of the sesamoids on both forelimbs. This was not accompanied by any detectable heat, pain, swelling, or history of lameness. It is possible that occasionally there is congenital imperfection in the bone, which would be termed *bipartite* sesamoids.

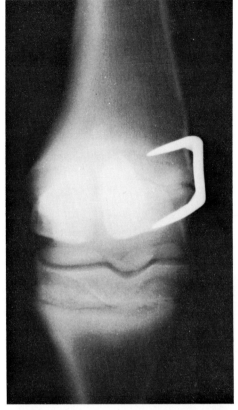

Fig. 6–51. Radiograph of vitallium staple placed in the lateral aspect of the distal epiphysis of the third metacarpal bone to correct lateral deviation of the fetlock. (Courtesy of Dr. J. Lebel.)

Signs

The medial or lateral sesamoid bones, or both, may be fractured. Lameness is very pronounced in acute stages: The horse is reluctant to bear weight on the limb and will not permit the fetlock to descend to normal position. Swelling, heat, and pain are marked in the fetlock area. Tendosynovitis, which also may be present, may confuse the diagnosis if radiographs are not taken. The horse evidences pain when pressure is applied to the affected bone or bones. Descent of the fetlock causes pain. Observation of the gait will reveal that the fetlock is held rigid so that it cannot descend as much as the opposite normal fetlock. The fracture in the bone may occur in any area of the sesamoids, but proximal fractures are more common than distal fractures; proximal fractures also are more amenable to treatment (Figs. 6-52, 6-53, and 6-54). Desmitis of the suspensory ligament and distal sesamoidean ligaments may occur concurrently with fractured sesamoids.

Diagnosis

Diagnosis is based on radiological examination of the affected fetlock and the physical changes described above. If a fetlock joint is severely swollen and the horse shows pain when pressure is applied over the sesamoid bone(s), radiographs should be taken to rule out the possibility of fracture. Cases of tendosynovitis also should be radiographed to eliminate the possibility of fractured

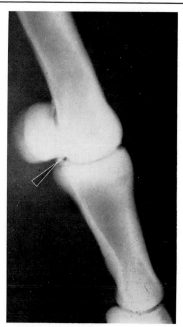

FIG. 6-53. Small distal fracture from the sesamoid bone, as indicated by the dark pointer. Removal of this fracture would be possible.

sesamoid accompanying this disease. Sesamoiditis causes similar signs, but radiographs will show no fracture.

Treatment

Treatment is based upon surgical correction and removal of the bone fragment, application of compression screws, or casting of the leg in an attempt to obtain union of the two fragments.

If the bone fragments are in close apposition and show very little displacement, it may be advisable to attempt a plaster cast or to apply compression screws, especially when a third or more of the bone is involved in the fracture. The horse should be tranquilized and the limb cast, in standing position, in as nearly normal a position as possible. The cast should be left on for 12 to 16 weeks, with periodic changes to make sure that it will remain snug. If, after one or two weeks, the horse shows improvement in walking, confinement is necessary to keep

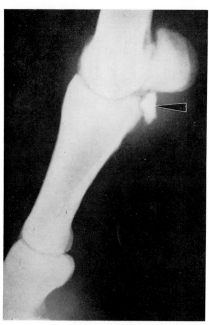

FIG. 6-52. Fracture from the base of a sesamoid bone is indicated by the dark pointer. With such a large fracture, the prognosis would be guarded to unfavorable for removal because the entire base of the sesamoid bone is gone.

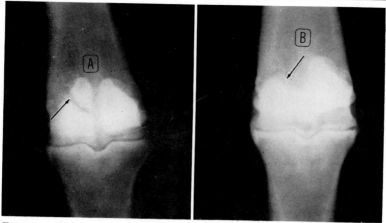

FIG. 6–54. *A*, Fracture of the apex of a sesamoid bone, as indicated by the arrow. This fragment is bordering on the largest piece that should surgically be removed from this area. The prognosis would be guarded. *B*, Arrow indicates the same sesamoid bone following removal of the fragment.

him from breaking down the cast and possibly reinjuring the area. Sesamoid bones are very slow to heal and the fracture line will be evident for a long time. The prolonged period in a cast is necessary because of the slow healing process. When casts are applied shortly after the injury, the results often are very gratifying.

If there is separation of the bone fragments, but the horse is not to be used again for racing, it is usually advisable to cast the limb. Surgical removal of the fragment is usually not necessary if the animal is to be used only for breeding purposes.

If a fractured portion of the bone is displaced, or if the bone was fractured some time before diagnosis and has not healed, it usually is advisable to remove the fragment if possible; however, this procedure is limited to fractures that constitute less than one third of the total size of the bone. Fractures constituting more than one third of the sesamoid bone should not be removed surgically because of poor results; plaster cast or correction with compression bone screws should be considered. Removal of a proximal fragment is more successful than removal of those in the distal portion of the

bone; small chips, though, may be removed from the distal portion of the bone with satisfactory results (Figs. 6–53 and 6–54). Removal of large fragments removes the attachment surface for either the suspensory ligament or the distal sesamoidean ligaments and will usually have an unfavorable result.

Operation is most easily performed when the horse is in lateral recumbency. The limb should be prepared for aseptic operation and the horse given a general anesthetic to control struggling. The volvar nerves may be blocked with local anesthetic to aid in reducing the amount of general anesthetic required. A tourniquet should be used to control hemorrhage. An Esmarch's bandage, used to force blood from the limb before the tourniquet is applied, will give one an almost bloodless field. An Esmarch's bandage may be fashioned from a piece of rubber inner tubing approximately 2″ wide or other suitable material.

When the fragment is in the apex of the bone, the incision should be made between the suspensory ligament and the posterior surface of the cannon bone (Fig. 6–54). The incision should be made proximal to the sesamoid bone and should extend into the collateral ligament as far as necessary. After the incision is made, the fetlock should be flexed slightly to reduce tension on the flexor tendons. This enables one to pull the suspensory ligament posteriorly so that the apex of the sesamoid bone can be seen. The fragment should be gently dissected away from the rest of the bone. Some authorities say sharp instruments cannot be used within the joint cavity, but they may, if caution is exercised. The fragment can be grasped with a small pair of rongeurs to permit dissection of the fibrous attachments from the bone. After the fragment is removed, tissue fragments are removed and the bone is smoothed with a curette. A layer of simple interrupted sutures should be placed in the fibrous joint capsule, the severed portion of the collateral ligament, and adjacent tissues, with 00 catgut or collagen with swaged-on taper-point needle. The point of the needle should not go through the synovial layer of the capsule. The severed portion of the collateral ligament can be sutured separately when necessary. A second layer of simple interrupted sutures should be placed in the subcutaneous tissues, and the skin closed with a noncapillary, nonabsorbable, plastic suture. One million units of crystalline penicillin may be injected into the joint capsule after the subcutaneous layer of sutures is finished. Do not inject a corticoid if they have previously been used in the joint. In this case, penicillin alone is used. The skin incision should be protected with a layer of sterile petrolatum gauze, and the limb heavily wrapped in supporting elastic bandages or placed in a plaster cast for approximately ten days. A plaster cast for 10 days is especially indicated if the joint has had previous surgery or if it has had corticoid injections. After ten days to two weeks, the horse should be walked daily for short periods. Supporting wraps should be kept on for a minimum of 30 days; they are especially important during the two weeks following surgery to prevent as much swelling as possible.

For fragments of the distal portion of the bone, the incision can be made directly over the fragment and extend through the distal sesamoidian ligaments. These fragments are somewhat more difficult to remove because of the ligamentous structure attached to the bone. The horse should be confined in the manner described above, and the area over the fracture should be prepared for aseptic operation. An incision directly over the fragment should be made after careful radiographic identification of its position. After the fractured bone has been identified, the fibrous adhesions joining it to the large fragment should be dissected away, as should the attachment of the sesamoidean ligaments to the bone. After removal of the fragment, the ligamentous tissue should be sutured with 00 catgut or collagen with swaged-on taper-point needle. The skin should be closed with a noncapillary plastic suture, and the incision line protected as mentioned above. A cast, or bandage, described above, also should be used. Large ventral fragments should not be removed, since this severs the attachment of the distal sesamoidean ligaments to this bone.

Distal fragments can also be removed by extending the incision made to remove proximal fragments between the suspensory ligament and cannon bone. If this incision is extended down through the collateral ligament of the sesamoid bone, some distal fragments that fracture cleanly through the articular surface can be reached. Those fragments that lie entirely on the posterior aspect of the sesamoid bone cannot be reached by this approach. These fragments can be removed by incision directly over the fragment or by the incision described below.

Another incision that can be used to remove basal sesamoid fractures is made on the posterior aspect of the fetlock on the medial or lateral side of the superficial flexor tendon depending on which side the fracture is located. The incision extends down through the volar annular ligament and tendon sheath, and the flexor tendons are pushed aside. This exposes the distal sesamoidean ligaments, which can then be incised horizontally in order to reach the basal portion of the sesamoid bone. The incision in the distal sesamoidean ligaments is sutured as a separate layer. The volar annular ligament and tendon sheath are sutured as one layer, then subcutaneous tissue and skin separately. It is best to use a plaster cast for approximately one week following surgery if this incision is used.

When a basal fracture involves a third or more of the sesamoid bone, it may be best to fix the fragment with a bone screw, using an ASIF cortical screw and a "lag" technique. A large basal fragment may be split in two pieces, and these fragments can be fixed into position in some cases by bone screws (Figs. 6–55 and 6–56). The incision is made directly over the area for drilling. All structures are severed (volar annular ligament, distal sesamoid ligaments) to expose the base of the bone. In order to evaluate the progress of the operation properly when placing the bone screws, it is necessary either to follow the technique closely with radiological examination or to open the volar pouch of the joint capsule between the suspensory ligament and the bone. The approximation of the fragments can be monitored through the incision in the volar pouch of the joint capsule by visualizing the fracture and by palpation. Radiographic examination is also helpful. The incision in the volar pouch is well worthwhile for a good end result. Drilling the bone should be done at a slow speed to avoid thermal necrosis caused by the drill. It is necessary to study the approach and to be thoroughly acquainted with the anatomy involved before placing the screw. If the fracture is of some duration, the distal fragment may be demineralized and eas-

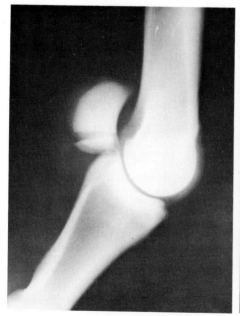 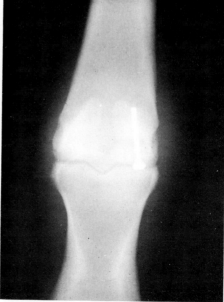

FIG. 6–55. Basal fracture of the medial sesamoid bone and repair using compression-screw technique. *Left.* Basal fracture before repair with screw (lateral view). *Right.* Basal fracture after repair with ASIF cortical screw (A-P view). (Courtesy Dr. W. A. Aanes.)

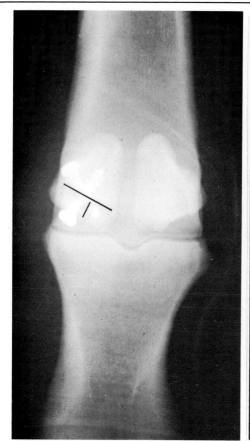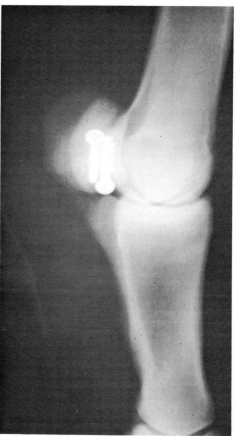

FIG. 6–56. Example of use of screws for a large basal fracture of the sesamoid bone. This type of repair is used when the fracture has split as indicated by dark lines.

ily fractured. One should exercise caution when tightening the screw to make sure that the fragment does not split as a result of demineralization or excessive pressure. The cancellous bone in the sesamoids is quite soft, and care must be used not to strip the threads in the cancellous and cortical bone. The cortex on the sesamoid bone is very thin and can also be easily damaged. Ideally, one would use an ASIF cancellous bone screw, and in some cases it can be used (Fig. 6–56). However, in most cases, the screw is too large and may itself fracture the fragment. Cancellous screws are difficult to remove after a period of time, should it become necessary. After the operation, the limb may be placed in a cast up to the carpus or up to the tarsus, or placed in Gelocast, Medi-copaste, or other suitable supporting bandaging. A plaster cast is helpful in supporting the fetlock postsurgically.

Before this type of surgery is done, one should be certain that all things possible are present to make it a possible success. The fragment should be in one piece and should involve at least 20 percent of the bone. Those approaching half of the bone are the most favorable. If the fragment is split, the prognosis is less favorable, and if additional fragments are present, it may make the operation impractical. A good radiological examination will help in anticipating any problems.

If desmitis is present in one or both branches of the suspensory ligament, surgery for the desmitis may be indicated. This technique is described on p. 214.

Prognosis

The prognosis is unfavorable if more than one third of the bone has been fractured, as it is for fractures of long standing that have not been cast or treated surgically. Small fragments of long duration may be removed successfully, but the sooner after acute inflammation subsides the better, as far as the outcome for the patient is concerned. Small fragments may be removed with a guarded to favorable prognosis. Those cases that are placed in a plaster cast soon after the fracture occurs often can return to racing if the fragments are in apposition. If both sesamoids are fractured, operation will not be as successful; fragments of both bones can be removed during the same operation.

SPECIFIC REFERENCES

BASSINGNANA, G. 1966. The use of neurotomy after fracture of the proximal sesamoids. 5th Ann. Cong. Brit. Eq. Vet. Assoc., 17–24.

CHURCHILL, E. A. 1962. Sesamoid fractures. Proc. AAEP, 206.

CHURCHILL, E. A. 1956. Surgical removal of fracture fragments of the proximal sesamoid bone. JAVMA 128: 581.

COPELAN, R. W. 1970. Bone screws as a method of immobilizing sesamoid fragments. Proc. AAEP, 207–231.

FRASER, J. A. 1971. Some conditions of the proximal sesamoid bones in the horse. Eq. Vet. J. 3(1): 20–24.

McKIBBIN, L. S., and K. N. ARMSTRONG. 1970. Bone screws as a method of immobilizing sesamoid fragments. Proc. AAEP, 203–206.

PETERS, J. E. 1949. Fractures of the third phalanx and sesamoids in the race horse. JAVMA 114: 405.

PROCTOR, D. L. 1963. *Equine Medicine and Surgery.* Santa Barbara, Calif.: American Veterinary Publications Inc. p. 694.

SEVELIUS, F., and G. TUFVESSON. 1963. Treatment for fractures of the sesamoid bones. JAVMA 142: 981.

WHEAT, J. D., and E. A. RHODE. 1958. Surgical treatment of fractures of the proximal sesamoid bones in the horse, JAVMA 132: 378.

WIRSTAD, H. F. 1963. Fractures of the proximal sesamoid bones. Vet. Rec. 75: 509.

WIRSTAD, H. F., G. TUFVESSON, and F. SEVELIUS. 1962. Fractures of the proximal sesamoid bones. Nord. Vet. Med. 14: 33 (suppl.).

Chip Fractures of the First Phalanx in the Metacarpophalangeal (Fetlock) Joint

Definition

Chip fractures of the proximal end of the first phalanx are relatively common in the forelimb of the horse. Most fractures of this type involve the anterior surface of the proximal end, just medial or lateral to the common digital extensor tendon. The medial side is affected more often than the lateral side. Other areas are not so commonly involved. Concussion and overextension of the joint are factors in the production of these fractures. Chip fractures from the distal end of the third metacarpal bone also occur but are less common.

Etiology

Trauma is the cause of these chip fractures of the first phalanx in the horse. From the appearance of the fractures, it seems that overextension of the joint is probably involved (Fig. 6–57). Overextension places stress on the anterior aspect of the proximal end of the first phalanx as it is pressed against the third metacarpal bone. Limb fatigue is a factor in overextension of the metacarpophalangeal joint (Fig. 6–28). Why the fracture most frequently occurs medial to the midline is not fully understood (Fig. 6–58).

Signs

Signs of chip fractures in the metacarpophalangeal joint are similar to those of osselets. There is arthritis in the joint, and permanent damage to the joint may result if the fragment grooves the articular surfaces. Serous arthritis of the fetlock joint indicated by distention of the joint

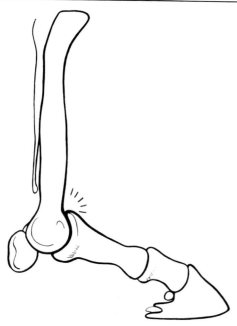

FIG. 6-57. Mechanism of chip fracture of the first phalanx. (Courtesy of Dr. W. Berkley.)

capsule (between the suspensory ligament and the volar surface of the cannon bone) is commonly found.

Lameness is most obvious in the trot. It is primarily a concussion lameness. Some horses have only a small amount of swelling or lameness to indicate that there is a chip fracture. There is often fibrous enlargement on the anterior surface of the fetlock joint that is easily palpated. However, anterior swelling is also often seen in osselets. Lameness will usually increase after exercise, and a workout or a race may cause the horse to be markedly lame. It is difficult to produce pain in the affected area by digital pressure, but some heat can usually be detected over the anterior surface of the joint. After prolonged rest, the horse may seem to be sound, only to go lame again when returned to training. Occasionally, there may be acute lameness followed by dramatic relief when a chip that was caught in the joint is dislodged.

Diagnosis

Diagnosis cannot be made without radiographic examination. The usual clinical case of chip fracture in the metacarpophalangeal joint has much the same appearance as a case of osselets. Affected horses are commonly blistered or fired when radiographs have not been taken.

The lateral radiograph is most revealing diagnostically (Fig. 6-59). Oblique radiographs should be taken to determine if the chip is on the medial or lateral side of the

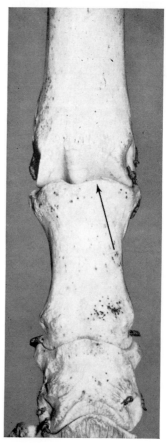

FIG. 6-58. Skeleton of the equine metacarpophalangeal joint revealing the most common area of occurrence for fractures of the first phalanx medial to the midline (arrow). These fractures occur less commonly lateral to the midline on the proximal phalanx. (From Adams, 1966; courtesy of JAVMA.)

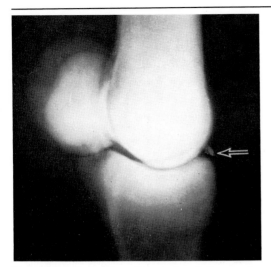

FIG. 6-59. Lateral radiograph of the metacarpophalangeal joint revealing a chip fracture (arrow) of the first phalanx. (From Adams, 1966; courtesy of JAVMA.)

midline. This is important, since the surgical approach must be made directly over the chip (Fig. 6-60). It is important to radiograph the opposite fetlock, since bilateral fractures are not uncommon, and clinical signs may not appear until the horse is back in training.

Differential Diagnosis

The lameness is most commonly confused with osselets. Radiographs will aid in differentiation. The lameness can be alleviated by injecting lidocaine hydrochloride* into the volar pouch of the joint capsule or by using a ring block above the metacarpophalangeal joint (Fig. 4-13). Local anesthesia of the volar nerves above the fetlock may not relieve the lameness without the use of a complete ring block.

Treatment

Surgical removal of the bone fragment is the only successful treatment. Once the

*Xylocaine, Astra Pharmaceutical Products Inc., Worcester, Mass.

exact location of the chip has been established (most chips are located medial to the midline), surgical removal is done if it is economically feasible. General anesthesia is administered and the area of incision prepared for aseptic surgery. The hair is clipped from the coronary band to the carpus. The area of incision is shaved and scrubbed, and skin antiseptics are applied. A tourniquet is placed in the metacarpal region to reduce hemorrhage. A plastic adhesive drape* is placed over the incision site. This is a self-adhering sterile drape that prevents fluid from soaking through and contaminating the area. The area is then prepared further by placing four sterile towels around the area of incision, plus two surgical muslin drapes. Using sterile gloves and instruments, a longitudinal incision is made to the side of the common digital extensor tendon. Since most fractures are medial

*Band-Aid Adhesive Drape, Vetco Division of Johnson & Johnson, New Brunswick, N.J.

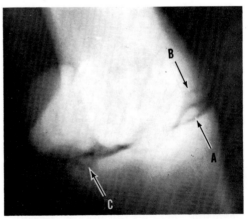

FIG. 6-60. Oblique radiograph of the medial aspect of the metacarpophalangeal joint showing the fracture fragment from the first phalanx (B). The articular surface of the metacarpophalangeal joint is shown (A). An additional lesion in the first phalanx is on the posterior aspect (C). The old lesion (C) may have been aseptic necrosis or a fracture that did not involve the articulation. (From Adams, 1966; courtesy of JAVMA.)

to the tendon, no other structures are involved. However, when the fracture is lateral to the tendon, the incision must be kept between the common and lateral digital extensors.

The incision over the fracture is made through the skin, fascia, annular ligament of the fetlock, and the fibrous and synovial layers of the joint capsule. The knife that is used to cut the skin and fascia is discarded, and a second knife is used to cut into the joint. The joint is flexed slightly to better reveal the chip. If the incision has been properly made, the chip is obvious once the joint is exposed. The incised area should be cleared of synovia and hemorrhage with sterile sponges so that the fracture line in the first phalanx can be seen. The chip is removed with a small periosteal elevator, and any rough portions on the joint cartilage or bone are curetted smooth. The fibrous portion of the joint capsule is approximated with 00 catgut or collagen* with a taper-point swaged-on needle. A simple interrupted suture pattern is used. Next, the subcutaneous fascia is approximated with a simple interrupted suture pattern of 00 catgut or collagen. At this point, a corticoid may be administered into the joint cavity if corticoids have not been used in the joint previously. One to five million units of crystalline penicillin are also injected.

The skin is then closed with 00 monofilament nylon or 00 dacron† using a simple interrupted pattern. A light bandage is then placed on the wound, and the foot is placed in a cast or strong supportive wrap that includes the hoof and extends to just below the carpal joint. The cast or supporting wrap is left in place for six to eight days, then removed and replaced by a pressure bandage. Pressure bandaging is used for at least two weeks, and the horse is confined for 30 days. Six months' rest is recommended before training is resumed. The cast prevents injury to the incision during recovery from anesthesia, acts as an effective pressure bandage, and seemingly prevents postoperative swelling. When a cast is not applied, a substitute such as Gelocast* or Medicopaste† may be used.

Prognosis

When the bone chip is removed before damage to the articular cartilage has occurred, excellent results can be expected. Some cases with articular damage of long duration recover after surgery, making the operation worthwhile in valuable horses.

SPECIFIC REFERENCES

ADAMS, O. R. 1966. Chip fractures into the metacarpophalangeal (fetlock) joint. JAVMA 148: 360.
CANNON, J. 1969. An investigation of healing following arthrotomy of the equine fetlock. Proc. AAEP, 233–235.
MILNE, F. J., et al. 1964. Equine lameness panel. Proc. 10th Ann. AAEP, 259.

Sesamoiditis

Definition

Sesamoiditis, or inflammation of the proximal sesamoid bones, is usually accompanied by a periostitis and osteitis of these bones. The suspensory ligament and the distal sesamoidean ligaments may also be affected and show calcified areas. Demineralization of the sesamoid bone(s) may result from inflammation and impaired blood supply (Figs. 6–61 and 62).

Etiology

Any unusual strain to the fetlock area may produce sesamoiditis. Most common in race horses, hunters, and jumpers, it

---

*Collagen Suture, Ethicon Inc., Somerville, N.J.
†Mersilene, Ethicon Inc., Somerville, N.J.

*Gelocast, Duke Laboratories, South Norwalk, Conn.
†Medicopaste, Graham Field Laboratories, Woodside, N.Y.

can affect any type of horse. It is caused by injury to the attachment of the suspensory ligament to the sesamoid bones. This injury to the suspensory ligament attachment may impair blood supply to the sesamoid bone(s). Injury to the distal sesamoidean ligaments may also occur at their attachment to the basilar portion of the sesamoid bones.

Signs

Symptoms are similar to those caused by fracture of the sesamoid bones—pain and swelling of the fetlock joint, especially at the volar aspect. Pressure over the sesamoid bones will cause the horse to flinch. When the horse is in motion the pain is most evident when weight is placed on the limb. The horse will not allow the fetlock to descend to normal level. After the disease becomes chronic, radiographs will show periosteal new bone growth on the convex surface of the sesamoid bones (Fig. 6-61). In addition, calcification of the suspensory ligament above the sesamoid bones, or in the distal sesamoidean ligaments below, may occur (Fig. 6-47).

Diagnosis

Diagnosis usually can be made by careful examination of the limb. Radiographs should be taken approximately three weeks after onset of the condition to determine if bony changes are occurring on the sesamoid bones. The radiologic changes of true sesamoiditis have been described as bony changes on the abaxial surface or basilar area with increased radiodense buildups, increased number and irregularity of the vascular channels, and increased coarseness and mottling of the bone trabeculation. The condition may occur with tendosynovitis, fracture of the sesamoid bones, and injury to the suspensory ligament from which it must be differentiated.

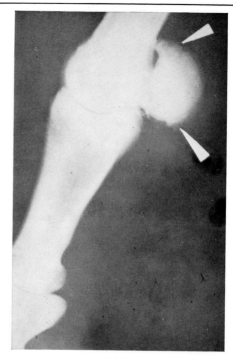

FIG. 6-61. Arrows indicate new bone growth on the sesamoid bones in sesamoiditis. This bone growth resulted from irritation of the periosteum caused by injury to the suspensory ligament, at the top, and to the distal sesamoidean ligaments, below.

Treatment

Efforts should be made to reduce the inflammation. Alternating cold and hot packs, as well as antiphlogistic packs, should be used. One of the best methods of therapy of early acute cases appears to be immobilization of the limb, from the hoof wall to just below the carpus, with a plaster cast. This cast should be left in place for two to three weeks and then removed and replaced, if necessary. In lieu of a cast, heavy supporting bandaging may be used. In chronic stages, volar neurectomy, firing, and blistering have been used but with only limited success. Volar neurectomy should not be used on a horse that will be ridden. X-ray and gamma-ray radiation are considered by some authors to be valuable therapy in this condition, as well as in the treatment of calcification in the suspensory ligament. Prolonged rest is essential to prevent possible sesamoid fracture.

Prognosis

The prognosis is guarded to unfavorable, depending upon the amount of periosteal reaction and new bone growth that occurs on the sesamoid bones and the extent of injury to the suspensory ligament and to the distal sesamoidean ligaments.

SPECIFIC REFERENCE

O'BRIEN, T. R. et al. 1971. Sesamoiditis in the Thoroughbred: A radiographic study. Am. J. Vet Rad. Soc. 12: 75–86.

Traumatic Arthritis of the Metacarpophalangeal (Fetlock) Joint (Osselets)

Definition

An osselet is a traumatic arthritis of the metacarpophalangeal joint. All other changes that occur are secondary to this fact. In addition to the arthritis present, there may be an inflammation of the periosteum at the distal end of the third metacarpal bone and/or the proximal end of the first phalanx due to stress on the fibrous portion of the joint capsule. The anterior surfaces of these bones are commonly involved. The fibrous portion of the joint capsule thickens dorsally as a result of the inflammatory process. In addition, the attachment of the lateral digital extensor, at the anterolateral surface of the proximal end of the first phalanx, is commonly involved. Ulceration of the joint cartilage often results from the chronic inflammation and causes recurring lameness. The term "green osselets" applies to early stages of the condition when it is limited to serous arthritis, and

before new bone growth has occurred. A similar condition rarely appears in the hind limb.

Osselets are most common in young Thoroughbreds and Standardbreds in early training; most cases appear in two-year-olds. Once the condition is established, it commonly affects the horse for several years, eventually causing the horse to be retired from racing.

Etiology

Concussion is probably the main factor responsible for osselets. A horse with upright pasterns is more apt to develop the condition than one with sloping pasterns because greater concussion is exerted on the fetlock joint as a result of the upright conformation. This same type of conformation also predisposes to navicular disease, which may be present along with osselets. New bone growth is caused by the periostitis that results from pulling of the joint capsule attachments or from pulling of the periosteum at the attachment of the lateral digital extensor tendon. It has also been suggested that pressure from the synovia may elevate the joint capsule attachments when the fetlock is flexed. This pressure would result from increased synovia caused by traumatic serous arthritis.

Signs

The traumatic arthritis causes distention of the volar pouch of the joint capsule between the suspensory ligament and cannon bone. The fact that arthritis is present should always be kept in mind. If work is continued after injection of corticoids, osteoarthritis will probably develop, damaging the articular cartilage.

Osselets result from concussion or a pulling of the attachment of the fibrous portion of the joint capsule at the distal end of the third metacarpal bone, or at the proximal end of the first phalanx, causing

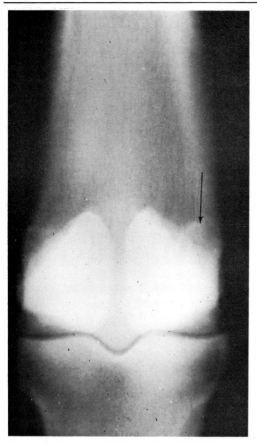

FIG. 6-62. Sesamoiditis with calcification extending into the suspensory ligament (arrow).

a disturbance of the periosteum and periostitis. In addition, or separately, the attachment of the lateral digital extensor may be pulled sufficiently to produce a periostitis in that area. The resulting periostitis in these areas often produces new bone growth that may affect the articular surfaces of the joint or that may be located in an area that does not involve the articular surfaces (Fig. 6-63). When new bone growth involves the joint, osteoarthritis is present.

There is swelling on the anterior surface of the metacarpophalangeal joint that varies in size, and in most instances it extends at least halfway around the joint. This swelling is due to thickening in the fibrous portion of the joint capsule. This swelling must be examined carefully be-

cause it is firm to palpation and may resemble new bone growth. Very often what is thought to be new bone growth will turn out to be soft tissue damage and fibrous tissue.

If both fetlock joints are involved, the horse moves with a short choppy gait. If only one fetlock is involved, the horse shows obvious lameness in that limb. Palpation will reveal pain, heat, and swelling over the anterior surface of the affected fetlock joint or joints. Pressure over the involved areas will cause the horse to flinch. Fibrous enlargement of the joint capsule on the anterior surface of the fetlock joint is present and is easily palpated. A choppy gait may lead one to believe that the shoulders are involved, but careful clinical examination will disclose the pathological changes at the fetlock joint. Lameness will increase with exercise, and, if only one limb is involved, the horse may point with the affected limb.

Radiographs should be taken to determine if new bone growth is present and if it is encroaching on the joint surfaces.

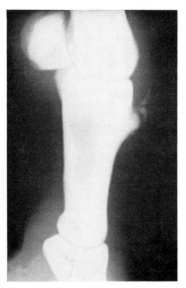

FIG. 6-63. Osselets resulting from periostitis at the insertion of the lateral digital extensor. Some calcification in the joint capsule also is present. (Carlson, *Veterinary Radiology*, Lea & Febiger.)

New bone growth is most common on the anterior surface of the proximal end of the first phalanx but may appear on the anterior surface of the distal end of the third metacarpal bone. Early cases show no radiographic bony changes. Calcification in the joint capsule may be present.

Diagnosis

Diagnosis is based upon the presence of hot, painful swellings on the anterior surface of the fetlock joint and upon other signs previously mentioned. Radiographs should always be taken to determine if periostitis is causing new bone growth, and if so, where and how much. Some cases show the presence of a joint mouse (a loose piece of bone within the joint capsule), which can be determined only by radiographs (Fig. 6–59). The possibility of chip fracture of the first phalanx should always be considered and eliminated, as should the possibility of concurrent navicular disease.

Treatment

Rest is absolutely necessary, so the horse must be removed from training. Antiphlogistic packs, ice packs, or cold water applications are commonly used to reduce acute inflammation. In addition, it is often helpful to inject the inflamed joint capsule with a corticoid (see Chap. 11). Corticoids decrease inflammation of the joint capsule and help prevent some new bone growth if used soon enough. The affected fetlock should be wrapped in supporting wraps for about two weeks, and the horse rested for at least 60 days. The corticoid therapy can be repeated at weekly intervals for three injections if necessary. The injections should be made using strict aseptic techniques. The fetlock may be fired after the inflammation has been reduced, but not following the use of corticoids.

After acute inflammation recedes, x-ray therapy is sometimes beneficial; x-ray therapy should not be combined with other methods, such as firing or blistering. When x-ray therapy is used, 700 to 1000 roentgens is the usual dose, given in two treatments of 350 to 500 roentgens each. Gamma-ray therapy with cobalt-60 (700-1000 roentgens) will produce similar results.

When osselets are in the chronic phase, firing and blistering are often used. Blistering is probably of little value, but firing is helpful in many cases because it creates an acute inflammation. When this process heals, the chronic osteoarthritis may disappear. In all cases, the horse must be rested approximately six months before being put back into training. Horses that receive corticoid therapy often are put into training too quickly because they appear to be normal. This results in a recurrence of the disease.

In horses that are affected with a chip fracture of the first phalanx, operation will be necessary to remove the bony tissue so that it will not catch between the articular surfaces of the cannon bone and the first phalanx and cause acute lameness. In some cases, bony tissue may be present in the wall of the joint capsule in a fixed position. This calcification of the joint capsule should not be confused with a chip fracture of the first phalanx. (See the discussion of chip fracture of first phalanx, p. 225.)

Prognosis

The prognosis is favorable when the condition is only a serous arthritis and when a periostitis has not resulted in new bone growth. When new bone growth is present, the prognosis may still be favorable, provided the bone growth does not encroach on the articular surfaces of the joint. Many horses can run normally even though much new bone tissue is present, as long as joint surfaces are not involved.

If the new bone growth involves the articular surfaces of the joint, the prognosis is unfavorable. The prognosis also is guarded if a chip fracture of the first phalanx is present, since major surgery is necessary to remove it and since the articular cartilage may have been damaged permanently by grooving if the chip has been caught repeatedly in the joint. Ulceration of the joint cartilage from any cause will cause chronic recurring lameness with a poor prognosis.

If the horse has steep conformation of the pastern, the prognosis is unfavorable, because this type of conformation increases concussion to the fetlock and thus increases the chances of recurrence of the injury. With this type of conformation, each case should be checked for navicular disease, since both types of lameness are commonly present in the same horse.

Desmitis of the Distal Sesamoidean Ligaments

Definition

Desmitis of the distal sesamoidean ligaments can occur as a result of the same stresses that cause damage to the suspensory ligament or the digital flexor tendons. Damage to the distal sesamoidean ligaments may also occur in conjunction with fractured sesamoids or desmitis of the suspensory ligament.

Signs

The middle distal sesamoidean ligament most often shows damage on radiographs at its bony attachment. Rodeo horses often have periosteal damage on the volar (palmar) aspect of the middle of the first phalanx and calcification in the middle ligament. However, this is not usually a primary cause of lameness and is only a radiographic change in some hardworking horses. Damage to the distal sesamoidean ligaments may result in a lesion that can be palpated. There may be damage to the digital flexor tendons below the fetlock, making palpation of the ligaments difficult, and lesions of bowed tendon may be evident above the fetlock.

Treatment

Treatment is very similar to that for desmitis of the suspensory ligament or bowed tendon. If acute desmitis of the distal sesamoidean ligaments is present with or without suspensory ligament damage or bowed tendon, a plaster cast plus parenteral injections of corticoids is very helpful. The area needs to be immobilized in early cases to promote healing. If the condition is allowed to go untreated or is aggravated, there will be considerable scar-tissue formation within the ligamentous tissue, making it subject to reinjury. A rest of one year is necessary to allow complete healing of these ligaments. Calcification often occurs in chronic injury of the distal sesamoidean ligaments.

Prognosis

Prognosis is guarded because of the possibility of reinjury. The ligaments probably never return to normal strength once severe injury has occurred.

Ringbone (Phalangeal Exostosis)

Definition

Ringbone is new bone growth that occurs on the first, second, or third phalanx. It is the result of a periostitis and may lead to an osteoarthritis or ankylosis of the pastern or coffin joints. This condition is seldom found in Thoroughbreds but is relatively common in other breeds.

Ringbone is classified in two ways:

High or Low Ringbone
a. High ringbone: This is new bone growth occurring on the distal end of the first phalanx and/or the proximal end of the second phalanx (Figs. 6–64 and 66).

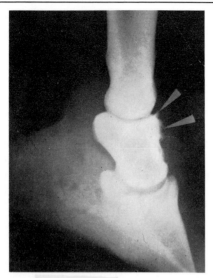

FIG. 6–64. High ringbone. The top pointer indicates new bone growth at the edge of the pastern joint. The lower arrow indicates new bone growth on the anterior surface of the proximal end of the second phalanx. These growths resulted from a pulling of the fibrous portion of the joint capsule or from a pulling of the attachment of the common digital extensor.

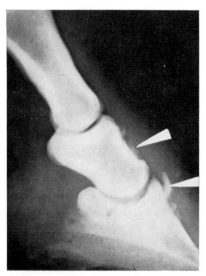

FIG. 6–65. Low ringbone. The upper arrow points to new bone growth on the distal end of the second phalanx while the lower arrow shows avulsion of a portion of the extensor process of the third phalanx. These changes are due to tension on the common digital extensor.

b. Low ringbone: This is new bone growth occurring on the distal end of the second phalanx and/or the proximal end of the third phalanx, especially at the extensor process of the third phalanx (Fig. 6–65).

Articular or Periarticular Ringbone

a. Articular ringbone: Articular ringbone means that the new bone growth involves the joint surface at the pastern or coffin joints (Figs. 6–68 and 70).

b. Periarticular ringbone: Periarticular ringbone means that the new bone growth is around the joint but does not involve a joint surface. It is most common in high ringbone (Fig. 6–67).

In describing ringbone, the following terminology is used: periarticular high ringbone; articular high ringbone; periarticular low ringbone; or articular low ringbone.

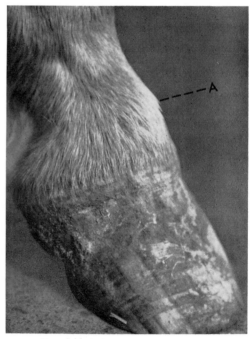

FIG. 6–66. Clinical appearance of high ringbone on the distal end of the first phalanx and proximal end of the second phalanx. Notice the bulging effect approximately 1″ above the coronary band (*A*).

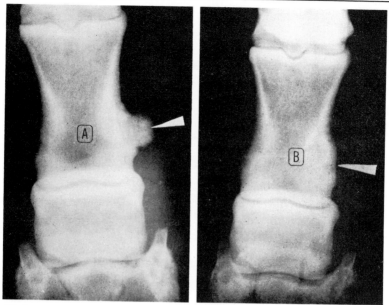

FIG. 6-67. *A*, High ringbone on the medial aspect of the distal end of the first phalanx as the result of an old wirecut. Periostitis produced by external trauma will produce ringbone, as shown. This growth was successfully removed surgically as shown in *B*. Removal was necessitated because the growth caused chronic lameness as the result of interference to the tendon of the superficial digital flexor.

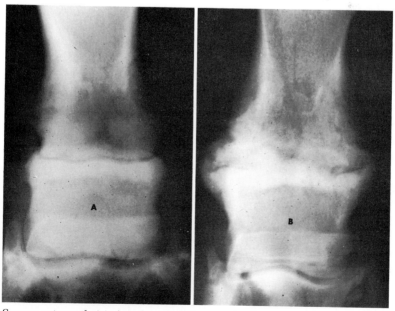

FIG. 6-68. *A*, Severe osteoarthritis (ringbone) of the proximal interphalangeal (pastern) joint. Note that joint spaces are still visible. *B*, Same joint six months after surgical arthrodesis. Note joint spaces are obliterated. The horse returned to full use.

Etiology

Trauma is the usual etiology of ringbone. A periostitis produced by pulling of the collateral ligaments of the joints involved, pulling of the joint capsule attachments to the bone, pulling of the attachment of the common extensor tendon to the first, second, or third phalanx, and direct blows to the phalanges are the most common causes of ringbone. Pulling of these structures does not cause rupture or tearing, although this can occur, but when these structures are "pulled," the periosteum is disturbed, and periostitis and new bone growth result. Wire cuts in the pastern region may cause periostitis that will cause ringbone, if the cut extends into the periosteum (Fig. 6–67). Ringbone also has been described as resulting from uneven spacing of the articular surfaces of the pastern joint and insufficient height of the ridge dividing the articular surfaces on the proximal surface of the second phalanx. Haakenstad (1954) made a study in Norwegian Dole horses and believes that all types of ringbone were inheritable in these horses.

In some cases, one of the phalanges will fracture in the area of the pastern, and this may lead to an ankylosis of the pastern joint and to severe ringbone. Fracture of the extensor process of the third phalanx results from tension on the common extensor tendon (Fig. 1–45, p. 31). Healing of this fracture may result in a large, low ringbone. If the insertion of the common digital extensor tendon is strained, but the extensor process of the third phalanx does not break, a periostitis still can result, causing new bone growth and low ringbone. This type of damage is commonly termed "buttress foot" (see p. 240).

Poor conformation may predispose to pulling of the collateral ligaments, joint capsule, and tendon insertions. Horses that are base-narrow and toe-in or toe-out are predisposed to ringbone on the lateral side of the joints, while horses that are base-wide and toe-in or toe-out are predisposed to ringbone on the medial side of the joints because the foot and leg conformation exerts greater stress on these areas. Ringbone is considered to be inheritable by some authors (Stecher, 1962), but it is probably inheritable through poor conformation. Pasterns that are overly upright will result in increased concussion to the pastern joint. The inheritability factor would not affect all forms of ringbone, because some result from trauma. Poor conformation increases stress on ligamentous and tendinous attachments to the phalanges and may cause ringbone resulting from an osteoarthritis caused by uneven pressures on the articular surfaces.

Signs

Ringbone may occur in either the front or hind feet, but it is more common in the forefeet.

Signs of lameness are not specific. Lameness is usually evident in all gaits and upon turning. Heat and swelling will be present over the involved areas, and the horse will sometimes flinch when finger pressure is applied to the area of the active ringbone. In a case of low ringbone, where the distal end of the second phalanx or the extensor process of the third phalanx is involved, the hair on the coronary band will stand erect at the front of the foot. There also will be heat and pain present in this area, and after the condition becomes chronic, there will be a change in shape of the toe of the hoof wall (Fig. 6–69). When there is bilateral osteoarthritis of the distal interphalangeal joints the horse may point the feet and shorten the anterior phase of the stride much as in navicular disease, but more often the gait is characterized by excessive landing on the heel.

Some cases of ringbone are relatively

asymptomatic, especially if they are peri-articular. Those cases of ringbone that are nonarticular may have little if any lameness, and no heat or pain is present after they are healed. Articular ringbone is accompanied by arthritis (usually osteoarthritis) of the affected joint, but ankylosis of the pastern joint may occur (Fig. 5–6, p. 126). Radiographic examination of ringbone will show minor to extreme bony changes on the first, second, and third phalanges.

Early cases of high ringbone, especially those involving the proximal end of the second phalanx, may show periodic swelling and lameness that will disappear with corticoid injections. This will reappear after the horse is put back to work until the firm swellings of ringbone are recognized. Radiographic changes showing periosteal new bone growth will then be present. The gait in these cases often resembles that of laminitis, with the heel landing long before the toe.

Diagnosis

A positive diagnosis of ringbone cannot be made without radiographic examination. In early cases, when swelling is not marked, the diagnosis is based on finding heat and pain in the involved areas. Careful comparison with the opposite limb should be made. One must be exceedingly cautious when bilateral swellings that are cold are present. Some horses will demonstrate this, but radiographic examination will reveal normal bones with only an enlarged distal epiphysis on the first phalanx.

Treatment

If a case is diagnosed in the very early stages before new bone growth begins, limiting motion of the joints by placing the limb in a plaster cast from the hoof wall to just below the carpal joint is a

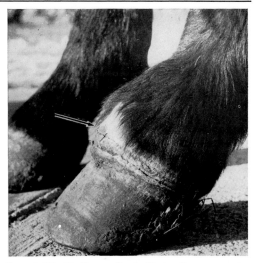

FIG. 6–69. Buttress foot. Note the extensive swelling at the anterior portion of the coronary band as the result of low ringbone. This is the same foot as shown in Figure 6–70.

good method of treatment. The foot should remain in a cast for a minimum of four weeks and should be rested for a minimum of four months. Injection of the area with a corticoid is indicated before application of a plaster cast (Chap. 11, p. 447).

When the pastern joint has become ankylosed, signs of lameness may not be present. This is especially true in the hind limb, where fractures of the phalanges may heal by ankylosing the pastern joint (Fig. 5–6, p. 126). If high ringbone is articular in nature, the horse will be lame until the pastern joint is ankylosed. Too often, the joint refuses to ankylose; this results in massive deposits of new bone growth around the joint with a hairline articular space shown on radiographs.

In chronic cases, a plaster cast is of little value, and the area is commonly fired or blistered. Neither of these methods of treatment is of value in articular ringbone, but firing is indicated and will usually help in periarticular ringbone. Ankylosis may be stimulated by surgically stripping the pastern joint of its articular cartilage, after which the limb is placed in a plaster cast for eight weeks to allow complete ankylosis of the pastern joint. (Fig. 6–68). Ankylosis of the proximal interphalangeal joint may be done under general anesthesia by means of a drill bit or an osteotome. The method that I prefer is as follows: After a general anesthetic has been administered and the skin area prepared, an incision is made on the anterolateral aspect of the proximal interphalangeal joint, between the lateral collateral ligament and the common digital extensor tendon. After identification of the proximal interphalangeal joint, a $\frac{3}{16}''$ drill is introduced between the collateral ligament and the common digital extensor tendon, between the first and second phalanges. The drill is introduced from one hole but is used to strip as much cartilage and subchondral bone as possible. The drill from the one hole is moved anteriorly, posteriorly, and medially many times to ensure as much destruction of the joint as possible. Subchondral bone as well as articular cartilage must be removed to get a good ankylosis. Caution should be exercised so as to prevent the drill bit from becoming hot and causing bone necrosis. The drill bit should not encounter the medial digital artery, vein, or nerve. In addition, the tendons behind should not be injured. It is not important to remove bone fragments left by the drill, since they will help to fuse the joint. The arthrodesis procedure can also be done utilizing a dorsal midline incision, dividing the long or common extensor longitudinally, and using the $\frac{3}{16}''$ drill bit as described.

Cancellous bone graft from the tuber coxae may be helpful in shortening the time required for ankylosis. The procedure is as follows: after proper surgical preparation of the tuber coxae, a piece of bone $\frac{1}{2}''$ by $\frac{1}{2}''$ by 2'' is removed by osteotome or surgical saw. The bone is cut into pieces small enough to go into the $\frac{3}{16}''$ drill hole. A piece of Steinmann pin 4''

long and with the ends cut off squarely is used to tamp the graft tightly into the joint. An orthopedic hammer is used to tap the Steinmann pin punch. Only enough bone is used to completely fill the cavity. The suturing procedure is the same as described below. The donor graft area is sutured with #1 catgut in the soft tissue and #1 vertical mattress sutures in the skin. A Penrose* drain is employed to facilitate drainage of serum.

Similar destruction of the joint can be done using an osteotome. In this case, the articular cartilage and cancellous bone adjacent to the joint are chiseled away. Caution must be used not to destroy the collateral ligaments, tendons, or vessels. After destruction of cartilage and subchondral bone is done, the subcutaneous tissues are sutured with 00 catgut or collagen with a simple interrupted pattern. The skin is then closed with 00 monofilament nylon with a simple interrupted pattern. Dry gauze sponges are placed over the wound prior to application of stockinette for the cast. The use of ASIF† cortical screws to aid in compression of the pastern joint after drilling to destroy the joint cartilage has been reported (von Salis, 1972). The screws are inserted above the pastern joint in the first phalanx on the dorsal surface and imbedded in the proximal end of the second phalanx; the joint is then compressed by the "lag" method (Müller, 1970).

The limb is then immobilized to just below the tarsus or carpus in a plaster cast. The foot must be included in the plaster cast. The cast has no padding except stockinette and a ring of $\frac{1}{4}''$ orthopedic felt just below the carpus or tarsus. The first layers of plaster are merely laid on without pressure. After two or three rolls of 6'' plaster have been put on, plaster splints 4'' wide and 18'' long are used

*Davol Rubber Co., Providence, R.I.
†Smith Kline Surgical Specialties, Philadelphia.

to reinforce the front and back of the cast. Then an additional three or four rolls of 6″ plaster are used to thoroughly immobilize the joint. Some pressure can be put on these latter rolls because the original plaster and splints are beginning to harden somewhat by this time. If Zoroc* plaster is used, fewer rolls are necessary. After the cast is finished, it is well either to paint the cast with fiberglas or a quick-drying enamel or to enclose the foot of it in a piece of rubber tubing to prevent moisture from seeping through the bottom part of the cast. The cast is changed if any increased lameness is shown or if any part of it cracks. It is usual to have to change the cast once or twice during the ten weeks the foot is immobilized. Each time the cast is changed, the horse should be restrained with general anesthesia. A radiograph can be taken when the cast is removed to check progress of the ankylosis. The foot should be cast in as normal a position as possible. After final removal of the cast, a 3″ trailer shoe is used to support the fetlock. This shoe is worn for approximately four weeks.

If the coffin joint is involved, there is little hope of ever obtaining a sound horse (Fig. 6–70). A neurectomy is sometimes performed to remove the pain. If a bilateral volar neurectomy is done, the same precautions should be used as described for posterior digital neurectomy for navicular disease (p. 271). Stumbling and loss of hoof wall are described as complications but are probably due to loss of blood supply rather than nerve supply; this loss of blood supply results from connective tissue and nerve regeneration that surround and occlude the volar arteries. In some cases, the anterior or posterior branch of the digital nerve may be cut to relieve pain. X-ray and gamma-ray therapy are used for treating ringbone, but without outstanding results. Periarticular

*Johnson & Johnson, New Brunswick, N.J.

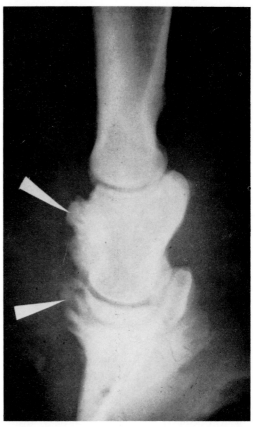

Fig. 6–70. Buttress foot changes on radiograph. The new bone growth is extensive as shown by the upper pointer on the second phalanx. The lower pointer shows new bone growth on the extensor process of the third phalanx. This is the same foot as shown in Figure 6–69. Since the proximal end of the second phalanx is involved, the horse actually had both high and low ringbone.

ringbone may respond favorably to this therapy.

Horses with ringbone are usually shod with full roller motion shoes (see Chap. 9), which aid in removing some of the action from the ankylosed or involved joints.

In some cases of nonarticular ringbone, removal of the new bone growth is indicated because it is causing lameness by encroaching on adjacent structures (Fig.

6–67). This is successful in about half the cases.

Prognosis

The prognosis is always unfavorable if the ringbone is articular. It is guarded if the ringbone is periarticular.

SPECIFIC REFERENCES

HAAKENSTAD, L. H. 1954. Investigations on ringbone. Nord. Veterinaermed. 7: 1.

MÜLLER, M. E., et al. 1970. Manual of Internal Fixation. J. B. Schatzker et al., trans. New York: Springer-Verlag.

STECHER, R. M. 1962. Discussion of osteoarthritis. JAVMA 141: 1249.

VON SALIS, B. 1972. Internal fixation in the equine: Recent advances and possible applications in private practice. Proc. 18th AAEP.

Pyramidal Disease (Buttress Foot)

Definition

Pyramidal disease, due to new bone growth in the area of the extensor process of the third phalanx, is a form of low ringbone. This new bone growth may be due to fracture or periostitis of the extensor process. Healing of the pathological changes produces new bone growth, causing an enlargement at the coronary band at the center of the hoof (Fig. 1–44, p. 30; Fig. 6–69). The same bony enlargement occurs in periostitis of the extensor process, making the clinical picture identical to that for fracture of this process.

Etiology

Pyramidal disease is caused by excessive strain on the long or common digital extensor as it inserts on the extensor process of the third phalanx. This results in a periostitis that causes new bone growth or in a fracture of the extensor process of the third phalanx that heals with excessive callus (Fig. 1–45, p. 31; Fig. 6–70).

Signs

Signs of lameness are not specific, but the horse often will show a tendency to point with the affected foot, and the anterior phase of the stride will be shortened. There often is a tendency to land heavily on the heel. In early stages, heat, pain, and some swelling are evident at the coronary band in the center of the wall, and lameness is present in all gaits. The hair shows a tendency to stand upright at the center of the coronary band (Fig. 6–69) and the horse flinches when finger pressure is put on the affected tissues. Arthritis of the coffin joint results and usually becomes chronic in the form of an osteoarthritis (Fig. 6–70). After some time, a change takes place in the shape of the front of the hoof wall, with a bulging from the coronary band to the bearing surface of the wall. Radiographs reveal variable changes in the second and third phalanges and in the coffin joint (Fig. 6–70).

Treatment

No treatment is of particular value in relieving this disease. Firing and blistering have been used, but these are of doubtful value. In early cases, injection of corticoids and immobilization of the part with a plaster cast may be of some help. Anterior digital neurectomy may relieve signs of lameness and allow limited use of the horse. Corrective shoeing consists of using full roller motion shoes on the affected foot to take as much motion as possible from the coffin joint.

Prognosis

The prognosis is unfavorable in all cases.

SPECIFIC REFERENCE

FRANK, E. R. 1935. Pyramidal disease. N. Amer. Vet. 16: 34.

Fracture of the Extensor Process of the Third Phalanx

Definition

Fracture of the extensor process may occur unilaterally or bilaterally in the forefeet of horses. It is seen more rarely in the hind feet. It may or may not be accompanied by buttress foot, which is produced by periosteal new bone growth (see above).

Etiology

The apparent etiology is excessive pressure on the common digital extensor tendon. This could produce enough pressure to fracture the process. It can also occur from overextension of the coffin joint. Bilateral cases could be due to congenital fractures (Fig. 6–71). In this case, it may be that the process has attempted to ossify from a separate ossification center, weakening the process and allowing it to be separated from the rest of the bone. Cases of this type do not have large amounts of periosteal new bone growth or the appearance of buttress foot.

Signs

Lameness signs are relatively obscure. The anterior phase of the stride is shortened, and the horse shows a stride similar to that seen in navicular disease. However, there is no reaction to the hoof tester over the frog or other parts of the foot. After the condition has been present for some time, there is a change in the shape of the hoof wall, with a tendency for V-shaped foot (Fig. 6-72). If the condition has been present a year or longer, this

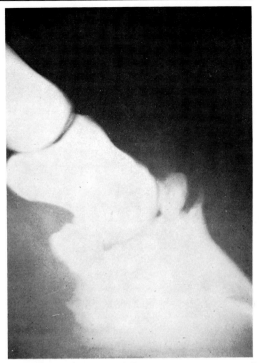

FIG. 6–71. Fracture of the extensor process of the third phalanx. This horse was affected with fracture of the extensor process on both forelimbs. It is possible that such a condition has a congenital origin when bilateral and not accompanied by periosteal new bone growth. Such fragments can be removed surgically.

shape will extend the full length of the hoof wall. Lateral radiographs of the foot reveal the fracture or a separated extensor process (Figs. 6-71 and 6-73). If extensive amounts of periosteal new bone growth are present, the foot assumes the typical appearance of buttress foot, which has been discussed above as a separate condition. Pain may be shown when pressure is applied over the center of the coronary band.

Diagnosis

Diagnosis is established by the changes in the shape of the hoof wall, pain on pressure over the extensor process (which

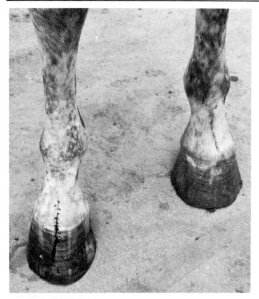

FIG. 6–72. Appearance of foot after removal of fracture of extensor process of the third phalanx. Notice the triangular appearance of the affected foot on its dorsal surface as compared to the normal foot. This change is characteristic of long-standing fracture of the third phalanx.

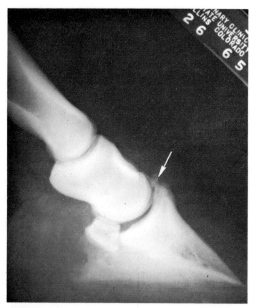

FIG. 6–73. An example of a small fracture of the extensor process of the third phalanx.

may or may not be present), and radiographs (Figs. 1–45, 6–71).

Treatment

Fragments of the extensor process can be removed surgically, or an attempt can be made to fix large fragments with a bone screw. The surgery is done under general anesthesia and with accepted aseptic technique. A midline incision is made over the center of the common digital extensor tendon, just above the coronary band. The incision need not extend the full depth of the coronary band. The common digital extensor tendon is separated longitudinally, and the fragment can be palpated and grasped with forceps. Alligator-type forceps work very well. Adhesions to the fragment are dissected and the fragment removed. The tendon is sutured with simple interrupted stitches of 00 catgut or collagen. The subcutaneous tissues are closed in a similar fashion, and the skin is closed with a 00 monofilament nylon with a simple interrupted suture pattern. The foot is placed in a cast that extends to below the carpus for one week. The cast is removed and the foot kept in supporting bandage for thirty days. A rigid supporting bandage can be substituted for a plaster cast. The horse should not be worked for at least six months.

When a large fracture of the extensor process is present, with little separation, an attempt may be made to fix the fragment surgically with a bone screw (Haynes and Adams, 1973). The same operative approach is used as for removal of the fracture. It is usually best to insert a small Steinmann pin to act as a radiographic guide for the placement of the screw (Fig. 6–74B). The screw preferred is an ASIF navicular screw.* A hole 3.6 mm in diameter is drilled and tapped for the navicular screw. The screw depth will

*Smith Kline Surgical Specialties, Philadelphia.

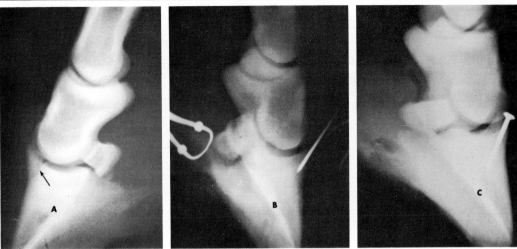

FIG. 6–74. A, Large fracture (arrow) of extensor process of third phalanx. B, Steinmann pin guide to check angulation for drilling. C, ASIF navicular screw in place.

usually vary between 24 and 28 mm. One must be careful not to go through the bottom of the third phalanx. The navicular screw has no threads on the proximal portion and will tend to pull the fracture fragment into position (Fig. 6–73C). The foot, including the hoof wall, should then be placed in a cast up to the carpus (or tarsus). The cast is left in place for approximately four weeks, with the horse in box stall confinement, followed by an additional four weeks of confinement in a stall after removal of the cast. Hand walking is then begun, but the horse should be rested at least six months before any hard workouts. Only selected cases should be attempted for screw fixation since the fragment must be large and in proper position to make the operation feasible.

Prognosis

Prognosis is guarded because osteoarthritis of the distal interphalangeal joint is present and may persist. New bone growth involving the joint makes for an unfavorable prognosis.

SPECIFIC REFERENCES

DUNKIN, D. B., and J. S. DINGWALL. 1971. Surgical removal of avulsed portions of the extensor process of the third phalanx in the horse. JAVMA 159(2): 201–203.

HAYNES, P. F., and O. R. ADAMS, 1974. Internal fixation for repairs of fractured extensor process in the horse. JAVMA 164(1): 61–63.

NUMANS, S. R., and H. F. WINTZER. 1961. Surgical treatment of apophysial and chip fractures. Berl. Munch. Tieraerztl. Wschr. 74: 205.

PETTERSSON, H., 1972. Conservative and surgical treatment of fractures of the third phalanx. Proc. AAEP.

Quittor

Definition

Quittor is a chronic purulent inflammation of a collateral cartilage of the third phalanx characterized by necrosis of the cartilage and sinus drainage through the coronary band. It is most common in the forelimb (Fig. 6-75).

Etiology

Injury near the coronary band over the region of the collateral cartilages may

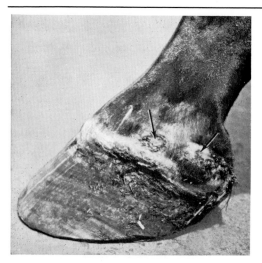

FIG. 6–75. Clinical appearance of typical quittor. Arrows point to two draining tracts. This case was cured through the surgical procedure described, making an elliptical incision above the coronary band. The anterior tract led posteriorly, and only the posterior tract had to be followed to necrotic cartilage.

cause quittor by producing a subcoronary abscess. Quittor can be secondary to a penetrating wound through the sole where infection has gained access to the collateral cartilage or to trauma of the cartilage resulting from wire cuts or bruises that damage the cartilage and reduce circulation in the area. Interfering may cause quittor by damaging a medial collateral cartilage.

Signs

The condition may occur over either the medial or lateral collateral cartilage. Swelling, heat, and pain over the coronary band, in the region of the affected collateral cartilage, and chronic suppurative sinus tracts that tend to heal and then break open at intervals characterize quittor. Lameness occurs in acute stages but may show remission when the lesion appears to be healing. Some sidebone may occur with the lesion, and permanent swelling usually results over the area of

the involved collateral cartilage. Permanent damage and deformity of the foot may result, causing persistent lameness.

Diagnosis

Enlargement over the affected collateral cartilage, characterized by one or more sinus tracts that show chronicity and recurrence, is diagnostic of quittor. It can be differentiated from shallow abscesses by using a probe. Drainage at the coronary band occurs with "gravel" (p. 370) and other foot infections; these should be differentiated from quittor.

Treatment

A few early cases of quittor will respond to irrigation of the tract with an escharotic agent, such as 20 percent silver nitrate, followed in ten minutes by saline injections that neutralize the silver nitrate. These injections may be repeated daily until all necrotic tissue is removed. A follow-up therapy to the above treatment is to apply an enzyme solution or ointment,* which aids in the removal of necrotic tissue. The lesion should be cleaned, shaved, and bandaged before and after therapy. Surgical removal of the necrotic cartilage may be necessary in long-standing cases; some veterinarians prefer surgical correction to routine treatment. A number of surgical procedures that are quite radical and involve sectioning of the coronary band have been recommended; however, I have found that elliptical incision over the sinus tract above the coronary band (Fig. 6–76), approximately 2″ to $2\frac{1}{2}$″ long and $\frac{1}{4}$″ to $\frac{1}{2}$″ above and parallel to the coronary band, facilitates removal of all necrotic tissue and cartilage. The advantages of this incision are shorter healing time and lack of involvement of the coronary band, which would result in cracks in the hoof

*Varidase, Lederle Laboratories; Elase Ointment, Parke, Davis Co.; Kymar Ointment, Armour Labs.

wall. The elliptical portion of skin should be removed, and all necrotic cartilage curetted out. Necrotic cartilage can be recognized by its dark blue color. All tracts should be followed to their end, and all involved tissues removed. A tourniquet is necessary to adequate visualization of the operative field. The incision should not be sutured but is bandaged with a topical antibiotic and later a poultice such as Denver Mud.*

Prognosis

The prognosis is guarded to unfavorable depending on the duration.

SPECIFIC REFERENCE

PROLIC, I. 1962. Treatment of quittor. Veterinaria (Sarajevo) 11: 27.

Sidebones

Definition

Sidebones, an ossification of the collateral cartilages, are usually found in the forefeet and are most common in horses having poor conformation. The condition is not common in Thoroughbreds.

Etiology

Concussion of the quarters of the foot causing trauma to cartilages is probably the cause of most cases. Some authorities believe that there is a hereditary predisposition, but this is probably through poor conformation. Horses that are base narrow are prone to develop lateral sidebone, while horses that are base wide are prone to develop medial sidebone. However, in both these conformations, sidebone may eventually develop in both cartilages.

Poor shoeing may cause increased concussion, resulting in sidebone. Shoeing with long heel calks for a prolonged pe-

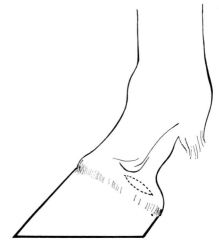

FIG. 6-76. The dotted lines show the site of a quittor operation for removal of necrotic cartilage.

riod may cause the condition by increasing concussion. Shoeing a horse off level may throw more stress on the inside or outside of the hoof wall, thereby increasing concussion to one of the cartilages. Such trauma can produce sidebone. Some cases of sidebone are produced by traumatic lesions, such as wire cuts that damage the cartilage.

Signs

Lameness may or may not be present. Lameness is often blamed on sidebones when they are not actually implicated. Lameness resulting from sidebones is rare, usually being present only when the cartilages are in the process of becoming ossified and when inflammation is present. Lameness may be evident when the horse turns, but seldom are the signs acute. Massive bone formation may cause mechanical interference with foot action.

If sidebones are a cause of lameness, there will be heat and pain over one or both of the cartilages. Careful examination of the cartilages will reveal that hardening is present. Pressure on the area will cause the horse to flinch if the cartilage is in the active stages of bone forma-

*Demco Corp., Denver, Colo.

tion. In some cases there will be a visible bulging of the quarters at the coronary band. Sidebone may accompany other lamenesses, such as navicular disease, and may be mistaken for the cause. Radiographs will reveal that the cartilages have partially or completely ossified (Fig. 6–77). After ossification stops, there usually are no signs of lameness, although the involved cartilages no longer function in the normal physiological processes of the foot (Chap. 2). Occasionally a sidebone is fractured, causing a small proximal fracture that can be surgically removed or a fracture through the third phalanx (Fig. 6–104).

Diagnosis

A diagnosis of sidebones as the cause of lameness should not be made unless pain and heat are present over the involved cartilage or cartilages. Radiological examination will reveal bone formation in the cartilages, but this does not

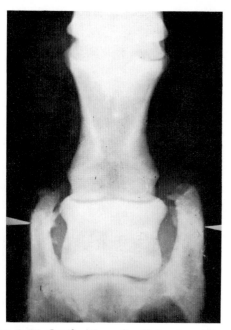

FIG. 6–77. Ossification of collateral cartilages of the third phalanx (sidebones).

necessarily mean that sidebones are the cause of lameness. Most cases of sidebones can be palpated, but again, their presence does not mean they are the cause of lameness. If sidebones are truly the cause of lameness, a volar nerve block above the fetlock on the affected side should relieve signs of lameness.

Treatment

If the sidebones are definitely the cause of lameness, the quarters may be grooved or thinned as prescribed for contracted foot (Fig. 9–18). This permits expansion of the foot and relieves the pain. The horse should be shod with full roller motion shoes (Chap. 9, p. 412) to decrease the action in the coffin joint area.

When fractured sidebones cause more acute signs of lameness, small proximal chips can be removed, but large fractures should not be surgically removed. If the fragment involves the proximal end of a sidebone, it can easily be removed by surgical incision over the area (Lundvall, 1965). The incision is made through skin and connective tissue down to the fragmented portion of bone. The fragment is dissected loose, and the subcutaneous tissue and skin are closed with sutures. A pressure bandage is kept in place for two weeks. One must not confuse proximal fractures of sidebones with separate ossification centers (Fig. 6–78). No attempt should be made to remove large proximal fragments, and when fractures of the third phalanx result, the foot should be immobilized in the third phalanx fracture shoe until healing has occurred (see the section on fracture of the third phalanx, p. 276, and Fig. 6–104).

Rest should be enforced until the inflammatory process resolves. The area commonly is fired or blistered, but these methods of treatment are probably of little, if any, value. In some cases where it is felt that a sidebone causes chronic and persistent lameness, a posterior digital neurectomy can be done on the affected side or sides.

Prognosis

The prognosis is guarded to favorable unless exostosis is extensive, in which case it is unfavorable.

SPECIFIC REFERENCE

LUNDVALL, R. L. 1965. Surgical removal of fractured sidebones. Proc. 11th Ann. AAEP.

Laminitis (Founder)

Definition

Laminitis is an inflammation of the laminae of the foot. It may be caused by either infectious or noninfectious agents and is characterized by passive congestion of the laminae with blood. Severe pain results from the inflammation caused by pressure on the sensitive laminae. Laminitis due to systemic causes may be acute or chronic and may involve two feet or all four; usually it affects both forefeet. Laminitis often results in changes in the hoof wall (founder) caused by inflammation in the coronary band. Changes in the third phalanx such as rotation and osteitis are common sequelae.

Laminae are classified as follows:

Dermal laminae. These laminae are formed from the corium or dermis. Their base is adherent to the third phalanx, and they contain blood vessels that nourish both the dermal and epidermal laminae. The epidermal laminae are nourished by diffusion.

Epidermal laminae. The hoof proper is a cornified epidermis, and the deeper layers of this cornified epidermis form the epidermal laminae. The epidermal lami-

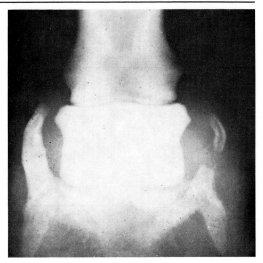

FIG. 6–78. Sidebones. On the left, note the large sidebone. On the right, note the separate ossification center in the sidebone. This should not be confused with fracture of a sidebone, which is sometimes surgically removed. This type of ossification does not require surgical removal.

nae intermesh directly with the dermal laminae.

There is some confusion in the use of the terms "sensitive" and "insensitive" laminae and "dermal" and "epidermal" laminae. The sensitive laminae and the dermal laminae are not synonymous. When the horny hoof is removed by maceration, the cornified and uncornified layers of the epidermis separate (Trautman and Febiger, 1962). The stratum germinativum is left on the dermal laminae, and these two tissues make up the sensitive laminae. Therefore, the insensitive laminae are composed of the layers of epidermis remaining, without the stratum germinativum of the epidermis.

Etiology

Laminitis is caused by numerous circumstances, not all of which are fully understood. Horses differ greatly in their susceptibility to laminitis, and some of this difference may be due to genetic factors. Laminitis may be induced by factors such as ingestion of grain or grazing on lush grass pastures, or it may follow infectious conditions, such as endometritis from membranes retained after parturition. Laminitis also occurs from completely unknown factors that may cause the third phalanx to rotate within three days and to protrude through the bottom of the sole within ten days. Since the etiology is not definite, numerous causes must be considered, such as organic toxins from feed, hormonal causes, bacterial endotoxins, histamine reaction, and lowering of the concentration of certain amino acids, such as methionine and cystine. Until experimental work can identify some etiological factors with certainty, the following etiological outline will be used. Laminitis may result from one of the following causes, but other circumstances not listed here may also produce laminitis.

Causes commonly recognized include

Laminitis Resulting from Ingestion of a Toxic Amount of Grain (Grain Founder). Grain founder is caused by ingestion of greater quantities of grain than can be tolerated by the horse. The amount varies, since a certain degree of tolerance develops in those horses accustomed to eating large quantities of grain. Signs of laminitis may occur suddenly in a horse that has been eating considerable quantities of grain as a daily ration, or the laminitis may result from accidental exposure of the horse to excessive amounts of grain, as when the horse gains access to open grain bins. This type of laminitis is associated with gastroenteritis, and the grains most commonly involved are wheat, corn, and barley. Ingestion of oats usually is not as serious, and signs of laminitis from overeating oats will be mild or may not appear at all. Many other grains and grain-based feeds are capable of causing the disease, including rabbit feed, chicken feed, and pig feed. Signs of laminitis do not usually appear until twelve to eighteen hours after ingestion of toxic amounts of grain, which often causes a delay in treatment. The toxin histidine, known to be formed in grain during digestion, is decarboxylated to histamine, which may cause the laminitis. This toxin is not present in cooked grain. The role of bacterial endotoxins is not known, and they may be a factor in the cause of this type of laminitis. Endotoxins have vasomotor influences and theoretically could be partially responsible for laminitis. Increased permeability of capillaries is another effect of endotoxins that could contribute to signs of laminitis.

Laminitis Due to Ingestion of Large Amounts of Cold Water (Water Founder). Ingestion of large amounts of cold water by an overheated horse is considered to be a cause of laminitis. Although the phenomenon is not fully understood, it may be due to gastroenteritis or possibly to histamine formation. Horses that are overheated should be allowed only small amounts of water until they have cooled.

Laminitis Due to Concussion (Road Founder). This type of laminitis is the result of concussion to the feet from hard work or fast work on a hard surface. Unconditioned animals are especially subject to this type of laminitis, as are those horses having thin walls and soles. This is a traumatic laminitis, and pedal osteitis and sole bruising will also result if the cause persists.

Laminitis Resulting from Endometritis or Severe Systemic Infections (Postparturient Laminitis). A mare may develop this type of laminitis shortly after foaling as a sequela of infection arising from retention of part of the fetal membranes or of a uterine infection without retention of fetal membranes. Always a serious form of laminitis, it also may occur as a sequel to severe pneumonia or other systemic infections.

Laminitis Resulting from Obesity and

Ingestion of Lush Grass Pasture (Grass Founder). Grass founder is common among horses grazed on summer grass pastures. Pastures containing clover and alfalfa apparently are more likely to cause the condition than grass pastures. However, cases resulting from grass pastures, usually lush pastures, have been recorded. Horses that develop grass founder usually are overweight, and affected horses have a heavy crest on the neck caused by fatty tissue. Shetland ponies, Welsh ponies, and fat horses of other breeds are especially subject to the disease. It appears that geldings are more susceptible than mares; however, this has not been proven statistically. The cause of this type of laminitis is unexplained. It is not uncommon for horses that previously have been affected with grass founder to show recurrence of laminitis in winter when fed legume hay. However, laminitis can occur in obese horses fed legume hay during the winter with no previous history of grass founder. Hormonal factors may be an etiologic agent in some cases, if the grasses or legumes contain estrogens. Such estrogens, if present, especially affect geldings, causing obesity. It could also be due to histamine release. Hypothyroidism has been considered a possible cause of this type of laminitis.

Miscellaneous Causes. Laminitis has been recorded in mares that had absolutely no exposure to any of the above causes. In some cases, these mares did not show estrus; once brought into heat, the laminitis ceased almost immediately. In other cases, mares that were in continuous estrus developed laminitis. It has been noted in a few cases that if this persistent heat was corrected, the laminitis ceased. It is possible that in some cases hormonal influences, other than those in grass founder, are an etiological factor. In these types of laminitis, permanent changes in the feet do not occur as rapidly as from other causes. There are other miscellaneous causes of laminitis, one of which is overeating of beet tops. It is common practice in some areas to turn horses into beet fields following harvest. It is not uncommon for these horses to develop "beet top founder." The pathogenesis is similar to that of grain founder.

Laminitis may be seen following viral respiratory disease or following administration of some drugs. Neither of these types of etiology has been proven. However, they are suspect, and research is necessary to determine if these causes are factual. In these cases, the overall wall changes are not as marked as they are in other types of laminitis. The sole shows extensive changes, and rotation of the third phalanx may occur within 72 hours. In some cases, portions of the sole slough out, exposing the third phalanx in as little as ten days. Some horses lose the hoof wall completely before typical laminitis rings are present. This begins as a crack at the coronary band, eventually extending completely around the hoof wall; the hoof wall loosens and comes off. Several weeks may elapse before slough of the hoof finally occurs.

Some horses showing this type of laminitis have a history of viral respiratory disease two to six weeks before onset of the laminitis. Study needs to be done to see if these viruses cause an endarteritis. Others have a history of having been wormed or having received large doses of corticoids or phenylbutazone derivatives. Whether these causes are valid is not truly known. Regardless of cause, this is one of the most severe and most difficult types of laminitis to treat.

Pathogenesis

Since the exact cause of laminitis has not yet been identified, one can only examine the end result. The factor or factors involved cause separation of the sensitive and insensitive laminae (see definition). The separation of the sensitive and insensitive laminae results from a passive congestion of this area. This would result in edema and separation of the laminae. No one has yet described the exact site of separation, so it is merely an assumption that it is at the junction of the sensitive and insensitive laminae (junction of the stratum germinativum and stratum corneum) rather than at the junction of the dermal and epidermal laminae (Trautman and Febiger, 1962) (see definition). Work on laminitis in lambs by Morrow et al. (1973) would tend to confirm this hypothesis. Larsson et al. (1956) theorized that the laminae separate because of the disappearance of the "onychogenic substance" in the deeper layers of the keratogenous zone in the lamellar region. Nils (1948) believed on the basis of his studies that, in the early stages of acute laminitis, histopathological changes occur only in the epidermis. Larsson et al. (1956) attribute this to a blocking of the metabolism of the sulfur-containing metabolites (methionine and cystine). However, it remains to be determined whether this blocking is an actual cause or whether it is the effect of a toxin, histamine, or of passive congestion. A logical question is why changes would occur only in the epidermal laminae without affecting the dermal laminae. The intimate adhesion between these structures and the fact that the sensitive laminae contain the vascular system that nourishes the insensitive laminae indicate that changes must occur in both structures. Whatever factors are involved—whether they are passive congestion, edema, or the work of toxins and/or histamine—once the laminae have separated, the pull of the deep flexor tendon, plus the weight on the phalanges, causes rotation of the third phalanx (Coffman, 1970). Rotation is also probably enhanced by pressure from the digital cushion below.

Once rotation of the third phalanx has occurred, it is of primary importance to correct it. Correction for rotation of the third phalanx should begin early in the course of the disease, because marked rotation can occur in as little as 72 hours. After rotation of the third phalanx is present, there is danger of penetration of the sole by the third phalanx.

It has been said (Coffman et al., 1970) that in the initial stages of laminitis there is a vasoconstriction. On this basis, it was theorized that laminar separation was due to lack of nourishment. However, experimental work by the author on vascular changes in acute laminitis has not confirmed this finding. Technical errors in studying the vascular bed in laminitis are frequent, and great caution must be used in interpreting radiographic findings using radiopaque material.

Demineralization of the third phalanx (pedal osteitis) may occur in chronic laminitis because of persistent inflammation of the foot.

Signs

Signs of laminitis from all causes are similar; therefore, they will be described here as acute and chronic. Signs for a specific type of etiology will be described in detail.

Acute Laminitis. Acute laminitis may affect both front feet or all four feet. If all four feet are affected, the horse tends to lie down for extended periods. When standing, the horse carries his hind feet well up under him and carries the forefeet caudally so that there is a very narrow base of support. Most commonly, only the two front feet are involved. In this case, the hind feet are carried well up under the body and the front feet are placed forward with the weight on the heel of the foot (Fig. 6–79). The horse shows great reluctance to move.

Radiological examination may show rotation of the third phalanx in as little as three days, and the toe of the third phalanx may protrude through the sole in as little as ten days.

Heat is present over the sole, the wall,

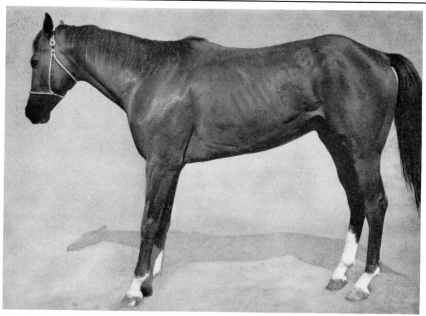

FIG. 6–79. Typical attitude of a horse with laminitis. The rear feet are carried up farther forward to help take more weight off the forefeet, which are extended anteriorly. This horse had laminitis following a respiratory infection. He was beginning to lose the hoof walls, as evidenced by cracking at the coronary band. Hoof wall changes were minimal, but the sole had dropped and the third phalanges were protruding through the soles of the forefeet.

and the coronary band. There is an increased digital pulse as palpated on the digital vessels over the fetlock joint. Many horses show anxiety, trembling of the musculature from severe pain, increased respiration, and variable elevation of temperature. The mucous membranes are injected as the result of toxemia. It is often difficult for the horse to lift one foot from the ground as he throws additional weight on the other affected foot or feet. If a person uses a hoof tester, a uniform tenderness will be noted over the entire area of the sole.

Signs of grain founder usually do not appear for twelve to eighteen hours after ingestion of the grain, often leading the owner to believe that the horse will not be affected. After this interval, however, laminitis, diarrhea, toxemia, muscular tremors and increased pulse and respiration appear, and there is a variable rise in temperature.

In mares suffering from laminitis re-sulting from metritis, the temperature will often be high (104° to 106°F), the mucous membranes will be injected, and considerable increase in pulse and respiration will be present. Uterine examination will reveal a dark watery fluid in variable quantities, and portions of the fetal membranes may be found.

Death may result from acute laminitis, but it is not common. In severe laminitis, the hoof may slough.

Chronic Laminitis. In chronic laminitis, rotation of the third phalanx will occur (Fig. 1–41, p. 28), as demonstrated by radiographs (Fig. 6–80). This rotation may cause the toe of the third phalanx to push out through the sole of the foot. Rotation of the third phalanx may be caused partially by the inflammation that causes some separation of the sensitive and insensitive laminae. The pull of the deep flexor tendon at its attachment on the semilunar crest of the third phalanx may also aid in displacement of the bone. Once

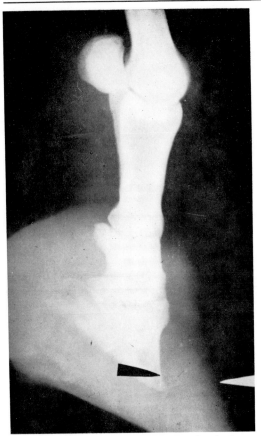

FIG. 6–80. Rotation of the third phalanx, caused by laminitis. Note the difference in distance between the anterior border of the third phalanx and the anterior aspect of the hoof wall, between the arrows, and the proximal areas of these two structures.

rotation of the phalanx has occurred, it cannot be returned to normal position without trimming the foot to make the distal border of the third phalanx parallel to the ground and using corrective shoeing or plastics to change the hoof shape (Fig. 6–83).

Horses suffering from chronic laminitis exhibit a tendency to land on the heel in an exaggerated motion. The sole is dropped and flat, showing excessive quantities of flaky material (Fig. 6–81). The hoof wall grows more rapidly than normal because of chronic inflammation, and the feet may develop a long toe that

curls up at the end (Fig. 6–82). Chronic laminitis causes heavy ring formation on the wall; these rings, usually present throughout the life of the horse, are caused by inflammation in the coronary band (Fig. 1–40, p. 27).

Once the horse has suffered an attack of laminitis, he seems more subject to recurrent attacks regardless of the etiology. Horses that develop grass founder one year may develop it in subsequent years and often are rendered useless by a second attack even if they recover from the first. They are also subject to laminitis if fed on legume hay.

"Seedy toe," resulting from separation of the sensitive and insensitive laminae, is usually present in chronic laminitis. Enough separation of the white line may occur to allow infection to penetrate the sensitive laminae (see Gravel, p. 370). An infection similar to thrush may invade the flaky sole in chronic laminitis and destroy all protection of the third phalanx.

When trimming the feet of a horse that has been affected with laminitis, it is easy to cause reddening and bleeding of the

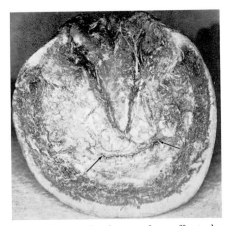

FIG. 6–81. Dropped sole on a foot affected with chronic laminitis. Note the excessive flaking of the sole, and the area, between the two arrows, that has broken through into the sensitive tissues. This type of crack often indicates impending protrusion of the third phalanx through the sole. The white line is widened and is affected with "seedy toe."

sole, because the vascularity of these areas increases with laminitis. This increased tendency toward hemorrhage remains for many months after an attack of laminitis.

Diagnosis

The observable signs make diagnosis of laminitis relatively easy. The typical attitude of the animal, the increased pulsation of the digital arteries, the heat in the foot, and the pain evidenced by hoof testers should furnish adequate proof of laminitis. Chronic laminitis shows characteristic changes in the foot and a typical gait. In some cases, the etiology is difficult to determine; occasionally, the cause is never determined.

Treatment

Grain Founder. In this type of laminitis, the treatment is directed at neutralizing the effects of the ingested grain and at controlling the laminitis. Since the signs of laminitis from this cause often do not appear for twelve to eighteen hours after ingestion of the grain, the treatment to clear the intestinal tract is used regardless of whether signs of laminitis have yet appeared. To clear the intestinal tract of the ingested grain, mineral oil is commonly used. Mineral oil acts as a bulk laxative and also coats the wall of the intestine, perhaps inhibiting absorption of toxins. Magnesium sulfate or sodium thiosulfate may be used instead of mineral oil as purgative drugs. Sodium thiosulfate may have some detoxifying action, as well as acting as a purgative in cases of overeating of grain. The two drugs work more rapidly than does mineral oil in most cases. Mineral oil can be repeated at four- to six-hour intervals until all grain has been removed from the intestinal tract. The mineral oil can be moved more rapidly through the intestinal tract by the use of peristaltic stimulant drugs, such as

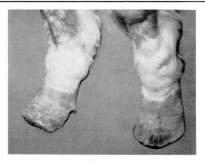

FIG. 6–82. Long curled feet affected by chronic laminitis. Due to chronic inflammation of the feet, the wall grows at a more rapid rate than normal. This often causes a curling of the toes, as shown.

carbachol. It is usually best not to use maximum doses of peristaltic stimulant drugs, but rather smaller doses repeated at intervals. Antihistamines are used to counteract the effects of histamine. Since bacterial endotoxins may play a part in causing laminitis, oral antibiotics are indicated. Oral neomycin* (10–20 gm) or nitrofurantoin† is commonly used once daily as an aid in preventing endotoxin production. Urmas (1968) has advocated the administration of methionine intravenously, giving 10 to 15 gm at intervals of 1 to 3 days. The larger doses of methionine may cause temporary intoxication and should be administered carefully. The dosage of methionine may be varied and given as 10 gm intravenously the first day followed by 10 to 15 gm orally for 10 to 15 days and 5 gm daily for an additional five days. In addition, sulfate ions are indicated because of the possibility of a total sulfate-ion reduction. Magnesium sulfate (20 mg per kg) or sodium thiosulfate (30 mg per kg) can be used intravenously for this purpose.

To aid in promoting venous blood flow, forced exercise of the horse is used. Whatever means required to make the horse walk are used. If pain is so severe the horse cannot move, the volar nerves

*Bisol, Upjohn Laboratories, Kalamazoo, Mich.
†Dantafur, Eaton Laboratories, Norwich, N.Y.

are blocked with local anesthetic. If possible, the horse should be walked for three hours a day, at one-hour intervals. In addition, hot-soaking of the feet is used to further promote circulation. Alternating ice-packing the feet and hot-soaking also may be of value. Hot-soaking the feet appears to be of more value than prolonged cold soaking. The increase in circulation may help remove toxic products and edema from the laminar area. Parenteral therapy with phenylbutazone or corticoids may be used to reduce inflammation in the feet. These are of most value in the acute phase of laminitis. Intravenous therapy with electrolytes and dextrose is used to aid in replacement of fluid and electrolyte loss resulting from diarrhea caused by the ingestion of the grain and the effects of laxatives used. Diuretics and 50 percent dextrose given intravenously may be helpful in reducing congestion in the feet. Prügelhof (1962) claims good results in treating acute laminitis using either forced exercise or a plaster-of-paris pad applied under a treatment shoe plate so that the sole has a firm support. He also advocates the use of 40 gm of sodium bicarbonate intravenously.

Prevention of rotation of the third phalanx is of primary importance in acute laminitis because of the difficulty in correcting rotation once it has occurred. In the early stages, lowering the heel, exercise, and standing the horse in sand are helpful. Once rotation has occurred, it is treated by corrective shoeing. Rotation of the third phalanx can occur within 72 hours, so immediate steps should be taken for prevention.

Water Founder. Mild purgation at repeated intervals, antihistamines, intramuscular blood, phenylbutazone, and corticoids parenterally are used to treat water founder. Cold-packing or hot-soaking of the feet also may be employed.

Postparturient Laminitis. In postparturient laminitis, the mare must be treated for metritis as well as for laminitis. If retained membranes are still present in the uterus, they should be removed manually and the uterus packed with antibiotics and/or sulfonamides. A drug, such as purified oxytocic principle (POP), 5 cc injected intramuscularly, may be used to constrict the uterus. The infection in the uterus should be treated parenterally with intravenous or intramuscular broad-spectrum antibiotics or intravenous sulfonamides. This therapy should be continued for at least three to five days. Antihistamines, phenylbutazone, or corticoids (Chap. 11) also are useful after the infection is under control. Local treatment of the feet, including forced exercise, as described for grain founder, should be used.

Grass Founder. In grass founder, there is probably no gastroenteritis present; however, the horse is often treated with purgation at repeated intervals. Antihistamines, phenylbutazone or corticoids, and diuretics are all used to treat this type of laminitis. The feet may be soaked in hot packs and the feed restricted to dry grass hay only. Forced exercise and measures to try to prevent rotation of the third phalanx are used as described above for grain founder. In a limited number of cases, it appears that testosterone used intramuscularly in fat geldings is necessary to counteract effects of possible estrogens in the forage in the pastures. A drastic reduction of food intake for the first 72 hours and limited diet for an indefinite period are necessary to aid in weight loss.

Iodinated casein and thyroid extract have been recommended for grass founder, on the theory that they increase metabolism and aid in reducing the weight of the horse. Obesity accompanies many cases of grass founder, but not all obese horses have laminitis. Iodinated casein does not give spectacular results but may be worthwhile in reducing weight. Thyroid subcutaneous implants (Cytobin*) or thyroid tablets (six to ten 5 grain tablets daily) in a small amount of grain can be used to increase the metabolism. In geldings this implant can be combined with the use of repositol testosterone (100 mg) at three-week intervals for three injections.

Coffman et al. (1966) claim good results in treating chronic laminitis in obese horses, such as caused by grass founder, with adrenocorticotropic hormone (ACTH), intravenous 50 percent dextrose, and intravenous amino acids with B-complex vitamins. This treatment was not effective in horses with normal SGOT and cholesterol levels. The regimen of treatment was as follows: Horses with SGOT levels of 400 Reitman-Frankel (RF) units or above were treated with 50 ml of 50 percent dextrose per 100 pounds body weight (up to 500 ml), IV protein hydrolysate (500 ml of a 5 percent solution) containing 10 ml vitamin B complex, and ACTH intramuscularly. Four hundred units of ACTH† were given on the first day of treatment, and two hundred units were given on the second, third, and fourth days. Intravenous therapy was continued for four to six days. Obese horses with SGOT levels of less than 400 RF units were treated with analgesics and a reducing diet. If the history revealed that the onset of laminitis occurred while the horse was on lush pastures, thyroid extract was given orally at the rate of 1,200 to 1,800 mg daily. Thyroid extract was given at those levels for 30 days, then gradually reduced to zero over a period of 60 days by giving 600 mg daily for 30 days, then 300 mg daily for 30 days.

For mares that develop laminitis accompanied by prolonged anestrus, it often is beneficial to infuse the uterus with 500 cc of sterile saline solution to bring them in estrus. In some cases, laminitis symptoms disappear with the onset of estrus. For mares that are in heat for prolonged periods with accompanying laminitis, repositol progesterone (500 mg), or other appropriate drugs, should be used intramuscularly.

Chronic Laminitis. Grooving the hoof wall by various methods, or rasping the quarters to thin the wall and provide expansion of the quarters, as described for contracted heels and laminitis in Chapter 9, page 412, is often of value if combined with corrective shoeing (p. 258). Neurectomies or alcohol block of the median or volar nerves are sometimes used to alleviate pain, but this should be discouraged because of the potential danger to a rider of the horse. Testosterone injections may be valuable in fat geldings affected with recurring chronic laminitis.

When infection is present in sensitive tissues as a result of a defect in the white line, the defect should be opened to allow drainage. The foot should be treated locally with tincture of iodine and the foot bandaged. Tetanus antitoxin should be administered. If the sole becomes infected with *Spheropherus necrophorus*, the sole should be thoroughly trimmed and treated locally with 10 percent sodium sulfapyridine solution and bandaged. Tetanus antitoxin should be administered.

When the sole of the foot has opened at the toe of the third phalanx, infection undermining the sole is usually extensive. Soaking the foot in sodium sulfapyridine (10 percent) solution is helpful in controlling the infection. The foot is then bandaged and the treatment repeated daily until the infection is overcome. Intravenous administration of sulfonamide mixtures containing sodium sulfapyridine is combined with local therapy.

Jenny et al. (1962) have described the use of foot trimming and plastics for correction of third phalanx rotation. The

---

*Smith Kline & French Laboratories, Philadelphia.
†Adrenomone, Armour-Baldwin Laboratories, Omaha, Neb.

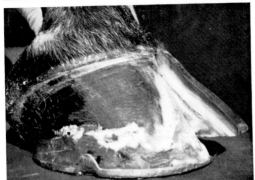

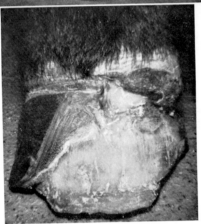

FIG. 6–83. *Above,* A foot affected with laminitis that has been cut in half, showing how the foot appears after shaping and shoeing, in comparison to the half that is untreated. *Below,* A foot affected by laminitis after reshaping and before plastic is applied. (From Jenny, 1962; courtesy of Dr. Jacques Jenny, Dr. Loren Evans, and AAEP.)

changed as much as possible to resemble a normal hoof, and the heel is lowered as far as possible to drop the distal border of the third phalanx. Hemorrhage is controlled, if encountered while trimming, by cauterization. The sole is thoroughly cleansed and trimmed. The foot is then

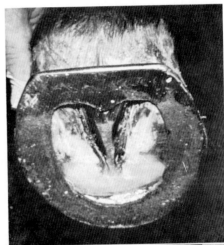

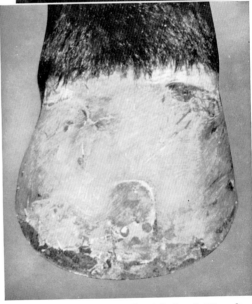

FIG. 6–84. Foot affected with laminitis after reshaping and application of a shoe with toe and quarter clips and plastic to reshape the foot. The clips on the shoe help the plastic to anchor it to the foot. (From Jenny, 1962; courtesy of Dr. Jacques Jenny, Dr. Loren Evans, and AAEP.)

fundamental principle of this treatment is to lower the heel so that the distal border of the third phalanx will parallel the surface of the ground when the foot is bearing weight. The changes in the hoof wall caused by chronic laminitis are corrected by trimming and rasping (Fig. 6–83). A shoe is then placed on the foot and held by means of the plastic and clips (Fig. 6–84). The front of the hoof wall is rasped down until, in some cases, one actually encounters blood at the toe. The junction of the normal and abnormal wall is undermined with a motorized burr to give an anchor to the plastic. The foot is painted with some of the plastic catalyst to facilitate adhesion. The plastic is then mixed with its catalyst and applied to the foot. The plastic incorporates a shoe that has toe and quarter clips on it to aid holding it to the foot. Plastic is also applied to the sole to protect the areas where dead sole has been removed. It is important to raise the toe with a layer of plastic to return the third phalanx to a more normal position (Fig. 6–85). The area is then covered with aluminum foil to facilitate shaping the plastic (Fig. 6–86).

This type of treatment is repeated approximately every six weeks until the foot resumes a more normal appearance and the third phalanx has begun to resume its normal position. This type of treatment must be done for as long as a year before the foot assumes a normal shape. Each time the plastic is reapplied, the foot is reshaped and the heel lowered to accomplish the desired results. Several kinds of plastics are available: Hoof repair material* is available, but the cost is prohibitive for most horses. The advantages of this plastic are that it is available in two consistencies, one approaching the consistency of the frog and another, that of

*H. D. Justi Co., Philadelphia.

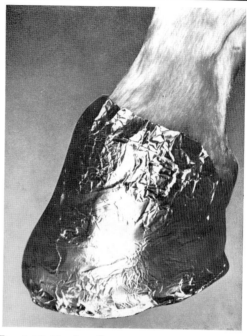

FIG. 6–86. Hoof wall wrapped in aluminum foil to aid in holding and shaping the plastic while it hardens. (From Jenny, 1962; courtesy of Dr. Jacques Jenny, Dr. Loren Evans, and AAEP.)

the wall; it also sets up quite rapidly. Ordinary fiber glass can be used at a much more reasonable cost, but good results are not as consistent. Fiber glass is available in a powdered form and adding extra

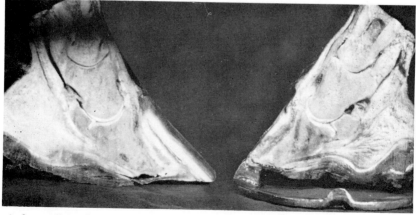

FIG. 6–85. A foot affected with laminitis cut in half. The left half shows appearance before reshaping and plastic application. The right half shows the same foot after reshaping, plastic and shoe application. Note raised toe and realignment of third phalanx with the hoof wall. (Courtesy of Dr. Jacques Jenny.)

catalyst can force it to harden more rapidly. When using fiber glass, one should mix the catalyst with the fiber glass before the hoof wall is prepared because it takes longer to set. It also dries to a harder consistency, but is satisfactory.

The disadvantages of a plastic repair of the foot in laminitis include destruction of underlying tissues from heat generated by polymerization of the material, the radical deformation of the foot in preparation for plastic repair, and the high cost of repair due to cost of materials and time spent in repair. Polymerization of plastic materials of this type may generate temperatures as high as 280° F. These high temperatures destroy underlying hoof wall and sole tissue, and infection of the foot may result. This is highly undesirable and may necessitate destruction of the horse. Any plastic repair of the foot should be watched closely for any sign of increased lameness and for draining tracts at the coronary band. The appearance of any ill effects from plastic repair necessitates immediate removal of the plastic material. The foot is then deformed enough from the repair that corrective shoeing cannot be used. This has led the author to use corrective shoeing.

Corrective shoeing can accomplish the objectives of plastic hoof repair at lower cost and with more safety. The objective of either plastic repair or corrective shoeing is to prevent or correct rotation of the third phalanx, and at the same time protect the bottom of the foot from pain of pressure. Rotation begins in a very short time in some types of laminitis and may be present in as short a time as 72 hours. Corrective shoeing should be begun as soon as possible if the acute case of laminitis does not show definite signs of improvement within 72 hours. Once the third phalanx has rotated, there is a tendency for the bone to come through the sole of the foot.

The correction used for rotation of the third phalanx is as follows:

1. Rasp all excess horn tissue from the toe of the foot to re-establish a normal relationship between the hoof wall and the dorsal border of the first phalanx (Fig. 6–87).

2. Trim the foot so that the heels are as low as possible in order to make the solar surface of the third phalanx parallel the ground.

3. Apply a wide web shoe with a wedge

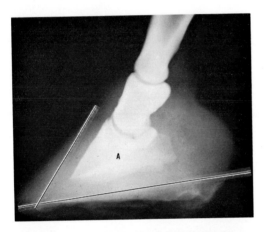

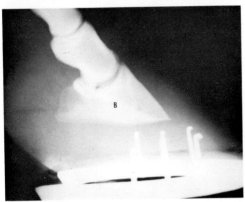

FIG. 6–87. Corrective shoeing for chronic laminitis. A, Radiograph of affected foot before corrective shoeing. Lines show desired correction of foot. B, Same foot after shoeing. Notice that the bottom of the third phalanx is more nearly parallel to the ground surface. Treatment used was: (1) Rasp off front of hoof wall; (2) trim heel down as far as possible; (3) place leather or plastic shim under toe of shoe to raise toe; (4) place silicone rubber and full plastic pad under shoe.

of leather or plastic* between the shoe and the toe of the hoof to further increase the effect of low heels so that the third phalanx will more nearly parallel the ground. A wide full bar (1½″ wide) is also helpful. In addition, during the more painful stages of laminitis, a pad of silicone rubber† or retread rubber can be applied as a pad to the foot. These rubber pads are covered with a hard plastic pad to hold them in place. This rubber padding eases pain from concussion, and the shoeing helps to prevent or correct third phalanx rotation. The shoe should be changed every four to six weeks, and the rubber pad can be left off when the painful phase has disappeared. Continual shoeing in the manner described may return the third phalanx to a normal position within one year. The shoeing must be done accurately and by one skilled in the profession. Failure to follow through with continual shoeing of this type will result in failure. Some cases will not respond because of infection, persistent laminitis, or recurring attacks of laminitis. The systemic effects of laminitis must be overcome before mechanical management of the foot will be effective.

Prognosis

The prognosis is always guarded in any case of laminitis. If the symptoms continue for more than ten days, the prognosis is unfavorable. However, some cases, such as those that seem to be associated with hormonal imbalances, may continue for prolonged periods without causing excessive changes in the foot, such as rings on the wall and rotation of the third phalanx. Some cases of laminitis continue for a long period and then disappear, leaving the feet distorted. The third phalanx often is rotated when viewed on radiographs (Figs. 6–80 and 6–87). Whenever

*Technovit, Kulzer & Co., Hamburg, West Germany.

†Hoof Cushion, Miller Harness Co., New York.

rotation of the phalanx has occurred, the prognosis is unfavorable. Occasionally, infection will enter the pododerm of the foot as the result of separation at the white line (seedy toe) caused by disunion of the sensitive and nonsensitive laminae; it may also enter through the sole. Any infection makes the prognosis unfavorable. If cracks appear in the coronary band, the hoof is likely to slough, making the prognosis more unfavorable.

SPECIFIC REFERENCES

ADAMS, O. R. 1972. Vascular changes in experimental laminitis. Proc. AAEP.

AKERBLOM, E. 1937. The etiology of laminitis. Aust. Vet. J. 13: 254.

BACKUS, W. O. 1937. Lameness in the horse with special reference to acute laminitis. JAVMA 91: 64.

BAIRD, J. 1933. Laminitis. JAVMA 83: 44.

BRITTON, J. W. 1959. Spontaneous chronic equine laminitis. Calif. Vet. 15: 17.

CHAVANCE, J. 1946. Histamine theory and treatment of laminitis. Vet. Med. 41: 199.

COFFMAN, J. R., et al. 1970. Hoof circulation in equine laminitis. JAVMA 156(1): 76–83.

COFFMAN, J. R. 1970. Biomechanics of pedal rotation in equine laminitis. JAVMA 156(2): 219–221.

COFFMAN, J. R., and J. H. JOHNSON. 1969. Management of chronic laminitis. JAVMA 155(1): 45–49.

COFFMAN, J. R., et al. 1966. The chronic laminitis-fatty liver syndrome. Proc. AAEP, 275–281.

COFFMAN, J. R., and H. E. GARNER. 1972. Acute laminitis. JAVMA 161(11): 1280.

GIBBONS, W. J. 1964. Chronic founder in ponies. Mod. Vet. Pract. 45(10): 86.

GROSS, D. R. 1961. Treatment of laminitis. Mod. Vet. Pract. 42: 58.

HALLET, C. S. 1936. Laminitis in horses. Vet. Med. 31: 339.

JENNY, J. 1962. Mechanical treatment of laminitis. Proc. 8th Ann. AAEP, 212.

KOCHAN, W. F. 1948. Antihistamine treatment of laminitis. Vet. Med. 43: 478.

LARSSON, B., et al. 1956. On the biochemistry of keratinization in the matrix of horses' hoof in normal conditions and in laminitis. Nord. Vet. Med. 8: 761–776.

LAWSON, M. R. 1958. Acute laminitis in the horse. Vet. Rec. 66: 615.

LUNDVALL, R. L. 1971. Diagnosis and treatment of laminitis. Biochem. Rev. (Fort Dodge) 33(1): 3–7.

MACLEAN, C. W. 1970a. A post mortem x-ray study of laminitis in barley beef animals. Vet. Rec. 86: 457–462.

MACLEAN, C. W. 1970. The hematology of bovine laminitis. Vet. Rec. 86: 710–714.

MARTIN, W. J.: 1916. Equine laminitis. Amer. J. Vet. Med. 11: 297.

MERILLAT, L. A. 1920. The treatment of acute laminitis. Amer. J. Vet. Med. 15: 535.

MOORE, R. C. 1916. Equine laminitis or pododermatitis. Amer. J. Vet. Med. 11: 281.

MORROW, L. L., et al. 1973. Laminitis in lambs injected with lactic acid. Amer. J. Vet. Res. 34(10): 1305–1307.

NILS, O. 1948. Studies on the Histopathology of Acute Laminitis. Uppsala: Almquist & Wiksells. Boktrycekeri Ab.

NILSSON, S. A. 1963. Clinical, morphological, and experimental studies of laminitis in cattle. Acta Vet. Scand. 4 (Suppl. 1).

PRÜGELHOF, F. 1962. Über die Hufrehe des Pferdes. Wein Tieraertzl. Mschr. 49(7): 589.

ROBERTS, W. D. 1964. The treatment of laminitis by intra-arterial infusion of adrenocorticoid steroids. Proc. 10th Ann. AAEP, 241.

RODEBAUGH, H. D. 1938. Surgical treatment of chronic laminitis. Vet. Med. 33: 288.

SELBY, O. C.: 1909. Acute laminitis. Amer. Vet. Rev. 35: 433.

STUMP, J. E. 1967. Anatomy of the normal equine foot, including microscopic features of the laminar region. JAVMA 151(12): 1588.

SULLIVAN, M. W. 1938. A complicated case of acute laminitis. JAVMA 93: 394.

THOMAS, E. F. 1945. Autogenous blood therapy in laminitis. N. Amer. Vet. 26: 278.

TRAUTMAN, A., and J. Febiger. 1962. Histology of Domestic Animals. Ithaca, N.Y.: Comstock Publishing Associates.

URMAS, PEKKA. 1968. Finsk Vet., Tidskr. '74: 11–20.

Navicular Disease (Navicular Bursitis, Podotrochleitis)

Definition

Navicular disease begins as bursitis of the navicular bursa between the deep flexor tendon and the navicular bone (Fig. 2–3, p. 36, and Fig. 6–88). As the disease progresses, degenerative and erosive lesions of the fibrocartilage begin on the tendinous surface of the bone. The degenerate fibrocartilage becomes frayed and pitted near the sagittal ridge. The articular surface of the navicular bone is affected occasionally. Pathological changes are usually confined to the tendinous surface of the bone, the bone substance, and the adjacent tendon of the deep flexor. Fibrils of the tendon are torn adjacent to the distal edge of the navicular bone. The surface of the tendon is progressively destroyed and may eventually rupture spontaneously, especially after neurectomy. Adhesions of the tendon to the navicular bone may begin early, before extensive radiographic changes are shown. As the disease advances, the bone becomes hyperemic, and rarefaction (osteoporosis) occurs. Rarely, fracture of the bone will occur. In advanced cases, calcification of the suspensory ligament of the navicular bone occurs, as well as extensive rarefaction of the navicular bone. That part of the navicular bone articulating with the coffin joint is occasionally involved, leading to arthritis of the coffin joint. Wintzer (1965a) describes changes in the distal ligament of the navicular bone and says pain is due to these changes.

This is an insidious disease that shows improvement upon rest in the early stages but reappears when the horse is put back into training. Navicular disease affects only the front feet, so no description is available of the disease in the hind feet. It is one of the most important causes of lameness in horses.

Etiology

Navicular disease has been described as an inheritable disease resulting from upright conformation and a weak navicular bone. Concussion also is a definite factor in the etiology. Horses that do hard work, such as racing, cutting, calf-roping, and barrel-racing, are especially subject to the disease. If the work is performed on rough or hard surfaces, concussion is greatly increased, so the likelihood of disease is greater. Upright conformation definitely increases concussion to the navicular area. The navicular bone transmits a portion of the weight, as distributed through the second phalanx, to the third phalanx. In doing this, the bone is forced posteriorly against the deep flexor tendon. An even greater pressure against the tendon occurs as the body weight passes over the foot during motion. The pressure of the navicular bone against the tendon may be an exciting factor in beginning bursitis. The small foot characteristic of some horses, which has been promoted by selective breeding, may be a factor in increasing concussion. The small foot does not have as large an area over which to distribute concussion and weight; thus, pressure per unit area is increased.

Pressure of the deep flexor tendon against the navicular bone is commonly increased by improper trimming and shoeing (see Fig. 1–23, p. 16). It is common to trim the heel too low on a horse that has upright pasterns. This breaks the pastern and foot axes and produces greater pressure of the deep flexor tendon against the navicular bone.

The hind limbs are not involved in navicular disease, unless caused by puncture wounds, because they are primarily the propelling agents, and the forelimbs receive most of the shock. Puncture wounds of the navicular bursa can cause the disease, but this usually is a suppurative condition and so will not be considered in this discussion. Senile decay of the bone may occur in some horses that have been used heavily for a period of years. In such a case, demineralization of the bone occurs as the result of chronic bursitis. Defective or irregular blood supply to the navicular bone also has been described as a cause. This could be brought about by hard work followed by prolonged periods of rest, at which time the blood supply to the bone may be reduced, causing gradual necrosis of the bone. The hyperemia that occurs with the bursitis of navicular disease is generally

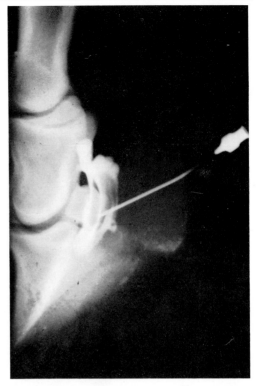

FIG. 6–88. An eighteen-gauge needle in position in the navicular bursa. A small amount of radiopaque material has been injected to outline the bursa, as shown.

blamed for the decalcification (osteoporosis) of the navicular bone.

Signs

The affected horse often has a history of intermittent lameness that decreases when he is rested. The lameness of the horse may be noticeably worse the morning after heavy work. In the early stages of the disease, rest will produce remission of the clinical signs, suggesting that the horse is cured, but as soon as hard work is begun, signs of the disease reappear.

Both front feet usually are involved in navicular disease; however, one foot often shows more lameness than the other, and it may not be until a nerve block has been used on that foot that it is noticeable that lameness also is present in the opposite forefoot. If both feet are painful, the horse often points alternately with one foot and then the other, or stands with both feet too far in front (camped in front). If only one foot is involved, or if one foot is more severely involved than the other, the horse points with the more severely affected foot.

During movement, the horse tends to land on the toe of the foot to avoid concussion to the heel area. The navicular bone underlies the middle third of the frog, so the horse attempts to prevent pressure on this area. The attempt to protect the heel area hinders a roping horse in stopping and slows a race horse by shortening the anterior phase of the stride; it may also predispose to fetlock injury.

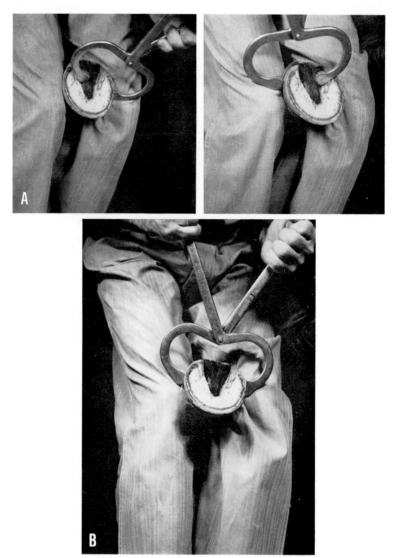

FIG. 6–89. A, Using hoof testers to check the medial and lateral sides of the center third of the frog for navicular disease. Sensitivity in this area should be checked against other feet to help determine the amount of pain that is present. B, Using hoof testers to check the ends of the navicular bone. This test is less reliable than the test of the center third of the frog. Reaction here should be compared with reaction in other feet that are sound.

The effort that the horse makes to land on the toe is most noticeable in the walk and trot and causes a shortened anterior phase of the stride. The toe may show signs of being excessively worn, and the horse may stumble in the walk or trot because of the tendency to land on the toe. Increased lameness will be evident if the horse is on irregular ground because of frog pressure caused by irregularities of the ground. Increased lameness also will be noted when the horse is turned in the direction of the affected foot or feet. Examination of the foot with a hoof tester will pinpoint the pain at the center third of the frog and to a lesser extent over the ends of the navicular bone (Fig. 6–89). Normal horses will show some variation in reaction to the hoof tester over the ends of the navicular bone and over the center third of the frog. The lame foot should be compared with the opposite forefoot, if it is sound, and, if not, compared with the reaction of the rear feet.

It is not uncommon for a horse with navicular disease to develop bruising of the sole at the toe. This may be misleading in examination, both clinically and with a hoof tester. If the bruising of the sole at the toe is severe enough, the horse will begin to walk back on the heel, a situation similar to that seen in laminitis. With a hoof tester there is considerable sensitivity in the bruised area. Peeling the sole with a hoof knife will show increased vascularity of the sole. One must be careful not to allow this to confuse the diagnosis. If pain is shown over the center third of the frog, the horse shows some improvement following blocking of the posterior digital nerve, and if radiographs aid in positive identification of navicular disease, the condition should be treated as navicular disease. Sole bruising will disappear after several months as the horse begins to use a more normal gait. Early cases of bilateral low ringbone may cause signs similar to those of navicular disease, but typical findings on hoof tester examination and relief of lameness by posterior digital nerve block are not obtained.

The shuffling gait exhibited in navicular disease often causes the owner to believe his horse is lame in the shoulders. The shortened anterior phase of the stride causes a very disagreeable ride, and to the inexperienced observer, the horse appears to be favoring the shoulder areas.

Arthritis of the coffin joint may be caused by changes in the navicular bone that extend to the articular surface of the distal interphalangeal (coffin) joint.

Over a period of time, the foot gradually changes shape. The effort to avoid frog pressure causes the heels to contract and to rise. The sole becomes more concave both anterior to posterior and medial to lateral, and the foot narrows across the quarters. If the navicular disease is unilateral, the foot will become smaller due to contraction (Fig. 6–90). Fetlock injury, such as osselets, may be present at the same time, because upright conformation of the pasterns predisposes to both diseases.

Radiological examination of the navicular bone reveals changes in less than half of the early cases. Some authors claim that navicular disease is not present if

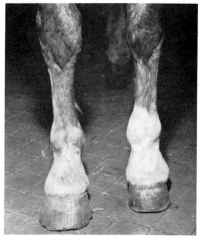

FIG. 6–90. Contracted left foot resulting from chronic navicular disease.

radiological changes are not evident, but this cannot be true, for such changes are evident only after the condition has become well established. Radiological changes occur in the form of osteoporosis, exostosis, enlarged vascular channels, narrowing of the articular space, sclerosis, and osteolysis (Figs. 6–91, 6–92 and 6–93).

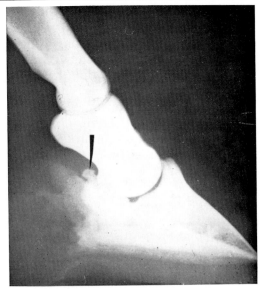

FIG. 6–93. Calcification of the navicular suspensory ligament in a long-standing case of navicular disease.

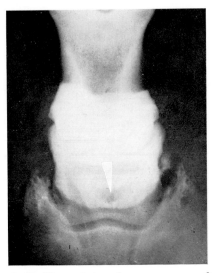

FIG. 6–91. The pointer shows an area of demineralization in the center of the navicular bone. Changes of this type indicate a long-standing case of navicular disease.

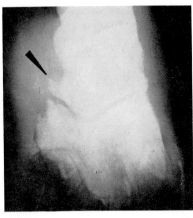

FIG. 6–92. The pointer shows a spur on the end of the navicular bone, in an oblique view of the bone. This spur indicates a long-standing case of navicular disease and is the result of calcification in the suspensory ligament of the navicular bone.

These changes indicate a well-advanced case. Radiological changes often can be demonstrated in the navicular bone after it has been removed and all extraneous tissues scraped away. This, however, is of no value in diagnosis of the disease. Technically high-quality radiographs are necessary for identification of the disease if changes are to be shown. Adhesion of the deep flexor tendon to the navicular bone can occur before extensive radiographic changes are present.

Changes in the navicular bone and bursa found at necropsy are erosions of the cartilage of the bone, discoloration of the tendon and bone, fibrous adhesions between the deep flexor tendon and the bone, osteoporosis, exostosis of the bone, enlargement of the nutrient foramina of the bone, changes in the articular surface, and, in some cases, fracture of the navicular bone.

Diagnosis

Signs of lameness are reasonably characteristic, and one should watch closely to see if the toe lands before the heel and if the anterior phase of the stride is short. Other signs that are very helpful are the reactions of the horse to a hoof tester applied to the center third of the frog. Considerable pressure must be put on this area, since the foot takes great pressure when the foot is put down. A good set of hoof testers will cause the horse to flinch when pressure is applied over the center third of the frog (Fig. 6–89). However, this reaction should be compared with the reaction of the hind feet or the opposite forefoot, if sound. One should keep in mind that in most cases there is at least some degree of involvement in the opposite forefoot. Sole bruising from constant landing on the toe is a factor that should be kept in mind in using hoof testers. Pain may be shown over the toe area of the sole in chronic navicular disease. As mentioned previously, this pain may be so severe as to force the horse to walk back on the heel. Radiographs, blocking the posterior digital nerve, and good judgment will aid in deciding whether sole bruising is primary or secondary.

In a small number of cases, changes in the navicular bone are shown radiographically when there are no signs of navicular disease lameness. This must be kept in mind in diagnosis of other types of lameness.

Blocking of the posterior digital nerves can be an aid in diagnosis. The landmark for blocking these nerves is located between the posterior edge of the first phalanx and the anterior edge of the superficial flexor tendon. The nerve lies closer to the edge of the tendon than to the first phalanx and runs parallel to the edge of the deep flexor tendon. A small amount (1 to 2 cc) of 2 percent lidocaine hydrochloride* should be placed over the area of the nerve on the medial and lateral sides, about one third of the way between the fetlock and the coronary band. A 25-

gauge $\frac{5}{8}''$ needle should be used to deposit the local anesthetic over the nerves, and the horse should be twitched to facilitate the nerve block. After allowing five to ten minutes for the block to take effect, the horse should tend to show improvement if affected by navicular disease. This nerve block also is an indication of the amount of relief that can be obtained from posterior digital neurectomy.

When doing a posterior digital nerve block for diagnostic purposes, one can expect approximately the same relief from a posterior digital neurectomy as obtained from using a small amount (1 to $1\frac{1}{2}$ cc) of a local anesthetic over the posterior digital nerve. If there is only a partial response to this block, one can expect that whatever lameness is evident after the posterior digital nerve block will still be present after a posterior digital neurectomy. There are several reasons that a horse with navicular disease may not respond completely to a posterior digital nerve block.

Fibrous Adhesions between the Navicular Bone and the Deep Flexor Tendon. When adhesions are present between the deep flexor tendon and the navicular bone, it is nearly impossible for the horse to modify his gait. The gait will improve slightly after posterior digital nerve block because of some pain relief, but the foot will still hit toe first with a short anterior stride. This is a mechanical interference to the gait and cannot be modified by nerve block.

Possible Arthritis of the Coffin Joint. In severe cases of navicular disease, the changes in the navicular bone may extend into the coffin joint. In this case, there is a coffin joint arthritis present, and posterior digital neurectomy will give only partial relief to the lameness. One can then put a local anesthetic into the coffin joint as described on page 451 to desensitize the coffin joint. If complete relief of the lameness is obtained, it is reasonably certain that there is arthritis in the coffin joint.

---

*Xylocaine, Astra Laboratories, Scotia, N.Y.

This means that a posterior digital neurectomy would be only partially successful for treatment, since the coffin joint would still be painful.

Accessory Nerve Supply from the Anterior Digital Nerve or from the Posterior Digital Nerve (Fig. 2-7). Sometimes the accessory branches from the posterior digital nerve will be separate enough from the main posterior digital nerve to escape blocking by a differential diagnostic block. In other cases, the anterior digital nerve will bifurcate and send a posterior branch back to the navicular area. In either case, this accessory nerve supply will be responsible for only a partial response to the posterior digital nerve block. Unless all nerve supply is severed to the navicular area, there will be poor response to the posterior digital neurectomy. Accessory branches of the posterior digital nerve can usually be found during surgery, but a posterior branch from a bifurcation of the anterior digital nerve must be searched out (Fig. 2-7). In racing horses, the anterior digital nerve should not be cut.

Sole Bruising. In severe cases of navicular disease, the horse bruises the soles in the toe areas from landing on the toe. In this case, the hoof tester examination should reveal pain over the toe area of the sole, and this should be taken into consideration when doing posterior digital neurectomy. The lameness caused by the sole bruising at the toe will still be present after the posterior digital nerve block.

Concurrent Traumatic Arthritis of the Fetlock. Pasterns that are too straight also predispose to traumatic arthritis (osselets) of the metacarpophalangeal (fetlock) joint. Navicular disease and traumatic arthritis of the metacarpophalangeal joint may both be present at the same time. Injection of the volar pouch of the metacarpophalangeal joint with local anesthetic after blocking the posterior digital nerves will reveal how much lameness is due to each condition.

Improper or Incomplete Anesthesia.

Skin sensation can be checked medially and laterally on the same foot, and one foot can be compared to the other. A hoof tester may also be used, and if sensation is still evident over the center third of the frog, the anesthesia is inadequate. In this case, the block should be repeated after confirming the landmarks.

Local anesthesia of a navicular bursa can be accomplished by injecting it with 2 percent lidocaine hydrochloride. A topical anesthetic of some type must be used to produce local anesthesia in this area. Only 5 cc should be used, since the fluid of the bursa may be diffused to other areas by osmosis. The procedure for injecting the navicular bursa is as follows:

The fossa of the heel should be shaved and prepared with skin antiseptics for passage of an 18-gauge 2″ needle into the navicular bursa. A small area of skin $\frac{1}{2}$″ in diameter should be blocked with 2 percent lidocaine hydrochloride using a 25-gauge $\frac{5}{8}$″ needle between the heels (Fig. 11-8, p. 452). The foot should be placed on a wooden block and an 18-gauge 2″ needle passed through the skin at the anesthetized fossa of the heel in a line paralleling the angle of the coronary band (Fig. 11-9, p. 452). When the needle encounters bony tissue, it is in the navicular bursa (Figs. 11-10 and 11-11, p. 453). The digital cushion seems to be relatively insensitive, so the horse usually offers no resistance to passage of the needle, even without deep injection of a local anesthetic. Once the needle is in the bursa, 5 cc of 2 percent lidocaine hydrochloride should be injected. If the needle is not in the bursa, difficulty will be encountered in trying to inject the fluid. One can feel the bursa fill with fluid; when it is tense, injection should be stopped. The suspected area of foot pathology must be well localized before this type of block is used, because the spread of the local anesthetic fluid will block some third phalanx fractures or possibly other foot pathology. If extensive adhesions between the deep flexor tendon and the navicular bone are present, this block is ineffective.

Following nerve block of the posterior digital nerves, or injection of the navicular bursa with a local anesthetic, the horse should be checked to see if there is improvement of the gait. Improvement signifies that navicular disease is present, if other lamenesses have been ruled out. This improvement is gradual, so the horse should be worked for ten to twenty minutes to achieve the best diagnostic results. If only partial improvement is noted, coffin joint arthritis as a complicating factor, and accessory nerve supply from the anterior digital nerve should be considered. If extensive adhesions are present between the deep flexor tendon and the navicular bone, the horse cannot show a normal gait, since the short anterior stride is mechanical. Radiographs are helpful in diagnosis of some cases of navicular disease (Figs. 6–91 and 6–92), but since most early cases are not advanced enough to show changes, negative findings are not significant. The best diagnostic radiographs are taken through water to eliminate lines from the sulci of the frog (Figs. 6–94 through 6–98).

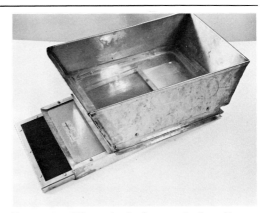

FIG. 6–95. Water bath for navicular disease radiography showing grid and cassette in place underneath container of water. (Courtesy of Dr. J. Lebel.)

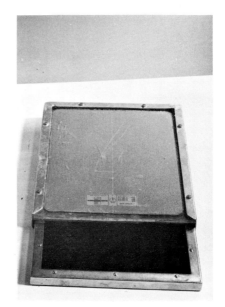

FIG. 6–96. Grid and cassette holder from water bath. (Courtesy of Dr. J. Lebel.)

Differential Diagnosis

Differential diagnosis should include puncture wounds of the sole and frog, fractured navicular bone, fractured third phalanx, laminitis, sole bruising, corns, pedal osteitis, and ringbone. Careful physical examination and radiographs can quickly narrow the considerations. In laminitis, the action of the shoulders is

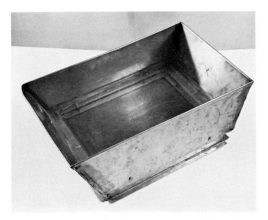

FIG. 6–94. Water bath set complete for taking radiographs in navicular disease. The box is metal with a watertight plexiglass bottom. (Courtesy of Dr. J. Lebel.)

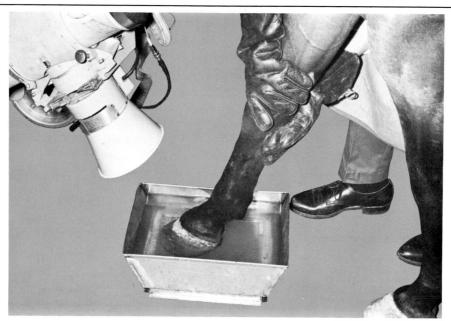

FIG. 6-97. Water bath in use with x-ray grid and cassette underneath. Radiograph being taken. (Courtesy of Dr. J. Lebel.)

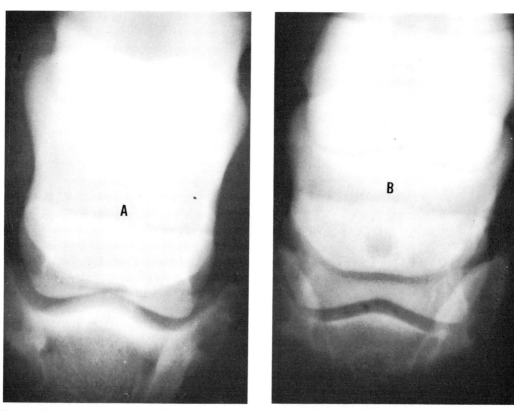

FIG. 6-98. Comparison radiographs of navicular bone on the same horse showing view without water bath (*A*) and with water bath (*B*). This comparison shows the importance of this technique in diagnosis of navicular disease. (Courtesy of Dr. J. Lebel.)

similar to that in bilateral navicular disease, but the foot lands on the heel and not the toe. Navicular disease is the most common of this group of lamenesses. Osteoarthritis of the distal interphalangeal joints can cause similar signs but can be differentiated on hoof tester, nerve block, and radiographic examinations.

If complicating coffin joint arthritis is present, it can be determined by local anesthesia of this joint (see p. 265). When accessory nerve supply is present from the anterior digital nerve (see p. 266), it can be blocked by a ring block. This type of accessory nerve supply will render posterior digital neurectomy only partially effective.

Treatment

Injection of the navicular bursa with a corticoid can be done in the same manner as an injection of a local anesthetic. Intrabursal corticoids give temporary relief, but are of little value as a permanent cure. Injection of the navicular bursa with irritants, such as Lugol's iodine, has been described in some of the older literature. This is not now recommended since it causes the horse pain but seldom effects a cure. Such injections are nearly impossible if adhesions are already present. Treatment with x-ray therapy has not given consistent results. Bilateral posterior digital neurectomy is the only method of achieving any degree of permanent relief. Corrective shoeing may relieve symptoms temporarily, but posterior digital neurectomy usually has to be done eventually. Complications of posterior digital neurectomy are as follows:

Neuroma Formation. All severed nerve endings develop neuromas. It is the painful neuroma that causes a problem. The cause of painful neuromas is not definitely known. However, irritation of the nerve produced by injection of local anesthetic and trauma during surgery may be contributing causes. Exercising the horse too soon after surgery may be an additional irritant. In the experience of the author, the following are helpful in avoiding some of the causes of neuroma.

a. Inject the posterior digital nerve at the level of the proximal sesamoid bone for the neurectomy. This will block both the anterior and posterior digital nerves but will keep the irritation of the local anesthetic away from the surgical site.

b. Incise the tissues cleanly with a knife and avoid trauma to the subcutaneous tissues and deep fascia as much as possible.

c. Stretch the nerve slightly before it is cut and incise it with a clean guillotine cut. This allows the cut end to retract proximally for a short distance. Epineural capping is more effective than transection in preventing painful neuromas. Ligation of the distal nerve end is recommended.

d. Keep a pressure bandage on the wound until it is completely healed.

e. Postoperative injections of butazolidin and/or corticoids parenterally are probably helpful in preventing inflammation at the surgical site.

f. Wait at least six weeks before returning the horse to active use. If painful neuromas appear to be developing following neurectomy, local injection of 0.5 cc of a corticoid into each surgical site every three days, accompanied by parenteral injections of a corticoid or phenylbutazone and poulticing of the wound area, may be helpful in preventing their further development.

Rupture of the Deep Digital Flexor Tendon. This occurs when posterior digital neurectomy has been done and the deep flexor tendon is weakened by degeneration and is attached to the navicular bone by fibrous adhesions. As soon as the horse starts using the foot in a normal fashion, these adhesions are torn, and the weak necrotic deep digital flexor tendon ruptures. This may not occur for several weeks following the surgery. It is recognized by the fact that the toe of the foot is raised from the ground on weight-bearing. There is no treatment.

Loss of the Hoof Wall. When a posterior digital neurectomy has been done and follow-up surgery must be done for removal of painful neuromas, a hoof wall may slough (Fig. 6–99). Dissection of these specimens reveal that it is not due to loss of nerve supply but to the fact that the trauma produced by surgery plus the efforts of the nerve to regenerate surrounds the posterior digital artery with tissue that occludes its lumen. This leads to a dry gangrene of the hoof, and it

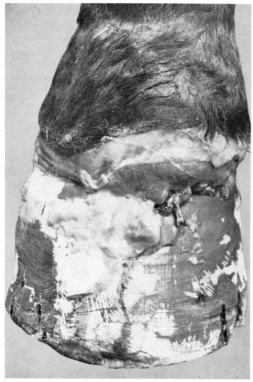

FIG. 6–99. Appearance of a foot that sloughed after two operations for neurectomy. The first one was for posterior digital neurectomy and the second for removal of neuromas. Several weeks later, the foot presented the above appearance. At necropsy the vessels and nerves were dissected out, and it was found that neurofibers and scar tissue had completely occluded and even invaded the digital arteries. Water could not be forced through the arteries by syringe.

sloughs off. Whenever more than one operation must be done in the same site, great care should be taken to avoid tissue injury. Less trauma is caused if the neuroma is left and the nerve is operated on just above the neuroma, leaving the neuroma without dissection, and removing a segment of nerve above it.

In all cases, the owner should be warned of the possibility of hoof slough, especially when a second or third operation is required.

Regeneration of the Posterior Digital Nerves. Regeneration of the posterior digital nerves may occur any time after six months following posterior digital neurectomy. This is evidenced by recurrence of symptoms. If half an inch or more of the nerve is removed at time of surgery, this is considered adequate. However, in some cases this gap is bridged by the regenerative efforts of the nerve or new nerve channels are established. Reoperation is the only effective treatment.

Incomplete Desensitization of the Heel. Approximately 50 percent of the horses will show nerve pattern variations. These include small branches coming from the posterior digital nerve high up at its origin. These small branches come down subcutaneously and often follow the ligament of the ergot. Careful examination should be made for these branches during the posterior digital neurectomy. If accessory branches are not found and removed, partial sensation to the heel remains, making the operation only partially successful. Another nerve variation sends a branch from the anterior digital nerve back to the heel area low down in the foot. In this case, posterior digital neurectomy would not be effective (Fig. 2–7).

Ordinarily, neurectomy of the volar nerves is not recommended. Loss of the hoof wall has been described, with loss of nerve supply blamed. In my opinion, the hoof wall is not lost because of the loss of nerve supply, but because of the encroachment on the volar arteries by fibrous tissue and nerve tissue resulting from scar formation and nerve regeneration efforts. Once the blood supply is limited or shut off to this area, the hoof wall will slough. This points again to the importance of minimal trauma during surgery and adequate rest after surgery in preventing this type of complication. Many horses are not lame following volar neurectomy, but in general its use should probably be discouraged.

Neurectomy of the posterior digital nerves without capping is performed as follows: The horse should be tranquilized with Promazine* or other suitable tranquilizer, and the area for neurectomy clipped and shaved. The skin should be prepared for operation about half the distance between the fetlock and coronary band, just in front of the tendon of the superficial digital flexor. Two to 3 cc of lidocaine hydrochloride or other suitable anesthetic should be injected through a 25-gauge $\frac{5}{8}''$ needle over the nerve on the abaxial surface of the medial and lateral sesamoid bones. One can palpate the artery as it crosses this area, and the nerve lies just behind it. By infusing the anesthetic around the artery, local anesthesia of both posterior and anterior digital nerves can be accomplished. This aids in keeping the irritating effect of the anesthetic away from the surgical site. However, if neurectomy is to be done soon after a diagnostic block of the posterior digital nerve has been done a third of the distance between the fetlock and the coronary band, this same block can then be utilized for the surgical procedure. A nose twitch should be applied to the horse during these injections. After checking the volar aspect of the foot with a needle to be sure that the nerves have been anesthetized, an incision $1\frac{1}{2}''$ long should be made at the anterior border of the super-

---

*Promazine, Fort Dodge Laboratories; Sparine, Wyeth Laboratories.

ficial flexor tendon. The incision is made through the skin and subcutaneous tissues. At this point the tissues may be separated by the jaws of a hemostat or by careful knife dissection. It is essential not to do any more damage to the tissues than necessary. The ligament of the ergot, which lies subcutaneously, can be removed or pushed aside. It is preferable to leave it in order to minimize scar tissue formation. A careful check is made for accessory branches of the posterior digital nerve, which are often near the ligament of the ergot. The nerve will be found lying just posterior to the artery at about $\frac{1}{2}''$ depth. One should positively identify the nerve before cutting it. The relationship of the structures are: vein in front, artery in the center, and nerve behind. The nerve can be identified by placing a hemostat under it, and then, with the thumbnail, identifying the longitudinal strands of the axons. The nerve should first be cut proximally and then a $\frac{1}{2}''$ section removed. Ligation of the distal nerve ending with 4-0 silk is recommended to help prevent reinnervation. The incision area should be sutured with 00 monofilament nylon and the procedure repeated on the opposite nerve, and, if necessary, the opposite foot. A pressure bandage should be applied and changed every other day for seven days. The sutures should be removed in ten days; the horse can be put back to work in four to six weeks. This operation is not optimal because about 25 percent of the horses treated in this manner will develop painful neuromas. The best surgical method to prevent painful neuromas at this time appears to be the use of epineural capping as described by Evans (1970).

The horse is confined in lateral recumbency with general anesthesia. The surgical sites are prepared for aseptic surgery. All four sites of incision should be prepared at the same time so that after the first two have been operated and the horse is rolled over for the other two incisions, time will not be consumed with additional preparation.

The medial posterior (palmar) digital nerve on the forelimb that is down and the lateral posterior (palmar) digital nerve on the forelimb that is up are neurectomized first. An incision 2″ to 3″ long is made on the anterior border of the superficial flexor tendon starting below the base of the sesamoid bone. The skin and fascia are incised and the ligament of the ergot identified. The area near the ligament of the ergot is carefully examined for possible accessory branches from the posterior digital nerve. Approximately 50 percent of the horses operated will show an accessory branch near the ligament of the ergot. If an accessory branch is found, a long section of it ($1\frac{1}{2}$″) is removed and exploration continued for the main branch of the posterior digital nerve. The nerve lies behind the digital artery and beneath the ligament of the ergot. Once the nerve is exposed, a section approximately 2″ long is freed from all fascia and connective tissue. The nerve is then cut as distally as possible and raised from the incision (Fig. 6–100A). Using ophthalmic thumb forceps or an iris spatula (Fig. 6–100B), the axons of the severed nerve are held with the forceps while the epineurium is carefully reflected. After approximately $\frac{1}{4}$″ of the axons is freed from epineurium, a small curved mosquito

hemostat is placed on the axons for holding purposes. While an assistant holds the forceps and straightens the nerve, the surgeon reflects the epineurium with two ophthalmic thumb forceps or an iris spatula for a distance of 1″ to $1\frac{1}{2}$″. At the proximal part of the bare axons, an incision is made halfway through the axons on one side of the nerve, and another incision halfway through the nerve is made on the opposite side $\frac{1}{8}$″ distally (Fig. 6–100C). The nerve is then completely severed $\frac{1}{8}$″ distally to this last cut (Fig. 6–100D). The epineurium is then pulled back over the severed end and ligated in two places with 00 silk just distal to the cut end of the nerve (Fig. 6–100E). The excess epineurium is then cut off and the nerve replaced behind the digital artery. The end of the distal fragment is ligated with 4-0 silk to help prevent reinnervation. The fascia and ligament of the ergot are sutured over the nerve without the needle penetrating into the nerve, with simple interrupted stitches of 00 Dexon,* 00 collagen, or catgut using a tapered-point atraumatic needle. The skin is then sutured with simple interrupted stitches of 00 monofilament nylon or silk. A pressure bandage of elastic gauze† and elastic

*Davis and Geck, Danbury, Conn.
†Kling, Johnson & Johnson, New Brunswick, N.J.

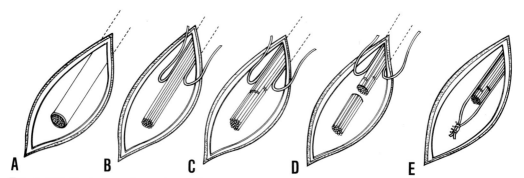

FIG. 6–100. Technique for epineural capping of posterior digital nerve. A, Incision of skin with posterior digital nerve isolated and sectioned. B, Epineural cuff reflected. C, Axons of posterior digital nerve cut halfway through from two sides. D, Removal of distal segment of posterior digital nerve, leaving partially cut segment. E, Replacement of epineural cap over the nerve, with two 4-0 silk ligatures in place on the distal end of the cuff.

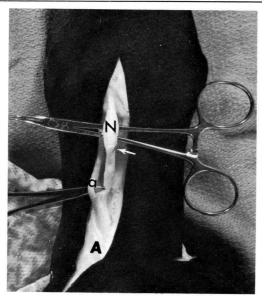
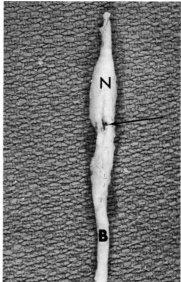

FIG. 6–101. Example of regeneration of the posterior digital nerve one year after epineural capping. A, Dissected specimen showing neuroma (N), point of ligature on cap (arrow), and artery (a). B, Nerve specimen showing neuroma (N), silk ligature (arrow) and normal nerve structure below the ligature.

tape* is then applied. Tetanus antitoxin is administered unless the horse is on a permanent tetanus-immunizing program, in which case tetanus toxoid is given. The bandage is changed in approximately four days and the stitches removed in seven to ten days. A pressure bandage is maintained for at least ten days. The horse is rested for approximately six weeks.

This method of neurectomy is apparently much more successful in preventing painful neuromas than other neurectomy methods (Evans, 1970). During surgery, one must be careful not to shred or tear the epineurium at any time. Any tears in the epineurium will allow axons to escape, and a painful neuroma will often result. As the epineurium is reflected, it is not uncommon for one or more axons to cling to the epineurium. These are not cut loose until all epineurium has been reflected and the axon is allowed to come down with the reflected epineurium. The axons, enclosed in the epineurium, are

less likely to escape to form a painful neuroma. They are also not as likely to regenerate and form new innervation channels. However, the nerve can regenerate in spite of the best technique (Fig. 6–101). This surgical technique is less likely to cause encroachment on the digital artery and consequent loss of blood supply to the hoof.

Whenever the nerves do not seem to be the proper size, careful checking should be done for accessory branches. About 50 percent of horses operated will show some degree of nerve variation. Commonly there is a subcutaneous branch traversing with the ligament of the ergot. It is found subcutaneously and not so deep as the posterior digital nerve. It is a small branch, but enough to prevent full effectiveness of posterior digital neurectomy.

Corrective shoeing for navicular disease will sometimes alleviate pain in the foot enough to allow use of the horse for many types of work. However, this type of corrective shoeing is usually not successful for race horses because of the extra

*Elasticon, Johnson & Johnson, New Brunswick, N.J.

weight of the shoe. When the hoof is trimmed, it should be trimmed at the angle normal for the particular horse, making sure that the axis of the hoof is steep enough to match the pastern axis. Many of these horses have an upright hoof and pastern, and as long as the hoof and pastern axes are continuous, one should not change the angle.

Corrective shoeing consists of raising the heels by building them up, rolling the toe, and using a bar across the center one-third of the frog. In addition, the branches of the shoe are slippered from the quarters through the heels to aid the hoof wall in expansion. The slippering effect is done by tapering the branches of the shoe so that the wall will slide outwards (Chap. 9, Fig. 9–16). The rolled toe and raised heel aid quick breakover. The raised heel and bar across the frog protect the frog from ground pressure. The raised heel also helps to bring the hoof back to proper angulation. The slippered quarters and heels of the shoe allow expansion of the hoof wall to help counteract the effect of the bar on the shoe. Rasping the quarters of the hoof wall or putting in vertical or parallel grooves on the quarters also aids foot expansion and helps overcome foot contraction (Chap. 9, Fig. 9–18). In addition to this, the application of silicone rubber* or rubber used for retreading tires can be used as a pad for the foot. This rubber material is covered with a hard plastic pad to hold it in place. Rubber cushioning of the foot is effective in many cases in relieving pain. When the hoof is reshod, the rubber pads can be reused if care is used in removal of the shoe and pad. Use of these shoeing methods can sometimes avoid neurectomy for a long time. In most cases, corrective shoeing is not necessary if neurectomy is done (if pedal osteitis is not present), but it can be tried first to see if it will obviate the need for neurectomy.

*Hoof Cushion, Miller Harness Co., New York.

Prognosis

The prognosis is unfavorable in all cases, but neurectomy can aid in providing several years of useful service from the horse. Posterior digital neurectomy is not legal in all states on race horses so the veterinarian should check with his state racing commission before performing the operation. In addition, the state may regulate the site of incision. As long as only the posterior digital nerve is neurectomized, the horse will have good prehension with the foot. Although the heel area is desensitized, nail punctures in this area will cause the inflammation to spread to sensitive areas in a very short time. Complications of neurectomy have already been described and include painful neuroma formation, rupture of the deep digital flexor tendon, regrowth of the nerve, accessory branches of nerve supply to the heel, and loss of the hoof wall. For painful neuroma formation and regeneration of the nerve, the neurectomy is redone, and if a neuroma is present, it is dissected out or the nerve is cut above the neuroma, preferably with an epineural cap. If it is suspected that accessory nerve supply is present, surgery should be done with a careful check for the small branches that lie subcutaneously near the ligament of the ergot. Methods of attempting to prevent neuroma have already been discussed. There is no satisfactory way to prevent innervation by the anterior digital nerve without actually cutting it.

SPECIFIC REFERENCES

BRYDEN, W. 1892. Navicular disease. Am. Vet. Rev. 16: 19.

CALISAR, T., and L. E. ST. CLAIR. 1969. Observations on the navicular bursa and the distal interphalangeal joint cavity of the horse. JAVMA 154(4): 55–59.

DONAHUE, M. 1935. Navicular disease in horses. Vet. Med. 30: 244.

DRAKE, H. S. 1897. Navicular arthritis. Am. Vet. Rev. 20: 476.

EBERT, E., and L. D. KINTNER. 1969. The effects of ligation on neuroma development following neurectomy. Berl. Munch. Tieraerztl. Wschr. 82(13): 244–247.

EVANS, L. H. 1970. Procedures used to prevent painful neuromas. Proc. AAEP, 103–115.

GIBBONS, W. J. 1966. Authorization for neurectomy. Mod. Vet. Pract. 47(13): 82.

GORMAN, T. N., M. M. NOLD, and J. M. KING, 1962. Use of radioactivity in neurectomy of the horse. Cornell Vet. 52: 542.

HICKMAN, J. 1964. Navicular disease. 3rd Ann. Cong. Brit. Eq. Vet. Assoc., 13.

HOLLINGSWORTH, J. B. 1904. Navicular disease. Am. Vet. Rev., 28: 263.

HUME, W. 1913. Neurectomy in foot lameness. JAVMA 8: 115.

JOHNSON, J. H. 1973. The navicular syndrome. VM/SAC. 54(12): 69–74.

JUBB, K. V. F., and P. C. KENNEDY. 1963. *Pathology of Domestic Animals.* New York: Academic Press. Vol. 2.

KELLER, H. 1969. Sequelae of volar neurectomy. Berl. Munch. Tieraerztl. Wschr. 82(13): 244–247.

KOCH, T. 1940. Termination of the volar nerve in the horse. Vet. Rec. 52(2): 26.

LIAUTARD, A. 1906. What is navicular disease? Am. Vet. Rev. 30: 1.

MUNRO, D. 1962. Prevention of amputation neuromas. Norden News, 14–15 (November).

NUMANS, S. R., and VAN DER WATERING, C. C. 1973. Navicular disease: Podotrochlitis chronica aseptica podotrochlosis. Eq. Vet. J. 5(1): 1–7.

OLSSON, S. E. 1954. On navicular disease in the horse: A roentgenological and patho-anatomical study. Nord. Veterinaemed. 6: 547.

OXSPRING, G. E. 1935. The radiology of navicular disease, with observations on its pathology. Vet. Rec. 15: 1433.

ROBB, A. H. 1958. Navicular disease in the horse. Vet. Rec. 70: 962.

ROONEY, J. R. 1967. Navicular disease. Proc. AAEP, 263–272.

SCHEBITZ, H.: 1964. Podotrochleosis in the horse. Proc. 10th Ann. AAEP, 49.

SCHEBITZ, H. 1965. Zur Podotrochlase, Spotergluis nach Neurektomie der Rami Volares. Berl. Munch. Tieraerztl. Wschr. 78, Jahrgang, Heft 2, S21–26.

SCHEBITZ, H. 1965. Podotrochleosis, results of neurectomy of rami volares. Tieraerztl. Wschr. 78(2): 1–18.

ST. CLAIR, L. E., and H. J. HARDENBROOK. 1969. Observations on the navicular bursa and the distal interphalangeal joint cavity of the horse. JAVMA. 154(4): 410.

VAN HOOSEN, N. W. 1965. Corrective shoeing for navicular disease. AAEP Program for AVMA meeting, Portland.

WILKINSON, G. T. 1953. Pathology of navicular disease. Brit. Vet. J. 109: 55.

WILKINSON, G. T. 1959. The pathology of navicular disease. J. Mammal. 40: 55–59.

WINTZER, H. J. 1965a. Navicular disease. Vet. Rec. 77(6): 162, 163.

WINTZER, H. J. 1965. Studies on navicular disease in horses. Tijdschr. Diergeneersk. 90: 1111–1115.

WINTZER, H. J., and K. DAMMRICH. 1971. Research into the pathogenesis of so-called navicular disease in horses. Tieraerztl. Wschr. 84(12): 221–225.

Fracture of the Navicular Bone

Definition

Fracture of the navicular bone is rare, but it may follow navicular disease or result from trauma to the foot.

Etiology

Violent concussion to the foot may cause fracture of the navicular bone, or the condition may follow a chronic case of navicular disease. When a navicular bone has been demineralized by chronic inflammation, adhesions between the deep flexor tendon and the navicular bone may fracture the bone after posterior digital neurectomy when the horse starts to use the foot normally. The demineralized bone breaks because of stress from the adhesions.

Signs

The signs are identical to those caused by navicular disease, but they may be more acute. Unilateral contraction of a front foot may be evident, especially if only fracture is present and not a bilateral navicular disease. Radiographs will reveal the fracture (Figs. 6–102 and 6–103).

Differential Diagnosis

Great care must be used in diagnosing fracture of the navicular bone because lines from the lateral sulci of the frog

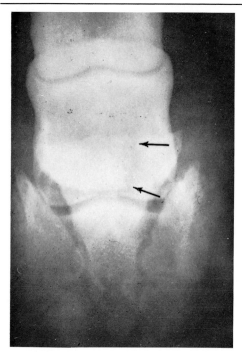

FIG. 6-102. Fracture of the navicular bone (arrows). Caution should be used not to confuse the lines of the lateral sulci of the frog with navicular fractures (see Chap. 12).

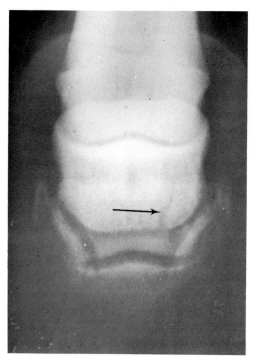

FIG. 6-103. Fracture of the navicular bone (arrow).

cross the area and commonly appear as fractures in the navicular bone or second phalanx. If these lines extend above or below the navicular bone, it is not a fracture line. When in doubt, retake the radiograph at a slightly different angle, and if what appears to be the fracture line extends above or below the bone in this new view, it is not a fracture (see Chap. 12). Taking the radiographs with the foot in a water bath will eliminate most of this problem (Figs. 6-94 through 6-97).

Treatment

Posterior digital neurectomy is the only treatment that will permit the horse to be used or to travel without pain.

Prognosis

The prognosis is unfavorable, but posterior digital neurectomy will permit limited use of some horses.

SPECIFIC REFERENCES

SMYTHE, R. A. 1961. Fracture of the navicular bone. Vet. Rec. 73: 1009.
VAUGHN, L. C. 1961. Fracture of the navicular bone. Vet. Rec. 73: 95.

Fracture of the Third Phalanx (Pedal Bone, Os Pedis, Coffin Bone)

Definition

Fracture of the third phalanx can occur in any class of horses and is not uncommon in either race horses or working Quarter Horses. Fracture of the third phalanx, though, is more common in the forefeet than in the hind feet.

Etiology

Trauma, especially when accompanied by a twisting action as the foot lands, is the predominant cause of fracture of the

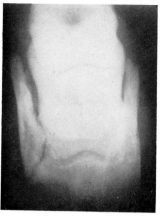

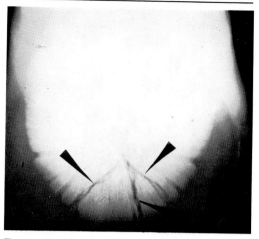

FIG. 6-104. Fracture of the third phalanx through one of the lateral wings. This horse had large sidebones. A cow stepped on the horse's foot, causing fracture of the third phalanx on the left side. (Carlson, *Veterinary Radiology*, Lea & Febiger.)

FIG. 6-105. Fracture of the third phalanx. This fracture occured in three places, as indicated by the pointers, and extends into the coffin joint.

third phalanx. Occasionally, the third phalanx may be fractured as a result of the penetration of a foreign body through the sole. The third phalanx also may be fractured as the result of trauma to a large sidebone (Fig. 6-104). In such a case, the phalanx usually breaks through one of the lateral wings.

Signs

If the third phalanx is fractured through the center of the bone and the fracture involves the articular surface, the lameness is an acute supporting-leg lameness. In some such cases, the horse may refuse to place the affected foot on the ground for as long as 72 hours. The history will often reveal that the lameness occurred suddenly during work and that no known trauma had occurred. There will be increased pulsation and heat in the affected foot, and examination with hoof testers will reveal uniform pain over the entire sole area (Fig. 6-105). Sometimes the bone will be fractured near one of the lateral wings of the phalanx and the lameness will not be so severe (Figs. 6-104 and 6-106). Hoof testers will cause less pain over the entire area of the sole but consid-

erable pain over the affected quarter. If the fracture has been present for some time, signs of lameness will not be as evident, and the history, hoof testers, and radiographs will be necessary to diagnose it.

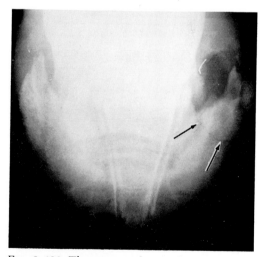

FIG. 6-106. The arrows show a fracture of the lateral wing of the third phalanx. The fracture line is not distinct, so careful radiography must be used. When the hoof tester is used, a horse affected with such a fracture would show the greatest pain over the affected area, rather than the diffuse pain caused by the injury pictured in Figure 6-105.

Fractures of the third phalanx in the hind limb can be overlooked because the attitude of the limb may resemble that in injuries further up the limb. Any acute weight-bearing lameness should be examined for the possibility of third phalanx fracture.

Diagnosis

The diagnosis can be positively confirmed only by use of radiographs. These should be taken to determine not only if the fracture is present, but also where it is. In some cases it may be necessary to take special views of the lateral wings to find the crack in the third phalanx. The defect in the bone may remain for a long time and, in some cases, never show clinical union. Horses so affected may be sound even though union is not obvious on the radiographs. Caution must be used so that normal vascular channels are not confused with fractures during interpretation of radiographs (see Chap. 12).

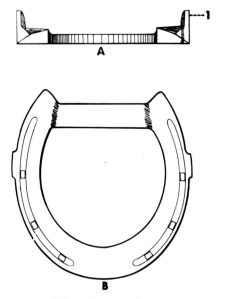

FIG. 6–107. Full bar shoe used in case of fracture of the third phalanx. *A*, Rear view of shoe showing quarter clips (1). *B*, Ground surface view of the shoe showing full bar and quarter clips welded to shoe.

Examination of the foot with hoof testers, along with the history, is often the most accurate way of establishing a diagnosis before radiographs have been taken.

Treatment

In treatment of this condition, the third phalanx should be immobilized as effectively as possible by use of a full bar shoe with quarter clips (Figs. 6–107 and 6–108). The bar should be placed on the shoe so that it is recessed from the frog and no frog pressure results. The quarter clips should be welded to the outside of the branches of the shoe near the junction of the heel and quarters. This prevents the quarters from expanding and, when combined with the bar to prevent frog pressure, reduces movement of the phalanx. The foot should be kept in this type of shoe for three to six months, with the shoe reset every four to six weeks. After clinical relief of the symptoms, the horse should be shod with either quarter clips or a bar for a time before both are removed. Some horses require constant use of clips or bar to ensure working soundness. The affected horse should not be worked for approximately six months, and in some cases, one year of rest may be advisable if symptoms do not disappear at the end of six months.

If the fracture has been caused by a puncture wound, the wound must be treated as discussed below in the section on puncture wounds of the foot. In such a case, tetanus antitoxin always should be administered. A bone abscess or demineralization of the third phalanx may result from such a fracture (Fig. 6–109). A corrective shoe may be necessary.

In some cases of persistent lameness resulting from fracture of the third phalanx, neurectomy of the posterior digital nerves may afford enough relief that the horse can be returned to full use. The success of this operation can be deter-

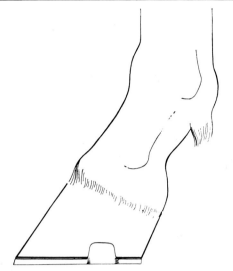

FIG. 6-108. Side view of shoe used for third phalanx fracture showing quarter clip in place.

ticular surface of the coffin joint. If small splinters of bone separate from the third phalanx, a sequestrum may result, causing prolonged lameness even after being removed. Radiographic evaluation of the fracture line is difficult because it will be apparent after the bone is clinically healed. Fibrous union occurs long before calcification.

SPECIFIC REFERENCES

PETERS, J. E. 1949. Fracture of the third phalanx and sesamoids in the race horse. JAVMA 114: 405.

PETTERSSON, H. 1972. Conservative and surgical treatment of fractures of the third phalanx. Proc. AAEP. 183-192.

WEAVER, A. D. 1969. Fracture of the equine pedal bone. Equine Vet. J. 1(6): 283-286.

mined beforehand by blocking the posterior digital nerves with a suitable local anesthetic.

Pettersson (1972) has used compression bone screws* to repair fractures of the third phalanx. In four of six cases he found it necessary to remove the screws after healing because of bone atrophy. He used both cortical screws and cancellous screws for repair. If cancellous bone screws are used, he stresses the need to use screws threaded all the way to the head of the screw so that they can be removed if necessary.

Prognosis

The prognosis is always guarded, but most horses can be returned to working soundness if treatment is instituted soon after the fracture. Fractures through the wings of the third phalanx are most favorable. A greater chance of chronic lameness exists if the fracture is through the center of the bone, involving the ar-

*ASIF screws, Smith Kline Surgical Specialties, Philadelphia.

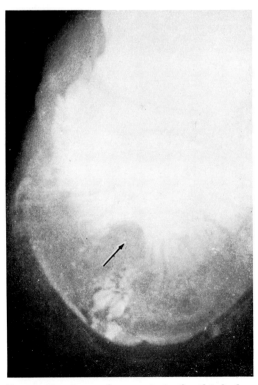

FIG. 6-109. Area of necrosis in the third phalanx caused by an old puncture wound. Pedal osteitis is present. This should not be confused with the normal notch that occurs at the center of the toe of the third phalanx in some horses.

Pedal Osteitis

Definition

Pedal osteitis is a demineralization of the third phalanx resulting from inflammation. It may also manifest itself as a roughness on the borders of the third phalanx, most commonly on the lateral wings.

Etiology

Persistent inflammation of the foot, due to numerous causes, may cause rarefaction of the third phalanx. Chronic bruising of the sole (as in navicular disease), persistent corns, laminitis (especially from concussion, or road founder), puncture wounds, and other inflammations over a long period of time may cause the disease. In some cases of osteitis there is actually an infection present. Whenever an infected corn or a puncture wound causes damage to the third phalanx, this is the case. Other causes, such as laminitis

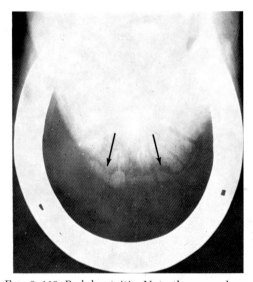

FIG. 6–110. Pedal osteitis. Note the ragged appearance of the tip of the third phalanx indicating osteitis and fragmentation. This was caused by a sole abscess at the toe, and osteitis resulted.

or persistent sole bruising, are not infectious. Nutritional and heritable causes must also be considered.

In some cases, the osteophytic development may be the result of local periostitis due to detachment of a few sensitive laminae. However, osteophytic outgrowths of this type are not uncommon in horses that show no lameness, and great care must be used in evaluating their significance.

Signs

Lameness is obvious in all gaits, and examination with a hoof tester will reveal pain at the bottom of the foot. This pain may be diffuse or localized. Pedal osteitis may merely be a sign of one of the diseases mentioned in the discussion of etiology. Radiographs indicate demineralization at one or more points in the third phalanx (Figs. 6–110 and 6–111), but a veterinarian must be careful not to confuse the normal notch of the toe of the third phalanx, that occurs in some horses, with rarefying osteitis (Fig. 6–109). Roughened areas along the distal border of the third phalanx may appear anywhere from the toe to the lateral wings. These ridges are not normally smooth because of vascular patterns in the bone, and careful evaluation must be made when they are present.

Treatment

Treatment of this disease is dependent upon the cause. Shoeing may help by keeping the sole away from the ground and preventing pressure on it. Pads of leather or Neolite under the shoe also may be helpful, as may padding of retread rubber or silicone rubber* covered by a full pad of plastic or leather. When pedal osteitis affects the lateral wings of the

*Miller Harness Co. Inc., New York.

distal border of the bone, neurectomy of the posterior digital nerves may be helpful, provided soundness occurs after blocking these nerves with a local anesthetic.

Prognosis

The prognosis is unfavorable because demineralization indicates that the disease is chronic; such a condition is difficult to reverse.

SPECIFIC REFERENCE

LUNDVALL, R. L. 1969. Pedal osteitis in horses. Norden News 44(3): 16–18.

Puncture Wounds of the Foot

Definition

Puncture wounds of the foot are quite common in horses. A variety of objects may produce the wounds. Some puncture wounds are extremely difficult to find, especially if they occur in the frog and the foreign body is missing. Puncture wounds in the middle third of the frog are most serious because of the possibility of puncture of the navicular bursa. Puncture wounds of the sole may cause osteitis fracture, and necrosis of the third phalanx or of the digital cushion.

Signs

In some cases, the foreign body will still be in the foot, making the diagnosis relatively simple. In such a case, the type of foreign object and the damage that has occurred to underlying structures should be determined. The attitude of the gait of the horse often is very helpful in determining the location of the puncture wound, if it is not obvious. If the wound is in the toe area of the sole, the horse

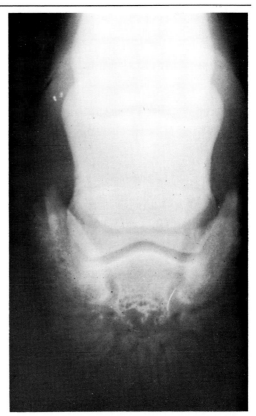

FIG. 6–111. Example of severe pedal osteitis. Notice demineralization of toe portion of the third phalanx. This condition usually results from a chronic inflammatory condition of the foot, such as laminitis, sole bruising, or persistent infection of the foot.

tends to land too heavily on the heel. If the puncture is in the heel area of the sole, the horse attempts to land on the toe. If the wound is in the medial side of the sole, the horse attempts to put most of his weight on the lateral side of the foot. If the wound is on the lateral side of the sole, the horse attempts to carry most of his weight on the medial side of the foot. Because of variation in this type of lameness, no characteristic signs can be described. The foot always should be checked thoroughly with a hoof tester to localize the site of the wound. Cracks in the white line, nail punctures, and shoe-nail punctures can be identified as black spots in the sole. These black spots should be probed until their full depth is determined, or until it is determined that they lead into sensitive structures.

Lameness may not be evident until after infection has caused a pododermatitis. If infection is present in the foot and the puncture wound has no drainage, the infection will force drainage at the coronary band near the heel. (Occasionally, drainage will occur slightly forward of the heel, and drain near the puncture wound, e.g., toe puncture draining at front of coronary band. A veterinarian should avoid the mistake of believing that drainage at the coronary band is the entire pathology; the bottom of the foot always should be checked for puncture wound. Supporting-leg lameness is usually evident because of the pain in the foot.

It is not uncommon to find that puncture wounds of the foot cause distention of the flexor tendon sheath just above the fetlock joint. Again, a veterinarian should not be confused by this swelling. Careful examination of the tendon sheath usually will reveal that there is no pain on pressure, although heat may be evident. Examination of the foot with the hoof testers will reveal a painful spot; this spot should be investigated to determine the position of the puncture wound.

Some cases of puncture wound in the foot will cause a septicemia and phlegmon of the limb with elevation of temperature and severe systemic manifestations. Other conditions that may occur as the result of puncture wounds include infectious laminitis, necrosis of the third phalanx (Fig. 6–109), fracture of the third phalanx, infection of the navicular bursa or digital cushion, fracture of the navicular bone, and tetanus.

Puncture wounds of the hind foot may cause a stringhalt attitude to the gait. The horse will move the limb in a hyperflexed manner, arousing suspicion of lameness involving structures farther up the limb.

A lameness in any limb warrants full examination of the foot and sole for pathological changes.

Diagnosis

If a veterinarian is conscientious about examining the bottom of the foot for any lameness, very few puncture wounds will be overlooked. One should always be sure that a shoe nail or separation of the white line (gravel, p. 370) does not cause the lameness. These conditions cause the same pathological changes and signs as direct puncture wounds. A hoof tester is essential for diagnosis of puncture wounds. Radiographs should be taken to determine damage, if any, to bony structures. Puncture wounds of the frog are the most difficult to locate, because once the foreign body has been pulled out, the spongy frog closes over the wound, making it difficult to find.

Treatment

To treat a puncture wound, establish drainage of the lesion, keep the area clean until protective healing occurs, and prevent tetanus. The entire sole, frog, and sulcus should be cleaned and washed. The area of the puncture wound should be drained so that there is at least a $\frac{1}{4}''$ opening into the sensitive laminae. The walls of the drainage hole should not be vertical but should widen toward the ground surface of the sole so that it is not apt to become occluded. If the wound is in the frog, the tract should be trimmed away until adequate drainage is established.

Following drainage, the wound should be cleaned with hydrogen peroxide or an enzyme preparation. The opening of the wound should be packed with tincture of iodine, and the foot bandaged thoroughly. The foot should be bandaged to protect it from moisture and filth, and the horse should be kept stalled, if possible, or at least in as dry an area as possible. Tetanus antitoxin should always be administered unless the horse is on a permanent immunity program with tetanus toxoid, in which case a booster of toxoid should be given, and antibiotics should be used as indicated.

When the infection causes drainage from a sinus at the coronary band, it is advisable to soak the foot daily in a magnesium sulfate solution. The foot should be checked carefully so the original puncture site can be located and drained as described above. Following soaking, tincture of iodine should be applied to the drainage established in the sole and the foot should be bandaged. Once healing begins, it is not essential that soaking and bandaging take place daily; every three to four days should be sufficient. It is essential to keep the wound clean until protective healing occurs.

If the puncture wound penetrates the navicular bursa, the bursa may require drainage through the center third of the frog. The foot is thoroughly cleansed and soaked in an antiseptic for 24 hours. The volar nerves should be blocked with local anesthetic and the center third of the frog trimmed out. When the plantar aponeurosis of the deep flexor tendon is exposed, a window should be cut in it to provide drainage to the bursa. The foot should be kept bandaged with antiseptics until healing has occurred. The navicular bursa also can be treated by injecting antibiotics and corticoids as described for treatment of navicular disease (pp. 266 and 269).

Emergency treatment for puncture wounds when the horse must be used for a time after treatment, such as on a trail ride, consists of establishing a small drainage hole with straight walls at the site of the puncture, and packing it tightly with tincture of iodine and cotton. Additional treatment can be done after the horse has been moved to a more suitable place.

Prognosis

The prognosis is favorable in early cases when the puncture wound has not damaged underlying structures. If the underlying bone or navicular bursa is damaged, the prognosis is guarded to unfavorable.

Corns and Bruised Sole

Definition

A corn is an involvement of the sensitive and insensitive tissues of the sole at the angle formed by the wall and the bar (Fig. 1–38, p. 26). Corns occur most frequently on the inner angle of the front feet and are rarely found in the hind feet. This may be due to the fact that the front feet bear more weight than the hind feet. Flat feet (*see* Chap. 1) predispose the sole to bruising.

Etiology

Corns usually are due to improper shoeing. When shoes are left on the feet too long, the heels of the shoe are forced inside the wall and cause pressure on the sole at the angle of the wall and the bar. Heel calks will enhance this effect. This pressure bruises the sole and causes corns. Improper trimming of the feet, making the heels too low, increases pressure at the angle of the wall and bar and also may cause corns. If a horse is shod too closely at the quarter, corns may result. Lack of frog pressure, causing bruising of the buttresses, and overreaching, also may cause corns. A long, weak fetlock and a narrow foot may cause corns to appear at the bars, while in a wide foot, corns are more likely to occur in the sole.

Corns are rare among horses that are used barefooted but sole bruising does occur as a result of trauma to the sole from rocks and other objects. Horses with thin soles are more subject to the disease, as are horses that have been affected previously with laminitis.

Signs

Three types of corn lesions may be evident:

Dry Corn. In this case, hemorrhage on the inner surface of the horn resulting from bruising of sensitive tissue usually causes red stains in the corn area.

Moist Corn. This is caused by severe injury that results in serum beneath the injured horn.

Suppurating Corn. The corn becomes infected, resulting in necrosis of the sensitive lamina, of the plantar aponeurosis, or of the digital cushion.

Pathological changes due to bruised sole are similar to those caused by corns but occur in the toe or quarter area of the sole rather than at the angle of the wall and bar. Bruised sole also may be of dry, moist, or suppurating types.

The horse will show varying degrees of lameness depending upon the severity of the bruise or corn, while the attitude of the lameness will vary according to the location of the bruise or corn. Hoof testers will reveal the location of the pathological changes. A cleaning of the flaky sole from the bottom of the foot with a hoof knife will reveal red stains in the sole indicating a bruised area. In some cases this area may show a bluish discoloration, especially if a sole abscess is developing.

The horse will tend to favor the heel, especially on the affected side. If the corn is present at the inside heel, the horse will tend to place more weight on the outside of the foot because of the pain. In some cases, the horse will tend to bear most of the weight on the toe and will rest the foot with the knee forward to decrease heel pressure. If the toe area of the sole is bruised, the horse will tend to land on the heel to protect the toe.

Treatment

In cases where shoeing is the cause, removal of the offending shoe may be all that is necessary. To prevent shoes from causing corns, the heels of the shoe always should extend well back on the buttresses and should fit full on the wall at the quarters and heels. Heel calks increase the chance of corns if a horse is shod too short at the heels or if the shoe is left on too long. Removal of some of the tissue over the corn helps relieve pressure, but sensitive tissue should not be exposed. The horse should be rested and should not be reshod until symptoms disappear.

In the case of a suppurating corn, the sole over the area should be removed until drainage into the sensitive tissues is established. The foot should be soaked daily in an antiseptic or in a solution of magnesium sulfate, after which tincture of iodine is applied. The foot should be bandaged and protected from contamination; tetanus antitoxin should be administered. Antiphlogistic packs can be used under the bandage for their ability to draw out infected fluids from the area.

If the horse must be used for some reason, the wall and bar in the area of the corn should be removed to prevent pressure by the shoe. Either a half- or full-bar shoe should be applied, as for quarter crack (Figs. 6–185, p. 368, and 7–8, p. 387). These shoes allow the frog to absorb the concussion that would normally be distributed to the corn area. When the shoe is applied, the half or full bar should press in against the frog about $\frac{1}{8}''$ to aid in preventing further contraction of the foot.

In cases of sole bruising, the horse should be rested from heavy work, especially if his soles are abnormally thin. When possible, the environment of the horse should be changed so that he is not worked on rough ground. If the horse must be used, the sole can be packed with silicone rubber or tire retread rubber and a pad applied under the shoe.

If the bruised area becomes a sole abscess, it should be drained by cutting away a portion of the diseased sole and exposing the sensitive laminae. The foot then should be soaked daily in magnesium sulfate solution, treated with tincture of iodine, and bandaged with an antiphlogistic paste until protective healing can occur. Tetanus antitoxin should be administered.

Prognosis

The prognosis is always guarded, since some such cases tend to become chronic, which eventually may cause osteitis of the third phalanx (pedal osteitis).

LAMENESSES IN THE HIND LIMB

Azoturia (Monday Morning Disease)

Definition

Azoturia is a severe destruction of muscle that occurs in horses kept on full feed when they are not worked. It is characteristically associated with a full diet of grain and a period of rest of one or two days or more while kept on full rations. When the horse is put back to work, signs appear even though the amount of work may be very light, consisting only of the act of a stallion breeding a mare in some cases. It also can occur as a sequel to casting for surgical procedures. This fact supports the contention that a horse should be starved for 24 hours before a surgical procedure that requires casting and anesthesia. The muscles most characteristically affected are the iliopsoas, quadriceps, and triceps. The gluteals and biceps femoris may be involved in severe cases.

Etiology

During the rest period, glycogen accumulates in the musculature. Upon exertion, this glycogen is broken down, and large amounts of lactic acid accumulate (Smith et al., 1972). Lactic acid causes muscle cell destruction and release of myoglobin. As the acid is formed, it cannot be eliminated fast enough, and the accumulation destroys the muscle. As a sequel to the muscular damage, renal lesions caused by the passage of the myoglobin through the kidney that are characterized by lower nephron degeneration, may cause death. Other unknown factors may be present.

Staron (1959a,b) claimed that his studies showed the causative agent of azoturia to be malonic acid, which blocks the enzyme system (succinoxidase).

Signs

Signs of azoturia usually occur within a few minutes after the horse is put to work. This is as compared to the tying up syndrome which usually occurs after severe muscular exertion has already been done. Usually within fifteen minutes or less after starting to walk or run, signs of pain, stiffness, incoordination, and muscular tremor occur. If exercise is continued, these signs increase until the horse may be unable to stand. They are accompanied by profuse sweating, and the eyes show evidence of acute pain. Palpation of the affected muscles causes pain and they are firm to the touch. If the horse goes down and is unable to rise, he may struggle and further aggravate the condition. Urine will be dark, almost black in severe cases. The dark color is due to myoglobin in the urine.

Diagnosis

Diagnosis can usually be established on the basis of the rapidity of the onset and clinical signs following work. Also, the history showing that the horse has been rested and kept on full feed is helpful. Azoturia must be differentiated from thromboembolism, which decreases circulation to the hind limbs and causes a very similar syndrome as far as incoordination, pain, sweating, and so on are concerned. In thromboembolism, some signs of poor circulation can usually be found, either by palpating the femoral arteries or by rectal examination of the iliac arteries (see p. 299). In thromboembolism there is no coffee-colored urine, and rest will relieve symptoms. In azoturia, rest will also usually produce a lessening of signs, but not nearly so rapidly. If a SGOT level is done on a case of azoturia, it will be found to be extremely high—over 1,000 units. Lactic acid dehydrogenase levels are also elevated. Blood urea nitrogen levels may be high if the kidney has been damaged.

Treatment

The horse must be stopped immediately from any work that he is doing. It usually pays to not even walk him back to a stall. The horse should be kept from moving and protected until treatment can be instituted. Treatment consists of reducing acidity by using intravenous and oral sodium bicarbonate. Two ounces of sodium bicarbonate can be administered intravenously in 2,000 cc of sterile saline solution, plus $\frac{1}{2}$ to 1 pound orally. Intravenous thiamine injections appear to hasten recovery. Calcium gluconate can be administered intravenously (250 to 500 cc of 20 percent solution) and may be of some help. Intravenous corticoids such as prednisolone sodium succinate* are indicated and very helpful. Tranquilization of the

*Solu-delta-cortef, Upjohn Co., Kalamazoo, Mich.

horse will decrease muscular activity and apprehension. The use of antihistamines may be beneficial.

Prevention

Each occurrence of azoturia produces muscular destruction and scarring in the muscles. If at all possible, subsequent attacks must be prevented by being very cautious about overfeeding during rest periods and using regular exercise instead of layoff periods. One attack seems to predispose the horse to further attack.

Injections of selenium and vitamin E are given for treatment and prevention of this condition. One cc of E-Se* per 100 pounds body weight is administered intramuscularly, and can be repeated. This product seems helpful in preventing recurrences. Sodium bicarbonate orally (2–4 oz) daily is also helpful in preventing the syndrome.

SPECIFIC REFERENCES

BAKER, R. H. 1962. Oxygen therapy. Proc. AAEP, 144.

DODD, D. C. 1963. *Equine Medicine and Surgery,* Santa Barbara, Calif.: American Veterinary Publishers Inc. p. 473.

FERRIOT, M. 1961. Treatment of myoglobinuria. Bull. Soc. Vet. Prat. 45(6): 214.

GERBER, H. 1968. The clinical significance of serum enzyme activities with particular reference to myoglobinuria. Proc. AAEP, 81–95.

GOLLNICK, P. D., and D. W. KING. 1969. Energy release in the muscle cell. Med. Sci. Sports 1(1): 23–31.

HERMANSEN, L. 1969. Anaerobic energy release. Med. Sci. Sports 1(1): 32–38.

Panel Report. 1960. Azoturia in the horse. Mod. Vet. Pract. 41(5): 45.

RICCI, B. 1967. Physiological Basis for Human Performance. Philadelphia: Lea & Febiger.

RIETHMULLER, H., and A. WELS. 1972. Effects of training on thoroughbreds—muscle specific enzymes. Zbl. Veterinarmed. 19(7): 537.

SMITH, H. A., T. C. JONES, and B. D. HUNT. 1972. Veterinary Pathology, 4th ed. Philadelphia: Lea & Febiger.

SMYTHE, R. H. 1964. Azoturia. Proc. Brit. Eq. Vet. Assoc., 37–43.

*H. C. Burns, Oakland, Calif.

STARON, T. 1959a. Pathogenesis and treatment of paroxysmal myoglobinuria in horses. Clin. Vet. 82: 169.

STARON, T. 1959b. Treatment of azoturia in the horse. Vet. Bull. 29: 700.

Tying-Up Syndrome (Cording Up)

Definition

The tying-up syndrome is a myopathy that occurs after active muscular exertion, such as racing. It is a painful condition of the iliopsoas, quadriceps, and gluteal groups of muscles that occurs within minutes after the exertion of a race is finished. The true physiological development of the condition is hypothetical at this time. Horses affected are usually on a high-grain ration and commonly have been rested one or two days from training. Studies by the author indicate that there is a marked rise in lactic acid dehydrogenase and SGOT levels in the presence of signs.

Horses that are highly susceptible to the disease may show the syndrome at the beginning of work rather than afterwards and often present a chronic problem. Those affected at the beginning of work are often nervous and hyperexcitable.

The condition can be seen after nervous exertion such as during transportation or following temperamental outbursts such as may occur when the horse is broken to saddle. Nervousness apparently can contribute to development of the disease, and this may be why it is seemingly more common in mares and fillies than in males. Although there is considerable disagreement among authorities, it appears that this disease is a mild form of azoturia, but relationship to azoturia has not been proven. Horses once affected with the condition seem to be subject to recurrence of the disease. Tying-up is not to be confused with complete muscular fatigue that occurs when a horse is overworked at one particular time.

Etiology

Etiology of the condition is controversial. However, it appears that, as in azoturia, lactic acid accumulates in the affected muscles, but it does not accumulate enough to cause the muscular destruction seen in azoturia. In tying-up, the horse is in better condition and builds up lactic acid levels more slowly. There probably is little, if any, actual muscular necrosis in the tying-up syndrome.

Briefly, there are two sources of energy in the body: anaerobic and aerobic. The anaerobic or glycolytic pathway utilizes carbohydrate exclusively and involves the breakdown of glycogen or glucose, with a subsequent production of lactic acid. No oxygen is consumed in these reactions, and the extent to which they contribute to muscular energy is estimated by the postexercise oxygen debt or by the difference between pre- and postexercise lactic acid concentrations. There is a direct relationship between oxygen debt and elevation of lactic acid levels in humans (Ricci, 1967). There is also an increase of blood lactate levels in humans to as much as thirty times normal during work. I assume that the same relationships exist in horses.

The aerobic or oxidative pathway utilizes carbohydrate, fat, or protein as substrate and yields energy on combustion of these products. The extent to which this pathway is utilized is measured by oxygen consumption during exercise and is known as the "oxygen uptake."

Our primary interest is in anaerobic energy because it is used in the severe exertion of racing (under 3 minutes of time). Through glycolysis, lactic acid is formed during exertion by anaerobic oxidation. If muscle circulation is sufficient to provide adequate oxygenation, lactic acid buildup is not a problem. However, in the tying-up syndrome, there apparently is a decreased blood flow in the affected muscles caused by a spasm of the arterioles supplying the involved muscles. This results in decreased blood flow at a time when a good supply is needed. Too much lactic acid is formed because of the increased anaerobic conditions, and little is removed because of the decreased circulation. The accumulation of lactic acid in the muscles and blood is the most common limiting factor of muscular activity and apparently results in cramping of the affected muscles, because they are firm on palpation.

Horses that are improperly conditioned will create a larger oxygen debt than those that are properly conditioned. There are inheritable differences between horses that will cause some to create a greater oxygen debt than others with the same degree of conditioning. Many horses are not properly trained for racing, and this factor probably also contributes to some cases of the tying-up syndrome. The horse is an athlete, and an athlete cannot train 1 hour a day and spend 23 hours in a $12' \times 12'$ room and expect to do well in athletic competition.

In recent years, vitamin E and selenium have been used with some success in the treatment and prevention of the tying-up syndrome. This brings to mind the possibility of deficiency of selenium and/or vitamin E as a cause of the tying-up syndrome. Deficiency of these has been incriminated in white-muscle disease of other species. The selenium-tocopherol mixture is said to be essential in some enzyme systems (Burns, 1968).

Signs

After severe exertion, such as racing, the horse shows stiffness, and the hind limbs do not flex normally. The back is rigid and the horse walks as though he has back pain. Pain can be produced by hand pressure over the loin region. It can also be produced by palpating the iliopsoas group of muscles by rectal palpation. The muscles are hard to the touch. In some cases, the muscular involvement may extend to the gluteals and the quadriceps. These are also hard to the touch, and pain is shown by the horse when these muscles are palpated. More commonly, only the muscles in the region of the loin and the iliopsoas group are involved. The SGOT level is usually elevated above 1,000 units (Cornelius et al., 1963) and there is a mild degree of myoglobinuria. Lactic acid dehydrogenase levels are also elevated. If the horse is walked for a time, the signs usually disappear.

Diagnosis

Diagnosis is made on the basis of the clinical signs and history. The syndrome usually manifests itself within a few minutes after exertion; however, some cases will exhibit signs soon after work begins, and this type of case is usually the most difficult to treat. Hand pressure over the longissimus dorsi in the region of the lumbosacral junction will produce pain. Rectal examination will also produce pain when the iliopsoas group of muscles is palpated. There is a rigidity of the back and stiffness of the gait in both hind limbs. In more severe cases, pain is shown over the gluteals and quadriceps.

Treatment

No specific drug treatment is necessary in the usual case of tying-up. Walking the horse for 30 to 40 minutes will usually relieve the signs. Treatments that are used to hasten recovery are intravenous corticoids, intravenous calcium gluconate 20 percent (250 to 500 cc), intramuscular Calphosan* (20 cc) and alkalinization of the bloodstream with sodium bicarbonate solution (one ounce in one liter of sterile water). Thiamine and tranquilizers are also used, as well as Robaxin† (20 cc) intravenously for muscle relaxation. For

---

*Carlton Corp., New York.
†A. H. Robbins Co., Richmond, Va.

prevention, selenium and vitamin E injections* are used at the rate of 1 cc per 100 pounds body weight. This can be repeated at weekly intervals for as many as four injections. Some horses respond to one injection, and others never respond. Oral calcium lactate, magnesium hydroxide, and vitamins A and D have been recommended as preventives of tying-up syndrome (Dodd et al., 1960). Therapeutic injections of ACTH† are also claimed to be of value in prevention. Results with these types of preventive therapy have been quite inconsistent. Grain ration should be cut in half 24 hours before a race or performance class.

Intravenous administration of 30 to 50 gm of sodium bicarbonate prior to work will usually prevent the syndrome. The author has also had success with the oral administration of 2 to 4 oz of sodium bicarbonate daily fed in the grain. This is perhaps the most effective single preventive for stubborn cases of tying-up syndrome. One should also be certain that the horse has adequate salt intake.

Prognosis

The prognosis for recovery from the syndrome is good. However, it may recur upon subsequent racing or exertion. Apparently, there is very little muscular damage with each attack, since atrophy and fibrosis of the muscles involved seldom occur. The prognosis is good if the horse stops showing signs of the condition after injection of selenium and vitamin E.

SPECIFIC REFERENCES

Blood-Horse. 1963. Prevention of tying up. 85(17): 780.
Bone, J. F. 1963. Equine Medicine and Surgery. Santa Barbara, California: American Veterinary Publishers. p. 475.

* E-Se, H. C. Burns, Co., Oakland, Calif.
† Adrenomone, Armour-Baldwin Laboratories, Omaha, Neb.

Brennan, B. F., et al. 1959. Proc. 5th Ann. AAEP, 157.
Burns, H. C. 1968. Data Book on Selenium-Tocopherol Mixtures. Oakland, Calif.
Cardinet, C. H., III, M. E. Fowler, and W. S. Tyler. 1963. Effects of training, exercise and tying-up on serum transaminase. Amer. J. Vet. Res. 24(102): 980.
Cornelius, C. E., L. G. Burnham, and H. E. Hill. 1963. Serum transaminase activities of Thoroughbred horses in training. JAVMA 142: 639.
Dodd, D. C., et al. 1960. Muscular dystrophy in New Zealand livestock. N.Z. Vet. J. 8: 45.
Fries, J. H. 1961. Treatment of the "tying-up" syndrome. Proc. 7th Ann. AAEP.
Gollnick, P. D., and D. W. King. Energy release in the muscle cell. Med. Sci. Sports 1(1): 23–31.
Haynes, P. F. 1973. Personal communication. Colo. State Univ.
Hartley, W. J., and D. C. Dodd. 1957. Muscular dystrophy in New Zealand livestock. N.Z. Vet. J. 5: 61.
Hermansen, L. 1969. Anaerobic energy release. Med. Sci. Sports 1(1): 32–38.
Hill, H. E. 1962. Selenium–Vitamin E treatment of tying up horses. Mod. Vet. Pract. 43: 66.
Miller, W. C. 1961. Atypical myoglobinuria. Irish Vet. J. 15: 154.
Ricci, B. 1967. Physiological Basis of Human Performance. Philadelphia: Lea & Febiger.
Steel, J. D. 1969. Abnormalities of gait in the racehorse referred to as tying-up syndromes. Aust. Vet. J. 45(4): 162–165.

Myositis of the Psoas and Longissimus Dorsi Muscles

Definition

Following severe muscular exertion such as racing or other work necessitating fast starts, the longissimus dorsi and psoas major and minor muscles may develop myositis. The area of pain in the loin region often causes the owner to think the horse has "kidney trouble."

Etiology

Trauma from muscular strain is the etiology. The psoas muscles are very important in the driving action of the hind limbs and are subject to injury when the horse is improperly trained. They are also involved in azoturia and the tying-up syndrome, and myositis may be one of the after effects of one of these diseases.

Signs

The horse carries himself with a stiffened attitude of the back. He will not exert normal propulsion of the hind limbs, and exhibits pain on pressure over the loin, which may cause him to groan and drop the back under hand pressure. Hand pressure on the psoas group of muscles by way of rectal examination will also produce pain. The action of the hind limb is not normal, in that the gait appears to be stiffened in both hind limbs. The abdomen may be held rigid as though intra-abdominal pain were present. SGOT levels are probably elevated in the active stage of the lameness.

Diagnosis

Diagnosis is made by the response of the horse to digital pressure over the loin and pressure to the psoas group of muscles on rectal examination. It must be differentiated from injury to the sacroiliac and lumbosacral junctions and overlapping of the thoracic and/or lumbar dorsal spinous processes. Disc injuries are rare in the horse, but if suspected must be differentiated. The latter four conditions seldom respond permanently to treatment. The signs are present for several days, or even weeks, differentiating it from the tying-up syndrome.

Treatment

Proper rest and training procedures are mandatory. The period of rest will vary with the severity of the injury. In most cases, a minimum of thirty days is required. In addition, injections of vitamin E and selenium* at the rate of 1 cc per

*E-Se, H. C. Burns Co., Oakland, Calif.

100 pounds are useful. These injections may be repeated at weekly intervals for three to four injections if necessary. Sodium bicarbonate in the grain (2–4 oz) daily will relieve symptoms in some cases. Some cases will not respond immediately, and others may require six weeks for evidence of recovery. Thiamine and corticoid injections are also useful. The horse should not be put back in training until all signs of pain have disappeared for three weeks after therapy is discontinued.

Prognosis

The prognosis is guarded because of the possibility of recurrence of injury. However, most horses return to full use.

Overlapping of Thoracic and/or Lumbar Dorsal Spinous Processes

Definition

Roberts (1968a,b) has described lameness due to overlapping of the thoracic and/or lumbar spinous processes. The lameness is due to pain caused by pressure on the vertical spines from enlargement of the proximal ends.

Etiology

The horse has usually suffered an injury to the back, although a clear history of this is not always obtained. This injury may be due to such mishaps as going over backwards, falling, or struggling in a casting harness. Signs may not be evident until two to three years after the injury.

Signs

Changes in behavior and temperament are common. The horse often resents saddling and grooming. Bucking and lying down after saddling may occur. As the cinch is tightened, the horse may groan and exhibit other signs of discomfort. Pressure along the back may cause signs of pain in some cases. Many other variations may result, as described by Roberts. The condition appears to be most prevalent in hunters and jumpers, and it is common for the horse to refuse jumps.

Diagnosis

Palpation along the back may reveal irregularities in the size of the summits of the spinous processes of the thoracic or lumbar vertebrae. Deep digital palpation is necessary in most cases to reveal these changes. Examination should begin forward at the withers and work backward. One will have to differentiate resentment shown by some horses to this examination from distress resulting from a pathological condition. Tests of the spine to show loss of flexibility are useful. This is done by compressing in the area of the last thoracic vertebra and the base of the tail. Alternate compression of these areas should produce the effect of dipping and arching the spine respectively. A horse with overlapping of the spinous processes will show little or no movement from these pressures. If satisfactory radiographs of the dorsal processes can be obtained, they will greatly aid diagnosis.

Differential Diagnosis

The above signs are by no means specific and may be shown in other types of lameness, especially subluxation of the sacroiliac joint. Tying-up syndrome and arthritis of the spine might also cause some similar signs. One must always be careful of the horse that has discovered that by malingering in some way, such as lying down when saddled, he may end the riding session. Diagnosis is best established with history and with positive changes on palpation and radiographs. A

positive radiographic examination will show diminished space between, and possibly overlapping of, the affected dorsal spinous processes.

Treatment

Surgical treatment as described by Roberts (1968b) will give satisfactory results in most cases, if the diagnosis is accurate. The summit of the affected spinous process is removed through an incision on either side of the midline. If there is pressure between as many as three spinous processes, removal of the center one will usually relieve symptoms. The supraspinous ligament is dissected free of the processes and not severed. The operative field is crowded by longissimus dorsi muscle, making complete exposure of the process difficult. Only enough of the process is removed to relieve pressure between processes. A bone saw or wire saw can be used for cutting. For a detailed description of the surgical procedure, the reader is referred to Roberts' (1968b) original discussion.

Aftercare consists of two months in a box stall and one month of hand walking before beginning riding. Some cases do not show full benefit for several months.

Prognosis

Prognosis is guarded. The expense involved in surgery will limit the number of cases operated on. Diagnosis is sometimes difficult because of the large x-ray machine required for adequate radiographs.

SPECIFIC REFERENCES

ROBERTS, E. J. 1968a. Amputation of a lumbar spinous process in the horse. Proc. AAEP, 115–117.
ROBERTS, E. J. 1968b. Resection of thoracic or lumbar spinous processes for the relief of pain responsible for lameness and some other locomotor disorders of horses. Proc. AAEP, 13–30.

Subluxation of the Sacroiliac Joint*

Definition

The sacroiliac joint in the horse is described by Sisson (1953) as a diarthrosis formed between the articular surfaces of the sacrum and the ilium (Figs. 6–112 and 6–113). The surfaces are not smooth in the adult, but are marked by reciprocal eminences and depressions covered by a thin layer of cartilage. The joint cavity is only a cleft and is often crossed by fibrous bands. The joint capsule is very close-fitting and is attached around the margins of the articular surfaces. The joint is reinforced by a ventral sacroiliac ligament that surrounds the joint (Figs. 6–112 and 6–113). This is a very stong ligament above, where it occupies the angle between the ilium and the wing of the sacrum, and it consists chiefly of nearly vertical fibers. Movement in the joint is inappreciable in the adult, with stability, not mobility, being desirable. In addition to the ventral sacroiliac ligament, there is

*This section is modified from Adams (1969).

a dorsal sacroiliac ligament, which is a strong band attached to the tuber sacrale and the summits of the sacral spines. There is also a lateral sacroiliac ligament, which is attached in front to the tuber sacrale and adjacent part of the medial border of the ilium above the greater sciatic notch, and below to the lateral border of the sacrum. It blends above with the dorsal sacroiliac ligament, below with the sacrosciatic ligament and behind with the coccygeal fascia. Since the sacroiliac joint is not meant to be mobile, stresses that produce motion may produce subluxation. Once the continuity of the joint is disturbed, there may be chronic pain resulting from the partial displacement. Pain is due to reflex muscular spasm and will usually be present until healing by scar tissue is sufficient to prevent any mobility in the joint. Ligament injury heals by scar tissue and therefore is subject to reinjury.

Etiology

Falls, slipping, and any other trauma that causes twisting or high stress to the sacroiliac joint can cause the lameness.

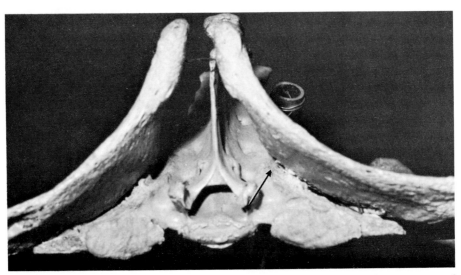

FIG. 6–112. Skeletal model of the sacroiliac joint. Arrow points between the sacrum and ilium. (From Adams, 1969; courtesy of AAEP.)

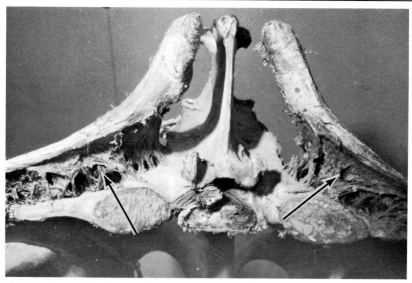

FIG. 6–113. Skeletal model of sacroiliac joint. Arrows point to dried and separated ventral sacroiliac ligament. (From Adams, 1969; courtesy of AAEP.)

Signs

Clinical signs of subluxation of the sacroiliac joint are highly variable. Usually stiffness and pain in the rear quarters are shown, with considerable variation in the signs. Pain may be produced when pressure is put on the tuber coxae to cause rotation of the pelvis and move the sacroiliac joint. Pain may also be present when finger pressure is put on the sacroiliac junction area. There often is some surrounding muscular pain, caused by spasm of the surrounding muscles in their attempt to re-establish the rigidity of the sacroiliac joint. The condition is most often chronic, and the tuber sacrale may become prominent, either unilaterally or bilaterally, depending on whether one or both sides are involved (Figs. 6–114 and 6–115). The prominence of one or both of the tubera sacrala (hunter's bumps) is due to subluxation of one or both sacroiliac joints. Crepitation can sometimes be produced by applying finger and thumb pressure over the sacroiliac joint, causing the horse to exhibit lordosis.

Rooney (1969) has described two acute cases in which the horses went down and were destroyed. He also describes shortening of the stride, limitation in hind-limb joint movement and reluctance to jump. The lameness may be unilateral or bilateral, depending on whether one or both sides are involved. The common complaint in the hunter-jumper type horse is that the horse is stiff and refuses to jump, or does a poor job of it. Apparently, the lameness in subluxation of the sacroiliac joint is caused by inflammation resulting from instability of the joint(s) and sympathetic muscular spasm. Dissimilarity or protrusion of the tuber sacrale, either unilaterally or bilaterally, may be present in a horse not now affected with the condition (Fig. 6–114). This can happen if a previous lesion has healed solidly and no motion is now present in the joint(s).

Rectal examination findings of sacroiliac subluxation will not be diagnostic unless enough motion is present in the joint to prouce some crepitation. Crepitation in the pelvis is difficult to pinpoint because of bone conduction. The rectal exam should be done while the horse is walking slowly, and while pressure is put

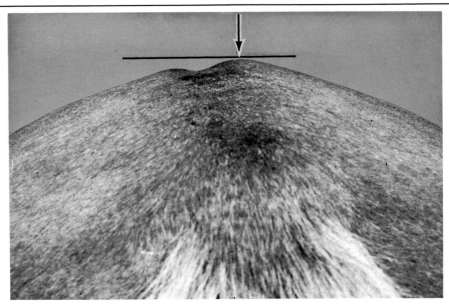

FIG. 6–114. Arrow points to upward displacement of tuber sacrale. The view is over the rump of the horse, looking forward. This area may move when the horse is walking and may show unilateral or bilateral displacement in subluxation of the sacroiliac joint.

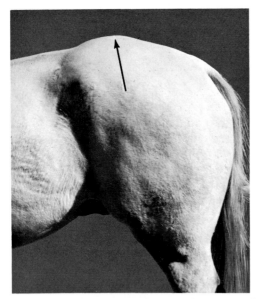

FIG. 6–115. Side view showing location of tuber sacrale (arrow). This point should be closely observed when a horse walks for signs of movement and, in old cases, for signs of unilateral or bilateral displacement. (From Adams, 1969; courtesy of AAEP.)

on the tuber coxae in an effort to produce rotation of the pelvis and crepitation. Rocking the horse back and forth, causing the horse to shift his weight from one hind limb to the other often produces the crepitation necessary for a diagnosis of the condition. The hand in the rectum should be held on the bottom of the sacrum as close to the sacroiliac junction as possible. When the horse is walking, movement of one or both tubera sacrala may be noticeable. In inactive cases, nonmovable displacement (hunter's bumps) will be present unilaterally or bilaterally.

Differential Diagnosis

Differential diagnosis of subluxation of the sacroiliac joint includes verminous aneurism of the posterior aorta or of one or more of the iliac arteries, azoturia, fracture of the ilium, myositis of the lumbar muscles, trochanteric bursitis, possible hormonal causes, and overlapping of the lumbar spinous processes. Verminous aneurysm, azoturia, fractures of the pelvis, lumbar myositis, trochanteric bursitis, and overlapping of the dorsal spinous processes of the lumbar vertebrae are described in this text.

In cattle, ligamentous relaxation causing separation of the symphysis pubis and/or subluxation of the sacroiliac joint is apparently mediated by hormonal factors. The hormone relaxin, produced by the corpus luteum, and/or estrogens are believed to be involved in causing the condition. It is possible that the same type of syndrome, producing relaxation of the supporting ligaments of the sacroiliac joint, might occur in older horses. It is not always possible to arrive at a positive diagnosis in such cases, but this possibility must be considered in differential diagnosis.

Overlapping of the vertebral spinous processes presents a highly variable clinical syndrome that has been described by Roberts (1968) and is discussed above.

Diagnosis

Diagnosis of sacroiliac subluxation is dependent upon elimination of the above lamenesses (these may not exhaust the list of alternatives). In some cases of sacroiliac subluxation, there may be slight motion of one or both tubera sacrala during walking, and close observation should be made on this point. Whenever there is unevenness or excessive prominence (hunter's bumps) of the tuber sacrale, one should consider that at least at one time there has been movement and partial luxation of this joint (Fig. 6–114). In humans, acute pain caused by sacroiliac subluxation is relieved by injection of a local anesthetic and steroids. This might be done in horses to aid in differential diagnosis. If pain were relieved by such injections, then one could be certain of the diagnosis. The injections would have to be rather extensive to cover the ligamentous attachments and the joint.

Treatment

Since subluxation of the sacroiliac joint(s) means that some ligamentous attachments are injured, time must be allowed for healing to occur. This means complete rest, preferably in a box stall for at least 30 days. The ligamentous attachments must be allowed to rejoin, and, if injury has been severe, the cartilaginous junction may be damaged enough to cause a bony fusion of the joint. Repeated injury may produce a chronic semimobile area that will cause persistent lameness. In chronic cases like this, it might be advisable to attempt to cause ligamentous reinforcement by scar-tissue formation, using irritants injected locally into the area of the ventral sacroiliac ligament. It might also be beneficial to attempt to get some of the irritant into the sacroiliac joint in the area of the joint capsule. Only by stabilization of the sacroiliac joint can lameness be reduced. Injections of any type should be done under only the strictest aseptic procedure. Infection in this area could be disastrous.

Prognosis

Prognosis is always guarded, and in those cases where there had been repeated injury and extensive weakening of the ligamentous attachments, healing might never occur. In horses that have obviously had past sacroiliac subluxation, but whose joint(s) now appears solid and who have no lameness, the prognosis would be favorable. A healed injury of this type is probably more subject to reinjury and damage than is the normal sacroiliac joint, and owners should be cautioned to avert such injury if at all possible.

SPECIFIC REFERENCES

ADAMS, O. R. 1969. Subluxation of the sacroiliac joint in horses. Proc. AAEP, 191–207.

ROBERTS, E. J. 1968. Resection of thoracic or lumbar spinous processes for the relief of pain responsible for lameness and some other locomotor disorders of horses. Proc. AAEP, 13–30.

ROONEY, J. R. 1969. Biomechanics of Lameness in Horses. Baltimore: Williams & Wilkins.

ROONEY, J. R., et al. 1969. Sacroiliac luxation in the horse. Proc. AAEP, 193–198.

ROONEY, J. R., et al. 1969. Sacroiliac luxation in the horse. Eq. Vet. J. 1(6): 287–290.

SISSON, S. 1953. Anatomy of Domestic Animals. 4th ed. J. D. Crossman, ed. Philadelphia: W. B. Saunders Co.

Fractures of the Pelvis

Definition

Fractures of the pelvis in horses are relatively common. They are most commonly found in the shaft of the ilium, but fractures of the tuber coxae, symphysis pubis, and obturator foramen also occur.

Etiology

Trauma is the etiology in all cases. Horses that slip and fall on their sides may fracture the pelvis. Horses also can fracture the ilium by fighting a sideline or struggling while the hind limbs are tied in a casting harness. The coxofemoral articulation of horses is rarely dislocated because of the strong formation of the hip joint; the ilium usually fractures instead.

Signs

Signs of fracture of the pelvis are variable because of the different sites of fractures (Fig. 6–116). If the tuber coxae is fractured, very little lameness will be present, but when the horse is observed from behind, the hip on the fractured side will be flatter than the hip of the sound side (knocked-down hip). In some cases, these fractured pieces of bone become sequestra and must be removed surgi-cally. In severe cases of fracture of the tuber coxae, the skin may be broken and the fractured ilium may protrude through the skin at the site of the tuber coxae.

If the shaft of the ilium is broken, it may break in front of, behind, or through the acetabulum. If there is overriding of the fragments, the limb of the affected side will appear shorter than the opposite limb. The horse will be very lame, often refusing to place the foot of the affected limb on the ground. The lameness will closely resemble hip-joint lameness when the horse walks, especially if the fracture has occurred through the acetabulum. The anterior phase of the stride will be short, and the horse will evidence pain as his weight passes onto the affected limb.

If the fracture occurs through the symphysis pubis or through the obturator foramen, the horse will often appear to be lame in both hind limbs, walking with a hesitating gait that is short in the anterior phase of the stride.

Diagnosis

Diagnosis is dependent on physical signs and examination by rectal palpation. The most accurate method of diagnosis is to move the horse while one hand is held in the rectum. Crepitation will be detected as the horse moves, and often the site of fracture can be pinpointed. In some fractures of the ilium, large hematomas that are easily palpable will be present. In other cases, one of the iliac arteries may be severed by the fractured ilium and the horse will die shortly after injury because of internal hemorrhage. Fractures of the symphysis pubis and obturator foramen may have no hematomas, so they should be detected by movement of bone fragments on rectal palpation. Grasping the tuber coxae and attempting to move it while keeping one hand in the rectum is helpful in distorting the pelvis and producing crepitation if fracture is present. Crepitation will not be obvious in all

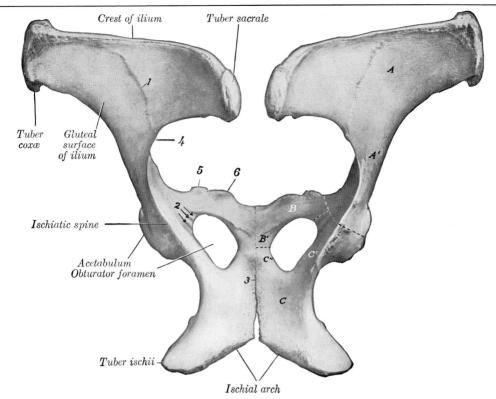

Crest of ilium   Tuber sacrale

A

A'

Tuber   Gluteal
coxæ   surface
         of ilium

1

4

5   6

B

Ischiatic spine

2

B'

C'

Acetabulum
Obturator foramen

C''

3

C

Tuber ischii

Ischial arch

FIG. 6–116. Ossa coxarum of horse; dorsal view. *A*, Wing of ilium; *A'*, shaft of ilium; *B*, acetabular branch of pubis; *B'*, symphyseal branch of pubis; *C*, body of ischium; *C'*, acetabular branch (or shaft of ischium); *C''*, symphyseal branch of ischium; *1*, gluteal line; *2*, grooves for obturator nerve and vessels; *3*, symphysis pelvis; *4*, greater sciatic notch; *5*, iliopectineal eminence; *6*, pubic tubercle. Dotted lines indicate primitive separation of three bones, which are potential fracture sites. (Sisson, *Anatomy of Domestic Animals*, courtesy of W. B. Saunders Company.)

cases, so careful and continued examination is necessary for an accurate diagnosis. Separation of the sacroiliac junction must be included in the differential diagnosis.

Treatment

At present, no surgical methods have been devised for correcting fracture of the pelvis of horses. The best treatment now appears to be to place the horse in a box stall and limit his movement. It is beneficial to sling the horse, whenever possible, for six to eight weeks. Healing of the pelvis, however, sometimes does not take place until a year after the original injury. So, if the horse is valued highly by the owner, it should not be destroyed until a year has passed, provided the horse is not suffering great pain. Close confinement will be necessary for long periods, and maximum space requirement will be a small paddock. Preferably, the horse should be box-stalled for three months or more. Surgical removal of a bone fragment from a fracture of the tuber coxae will be necessary if the fragments become sequestra.

Prognosis

The prognosis is guarded in all cases. Death may occur from internal hemorrhage as the result of a severed iliac artery.

SPECIFIC REFERENCES

COCHRAN, D. 1913. Lameness of the hip joint. Amer. Vet. Rev. 43: 491.

WHEAT, J. O. 1973. Lamenesses of the hip. AAEP Dec.

Thrombosis of the Posterior Aorta or Iliac Arteries

Definition

Thrombus formation in the posterior aorta, iliac arteries, or femoral artery as the result of damage by *Strongylus vulgaris* occasionally causes lameness in horses. Such thrombi cause lameness of the hind limb as a result of circulatory interference (Fig. 6–117). Thrombus formation also has been recorded in the brachial artery of the forelimb, causing lameness of that limb.

Etiology

The thrombi nearly always are caused by larval forms of *Strongylus vulgaris,* that cause damage to the intima of the arteries and subsequent thrombus formation. On the basis of his findings in 38 cases, Azzie (1969) believes that *Strongylus* sp. are not involved in aortic/iliac thrombosis. However, one should consider that larvae could damage the intima of these vessels and then be resorbed. Any damage, however slight, to the intima of these vessels could cause platelet adhesion and clot formation. Azzie proposes that trauma to the aorta and/or iliac from various causes and possible hormonal factors should be considered.

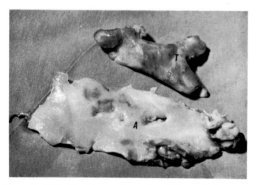

FIG. 6–117. Portion of aorta (*A*) and its enclosed thrombus (*T*). The bifurcation of the thrombus on the right shows how it had occluded not only the aorta but the iliac division. The horse afflicted with this thrombus was able to move only a few steps before incoordination and pain began. The limbs were cold and the condition was diagnosed by rectal examination, which revealed very weak pulsation in the iliac arteries.

Signs

Signs vary with the size of the thrombus and the amount of occlusion of the blood vessel. Signs also vary in time of their appearance after exercise. If the thrombus is small, and the occlusion of the vessel is not great, the horse may be exercised vigorously before lameness occurs; however, in most cases the lameness occurs shortly after exercise begins and so may be confused with azoturia. While at rest, the blood supply to the muscles may be adequate to prevent lameness, but some horses will be lame even when walking.

When lameness appears, profuse sweating, pain and anxiety occur if the horse is forced to continue the exercise. The affected limb will be cooler than the opposite member, and pulsation of the femoral artery will be less than that in the opposite limb, unless both limbs are involved. An outstanding characteristic of this lameness is its intermittent character; it appears with exercise and disappears with rest. If the thrombosis is bilateral in the aorta, the horse may have difficulty in supporting his hindquarters.

The veins on the affected limb will be more or less collapsed, while the veins on the normal limb will stand out. Another sign that may be present in a unilateral affliction is that the affected limb will not sweat, while the opposite normal limb does.

Diagnosis

Diagnosis is established by rectal examination of the aorta and the iliac arteries. If there is a noticeable decrease of pulsation in the iliacs of the affected side or if there is fremitus in these arteries, thrombosis should be suspected. In some cases, the thrombosis actually may be palpated. The femoral artery pulsation on the inside of the thigh may be compared in both limbs; this is helpful in diagnosis. Coldness of the affected limb or limbs is present, while in azoturia, the quadriceps muscles become hard, and urine is coffee-colored.

Treatment

Two cases successfully treated with sodium gluconate* appear in the literature (Tillotson, 1966; Branscomb, 1968). Both authors stress giving the drug slowly at an intravenous dosage rate of 500–600 mg/kg body weight. Alarming signs may occur during injection, and the rate must be slow (two hours and thirty minutes to administer the dosage in 1,500 ml of sterile water). These reports are encouraging and the methods merit trial, because other treatments usually are not successful. In addition, the horse should be wormed with thiabendazole† at the rate of 4 gm/100 lb (4 gm/45.4 kg) body weight once weekly for three weeks. This will aid in destroying migrating *Strongylus* larvae.

In the absence of treatment, the vessels may in time be able to establish collateral circulation that will overcome the effects of the thrombus. However, some horses become progressively worse, and destruction is necessary.

Prognosis

The prognosis, always guarded, is unfavorable if there is bilateral involvement

*Sodium gluconate, Chas. Pfizer Co., New York.
†Omnizole, Merck & Co., Rahway, N.J.

or if the horse seems to be getting progressively worse.

SPECIFIC REFERENCES

Azzie, M. A. J. 1969. Aortic iliac thrombosis of thoroughbred horses. Eq. Vet. J. 1(3): 113–116.
Branscomb, B. L. 1968. Treatment of arterial thrombosis in a horse with sodium gluconate. JAVMA 152(11): 1643–1644.
Miller, R. M. 1970. Thrombophlebitis of the external iliac vein in a horse. VM/SAC 65: 153–155.
Tillotson, P. J. 1966. Treatment of aortic thrombosis in a horse. JAVMA 149(6): 766–767.

Dislocation of the Hip Joint

Definition

Dislocation of the hip joint of horses is not common. In horses, the ilium tends to fracture before dislocation of the hip occurs; in cattle the opposite is true. However, the disease should be considered if hip lameness is present.

Etiology

Trauma is the etiology. A tethered horse that catches its foot in a rope may dislocate the hip in the struggle to free itself. The hip also may be dislocated if the horse fights a sideline or as a result of some other such trauma. The acetabulum is deep and the head of the femur is large, so a great trauma would be necessary to dislocate this joint.

Signs

The horse, which has both an accessory and a round ligament of the hip joint, must suffer a tear of the round ligament for the hip to dislocate (Fig. 6–119). The femur is usually displaced upward and forward when the hip luxates (Fig. 6–118). Signs that usually accompany dislocation are limited anterior stride, because of a pronounced shortening of the limb, and

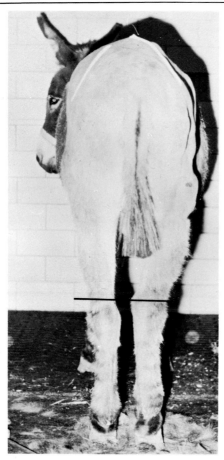

FIG. 6–118. Dorsal luxation of the right coxo-femoral joint in a burro. Notice the shortening of the right hind limb, as shown by the point of the right hock being higher than the point of the left hock.

more prominence of the greater tro-chanter of the femur. Soft-tissue swelling may make this prominence difficult to determine in early stages. Crepitation of the joint, as a result of the femur rubbing on the shaft of the ilium, may cause one to think the pelvis is fractured. A rectal examination should be made to eliminate such a possibility. By placing the hand on the posterior aspect of the greater tro-chanter and pushing forward, one often can move the femur farther than is normal when dislocation has occurred. The limb appears to dangle somewhat because of

shortening. The toe and stifle turn out-ward and the hock inward.

Treatment

Replacing the head of the femur in horses is very difficult without general anesthesia and a surgical approach. The horse should be anesthetized and the area over the greater trochanter prepared for surgical procedure. An incision 8″ long should be made anterior to the greater trochanter, and the muscles divided by

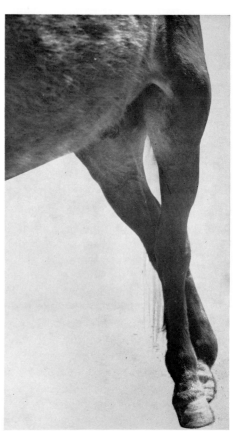

FIG. 6–119. Rupture of the round ligament of the coxofemoral joint. The stifle-out, toe-out, hock-in attitude of the limb typifies rupture of the round ligament. This same limb attitude is also present when the joint has luxated. When the round ligament ruptures, but the joint does not luxate, the limbs are the same length.

blunt dissection. Traction should be placed on the foot, using a block and tackle or a calf puller, and the limb pulled downward until the head of the femur rests in the acetabulum. This can be determined by exploring with the fingers while palpating the head of the femur and the acetabulum through the incision. This operation should be done soon after the dislocation occurs; otherwise contraction of the muscles will make it very difficult to reduce the dislocation. In addition, the acetabulum will tend to fill with connective tissue, making it difficult to identify. In some cases, muscles may be severed to facilitate relocation of the head of the femur.

In cattle, there is little possibility of the head of the femur remaining in the acetabulum, once in place. In horses, though, there is a better chance; if it remains in place for approximately three months, the muscles will usually keep it in place. An operation using a toggle pin to hold the hip in place is possible, as is done in cattle (Adams, 1957).

Prognosis

The prognosis is guarded to unfavorable. Horses may return to complete soundness after the head of the femur is replaced, but this is the exception and not the rule. Most horses, however, can be made sound enough for breeding purposes. If the animal is valuable, surgical correction is advisable and should be done; otherwise, destruction may be necessary.

SPECIFIC REFERENCES

ADAMS, O. R. 1957. Preliminary report on repair of coxofemoral luxation and coxofemoral subluxation in cattle. JAVMA 130: 515.

DAVIDSON, P. J. 1967. Coxofemoral subluxation in a Welsh pony. Vet. Rec. 80(14): 141–444.

JOGI, P., and I. NARBERG. 1962. Malformation in the hip joint of a standardbred horse. Vet. Rec. 74: 421.

MACKAY-SMITH, M. P. 1961. Fracture and luxation of the femoral head. JAVMA 145(3): 248–251.

ROTHENBACHER, H., and J. F. HOKANSON. 1965. Coxofemoral joint luxation in a quarterhorse. JAVMA 147: 148.

Rupture of the Round Ligament of the Coxofemoral Joint

Definition

The hip joint of the horse has several ligaments to help hold it together. The largest and strongest is the round ligament between the head of the femur and the acetabulum. Occasionally, stresses occur that cause rupture of the round ligament, but do not produce coxofemoral luxation. In this case, the head of the femur has greater motion than is normal, causing osteoarthritic changes in the joint.

Etiology

Trauma is the etiology of round ligament rupture. The same stresses that cause luxation of the coxofemoral joint can cause rupture without actual luxation.

Signs

Signs of round ligament rupture are very similar to those of luxation. The notable exception is that the limbs are of the same length. The signs that characterize round ligament rupture are toe-out, stifle-out, and hock-in appearance of the affected hind limb. This same appearance is also present in luxation of the coxofemoral joint, but the limbs are uneven in length (Fig. 6–119). Crepitation over the joint may be present because of the excessive motion of the femur allowed by rupture of the ligament or because of osteoarthritic changes that occur. Crepitation from these sources may be palpated either externally or per rectum. Comparison of the limbs will show that they are equal in length when the ligament is ruptured and luxation has not occurred. In cases of long duration, differential diagnosis from coxofemoral luxation may require radiographic aid.

Diagnosis

Diagnosis is based on the signs of stifle-out, toe-out, and hock-in appearance with equal length of the limbs. If the horse is anesthetized and laid on his back, a radiograph of the joint can be taken. If the condition is of long standing, radiography will show severe degenerative osteoarthritic changes. Otherwise, the abnormal position of the femoral head in the acetabulum can be identified.

Treatment

There is no effective treatment, except stabilization of the joint with a toggle pin apparatus. However, this is not practical in horses because the joint is never sound enough to permit galloping. This procedure is successful in cattle, but in cattle the gait seldom exceeds a walk.

Prognosis

Prognosis is unfavorable since the increased range of motion of the femoral head usually causes severe osteoarthritis before ligamentous regeneration can occur.

Trochanteric Bursitis (Trochanteric Lameness, Whorlbone Lameness)

Definition

This lameness, most common in Standardbreds, is an inflammation of the bursa beneath the tendon of the middle gluteus muscle as it passes over the great trochanter of the femur. The tendon of the middle gluteus muscle also may be involved, as well as the cartilage over the trochanter major. The deep portion of the gluteus medius muscle has a strong, flat tendon that passes over the convexity of the trochanter before it inserts into the crest. The trochanter is covered with cartilage and the trochanteric bursa is interposed between it and the tendon.

Etiology

Lameness is caused by bruising as a result of the horse falling on the affected side, by straining the tendon during racing or training, or by a direct kick on the trochanter. It also has been found following an attack of distemper. In most cases, bone spavin also exists in the affected hind limb, and hock lameness produces the bursitis.

Signs

Pain may be evident when pressure is applied over the great trochanter. Careful examination should be made for pain, because some horses naturally tend to shy away when pressure is applied over the hip joint. At rest, the limb may remain flexed; as the horse moves, weight is placed on the inside of the foot so that the inside wall of the foot wears more than the outside wall. This can be best seen when observing the horse from behind. From this observation it can be seen that the foot is carried inward and the horse sets the foot down on a line between the forelimbs. The horse tends to travel "dog fashion" since the hind quarters move toward the sound side because the stride of the affected limb is shorter than that of the sound side. After the condition has been present for some time, atrophy of the gluteal muscles occurs. In cases where the etiology has been a severe trauma, such as a direct kick, the cartilage or the bone of the trochanter may be fractured, causing persistent lameness.

Diagnosis

The foregoing symptoms should be used in diagnosis. The condition is difficult to differentiate from inflammation of the coxofemoral joint, or from a fracture through the acetabulum, if the fracture shows no crepitation. The lameness, which is not common, may be confused with spavin lameness. A lameness of unknown cause is sometimes ascribed to trochanteric bursitis. Injection of a local anesthetic into the area of the bursa is helpful in differential diagnosis.

Treatment

Injection of the bursa with corticoids apparently is the most effective method of treatment (see Chap. 11). Other treatments consist of injections of Lugol's solution of iodine into or around the bursa as a counterirritant. Hot packs applied to the affected area in the acute stages will relieve some pain. Phenylbutazone given orally may also relieve pain (p. 447). When the cartilage or bone has been damaged with fracture or periostitis, treatment is difficult. Surgery or injection of irritants may be indicated.

Prognosis

The prognosis is guarded to unfavorable. If the horse responds to therapy within four to six weeks, he may again become sound. However, if the injury is more severe, the lameness may remain indefinitely or may recur when the horse is put back into training.

Femoral Nerve Paralysis (Crural Paralysis)

Definition

Paralysis of the femoral nerve affects the quadriceps femoris group of muscles. This muscle group is composed of the rectus femoris muscle, the vastus lateralis muscle, the vastus medialis muscle, and the vastus intermedius muscle. This large muscular mass covers the front and sides of the femur and inserts into the patella.

Etiology

Femoral nerve paralysis may arise from trauma, from azoturia, or from unknown causes. Injury to the nerve may occur from overstretching of the limb during exertion, kicking, slipping, or while the horse is tied in a recumbent position.

Signs

The horse will not be able to bear weight on the affected limb. In standing position all joints of the affected limb will be flexed as a result of this condition. The horse will have difficulty advancing the limb, but can do so because the hock can be sufficiently flexed to pull the limb forward. During movement, the horse will not be able to bear weight on the limb, so compensation must be made in the gait. After the condition has been present for some time, atrophy of the quadriceps muscles occurs, causing these muscles to lose their normal softness and become more like tendinous structures.

Diagnosis

The signs listed above are characteristic and are used for diagnosis. The condition should be differentiated from lateral (true) luxation of the patella, rupture of the quadriceps femoris muscles, and avulsion of the tibial crest. Any of these conditions could cause a similar syndrome; however, all of these are rare. Lateral luxation of the patella can be diagnosed by palpation of the displaced patella; rupture of the quadriceps femoris muscle can also be palpated. Radiological examination can determine avulsion of the tibial crest where the patellar ligaments insert.

Treatment

No treatment is known. If the condition is due to injury of the femoral nerve, the animal should be stalled for a long time. The muscles should be massaged whenever possible, and, if some function returns, exercise should be used to minimize atrophy. If the cause is azoturia, exercise is a most important part of the treatment. Injections of selenium/vitamin E combinations and thiamine are indicated.

Prognosis

Prognosis is guarded to unfavorable. Prognosis should be withheld until sufficient time has elapsed to determine if any function will return. Thirty days is required, at a minimum, for function to return completely.

Upward Fixation of the Patella

Definition

Upward fixation of the patella occurs on the medial trochlea of the femur between the middle and medial patellar ligaments (Fig. 6–121). The fixation of the patella on the medial trochlea of the femur prevents flexion of the affected hind limb. It is sometimes called a luxation, although this is a misnomer. The terms "luxation" or "lateral luxation" of the patella should not be used for this condition; although true luxation may

occur, the signs are entirely different from those of upward fixation.

Etiology

It is generally considered that there may be a hereditary predisposition to upward fixation of the patella. This predisposition is brought about by conformation. A horse having a steep angle between femur and tibia, or so-called "straight hind leg" (Fig. 1–29, p. 19), with what appears to be a long tibia is more predisposed to the condition than is a horse of normal conformation. Some cases of upward fixation can be the result of trauma incurred when the limb was overextended. Long straight legs predispose the horse to upward fixation of the patella due to trauma. Debility and poor conditioning also can be predisposing factors. Once upward fixation occurs, the ligaments may be stretched, so recurrence is common. The condition may be visible in only one hind limb, but careful examination will often reveal susceptibility in both hind limbs. Shetland ponies probably are most often affected in this manner.

Signs

In acute upward fixation of the patella, the hind limb is locked in extension (Fig. 6–120). The stifle and hock cannot flex, but the fetlock can. The condition may temporarily relieve itself only to lock again in a few steps, or it may remain locked for several hours or even days. In some cases there is only a "catching" of the patella as the horse walks and the leg never truly locks in extension. This "catching" of the patella is most noticeable when the horse is turned in a short circle toward the affected hind limb. This intermittent upward fixation of the patella causes the lameness to be confused with stringhalt, and careful physical examination is required.

Upon palpation, when the limb is

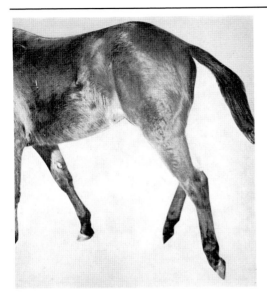

FIG. 6–120. Upward fixation of the patella. The limb is locked in extension as the horse attempts to pull the limb forward. Note that the left fetlock, pastern, and coffin joints are flexed while the stifle and hock joints are locked in extension.

locked in extension, the ligaments of the patella are tense and the patella is locked above the medial portion of the trochlea of the femur (Fig. 6–121). When the horse is forced to move forward with the limb locked, he drags the front of the hoof on the ground. In some cases, a snapping sound may be heard when the patella is released from the trochlea.

Diagnosis

The signs are typical, and, if the limb is locked, diagnosis is simple. In cases where the owner describes a partial locking, or complete locking, the limb should be checked by forcing the patella upward and outward with the hand (Fig. 4–6, p. 102). If the limb can be locked in extension for one or more steps, it is predisposed to upward fixation of the patella. In some cases, this condition is chronic, causing an inflammation of the stifle joint (gonitis) or chondromalacia of the patella. The arthritis or chondromalacia in the

joint may remain even though upward fixation is corrected. The joint capsule should be checked for distention by palpating between the lateral and middle patellar ligaments and between the middle and medial patellar ligaments. Excess fluid or thickening of the joint capsule indicates that gonitis is present.

When intermittent upward fixation of the patella is present, confusion with stringhalt sometimes exists. In this case, careful observation of the gait and stifle joint will reveal whether the patella is "catching." The patella should be forced upward and outward over the femoral trochlea to see if it can be temporarily locked, which would help to rule out stringhalt.

The condition is commonly bilateral, although it may be worse in one limb. In

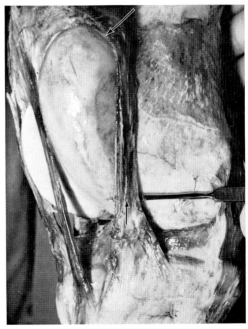

FIG. 6–121. Upward fixation of the patella. The lower arrow shows the approximate site for cutting the medial patellar ligament. The arrow above shows how the medial patellar ligament locks over the medial trochlea of the femur. The view is of the medial aspect of the left hind limb, and to reproduce locking, the patella must be pushed upward and laterally.

some vague cases it will be noted that the horse tends to drag the toe when advancing the limb. The flight of the foot has a low arc, and there is a short anterior phase to the stride. In such a case, the patella usually can be locked in upward fixation with the hand; if so, surgical treatment should be instituted. Radiographs of the stifle should be made on horses under 3 years of age to eliminate the possibility of concurrent osteochondritis dissecans.

Treatment

In acute upward fixation of the patella, a sideline may be applied to the affected limb so that as the limb is drawn forward, the patella is pushed medially and downward, which often disengages the fixed patella. Some authorities have advocated startling the horse with a whip so that the sudden jump will release the patella. In other cases, backing the horse while at the same time pushing inward and downward on the patella will release it. Blistering and firing the stifle also have been recommended, but only as temporary measures for preventing extension of the stifle joint through pain.

Surgical intervention (medial patellar desmotomy) is the best treatment for all cases. The area over the middle and medial patellar ligaments should be closely clipped and prepared for surgery by soap and water scrub and skin antiseptics. The horse should be tranquilized, and the tail wrapped to keep it from switching into the surgical sites. Two cubic centimeters of lidocaine hydrochloride* should be injected subcutaneously over the middle patellar ligament with a 25-gauge $\frac{5}{8}''$ needle. Then a 20-gauge 2″ needle should be inserted through this skin bleb to infiltrate the subcutaneous area over the medial patellar ligament and to infiltrate the medial patellar ligament itself just above

*Xylocaine, Astra Laboratories.

its tibial attachment. Care should be used to avoid damaging the bone, or periostitis may result. Five to 8 cc of lidocaine hydrochloride are used for this injection.

The operator should wear sterile gloves and use sterile instruments. A $\frac{1}{4}''$ to $\frac{1}{2}''$ incision should be made over the middle patellar ligament near the tibial attachment of the ligament. A Udall's teat bistoury, or other suitable blunt bistoury, should then be pushed underneath the *medial* patellar ligament close to its tibial attachment (Figs. 2-15 and 2-16, pp. 47 and 48; Figs. 6-121 and 6-122). The blade should be turned outward so that the cutting edge is against the ligament (Figs. 6-121 and 6-122). Then, using a sawing action, and pushing with the forefinger on the ligament, from the skin surface, the medial patellar ligament should be severed. All fibers of the ligament must be cut, but the surgeon should not go too far posteriorly. A definite cavity will be felt with the forefinger when the ligament is cut. One or two sutures then should be placed in the skin incision and the area covered with collodion and cotton. The horse should be given tetanus antitoxin and given box-stall rest for one week.

An improved method for medial patellar desmotomy is done as follows: After surgical preparation and infusion of local anesthetic as already described, a small incision ($\frac{1}{4}''$ to $\frac{1}{2}''$ long) is made through the skin on the medial aspect of the middle patellar ligament. Curved mosquito forceps are forced through the heavy fascia beneath the medial patellar ligament. When pushing the mosquito forceps through the heavy fascia, be sure that the curved portion gets completely beneath the medial patellar ligament (Fig. 6-122A). This tears the fascia so that a large bistoury can be inserted beneath the ligament (Fig. 6-122B). The blunt-pointed bistoury cannot be forced through the heavy fascia without first passing the mosquito forceps. The cutting edge of the bistoury is then turned outward and the ligament

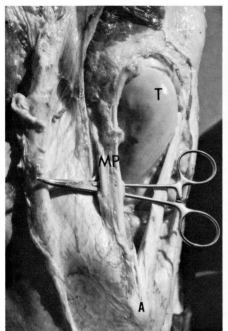

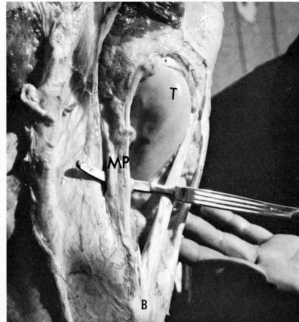

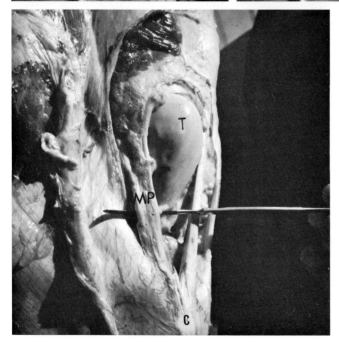

FIG. 6–122. *A,* Curved mosquito hemostat forced under medial patellar ligament (*MP*) to break fascia for bistoury; T, medial trochlea of femur. *B,* Large blunt curved bistoury under medial patellar ligament (*MP*); T, medial trochlea of femur. *C,* Cutting edge of bistoury turned for cutting medial patellar ligament (*MP*); T, medial trochlea of femur.

cut (Fig. 6–122C.) A careful check is then made to be sure that all fibers of the medial patellar ligament have been cut. Fibers next to the middle patellar ligament are those most commonly left, but will not be left if the hemostat and bis-toury have been manipulated properly. The advantages of the large bistoury are that there is less hemorrhage and the ligament can be cut in one stroke. This produces less trauma in the area and less postoperative swelling. One or two skin sutures are then placed in the skin incision.

No riding or training should be permitted for approximately six weeks so that full accommodation to the loss of the ligament can occur before stress is imposed on the joint. Both limbs may be done at the same time, if necessary. If surgical correction is carried out before gonitis or chondromalacia becomes evident, the method of treatment affords a high rate of recovery.

When upward fixation occurs in yearlings, it may be advisable to delay surgery to determine if the horse will grow out of the condition. However, if the limb, or limbs, locks in extension, surgery should be performed at once. Delaying surgery is advisable only for those young horses that show intermittent "catching" of the patella, since fixation may cease before they are two years of age.

Prognosis

The prognosis is favorable, provided surgery is done before gonitis becomes evident. Rarely the ligament will regenerate, necessitating another desmotomy.

SPECIFIC REFERENCES

COCHRAN, D. 1912–1913. Stifle lameness. Amer. Vet. Rev. 42: 308.

DELAHANTY, D. D. 1963. Medial patellar desmotomy in a pony. Sci. Proc. Amer. Vet. Med. Assoc., 81.

HICKMAN, J. 1964. Upward retention of the patella. Vet. Rec. 76(43): 1199.

RAO, S. V. 1965. Hey-Grove's knife for patellar desmotomy in the bovine. Nord. Vet. Med. 17: 172–173.

Chondromalacia of the Patella

Definition

Chondromalacia of the patella is a degeneration of the articular cartilage of the patella (Fig. 6–123). It may result from an inflammatory disease of the stifle joint or from a combination of inflammation and pressure exerted upon it from a partial or complete upward fixation of the patella.

Etiology

In most cases, the etiology is pressure produced between the patella and medial trochlea of the femur. This pressure is usually induced by a partial fixation of the patella between the medial and middle patellar ligaments (Fig. 6–121). Erosions in the surface of the cartilage are produced by the pressures, and consequent inflammation results in distention of the femoropatellar pouch, with excess synovia, and in the more chronic phases, a thickening of the capsule of the femoropatellar pouch. Traumatic injuries to the stifle joint will also produce chondromalacia. Ligamentous tears such as rupture of the anterior cruciate or medial collateral ligaments of the joint can produce inflammation that will result in accompanying chondromalacia of the patella.

Signs

Gonitis and stifle lameness are the primary signs of chondromalacia of the patella. The lameness is usually mild and may be difficult to diagnose. In the trot, the hip will elevate as it does with a hock or stifle lameness. Using the spavin test may cause the horse to show a mild reaction because of the arthritis that is present. This should not be confused with true bone spavin, in which the reaction is usually much more pronounced. Reduced flexion of the stifle and hock, shortening of the anterior phase of the stride, and possible dragging of the toe are the most common signs during movement. Careful palpation of the femoropatellar pouch will reveal distention of this pouch with synovial fluid between the patellar ligaments. In addition, there may be thickening of the femoropatellar pouch, and careful comparison between the unsound joint and the sound joint must be made. Chondromalacia can be bilateral. Pressing the patella upward and outward with the limb in an extended position may produce a partial locking of the joint or a soft-tissue crepitation between the patella and the medial femoral condyle. This crepitation is indicative of an inflammatory reaction and thickening of the synovium. It is regarded as a sign that chondromalacia of the patella is probably present.

Diagnosis

Diagnosis is based on the signs of lameness, palpation of the femoropatellar pouch for distention and thickening, palpation of crepitus as the patella is forced up over the trochlea of the femur, and diagnostic anesthesia of the femoropatellar pouch. The femoropatellar pouch can be injected with 30–50 cc of Xylocaine plus a steroid (see Chap. 11), and if lameness is relieved, this is good evidence that the site of lameness is in this joint. Radiographs of the stifle should be made on horses under three years of age to eliminate the possibility of concurrent osteochondritis dissecans (Fig. 6–129).

Treatment

Treatment is directed at removing the cause and reducing inflammation. Injection of the femoropatellar pouch with a corticoid will temporarily alleviate the inflammatory reaction (see Chap. 11). However, in most cases it is best to sever the medial patellar ligament as described for upward fixation of the patella. This relieves tension of the patella against the medial trochlea of the femur and aids in removing the cause of the chondromalacia. Following cutting of the medial patellar ligament, at least six months must be allowed for regeneration of the articular cartilage and relief of symptoms. In

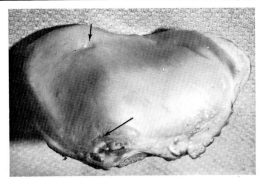

FIG. 6–123. Chondromalacia of the patella. Arrows show areas of chondromalacia on the articular surface and on the distal border of the patella. This type of injury to the patella takes several months to regenerate after the medial patellar ligament is cut.

some cases the disease is advanced to the point that no cure can be accomplished.

Prognosis

The prognosis is guarded, but if relief of symptoms occurs within six months after medial patellar desmotomy, the horse may remain sound.

Lamenesses of the Stifle (Femorotibial) Joint (Gonitis)

Definition

Gonitis is a vague term meaning inflammation of the stifle joint. The term does not really constitute a diagnosis; it merely describes a general area of involvement.

The most common involvement of the stifle is chondromalacia of the patella. This may result from upward fixation of the patella or by pressure between the patella and medial trochlea of the femur caused by near upward fixation without locking. The next most common cause of gonitis is damage to the medial meniscus, followed in occurrence by rupture of the medial collateral femorotibial ligament and/or the anterior cruciate ligament. In addition to occurring as a separate condition, damage to the medial meniscus occurs with or following injury to the above ligaments. Osteochondritis dissecans is relatively common in horses under three years of age, and the possibility should be considered and eliminated by radiographs in horses of this age group (Fig. 6–129).

Etiology

Gonitis may have many causes, and most are due to trauma. The following are conditions of the joint that may cause gonitis:

Partial or Complete Upward Fixation of the Patella. This is one of the most common causes of gonitis and, in addition, may produce chondromalacia of the patella. Irritation causes thickening of the synovium, and roughening of the patella

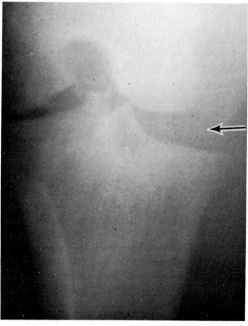

FIG. 6–124. Radiograph of stifle showing opening of medial aspect of femorotibial joint typical of rupture of medial femorotibial ligament (arrow). There is also a fracture of the tibial spine indicating sprain-fracture of the anterior cruciate ligament.

and medial trochlea of the femur may occur.

Sprain of the Medial or Lateral Collateral Ligaments. Sprain may occur to these ligaments in any of the categories listed in Chapter 5, page 147. Any form of sprain from mild to sprain fracture will produce gonitis. The medial collateral ligament is the one most commonly ruptured (Fig. 6–124). Rupture causes complete incapacitation because of resulting osteoarthritic changes. Damage to the medial meniscus will eventually occur, either when the medial collateral ligament is torn or from the resulting instability of the femorotibial joint.

Injury to the Anterior or Posterior Cruciate Ligaments. Sprain of these ligaments may occur to any degree described in Chapter 5. Sprain fracture also occurs (Fig. 6–125). If the ligament is sprained but not ruptured or a partial sprain fracture occurs, diagnosis is difficult. Radiographs may reveal separation of the tibial spine (Fig. 6–125). The anterior cruciate ligament is the one most commonly ruptured and may be damaged along with the medial collateral ligament. Damage to the medial meniscus will occur, either when the anterior cruciate ligament is damaged or from the resulting instability of the femorotibial joint.

Injury to the Menisci. Meniscal injuries occur in the horse but are difficult to diagnose. The medial meniscus is the one most commonly damaged. Persistent effusion of the joint and chronic lameness can be the result (Figs. 6–126 and 6–127).

Injuries to the Joint Capsule. The joint capsule may be injured and the fibrous portion partially torn from its attachment. This type of injury is rare.

Severe Trauma to the Joint. This may produce an injury such as a fractured trochlea of the femur or fracture of the patella (Fig. 6–128). This is also a rare type of injury.

Chondromalacia of the Patella (see p. 308). Chondromalacia of the patella is

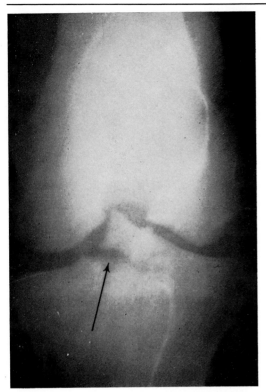

FIG. 6–125. Fracture of the tibial spine associated with rupture of the anterior cruciate ligament (sprain-fracture) in a horse. Fracture of this spine usually does not accompany rupture of the cruciate ligaments.

produced from partial or complete upward fixation of the patella. Even when the patella does not lock, there is tension of the patella against the trochlea of the femur, and chondromalacia occurs, causing persistent effusion of the joint and chronic lameness.

Infectious Arthritis. Infectious arthritis resulting from septicemia, especially in a foal, may leave residual damage that becomes evident when the horse is worked.

Osteochondritis Dissecans (aseptic necrosis). In young horses, this condition may damage the articular surfaces sufficiently to leave permanent damage (Fig. 6–129).

From the above, it can be seen that gonitis can be complex. Any one, or any combination, of the above structures, may

be injured. Sometimes small fractures of the joint are confused with inflammation from other causes and go undiagnosed. Several types of arthritis may affect the stifle joint, including serous arthritis, osteoarthritis, and suppurative arthritis. Navel ill of foals is the most common cause of suppurative arthritis (*see* Chap. 5).

Signs

The degree of lameness in gonitis varies according to severity of the injury. Involvements of the menisci and the cruciate or collateral ligaments usually produce severe lameness. Complete or incomplete upward fixation of the patella also can produce gonitis, but signs of lameness are less acute. If the patella partially or completely locks, irritation of the synovial structures occurs, and chronic distention of the joint capsule and persistent lameness eventually result. Thickening of the joint capsule can occur in con-

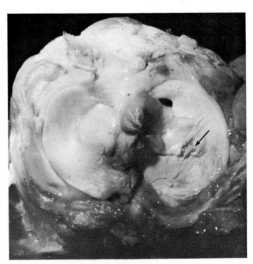

FIG. 6–126. Wrinkling and tearing of the medial meniscus (arrow). This type of injury can occur with or without tearing of the ligaments of the stifle. When chondromalacia of the patella and ligamentous injury can be ruled out, tearing of the medial meniscus should be considered in chronic gonitis.

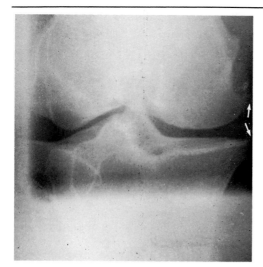

FIG. 6-127. Osteoarthritis of stifle joint caused by chronic medial meniscus damage. Notice lipping on medial aspect of joint (arrows).

junction with distention. The capsule should be carefully examined by palpation between the patellar ligaments to determine if either of these signs is present. In chondromalacia of the patella, soft-tissue crepitation can be palpated with

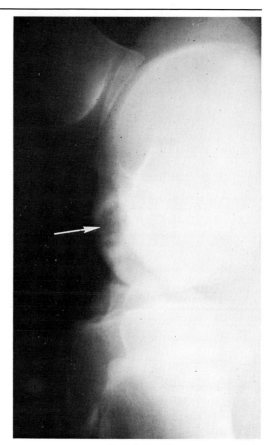

FIG. 6-129. Osteochondritis dissecans (aseptic necrosis) of medial condyle of femur (arrow).

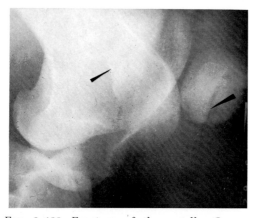

FIG. 6-128. Fracture of the patella. Severe trauma to the stifle joint accompanied by fractures can cause gonitis. In this case there was a fracture of the patella as shown by pointer and a fracture of one of the femoral trochlea indicated by the second pointer. Trauma to the anterior portion of the stifle causes this type of lesion.

the hand as the patella is forced upward and outward over the medial trochlea of the femur. This crepitation means that there is thickening of the synovium between the patella and the trochlea of the femur and is quite indicative of chondromalacia resulting from partial or complete upward fixation of the patella. If upward fixation of the patella is corrected by medial patellar desmotomy, lameness may persist as a result of chronic gonitis and chondromalacia of the patella. Involvement of the stifle joint with suppurative arthritis, as the result of joint ill in foals, usually affects both stifle joints. Aspiration of the contents of the swollen capsule will reveal suppurative material.

Some organisms, such as *E. coli,* may not produce pus but will produce infectious arthritis. A markedly swollen joint and elevated temperature accompany this disease.

Signs of gonitis, from whatever cause, include distention and thickening of the joint capsule between the middle and lateral patellar ligaments and between the middle and medial patellar ligaments. In severe cases, the capsule also is distended over the lateral surface of the joint. The horse will experience pain when moving the leg forward, causing him to shorten the anterior phase of his stride. The stifle joint often will be kept flexed as much as possible as the horse strives to keep the foot of the affected limb off the ground; at the very least, the heel will be raised and the fetlock joint pushed forward. The horse does this to prevent contact of the affected joint surfaces. The horse will put as little weight as possible on the limb when moving or standing; therefore, the lameness is classified as supporting-leg lameness, although it is swinging-leg lameness, in the sense that the horse attempts to protect the limb from concussion and thereby alters the stride of the limb.

If one or more of the collateral or cruciate ligaments are destroyed, movement can be produced between the femur and tibia, and crepitation may be present when moving the joint. This may be checked by locking one's hands around the anterior face of the tibia and pulling the tibia backward with a quick motion (Fig. 4–7, p. 103). Any movement between the femur and tibia in an anterior-posterior direction indicates definitely that a ligament, usually a cruciate ligament, is torn. The anterior cruciate ligament is most commonly involved. The limb should be abducted and adducted to check for rupture of the medial and lateral collateral ligaments. Lameness will be persistent and severe if any of these ligaments are ruptured.

Diagnosis

Diagnosis of gonitis can be made by careful observation of the gait, palpation of the joint, and elimination of other types of lameness. If no swelling of the joint capsule of the stifle joint is present, there probably is no gonitis. One must acquaint himself with the normal tension of fluid in the joint capsule, as palpated between the patellar ligaments, and carefully compare the two stifle joints. Determination of the structures involved can be difficult, but every effort should be made to do so.

Examine the femoropatellar pouch between the middle and lateral patellar ligaments and between the middle and medial patellar ligaments. This examination will disclose any distention of this pouch or thickening of the capsule. Distention or thickening of the pouch means that an inflammatory change is present either between the patella and femur or in the femorotibial joint. Both stifle joints are examined carefully for comparison. The finding of slight distention of the femoropatellar pouch in both hind limbs may or may not be serious. Prominent bilateral distention usually means that important changes have occurred in both stifles.

The next step is to force the patella upward and outward so that the medial patellar ligament will rest over the medial trochlea of the femur (Fig. 4–6, p. 102). This test will reveal whether the patella can be locked on the medial trochlea of the femur and may reveal crepitation as the patella is forced over the upper part of the trochlea. If crepitation is present as the patella is moved back and forth over the upper part of the trochlea, chondromalacia of the patella is probably present and could be the source of irritation. If the patella can be locked, chondromalacia of the patella may be present; in this case, the medial patellar ligament should be cut. Horses three years of age and under should have radiographs of the stifle to eliminate the possibility of concurrent osteochondritis dissecans (Fig. 6–129).

The stifle is then examined for looseness or tearing of the medial collateral or anterior cruciate ligaments. Facing cranially, the hand next to the horse is placed on the medial aspect of the hock joint, and the lower part of the limb is pulled outward while the stifle is forced inward with the shoulder. The other hand is held over the medial aspect of the stifle joint to detect opening of the joint (Fig. 4–7, p. 103). If one can detect opening of the medial aspect of the joint with this test, the medial collateral ligament is loosened or torn (Fig. 6–124). Next, the proximal aspect of the tibia is grasped between the hands, as in Figure 4–7, and given a quick backward pull. If the anterior cruciate ligament is ruptured, crepitation can be felt between the tibia and femur. This means that the anterior cruciate ligament is ruptured. Stretching or rupture of either of these ligaments is very unfavorable, and chronic lameness will result. If either the collateral or the anterior cruciate ligaments are ruptured, or stretched, there will be damage to the medial meniscus of the femorotibial joint. If both chondromalacia and ligamentous rupture can be ruled out, but there is distention of the femoropatellar pouch and a pronounced lameness, medial meniscus damage should be suspected. This can be arrived at only through a process of elimination. The posterior cruciate ligament may rupture with the anterior cruciate, which increases the mobility of the joint.

In the mature horse, the most common changes in the stifle joint are between the patella and femur in the form of intermittent upward fixation or chondromalacia from the patella riding too high. If this finding is negative, ligamentous rupture is differentiated as described. Medial meniscal damage is cause for an unfavorable prognosis, because at present there is no satisfactory surgical procedure for removal of the meniscus, and the constant irritation in the joint causes osteoarthritis (Figs. 6–126 and 6–127). Most changes in the femorotibial joint are limited to the medial side and take the form of ligamentous injury or meniscal damage to the medial meniscus. The lateral aspect of the joint is not commonly involved.

When examining a foal or a young horse (under three years of age), an additional change in the stifle joint that must be considered is osteochondritis dissecans of the joint. This is also known as aseptic necrosis and may involve either the femur or tibia. The change involves the articulation and can be diagnosed only on radiographic examination. This change may be present in very young foals and in horses up to three years of age. However, in most cases the change will be evident before the horse is one year old (Fig. 6–129).

If a suppurative or infectious arthritis is present in the joint, obvious heat, pain, swelling, temperature rise will be present, and one can aspirate abnormal synovial fluid. This type of arthritis usually occurs in the young foal and is one of the changes in navel ill.

Horses affected with gonitis may react to the spavin test. The reaction is usually not as severe as when the horse is truly affected with bone spavin. Any mild reaction to the spavin test should be viewed suspiciously, and the stifle joint given a complete examination for the signs mentioned above. Stifle and hock lameness can be difficult to differentiate because of the similarity of signs when the horse is in motion. When considering any lameness of the hind limb, puncture wounds of the foot and fractured third phalanx should always be ruled out. One tends to get careless about examination of these areas since the majority of lamenesses in the hind limb occur in the hock and stifle.

Treatment

If there is a rupture of one of the collateral or cruciate ligaments of the joint, or damage to the medial meniscus, treatment is unavailing, and chronic lameness will result. If radiological examination indicates that there are osteoarthritic changes or fractures within the joint, the prospects for treatment are also unfavorable (Figs. 6–124, 6–125, and 6–127). If the gonitis is believed to be due to sprain and injury to the joint capsule or to ligamentous attachments without rupture, absolute rest should be enforced for a long period. Confinement should consist of a minimum of thirty days in the box stall and then a minimum of two months in a small paddock; in some cases, three months in a box stall may be necessary. Injection of the stifle joint with a corticoid is recommended, if no infection is present. These injections should be repeated at least three times at one-week intervals (Chap. 11, p. 455). Injections can be made between the middle and lateral patellar ligaments, or between the middle and medial patellar ligaments into the femoropatellar pouch. Firing, blistering, and intraligamentous injection of irritants have been employed. Results of firing are inconsistent, and corticoids are of greater value. In Standardbreds, the collateral ligaments, patellar ligaments, and fibulotibial ligaments are commonly injected with irritants such as sodium morrhuate. Corticoid therapy should *not* be combined with a treatment that produces inflammation. In suppurative arthritis of the stifle joint, the joints should be treated with intra-articular antibiotics after antibiotic sensitivity of the organism has been determined. Parenteral antibiotics should also be given (*see* Chap. 5, p. 130).

Prognosis

If the gonitis is due to upward fixation of the patella, the prognosis is favorable, as long as chondromalacia is not extensive. For all other causes, the prognosis is guarded to unfavorable. Horses do not return to a sound condition if radio-graphic changes of osteoarthritis can be demonstrated.

SPECIFIC REFERENCES

COCHRAN, D. 1912–1913. Stifle lameness. Amer. Vet. Rev. 42: 308.

MACKAY-SMITH, M. P., and C. W. RAKER. 1964. Mechanical defects of the equine stifle: Diagnosis and treatment. Sci. Proc. 100th Meet. Amer. Vet. Med. Assoc.

VAN PELT, R. W., *et al.* 1970. Stifle disease (gonitis) in horses: Clinicopathologic findings and intra-articular therapy. JAVMA 157(9): 1173–1186.

Osteochondrosis of the Tibial Tuberosity

Definition

This condition is reported to affect horses. It is definitely known to occur in dogs and man; in man, the disease is known as Osgood-Schlatter disease. It appears to me that the diagnosis has been abused, as has "fracture of the fibula." Many of the so-called pathological changes of the tibial crest that appear on radiographs are normal for young horses. The tibial crest has an epiphyseal line of its own that is often irregular in outline.

Etiology

Trauma to the tibial crest resulting from tension on the patellar ligaments inserting into the tibial crest due to training of the young horse has been blamed for the condition. However, it is also possible that so-called "avulsion" of the tibial crest can occur from partial upward fixation of the patella. It is very possible that some mild cases of upward fixation of the patella are called osteochondrosis, without the careful examination necessary to determine partial upward fixation. Osteochondrosis is found in horses up to three years of age; this is the time that the tibial crest shows a normal epiphyseal line that makes it appear to be separated from the tibia.

Signs

Signs of this condition are vague. They include swelling, tenderness, and pain in the tibial crest following strenuous exercise. The horse will trot in "dog fashion" because of the short stride of the affected hind leg. If the lesion is bilateral, the stride will be shorter in both hind legs and the toe may be "dubbed off" as a result of the low arc of the foot in flight. Radiographic examination may show a partial avulsion of the tibial crest, and islets of bone in the cartilage that appear to suggest incomplete separation. These changes are difficult to differentiate from a normal epiphyseal line of the tibial crest (Fig. 6–130).

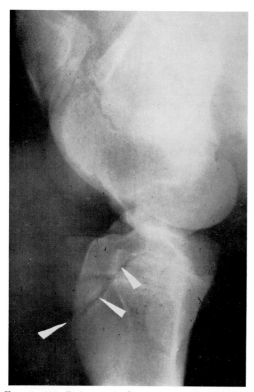

FIG. 6–130. Pointers indicate normal epiphyseal line of the tibial crest, which is often irregular; osteochondritis may be diagnosed, erroneously, if caution is not used. Variations from "normal" will appear in different horses.

Diagnosis

Diagnosis is based mainly on radiographic examination. Radiographs should be taken of both hind limbs for comparison purposes. Although osteochondrosis can occur, a careful examination should be made to eliminate other causes of lameness. A practitioner who has not examined numerous radiographs of young horses could easily be confused by the appearance of the epiphyseal line of the tibial crest. Tension on the patellar ligaments that attach to the tibial crest can occur as the result of intermittent upward fixation of the patella and can cause signs similar to those described for osteochondrosis.

Treatment

Subcutaneous injection of Lugol's iodine over the affected area has been used to hasten recovery. A treatment suggested as a result of work with humans is drilling of the tibial crest to produce inflammation. Corticoid therapy is not effective, and such cases are only mildly responsive to analgesics such as phenylbutazone. Stall rest or confinement in a small paddock for three months is essential. Rest is important because exertion may cause complete avulsion of the tibial crest; however, this is unlikely, since it is extremely rare to find avulsion of this process, even in cases of severe trauma.

Prognosis

The prognosis is guarded. The horse should be returned to work on the basis of the findings on the radiographs.

SPECIFIC REFERENCE

BAKER, H. 1960. Osteochondrosis of the tibial tuberosity of the horse. JAVMA 137: 354.

Fracture of the Fibula

In the past it was popular to diagnose obscure lameness of the hind limb as fracture of the fibula. This was a common diagnosis in Standardbreds and Thoroughbreds, but it has been misused greatly. Extensive radiological studies have revealed that what often appears to be a fracture of the fibula is merely a defect in the union of the proximal and distal segments of the bone (Fig. 6–131). No definite clinical symptoms have been propounded, and anything from sore back to undiagnosed ailments of the hind limb has been termed fracture of the fibula. This defect in union of the bone can be demonstrated in a high percentage of horses. When radiographs are taken of the opposite fibula, it usually is found that the defect is present here, too. Although fracture of the fibula undoubtedly can occur as a result of a direct trauma, it probably does not cause the lameness, and in most cases careful examination will reveal the true cause.

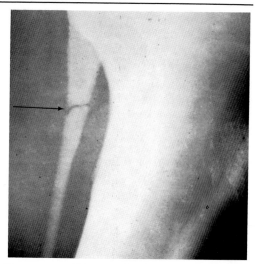

FIG. 6–131. "Fracture" of the fibula in the horse. The arrow indicates a normal fibrous junction in the bone found in many normal horses.

SPECIFIC REFERENCES

BANKS, W. C., and C. W. SCHULTZ. 1958. Additional studies of fibular defects in horses. JAVMA 133: 422.

DELAHANTY, D. D. 1958. Defects—not fractures—of the fibulae in horses. JAVMA 133: 258.

Editorial. 1957. A phenomenon in equine lameness. JAVMA 130: 51.

LUNDVALL, R. L. 1956. Fracture of the fibula in the horse. JAVMA 129: 10.

LUSK, N. D., and J. P. ROSBOROUGH. 1957. Fibular fracture in a filly. JAVMA 130: 4.

ZESKOV, F. 1959. A study of discontinuity of the fibula in the horse. Amer. J. Vet. Res. 78: 852.

ZESKOV, B., NAROLT, J., VUKELIC, E., and DOLINAR, Z. 1958. Fracture or congenital discontinuity of the fibula in the horse. Brit. Vet. J. 114: 145.

Rupture of the Peroneus Tertius

Definition

The peroneus tertius is a strong tendon that lies between the long digital extensor and the tibialis anterior muscle of the rear limb. It originates in common with the long digital extensor from the extensor fossa of the femur and inserts on the anterior surface of the proximal extremity of the third metatarsal bone and on the fibular and fourth tarsal bones. It is an important part of the reciprocal apparatus, mechanically flexing the hock when the stifle joint is flexed. When this muscle is ruptured, the stifle flexes, but the hock does not.

Etiology

Rupture of the peroneus tertius is usually due to overextension of the hock joint. This may occur if the leg is entrapped and the horse struggles violently to free his limb. Rupture may also occur during the exertion of a fast start, when tremendous power is transferred to the limb, causing overextension.

Signs

Signs of rupture of the peroneus tertius are well defined. The stifle joint flexes as the limb advances and the hock joint is carried forward with very little flexion. That portion of the limb below the hock tends to hang limp, giving the appearance of being fractured as it is carried forward. When the foot is put down the horse has no trouble bearing weight and shows little pain. As the horse walks though, it will be noted that there is a dimpling in the tendon of Achilles. If the limb is lifted from the ground one can easily produce a dimpling in the tendon of Achilles by extending the hock (Fig. 6–132). It will be noted that the hock can be extended without extending the stifle; this cannot be done in the normal limb.

Diagnosis

Diagnosis is easily made by the symptoms described above.

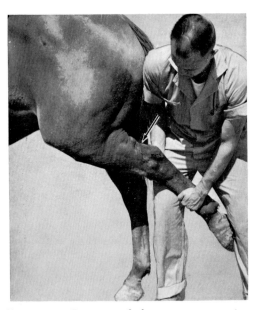

FIG. 6–132. Rupture of the peroneus tertius. The arrow indicates a dimpling in the tendon of Achilles when the limb is extended. Note that the hock is extended but the stifle is flexed; this cannot be done in a normal limb.

Treatment

Complete rest is the only known treatment. The horse should be placed in a box stall and kept quiet for at least four to six weeks. Then limited exercise should be given for the next two months. Most cases will heal and show normal limb action, and, if properly conditioned, most horses can return to normal work. Surgical intervention is not advisable. Hand-leading is advisable when exercise is first begun. This will help control the horse and prevent reinjury.

Prognosis

Prognosis is guarded to favorable. When the horse is properly rested by box-stall confinement, healing usually occurs. If healing is not evident at the end of four to six weeks, the prognosis is unfavorable, as the tendon may not unite. Final appraisal should not be made for at least three months following the injury.

SPECIFIC REFERENCE

SZABUNIEWIEZ, M., and R. S. TITUS. 1967. Rupture of the peroneus tertius. VM/SAC 62(10): 993–998.

Rupture of the Achilles Tendon

Definition

Rupture of the Achilles tendon includes the tendons of the gastrocnemius muscle and the superficial flexor of the hind limb. It is rare for both of these structures to rupture, but when they do, it is a very serious lameness.

Etiology

Trauma producing severe stress to these two tendons or lacerated wounds are the most common causes of rupture.

Signs

Signs of Achilles tendon rupture are characteristic. The hock of the affected limb is dropped to the ground or very near to it. The angle of hock deflection is greater than that in rupture of the gastrocnemius tendon alone. The horse has great difficulty in advancing the limb at all and is helpless, especially if both Achilles tendons are ruptured. The limb or limbs cannot support weight.

Treatment

The only treatment of value is a full-length leg cast including the hoof and extending as high on the limb as possible. This is usually up to the stifle joint. The horse must then be placed in a sling and kept in the cast and sling for six to ten weeks. If the horse will not tolerate these methods of treatment, euthanasia is usually required.

Prognosis

Prognosis is always unfavorable, and only an occasional case will make a recovery (Fig. 6–133).

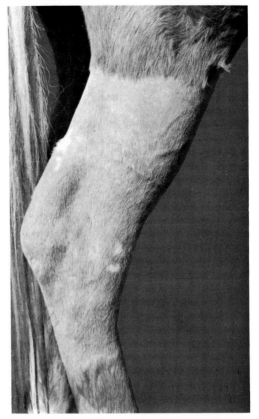

Fig. 6–133. Healed rupture of the Achilles tendon. Note fibrosis of the healed tendon. Treatment consisted of six weeks' immobilization of the limb in a plaster cast from the stifle down to and including the hoof. (Courtesy of Dr. J. T. Ingram.)

Rupture of the Gastrocnemius Tendon

Definition

Rupture of the gastrocnemius tendon may occur in one or both hind limbs. It is rare for both the superficial flexor tendon and the gastrocnemius tendon (Achilles tendon) to be ruptured at the same time. The gastrocnemius tendon apparently ruptures before the superficial flexor tendon.

Etiology

Trauma is the etiology in all cases. In some cases, the horse is found with the condition in one or both limbs, but the cause is not known. Rupture of this tendon can result from strenuous efforts at stopping or from any other exertion where great stress is applied to the hock in an attempt to extend it.

Signs

Signs of gastrocnemius tendon rupture are characteristic. The hock or hocks of the affected limb(s) are dropped so that there is an excessive angle to the hock joint. If the condition is bilateral, the horse appears to be squatting and he cannot straighten his hind limbs. The limb, or limbs, can be advanced and the horse can walk, but at no time do the hock joints assume a normal angle. If the entire tendon of Achilles is ruptured, the limb cannot support weight.

Treatment

No treatment is known at present. Because of the persistent flexion of the hocks, the muscle ends are unable to make contact, making recovery difficult. Placing the horse in a sling so that tension on the gastrocnemius tendon and superficial flexor tendon is eased may be beneficial if used for prolonged periods. A modified Thomas splint made from $\frac{3}{4}''$ electrical conduit or a plaster cast of the limb may be helpful if the horse will tolerate it.

Prognosis

Prognosis is unfavorable because of problems inherent with immobilization of the hind limb.

Fibrotic Myopathy and Ossifying Myopathy

Definition

Fibrotic and ossifying myopathy most commonly occur in the hind legs of horses. They result from old injuries to the semitendinosus, semimembranosus, and biceps femoris muscles. The fibrotic lesion in the semitendinosus muscle is most important because adhesions form between this muscle and the semimembranosus and biceps femoris muscles. These adhesions limit the action of the semitendinosus muscle, causing an ab-

normal gait. This lameness most often occurs in Quarter Horses because of the type of work they perform. Ossifying myopathy in the hind limb, which also results from previous injury to these muscles, is assumed to be an ossification of a fibrotic myopathy lesion. The signs of lameness are the same as with fibrotic myopathy because the adhesions extending from the bony lesion to the adjacent muscles cause a similar restriction of the limb. Ossifying myopathy has also been observed in the foreleg (Riley, 1957).

Etiology

Trauma is thought to be the cause of fibrotic myopathy and ossifying myopathy. Ossifying myopathy is a complication of the fibrotic lesion that also results from trauma. Involved muscles may be injured during sliding stops in rodeo work, or in other ways such as resisting a sideline or catching a foot in a halter. The lesions usually are unilateral, but a case of bilateral fibrotic myopathy resulting from a trailer accident has been recorded. In some cases the exact cause of the injury is not known, since clinical signs are not present during the myositis stage. When the injury heals and adhesions form between the involved muscles, these adhesions cause lameness.

When ossification of the fibrotic myopathy lesion occurs, it is presumed to be caused by osteoblasts that have developed from fibroblasts by metaplasia.

Signs

The signs are due to adhesions between the semitendinosus muscle and the semimembranosus muscle medially, and between the semitendinosus and the biceps femoris muscle laterally (Fig. 6–134). These adhesions partially inhibit normal action of the muscles. In the anterior phase of the stride, the foot of the affected hind leg is suddenly pulled posteriorly 3″

to 5″ just before contacting the ground (Fig. 6–135). Usually the lameness is most noticeable when the horse walks. The anterior phase of the stride is shortened, so consequently the posterior phase is lengthened. This abnormal gait, which is easily identified, may result from either fibrotic or ossifying myopathy. An area of firmness can be palpated over the affected muscles on the posterior surface of the affected limb at the level of the stifle joint and immediately above (Fig. 6–136).

Microscopic lesions of fibrotic myopathy consist of hyalinization of the muscle cell cytoplasm with loss of striations, and moderately pyknotic nuclei. No evidence of inflammation or neoplasia will be present. Bone tissue removed from an ossifying myopathy lesion will have normal structure.

Diagnosis

Diagnosis is based upon the altered gait and on palpation of a hardened area on the posterior surface of the leg at the level of the stifle joint. In making diagnosis, stringhalt also should be considered. In stringhalt the limb is pulled toward the abdomen, while in fibrotic myopathy the foot is pulled toward the ground in a posterior direction just before the foot contacts the ground. In fibrotic myopathy the limb is limited in the anterior phase of the stride by adhesions and by lack of elasticity in the affected area of the muscle belly, causing the limb to be pulled posteriorly before the full length of stride is reached.

Treatment

The most effective therapy is surgical removal of a 4″ portion of the semitendinosus tendon at the level of the stifle joint. The involved piece of tendon is removed at its junction with the muscle belly before the tendon divides. The operation includes separation of adhesions between

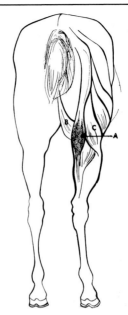

FIG. 6–134. Muscles involved in fibrotic myopathy. *A,* Fibrotic myopathy area in semitendinosus muscle; *B,* semimembranosus muscle; *C,* biceps femoris muscle.

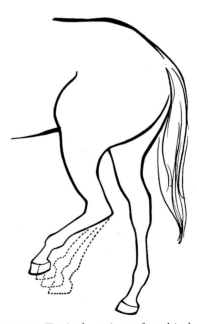

FIG. 6–135. Typical action of a hind limb affected by fibrotic or ossifying myopathy of the semitendinosus muscle. The foot jerks backward three to five inches just before it is put on the ground.

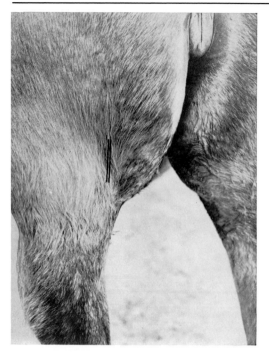

FIG. 6-136. The double lines indicate the area most commonly involved with fibrotic or ossifying myopathy. They also indicate the site of incision for surgical correction of the condition.

the semitendinosus muscle and the semimembranosus and biceps femoris muscles.

The horse should be tranquilized, cast with the affected side up, and surgical anesthesia administered. The caudal aspect of the leg, over the involved muscles at the level of the stifle joint and above, should be prepared for operation. The affected limb should be extended to facilitate surgical procedure. A vertical incision at least 6″ long should be made on the posterior aspect of the semitendinosus tendon (Fig. 6-136). The tendon should be identified and the adhesions from the semimembranosus and the biceps femoris muscles removed. The muscle belly of the semitendinosus muscle should be isolated and a 4″ portion removed. The part removed should comprise 2″ of tendon and 2″ of muscle belly when possible. Follow-

ing removal, the remaining muscle will contract immediately and a large cavity will result. The fascia should be closed over the cavity with No. 2 catgut. The skin should then be sutured with simple interrupted stitches with a noncapillary, nonabsorbable suture of adequate diameter. A quill suture (vertical mattress) of the same suture material is then placed to reinforce the suture line. Rubber intravenous tubing is used for the quill sutures (Fig. 6-137). A Penrose tube* drain is placed in the bottom of the incision line to allow drainage (Fig. 6-137). The wound can be flushed daily through the drain, which is removed in approximately seven days. The wound should be protected with collodion and cotton, and tetanus antitoxin should be administered. Antibiotics usually are not necessary, provided asepsis has been maintained during the operation.

If ossifying myopathy is present, presurgical treatment is the same, but after the incision is made, the skin should be reflected and the bony cover over the semitendinosus muscle dissected away. The adhesions on the medial and lateral sides of this muscle should be cut and the skin closed as described above.

Prognosis

Some relief will be evident in all cases. After healing, some cases develop characteristic, but less pronounced, signs, although limb function will be nearly normal and signs will not be noticeable except in the walk. Occasionally, it takes three to seven days for maximum benefits of surgical correction to become evident.

SPECIFIC REFERENCES

ADAMS, O. R. 1961. Fibrotic myopathy in the hindlegs of horses. JAVMA 139: 1089.

ADAMS, O. R. 1962. Lamenesses of rodeo horses. Vet. Scope (Upjohn Co.) (Spring).

*Davol Rubber Co., Providence, R.I.

ADAMS, R. D., D. D. BROWN, and C. M. PEARSON. 1953. *Diseases of Muscle.* New York: Harper and Brothers.

ANDERSON, J. G. 1966. Lameness due to myositis fibrosa. Southwestern Vet., 19(3): 240.

ARANEZ, J. B. 1969. Ossifying myopathy in a horse. A. U. Vet. Dig. Philippines. 3(1): 14, 23.

BISHOP, R. 1972. Fibrotic myopathy in the gracilis muscle of a horse. VM/SAC 67(3): 270.

LACKEY, S. H. 1968. Myositis fibrosa: Case report. Southwestern Vet. 22(1): 66–67.

RILEY, W. F. 1957. Personal communication, Michigan State University.

Stringhalt

Definition

Stringhalt is an involuntary flexion of the hock during progression and may affect one or both hind limbs.

Etiology

The true etiology is unknown, although the condition has been blamed on nervous diseases, degeneration of the sciatic and/or peroneal nerves, and affections of the spinal cord.

In most cases, the condition is considered to be an involvement of the lateral digital extensor. Some cases are observed following trauma to this tendon, and adhesions of the tendon may form as it crosses the lateral surface of the hock joint. Most cases show at least partial relief of signs following removal of the tendon of the lateral digital extensor, so it must be assumed that involvement of this tendon is at least partially responsible for the condition.

Signs

Signs of the disease are quite variable; some horses show a very mild flexion of the hock during walking, while others show a marked jerking of the foot toward the abdomen. The anterior surface of the fetlock joint may actually hit the abdominal wall in severe cases. Some horses show these signs at each step, while in others it is spasmodic. In nearly all cases, the signs are exaggerated when the horse is turning or backing. It usually is most noticeable after the horse has rested, but the signs may be intermittent and may disappear for variable periods of time. Any breed may be affected, and mild cases may not hinder the horse in use. Cold weather may cause an increase in signs, and usually there is a tendency to-

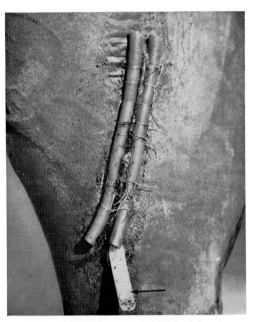

FIG. 6–137. Method of suturing used for operation on fibrotic myopathy. A quill-type suture (vertical mattress), using rubber tubing as the quill portion, reinforces the incision line so that it will not break open. A plastic drain (arrow) is placed into the wound and sutured to the skin. This plastic drain will allow serum and blood to drain from the wound. Even though this is second-intention healing, it is much faster than trying to obtain first-intention healing and having the sutures tear open from internal pressure. The tube is removed in seven days, and the quill sutures removed in approximately two weeks. The wound is rinsed daily through the plastic drain tube with sterile saline solution and an antibiotic solution of choice.

ward decreased intensity of signs during warm weather. Most horses affected have a nervous disposition, which may play a part in the etiology. The character of the lameness can be confused with intermittent upward fixation of the patella.

Diagnosis

The lameness is easily diagnosed, but in some cases signs may be absent at the time of examination. The condition must be differentiated from fibrotic myopathy, in which the foot is jerked suddenly downward and backward before being

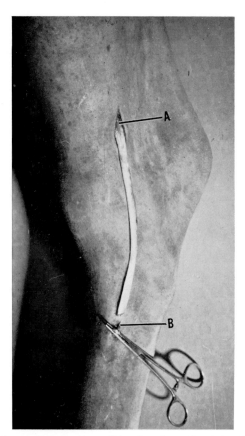

FIG. 6-138. Section of tendon from the lateral digital extensor removed to correct stringhalt. A, Site of the proximal incision just above the lateral malleolus of the tibia. B, Site of distal incision just before the lateral digital extensor joins the long extensor.

put to the ground (p. 320). It must also be differentiated from intermittent upward fixation of the patella, which resembles stringhalt more closely. In stringhalt, there is no locking and releasing of the patella, and the patella cannot be locked when forced upward and outward on the trochlea of the femur.

Treatment

The treatment is surgical and consists of removal of that portion of the tendon of the lateral digital extensor that crosses the lateral surface of the hock joint. Surgical correction can be performed in a standing position, with the horse cast on the ground, or on a surgical table. If the horse is to be operated on in the standing position, he should be tranquilized before preparation of the area for operation. If the horse is cast, the affected leg should be uppermost. The area should be prepared for surgical procedure by shaving the hair and applying skin antiseptics. A local anesthetic should be injected into the muscle of the lateral digital extensor starting about 1″ above the lateral malleolus of the tibia. A second injection of local anesthetic should be made over the tendon below the hock joint just before it joins the long digital extensor tendon. Lidocaine hydrochloride* is recommended as a local anesthetic. The addition of a corticoid will minimize the irritation caused by a local anesthetic (see Chap. 11).

An incision approximately 4″ long is made over the muscle of the lateral digital extensor just above the level of the point of the hock (Fig. 6-138). The muscle belly cannot be identified until several layers of fascia have been severed. Just overlying the tendon is a heavy layer of strong fascia. This is incised, and the muscle belly can be identified. An instrument is passed under the muscle belly so that it

*Xylocaine, Astra Laboratories.

can be properly identified and tension put on it. Pulling on the muscular portion will reveal movement in the distal portion just before it attaches to the long extensor. An incision approximately $\frac{1}{2}''$ long is then made over this distal portion before it joins the long extensor. The skin and subcutaneous tissues are cut with a scalpel and then a blunt pointed bistoury such as Udall teat knife is slipped under the tendon and it is severed. Rarely, there are variations in the insertion of the tendon, such as two tendons of insertion and insertion of the tendon on the first phalanx. Pressure is then exerted on the proximal portion, pulling out the tendon. Considerable tension is sometimes required to break adhesions that are formed around the tendon where it crosses the hock joint. If it seems as though undue pressures are required to pull it out, further dissection of the proximal portion of the tendon should be done to free it from adhesions and fascia. When the whole tendon is exposed, about 7″ of it has been pulled through the upper incision (Fig. 6–138). The tendon should be cut off, removing a 3″–4″ portion of the muscle belly with it. After removal of the tendon, the subcutaneous fascia should be sutured with No. 1 catgut sutures using a simple interrupted pattern. The skin incisions are closed with interrupted vertical or horizontal mattress sutures of a noncapillary, nonabsorbable suture of sufficient diameter to prevent tearing. The wounds are kept bandaged for ten days. Opening of the upper wound sometimes occurs because of the stringhalt action of the limb. In this case, the skin sutures are replaced. It is essential that the surgery be done aseptically or infectious tenosynovitis will result. Tetanus antitoxin should be used, but antibiotics are usually unnecessary. The incisions should be covered with collodion and cotton. Most cases show an almost immediate improvement, with complete recovery within two to three weeks. Other cases may take several months for any great improvement to occur, and still others may never show complete recovery. In those cases that recur after several months or a year, an additional portion of the lateral digital extensor muscle is removed. An incision is made at the previous proximal incision site, extending 2″ above the previous scar. The lateral digital extensor muscle is isolated and an additional 3″ to 4″ of the muscle removed. This will stop signs of stringhalt in come cases.

Some have recommended cutting the medial patellar ligament for stringhalt. This will give relief only when the surgeon has confused intermittent upward fixation of the patella with stringhalt.

The successful use of mephenesin* in one case of stringhalt has been reported (Dixon and Stewart, 1969). The drug was given in series of three injections both intravenously and intramuscularly. There was a relapse between the first and second series of injections. The drug merits further study on a significant number of cases.

Prognosis

Prognosis is guarded to favorable. Nearly all cases show some improvement after surgery, but the degree of improvement is not predictable beforehand.

SPECIFIC REFERENCES

Dixon, R. T., and G. A. Stewart. 1969. Clinical and pharmacological observations in the care of equine stringhalt. Aust. Vet. J. 45(3): 127–130.

Seddon, H. O. 1963. Sudden case of stringhalt in a horse. Vet. Rec. 75: 35.

Shivering

Definition

Shivering is characterized by involuntary muscular movements of the limbs

*Tolserol, Squibb Laboratories, Princeton, N.J.

and tail. Both hind limbs and the tail are usually affected, but sometimes the forelimbs may be involved.

Etiology

The etiology of shivering is unknown. Apparently, it is a nervous or neuromuscular disease.

Signs

In mild cases the signs may be difficult to detect, since they occur at irregular intervals, but in most cases the signs are characteristic. They usually are evident when an attempt is made to back the affected horse. As the horse attempts to back, he jerks a hind foot from the ground and holds it in a flexed position abducted from the body. The limb shakes violently, while the tail is elevated and quivers. After a short time the quivering ceases and the limb and tail return to a normal position. The symptoms usually recur if attempts are again made to force the horse to back. In some horses, the signs are most evident when the horse is turned or forced to step over an object or when his foot is raised from the ground by hand. The eyelids and ears may flicker, and the lips may be drawn backward.

If a forelimb is involved, the limb will be raised and abducted with the carpus flexed. The muscles above the elbow joint will quiver until signs disappear.

Treatment

No efficient method of treatment is known, but treatment with mephenesin* intravenously may be tried.

Prognosis

The prognosis is unfavorable since the signs usually tend to increase in severity over time. Horses that are affected with

*Tolserol, Squibb Laboratories, Princeton, N.J.

mild symptoms may be used for work in some cases.

Bone Spavin

Definition

An osteoarthritis, progressing to an ankylosing arthritis, with periostitis and osteitis, usually affecting the medial aspect of the proximal end of the third metatarsal bone and the medial aspect of the third and central tarsal bones (Fig. 6–139). The condition usually results in an ankylosis of the distal intertarsal and the tarsometatarsal joints (Fig. 5–12, p. 133). It causes an osteoarthritis of the involved joints and, in most cases, ankylosing arthritis of the distal intertarsal and/or tarsometatarsal joints. *Jack spavin* is a bone spavin of large proportions, and *high spavin* is a bone spavin located higher on the hock joint than ordinary bone spavin.

Etiology

Bone spavin commonly is due to poor conformation. Sickle hocks and cow hocks predispose a horse to bone spavin (Figs. 1–27 and 1–28, p. 18). These two malconformations, which often accompany each other, make some cases of bone spavin inheritable. Sickle and cow hocks tend to impose stress in the medial aspect of the hock joint. Bone spavin also may be caused by trauma, especially that trauma produced by quick stops during roping. Mineral imbalances or deficiencies, e.g., rickets, may predispose some horses to bone spavin. Horses with narrow, thin hocks are more subject to the disease than those with full, well-developed hocks.

Signs

Pain when the horse flexes the hock joint causes a reduction in the height of the foot flight arc (Fig. 4–2, p. 93) and a

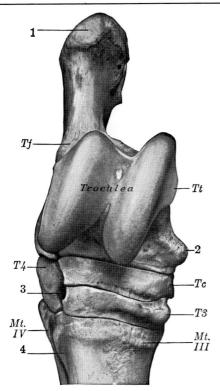

FIG. 6-139. Right tarsus and proximal part of metatarsus of horse, anterior or dorsal view. *Tt*. Tibial tarsal bone; *Tf*, fibular tarsal; *Tc*, central tarsal; *T3*, third tarsal; *T4*, fourth tarsal; *1*, tuber calcis; *2*, distal tuberosity of tibial tarsal; *3*, vascular canal; *4*, groove for great metatarsal artery; *Mt. III* and *Mt. IV*, metatarsal bones. The joints most commonly involved with bone spavin are the distal intertarsal joint between the central and third tarsal bones and the tarsometatarsal joint between the third tarsal and third metatarsal bones. Any spavin that involves the proximal intertarsal joint between the tibial tarsal bone and the central tarsal bone has a more unfavorable prognosis. (From Sisson, *Anatomy of Domestic Animals*, courtesy of W. B. Saunders Co.)

ness after working a short time; in severe cases, exercise may aggravate the lameness. Bone spavin causes an enlargement of variable size on the inner aspect of the hock (Fig. 6-140). This enlargement sometimes can be difficult to determine, especially if bilateral spavin is present or if a horse normally has large boxy hocks. When standing, the horse may flex the hock periodically in a spasmodic manner. Most cases of bone spavin react positively to the spavin test. The spavin test consists of flexing the hock for one to two minutes and then putting the horse into a trot (Fig. 6-141). A positive reaction to the test is for the horse to take several steps that show more lameness than before the test. Other conditions, though, may cause this same reaction, especially arthritis in older

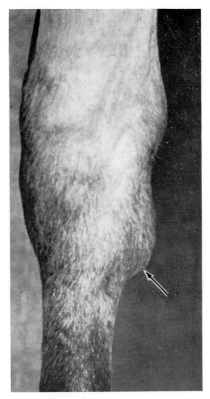

FIG. 6-140. Site of bone spavin on the right hind limb. The arrow indicates the prominence of new bone growth. (Reprinted from *Veterinary Scope* 7(1): 93, 1962; courtesy of Upjohn Company.)

shortening of the anterior phase of the stride. The foot lands on the toe, and over time, the toe becomes too short and the heel too high. Because of the lower arc of the foot flight, the horse tends to drag the toe, causing it to wear on its dorsal edge.

Bone spavin lameness tends to be worse when the horse is first used. Horses with mild cases tend to warm out of the lame-

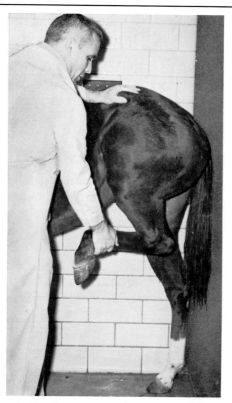

FIG. 6–141. Spavin test. The hind limb should be held in this position for one to two minutes and the horse should be observed for increased lameness in the first few steps he takes. Increased lameness is considered to be a positive reaction to the spavin test.

the muscles on the sound side may cause the hip on the sound side to look higher, but the unsound hip is pushed higher than it normally would be by this compensatory action. This is commonly called "hiking." This allows the horse to advance the affected limb with imperfect flexion. The foot or shoe may show more wear on the outside because the horse attempts to place most of his weight on the outside of the foot to relieve the pain of the spavin.

Diagnosis

The reduced arc of the foot flight, reduced flexion of the hock, wearing of the toe, and the spavin test are used in diagnosis. Blocking of the posterior tibial and deep peroneal nerves with a local anesthetic is a reasonably accurate diagnostic method for spavin. However, one must remember that other structures are blocked in addition to the spavin area. Local infusion of the lower tarsal joints with local anesthetics is helpful in localizing the joints involved (see Chap. 4, p. 115). Lamenesses of the hock and stifle cause practically identical symptoms. Therefore, careful examination must be given to the stifle as well as to the hock. An enlarged head of the second metatarsal bone may produce a swelling that looks similar to bone spavin. This can be differentiated by palpation, by its location, and by radiographs. The hocks must be examined carefully both from in front of the horse, comparing the two hocks by observing between the front legs, and from behind by observing the hocks straight-on and from oblique views. Uneven enlargements are easily detected (Fig. 6–140), but if the hocks are bilaterally involved it may be difficult without radiographs to determine if the swelling is normal or not. In most cases, radiographs show that the involvement is on the medial aspect of the proximal end of the third metatarsal bone and on the medial aspect of the third and

horses, but in general, the spavin test is considered accurate. It is often advisable to conduct the test on both limbs for comparison or for diagnosis of bilateral bone spavin. Gonitis from any cause can produce a reaction to the spavin test. Mild reaction to the spavin test should be viewed with suspicion, and the stifle joint should be carefully examined for pathological changes. The average bone spavin will cause a marked change in the gait, while stifle pathology usually causes milder reaction to the test.

As the affected limb is advanced, the sound limb pushes the hips upward so that the affected limb can be advanced with a minimum flexion. The tension in central tarsal bones, with ankylosis of the distal intertarsal and/or tarsometatarsal joints (Fig. 5–12, p. 133; Fig. 6–142); more involvement is present in some cases. Radiographs are essential to accurate diagnosis and prognosis. Radiographs also aid in determining tarsal bone fractures (Fig. 6–143). Standardbreds may have bursitis of the cunean tendon without spavin lesions (see p. 342).

Treatment

In spite of numerous types of therapy for treatment of bone spavin, many affected horses remain lame and resistant

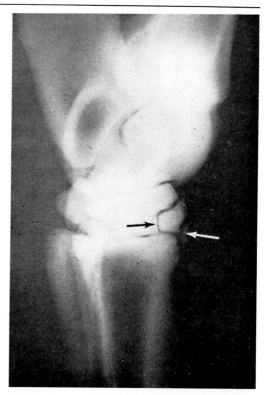

FIG. 6–143. Fracture of the third tarsal bone. Third tarsal bone is fractured (black arrow) and there is a small chip from this bone anteriorly (white arrow). Notice the abnormal shape of the third tarsal bone proximally. This horse showed clinical signs of bone spavin. The periosteal new bone growth on the proximal aspect of the third tarsal bone probably caused the fracture from downward pressure on it by the central tarsal bone. The horse recovered after ankylosis of the distal intertarsal and tarsometatarsal joints. Surgical intervention should not be used when there is a good possibility of natural repair.

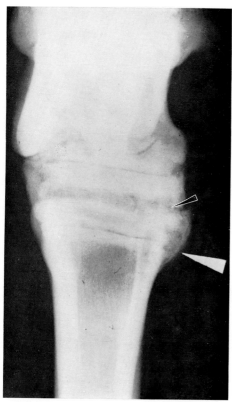

FIG. 6–142. Bone spavin. Dark pointer indicates ankylosis of the distal intertarsal joint. The white arrow indicates new bone growth on the medial aspects of the third and central tarsal bones. These are typical changes in bone spavin, but the tarsometatarsal joint is not yet ankylosed.

to all conventional methods of therapy. Common treatments used at the present time are cunean tenectomy; firing into the distal tarsal bones, with or without previous cunean tenectomy; Wamberg modification of cunean tenectomy, which includes cutting into the periosteal layer, theoretically destroying nerve supply to the spavin area; blistering; neurectomy of the posterior tibial and deep peroneal

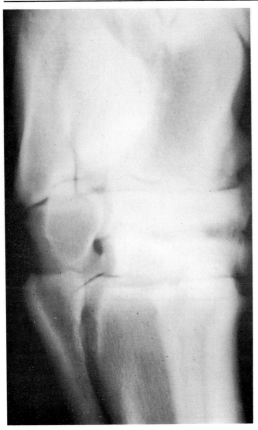

FIG. 6-144. Bone spavin involving the proximal and distal intertarsal joints as well as the tarsometatarsal joint. The involvement of the proximal intertarsal joint makes the prognosis more unfavorable.

the tendon and an incision $1\frac{1}{2}''$ long made over the center of the longitudinal axis of the cunean tendon where it crosses the medial aspect of the hock (Figs. 6-146 and 6-148). The incision can be made vertically if desired. The tendon should be isolated and a $1''$ to $1\frac{1}{2}''$ section removed (Figs. 6-147 and 6-148). The skin then should be sutured with a noncapillary, nonabsorbable suture, which should be removed in ten to fourteen days. Tetanus antitoxin should be administered, but antibiotics are unnecessary if aseptic techniques are used. The horse should be rested at least two months.

Cunean tenectomy removes a source of pain where the tendon crosses the spavin

nerves; and corrective shoeing, utilizing an open-medial-toe shoe in an effort to aid the horse in its way of going. In spite of these treatments, half of the affected horses do not respond and remain unserviceable.

Surgical arthrodesis appears to be a more effective treatment for bone spavin.

Cunean tenectomy is removal of a portion of the cunean tendon from the tibialis anterior muscle. The surgery can be performed with the horse in the standing or recumbent position. The area over the tendon should be clipped, shaved, and prepared with skin antiseptics. A local anesthetic then should be injected over

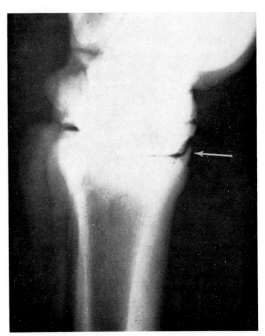

FIG. 6-145. A type of bone spavin in which most of the lesions are located anteriorly. Clinically the typical bone spavin swelling still occurs anteromedially. Arrow points at new bone growth extending from the third metacarpal bone. This new bone growth may later fracture. This type of fracture could then be treated by waiting for ankylosis of the tarsometatarsal joint to occur or by surgical removal of the fracture fragment.

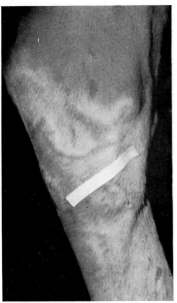

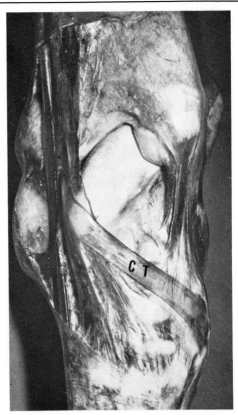

FIG. 6-146. The white tape indicates the course of the cunean tendon where it crosses the medial aspect of the tarsal joint. This is the site of incision for cunean tenectomy.

FIG. 6-148. Anteromedial view of the cunean tendon (CT). Approximately 1 inch of this tendon is removed to treat bone spavin.

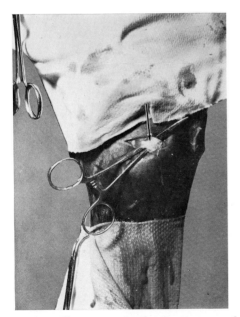

FIG. 6-147. The cunean tendon is seen over the hemostat which has been placed underneath it. One to one and one-half inches of this tendon is removed in cunean tenectomy.

area; the results of such an operation are variable depending on whether a bursitis of the cunean tendon is present.

Wamberg (1953a,b) uses a modified operation that he claims is superior to others. He states that most of the pain comes from the tissues around the bone and not from the bone itself. Under general anesthesia, he makes a rhomboid-type incision around the spavin exostoses. After loosening the skin from the subcutaneous tissue with dressing forceps, he uses a guarded knife to cut through all tissues in a more or less diamond-shaped pattern around the spavin. This blade goes through all tissues down to bone, regardless of the structures it encounters. It is his theory that the nerve supply to the spavin area is thus cut and the pain relieved. The horse is exercised daily for thirty days after the operation, and to adapt the scar tissue to movement, he recommends 50- to 100-yard dashes for the horse. The knife is forced underneath the saphenous vein at the forepart of the exostosis. Subcutaneous tissues and skin are sutured, the blood forced out through the incision, and then bandage is applied. He states he can get full working capacity from the horse as early as eighteen days after surgery.

In my hands, this type of operation has been no more successful than the type of surgery described above. As long as there is no ankylosis of the distal intertarsal and/or tarsometatarsal joints, pain will be present. Regardless of the type of surgery done, one must wait until ankylosis of these areas is complete before best results can be obtained.

Peter's spavin operation consists of cutting through the cunean tendon into the periosteum of the involved bones. Some persons modified this process by cutting the tendon and periosteum in two places. Neither of these methods is as effective as removal of a portion of the tendon. Cutting of the periosteum stimulates ankylosis of the intertarsal and/or the tarsometatarsal joints, but this usually occurs naturally in spavin without stimulation. Favorable results can be expected only in those cases that have definite involvement of the cunean bursa.

Firing and blistering of the area are often performed, though blistering is useless, since the inflammation produced is only superficial. Firing stimulates ankylosis of the above joints; the firing point is driven directly into the affected bones of the spavin area. The operator attempts to puncture the cunean tendon with the needle point in an effort to sever it if it has not already been cut. Firing is sometimes used after an unsuccessful cunean tenectomy in an effort to produce healing. Neurectomy of the posterior tibial and deep peroneal nerves also is sometimes used as a last-ditch effort to cure the lameness. This procedure, though effective in some cases, is not recommended.

If corrective shoeing is used, an effort should be made to force the foot of the affected limb to break over the medial aspect of the toe. This can be done by using two heel calks and two additional calks, one near the center of the outside toe, and one between the first and second nail holes on the inside. Another method of shoeing is to weld a $\frac{1}{4}''$ round steel rod on the inside edge of the ground surface of the branches of the shoe. On the inside branch, the rod should extend from the heel to midway between the first and second nail holes. On the outside branch, the rod should extend from the heel nearly to the center of the toe, leaving the inside toe open to stimulate breakover in that area (Fig. 9–20, p. 414). Another method of corrective shoeing is to raise the heels of the shoe and roll the toe. This simply aids the horse in his way of going. In Standardbreds the heel is commonly raised by turning the heels of the shoe back to form a swaged-up heel. The heels are turned completely back and blended with the shoe so they will not catch and stop the foot (Fig. 9–19, p. 413). A Memphis bar (Fig. 7–9, p. 387) is also used, as is an oval bar across the heels.

In an effort to find a method of producing satisfactory ankylosis in persistent cases of bone spavin, I developed a technique of surgical destruction of the joint surfaces (Adams, 1970). This method was based on my previous work with fusion of the pastern joint for ringbone. The method consists of destruction of at least 60 percent of the articular cartilage of the distal intertarsal and tarsometatarsal joints. Both joints are fused when necessary because many horses develop osteoarthritis in the second joint even if only one is involved originally. Most commonly, the distal intertarsal joint is involved first, and the tarsometatarsal joint may appear normal on radiographic examination (Fig. 6–149). As much as a year later, change may begin in the tarsometatarsal joint, so both the distal intertarsal and tarsometatarsal joints are surgically destroyed as a routine procedure if not already ankylosed. When there is damage in the proximal intertarsal joint, it too is destroyed surgically, along with the distal intertarsal and tarsometatarsal joints. Surgery is done only on those joints that are not solidly ankylosed on radiographic examination. For example, if radiographs show the distal intertarsal joint to be ankylosed and an early osteoarthritis present in the tarsometatarsal joint, only the latter joint is fused. It is very helpful to confirm the tarsometatarsal joint as the site of lameness by infusing a local anesthetic into this joint and noting a relief of lameness signs (see Chap. 4, p. 115).

The horse is anesthetized in lateral recumbency with the affected limb down, and the area is prepared for aseptic surgery. This is done by clipping and shaving the surgical area, scrubbing with antiseptic soap, and applying benzalkonium hydrochloride* and 70 percent alcohol, or other suitable skin antiseptic. Iodine† may be applied as the last application.

A 3″ (7.5 cm) incision is made over the anteromedial aspect of the distal intertarsal and tarsometatarsal joints, avoiding the saphenous vein, which is in the operative field. Depending upon the location of the vein, the incision is made either in front of or behind this vessel. The incision should be more anterior than posterior to avoid improper identification of the joints involved. At this time, a routine cunean tenectomy is done if it has not been performed previously (Figs. 6–150 and 6–151). The joints to be ankylosed are then identified with a needle (Figs. 6–152, 6–154, and 6–155). If there is partial ankylosis,

*Zephiran, Winthrop Laboratories, New York.
†Betadine, Purdue Fredrick Company, Yonkers, N.Y.

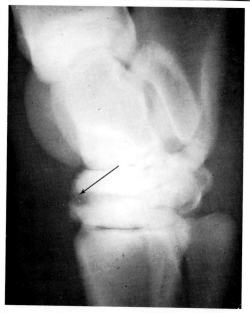

FIG. 6–149. Osteoarthritis of the distal intertarsal joint (bone spavin). Notice the porous appearance of the bone at this joint (arrow), indicating a poor bony union. The tarsometatarsal joint will usually become affected later if it is not affected early in the disease. (From Adams, 1970; courtesy of JAVMA.)

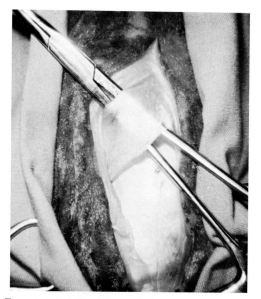

FIG. 6–150. Exposure of the cunean tendon during routine cunean tenectomy done prior to the arthrodesis procedure. (From Adams, 1970; courtesy of JAVMA.)

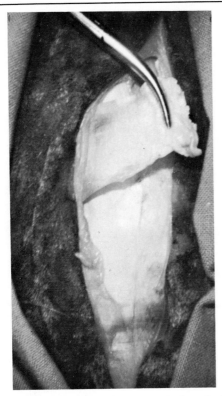

FIG. 6–151. Cut edge of cunean tendon during routine cunean tenectomy done prior to the arthrodesis procedure. (From Adams, 1970; courtesy of JAVMA.)

(Figs. 6–156 through 6–160). One starting hole is used, and the drill bit is moved in various directions from this one hole so that at least 60 percent of the cartilage and adjacent bone is destroyed in the individual joint. The drill bit should not go past the articular surface of the joint in any direction. The operator should also be aware that if the bit turns too fast, it can cause bone necrosis. It does not take long for the bit to heat and for the bone to be damaged. If the bone is burned, resulting bone necrosis could cause suppurative arthritis following surgery. The drill bit can be cooled by applying sterile saline solution to the bit during drilling. After drilling is completed, the drill hole is flushed with sterile physiologic saline solution. It is not imperative that all bone debris be removed from the drilled cavity.

the needle is probed more anteriorly to find a place where there is no bony tissue. For a preliminary identification of the joints, a 25-gauge needle is often used, followed by use of a 20- or an 18-gauge needle after the intra-articular space is located with a 25-gauge needle (Fig. 6–155). Reassurance as to the location of the needle can be obtained by taking a radiograph with the needles in place (Fig. 6–153). A person attempting this procedure for the first time should employ radiographic identification.

After the joint is positively identified, a $\frac{3}{16}''$ or $\frac{1}{4}''$ bit in either a manually operated or an electric drill is used to destroy the joints. The drilling of the joint spaces is done on the anteromedial aspect of the joint, parallel to the articular surfaces

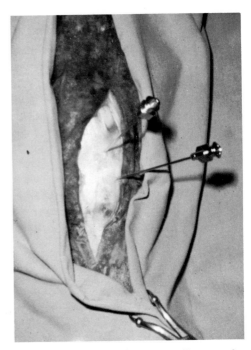

FIG. 6–152. Eighteen-gauge needles in place during joint identification for arthrodesis procedure. The upper needle is in the distal intertarsal joint, and the lower needle is in the tarsometatarsal joint. (From Adams, 1970; courtesy of JAVMA.)

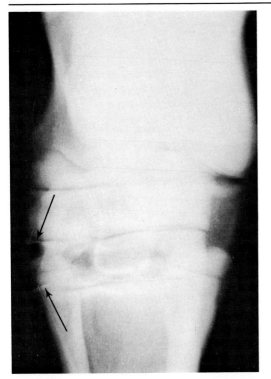

FIG. 6–153. Radiograph with 18-gauge needles identifying the joints (arrows). Present-day disposable needles are not of heavy metal and do not show up well on this radiograph. (From Adams, 1970; courtesy of JAVMA.)

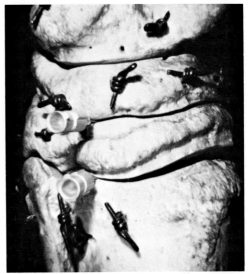

FIG. 6–154. Twenty-five-gauge needles in the distal intertarsal joint (upper needle) and in the tarsometatarsal joint (lower needle). This figure shows the need for staying on the anteromedial surface. If the needles are placed too far back, they will be placed between the second and third tarsal bones and possibly between the second and third metatarsal bones. (From Adams, 1970; courtesy of JAVMA.)

At this point, a cancellous bone graft from the tuber coxae may be used if desired. Under aseptic conditions, a piece of bone $\frac{1}{2}'' \times \frac{1}{2}'' \times 3''$ is removed from the tuber coxae. This graft is then cut into slender pieces small enough to go through the drill-bit hole. The bone graft is tamped firmly into place using a $\frac{3}{16}''$ Steinmann pin cut off squarely at both ends and about 4–5″ long. The pin is used as a punch, and by tapping it with an orthopedic hammer, the graft can be solidly embedded in the joint(s).

The subcutaneous tissues are sutured, using a simple interrupted pattern with 00 collagen or catgut, making sure that the suture needle does not enter the saphenous vein. The skin is sutured with 00 monofilament nylon with swaged-on cut-

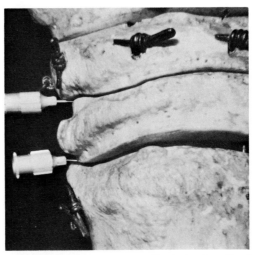

FIG. 6–155. The upper needle is in the distal intertarsal joint, and the needle below is in the tarsometatarsal joint. (From Adams, 1970; courtesy of JAVMA.)

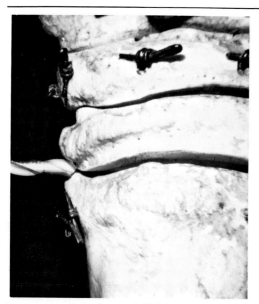

FIG. 6-156. A $\frac{3}{16}''$ bone drill bit in position on a bone specimen before drilling of the tarsometatarsal joint. (From Adams, 1970; courtesy of JAVMA.)

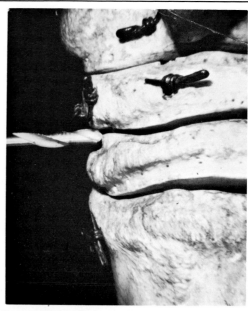

FIG. 6-158. A $\frac{3}{16}''$ bone drill bit in place before drilling the distal intertarsal joint. (From Adams, 1970; courtesy of JAVMA.)

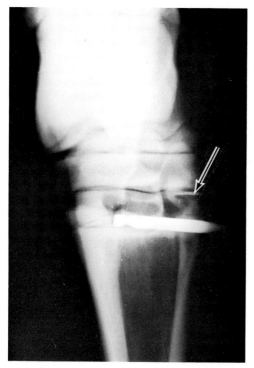

FIG. 6-157. Radiograph of a $\frac{3}{16}''$ drill bit in the tarsometatarsal joint. Identifying needle is in the distal intertarsal joint (arrow). (From Adams, 1970; courtesy of JAVMA.)

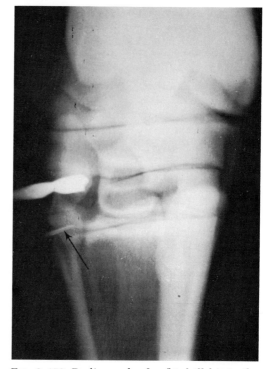

FIG. 6-159. Radiograph of a $\frac{3}{16}''$ drill bit in the distal intertarsal joint. Identifying needle is in the tarsometatarsal joint (arrow). (From Adams, 1970; courtesy of JAVMA.)

ting needle in a simple interrupted pattern. The sutures are tightened only enough to get apposition of the skin edges so that skin necrosis will not occur. The bone graft donor site is sutured with interrupted stitches of No. 1 catgut in the muscle tissue and No. 1 monofilament nylon in the skin using a vertical mattress pattern. A Penrose drain is used to facilitate drainage.

Horses that have bilateral bone spavin are operated on in both hocks during a single anesthetic period; the horse is rolled over and the procedure repeated.

The surgical area is bandaged by placing a sterile petrolatum gauze pad or dry sterile sponges over the wound and then applying elastic gauze* and elastic tape.† The bandage is examined after the horse assumes a standing position to be sure that the skin over the Achilles tendon is not wrapped too tightly. Antibiotics are optional, but tetanus antitoxin is routinely administered unless the horse is on a permanent tetanus immunity program, in which case a toxoid booster is given. Approximately one out of three horses is obviously in acute pain following surgery; these are given low dosages of phenylbutazone‡, 1 to 2 gm/day, intravenously, for three days, at which time the acute pain manifestations usually pass. Antibiotics are always given parenterally if phenylbutazone is administered.

The horse is rested in close confinement for 30 days and hand-walked only. The skin sutures are removed in 8 to 10 days and bandaging is discontinued after 14 days. Light riding exercise is begun after 30 days and gradually increased. Exercise seems to be important in production of the desired ankylosis.

Some horses take as long as one year

*Kling Elastic Gauze, Johnson & Johnson Company, New Brunswick, N.J.
†Elasticon Tape, Johnson & Johnson Company, New Brunswick, N.J.
‡Butazolidin, Jensen-Salsbery Laboratories, Kansas City, Mo.

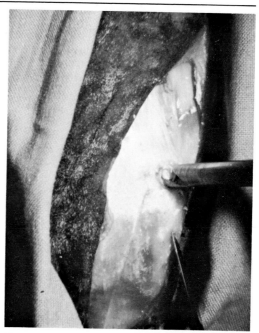

FIG. 6–160. A $\frac{3}{16}''$ drill bit drilling the distal intertarsal joint during surgical arthrodesis. (From Adams, 1970; courtesy of JAVMA.)

for recovery and complete ankylosis of the involved joints, but most recover in four to five months, if enough of the articular surface has been destroyed and if the horse is exercised sufficiently. The outlook for recovery is more favorable if only the distal intertarsal and tarsometatarsal joints are involved. If the proximal intertarsal joint is involved, the prognosis is less favorable, but it too should be treated, since this treatment offers the best hope of a complete recovery.

Prognosis

The prognosis of spavin is always guarded. In those cases that show bony changes in the tibiotibial tarsal articulation, the prognosis is unfavorable. A prognosis usually should be withheld until operation or other methods of therapy are used, especially in those cases showing ankylosis of the intertarsal and/or the tarsometatarsal joints. Complete recovery should not be expected, but a usable horse is often the result. The horse commonly will be slightly lame until warmed up, especially in cold weather.

Bog Spavin

Definition

Bog spavin is a chronic distention of the tibiotarsal joint capsule of the hock, causing a swelling of the anteromedial aspect of the hock joint.

Etiology

Bog spavin usually is caused by one of three etiological factors:

Faulty Conformation. A horse that is too straight in the hock joint is predisposed

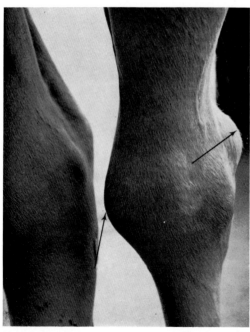

FIG. 6–161. Bog spavin. Arrows illustrate the swellings that occur in typical bog spavin. The anteromedial swelling is the largest. The swellings at the posterior aspect of the hock on the medial and lateral sides will vary in size.

to bog spavin (Chap. 1). If a horse with straight legs is not affected by bogs as a young horse, he may develop them after training begins.

Trauma. Injury to the hock joint as a result of quick stops, quick turning or other traumas, will cause bog spavin due to injury of the joint capsule or tarsal ligaments. Unilateral bog spavin can be caused by chip fractures in the tarsus or osteochondritis dissecans.

Mineral or Vitamin Imbalance. Deficiencies of calcium, phosphorus, vitamin A or vitamin D, alone or in any combination, apparently can produce bog spavin.

Bog spavin causes a blemish that is serious when due to conformational or nutritional causes; these causes should be considered strong possibilities in a bilateral condition. However, many yearlings show bog spavin in one or both hocks that disappears as they get older. Lameness is seldom present with bog spavin unless it is due to trauma or osteochondritis dissecans.

Signs

Bog spavin has three characteristic fluctuating swellings, the largest of which is located at the anteromedial aspect of the hock joint (Fig. 6–161). Two smaller swellings occasionally occur on either side of the posterior surface of the hock joint at the junction of the tibial tarsal and fibular tarsal bones. These swellings are lower than the swellings of thoroughpin. When pressure is exerted on any one of these swellings, the other enlargements will show an increase in size and an increase of tension of the joint capsule if held. Lameness, which usually accompanies only traumatic bog spavin, results in heat, pain, and swelling over the hock joint. No bone changes will be evident in uncomplicated bog spavin either upon palpation or on radiographs.

Diagnosis

Signs of bog spavin are diagnostic; the only variation is in the size of the three swellings. In most cases the anteromedial swelling is the largest, but in some cases the two posterior swellings are more prominent. These three areas are spots where the joint capsule is least inhibited by surrounding tissues. They must be differentiated from thoroughpin, which occurs posteriorly at the level of the point of the hock (see Chap. 5, p. 144). The most important factor in diagnosis is to determine the etiology. One should attempt immediately to establish whether the condition is due to conformation, trauma, or nutritional deficiency. When lameness is present, chip fractures in the tarsus should be ruled out with radiographic examination.

Treatment

Treatment is limited to bog spavins caused by trauma and nutritional deficiencies. Those bog spavins due to conformational conditions are exceedingly difficult to treat, since the cause cannot be eliminated. When trauma is the cause of bog spavin, injection of a corticoid into the joint capsule at weekly intervals for two to three injections is recommended if there are no radiographic changes (see Chap. 11, p. 454). Corticoids decrease inflammation of the synovial lining and help prevent formation of excess fluid. Corticoids should be injected into the anteromedial swelling at the most prominent portion of the swelling (Chap. 11, p. 454). The horse should be twitched and the skin shaved and prepared with antiseptics. A 20-gauge 2″ needle should be inserted into the capsule after a skin block (Figs. 11–19 and 11–20, p. 455), all fluid drained that will come out easily, and the corticoid injected. Counterpressure by bandaging, following injection of the capsule, is also recommended. Best results with counterpressure are obtained if elastic bandages or elastic braces are used. The horse should be rested approximately three weeks after all signs of lameness, if present, have disappeared. Van Pelt (1967) has recommended intra-articular injection of 6α-methyl, 17α-hydroxyprogesterone acetate alone and in combination with corticoids. These injections have not been helpful to the author in long-standing cases.

Chronic cases of bog spavin often are fired or blistered or injected subcutaneously with irritant drugs. In general, these methods are unsuccessful, though a few cases seem to respond. Injection of irritants increases the risk of suppurative arthritis. Irritation is already present in the joint capsule and producing more irritation usually is of no therapeutic value. At no time should blistering and firing be used in conjunction with corticoid therapy. These two treatments have opposite effects, and complications may result.

Treatment of bog spavin caused by nutritional deficiencies usually is of no avail unless proper corrections of diet are made. If the deficient mineral(s) and/or vitamin(s) are added to the diet, the overall nutrition regulated, and the horse freed from internal parasites, bog spavins usually disappear in four to six weeks. Bog spavin resulting from nutritional causes is most common in horses six months to two years of age. Some bog spavins will disappear in time without treatment. Synovectomy and destruction of the synovial lining of the joint capsule with nitrogen mustard have been used by the author on severe long-standing bog spavin without success.

Prognosis

Prognosis is guarded if the cause is traumatic or nutritional; it is unfavorable if due to conformation.

Blood Spavin

Blood spavin has no true definition. It usually applies only to an enlarged saphenous vein crossing a bog spavin. It will not be discussed here.

Occult Spavin (Blind Spavin)

Definition

Occult spavin is a disease that originates within the hock joint and causes typical spavin lameness but shows no palpable or radiological changes. Occult spavin is least common of the spavins. It is probable that the majority of those conditions diagnosed as occult spavin are truly in the stifle joint. Pathological changes in the stifle joint will cause a mild reaction to the spavin test. The stifle joint must always be examined carefully to determine if there is excess fluid and/or thickening in the joint capsule before a diagnosis of occult spavin is made.

Etiology

It is presumed that trauma is the etiology in nearly all cases of occult spavin. Most cases of this type of spavin lameness are presumed to be due to intra-articular lesions. This damage is usually in the form of ulceration of the articular cartilages. Other pathological changes may occur, however, such as injury to the small interosseous ligaments that bind the tarsal bones. These changes are not sufficient to be evident on radiological examination.

Signs

Signs of this disease are those of typical bone spavin lameness, with the exception of physical changes. The anterior phase of the stride is shortened because of the lowered arc of the foot flight resulting from incomplete flexion of the hock (Fig. 4–2, p. 93). The same type of rolling action of the hips occurs as in bone spavin. The horse tends to drag the toe of the hoof wall, or of the shoe, and it will wear excessively. The horse responds positively to the spavin test and shows all of the symptoms of spavin lameness, but there are no evident physical changes. The lameness usually continues throughout the life of the animal, even though there are no detectable physical changes other than lameness and reaction to the spavin test. Radiographic changes of bone spavin may become evident later.

Diagnosis

Bone spavin, bursitis of the cunean tendon, and gonitis must be differentiated from occult spavin. The use of the peroneal and tibial nerve blocks and local infusion of the lower tarsal joints is helpful in localizing the lameness in the hock (see Chap. 4, p. 115). Radiographs should be studied to detect early changes of bone spavin.

Treatment

Since pathological changes are difficult to determine, treatment too is difficult. One can only assume that some damage has taken place in the joint, since it is not evident on clinical or radiological examination. The prospects for treatment are unfavorable for these reasons. Some horses respond temporarily to intramuscular or intravenous injections of a corticoid or intravenous injections of phenylbutazone. Blistering and firing of the joint or cunean tenotomy are of no value in most cases.

When one is certain the lesion is localized in the hock, and early bone spavin is suspected, surgical arthrodesis of the distal intertarsal and tarsometatarsal joints, as described for bone spavin, will often give favorable results.

Prognosis

The prognosis is guarded to unfavorable.

SPECIFIC REFERENCES

ADAMS, O. R. 1970. Surgical arthrodesis for the treatment of bone spavin. JAVMA 157(11): 1480.

DYKSTRA, R. R. 1913. Bone spavin. Amer. J. Vet. Med. 8: 143.

GOLDBERG, S. A. 1918. Historical facts concerning pathology of spavin. JAVMA 53: 745.

LUTZ, W. H., and A. A. Gable. 1969. Spavin in standardbred racehorses. Mod. Vet. Pract. 50(6): 38–42.

MACKAY, R. C. J., and W. A. Liddell. 1972. Arthrodesis in the treatment of bone spavin. Eq. Vet. J. 4(1) 34–36.

MANNING, J. P. 1964. Diagnosis of occult spavin. Ill. Vet. 7: 26.

MARTIN, W. J. 1900. Spavin: Etiology and treatment. Amer. Vet. Rev. 24: 464.

McDONOUGH, J. 1913. Hock joint lameness. Amer. Vet. Rev. 43: 629.

SCHEBITZ, H. 1965. Spavin: Radiographic diagnosis and treatment. Proc. 11th Ann. AAEP.

SCHEBITZ, H., and H. WILKENS. 1967. Bone spavin diagnosis and therapy. Berl. Munch. Tieraerztl. Wschr. 80(20): 385.

VAN PELT, R. W., and W. F. RILEY. 1967. Therapeutic management of tarsal hydrarthrosis (bog spavin) in the horse by intra-articular injection of prednisolone. JAVMA 151(3): 328–338.

VAN PELT, R. W. 1967. Intra-articular injection of 6α-methyl, 17α-hydroxyprogesterone acetate in tarsal hydrarthrosis (bog spavin) in the horse. JAVMA 151(9): 1159.

WAMBERG, K. 1953. A new treatment for spavin in horses, p. 957. In Proc. 15th Int. Vet. Congress. Pt. 1, Vol. 2.

WAMBERG, K. 1953b. A new treatment for spavin in horses, p. 371. In Proc. 15th Int. Vet. Congress. Pt. 2.

WATTLES, J. H. 1895–1896. Injection of iodine in bone disease. Amer. Vet. Rev. 19: 51.

ZELLER, R. 1968. Wamberg's operation for spavin. Berl. Munch. Tieraerztl. Wschr. 81(19): 382–385.

ZUILL, W. L. 1894. Surgical treatment of diseases of the hock. Amer. Vet. Rev. 18: 247.

Chip Fractures of the Tibial Tarsal Bone

Definition

Chip fractures of the tibial tarsal bone may occur anywhere on the bone but are most common in one of the trochleae or in the portion of the bone articulating in the proximal intertarsal joint (Fig. 6–162). They also occur on the distal end of the tibia.

Etiology

Severe stress on the hock joint is undoubtedly the cause of most fractures. However, osteochondritis dissecans (aseptic necrosis) is responsible for some. Osteochondritis lesions most commonly occur on the trochlea, and motion may cause avulsion, the effects of which resemble a fracture.

Signs

Signs are usually those of bog spavin. Lameness is variable, from little or no

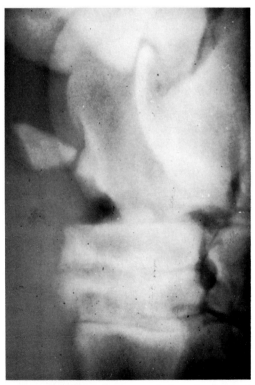

FIG. 6–162. Chip fracture of the tibial tarsal bone. Surgical removal is sometimes the treatment of choice.

lameness to a severe lameness. Any horse exhibiting signs of bog spavin accompanied by lameness should be radiographed for the possibility of fracture or osteochondritis dissecans lesions of the tibial tarsal bone.

Treatment

Depending on the site of the lesion, surgery may be indicated to remove the bony fragment. A large fragment near the distal aspect of the bone may be anchored in place with a bone screw in some cases. When lesions of osteochondritis dissecans are present without avulsion of the involved portion, the horse is confined and allowed to rest for several months.

Prognosis

The prognosis is most favorable when the fragment does not involve the articular portions of the trochlea. The prognosis should be guarded to unfavorable in all cases.

SPECIFIC REFERENCE

BIRKELAND, R., and L. H. HAAKENSTAD. 1968. Intracapsular bony fragments of the distal tibia of the horse. JAVMA 152(10): 1526–1529.

Thoroughpin (see Chap. 5, p. 144)

Bursitis of the Cunean Tendon

Bursitis of the cunean tendon is described as a separate entity in the Standardbred (Lutz and Gabel, 1969). Signs of lameness are the same as those for bone spavin. In some cases of hock lameness, most of the signs are due to bursitis of the cunean tendon and must be differentiated. Bursitis of the cunean tendon will usually exhibit swelling of the bursa over the cunean tendon. Injection of this area of a local anesthetic in and around the bursa

of the cunean tendon will reveal how much of the lameness is due to bursitis and how much is due to bone spavin. If injection of the bursa of the cunean tendon causes the signs of lameness to disappear, cunean tenectomy is indicated (see p. 330). If little or no relief is obtained by injection of the bursa with local anesthetic, little relief of any signs of lameness will be achieved with cunean tenectomy.

SPECIFIC REFERENCE

LUTZ, W. H. and A. A. GABEL. 1969. Spavin in standardbred racehorses. Mod. Vet. Pract. 50(6): 38–42.

Curb

Definition

Curb is an enlargement at the plantar (posterior) aspect of the fibular tarsal bone due to inflammation and thickening of the plantar ligament.

Etiology

Predisposing conditions include sickle hocks (curby hocks) and cow hocks. Such abnormal conformation imposes additional stress to the plantar ligament and thus tends to produce curb. Occasionally a foal is born in which curb appears soon after birth, as a result of faulty conformation of the hocks. Exciting causes include violent exertion, trauma from kicking walls or tailgates in trailers, and violent attempts to extend the hock. These causes can produce curb in hocks of normal conformation.

Signs

Curb is indicated by an enlargement on the plantar surface of the fibular tarsal bone (Fig. 6–164). If the condition is in the acute phase, there will be signs of inflammation and lameness. The horse will

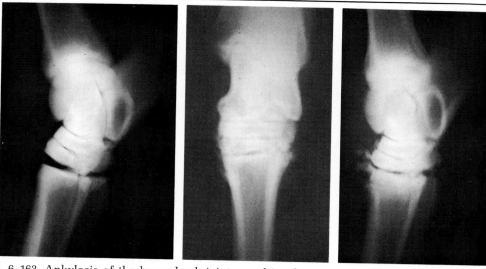

FIG. 6-163. Ankylosis of the lower hock joints resulting from complete ligamentous rupture of the tarsometatarsal joint. The limb was immobilized in a plaster cast from the stifle down to and including the hoof.

stand with the heel elevated when the leg is at rest, and heat and swelling can be palpated in the area. Swelling usually does not diminish with exercise, and exercise may actually increase lameness in acute curb. In a severe case, where trauma has been the exciting cause, periostitis on the plantar aspect of the fibular tarsal bone may result in new bone growth. If the inflammation is suppurative, extensive swelling and cellulitis may occur. In chronic cases, tissues surrounding the area often become infiltrated with scar tissue, and a permanent blemish results. Lameness may not be present even though a considerable blemish is evident. Occasionally, the proximal end of the fourth metatarsal bone is large and causes false curb. Careful examination will reveal that the swelling in this area is lateral to the plantar ligament and not on the ligament itself. This finding can be confirmed by radiological examination if necessary.

Treatment

In the early stages of curb, when acute inflammation is still present, the hair

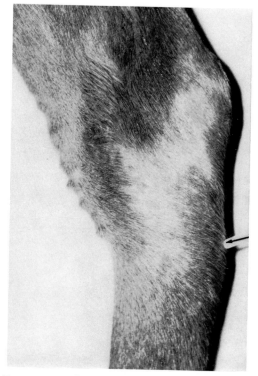

FIG. 6-164. The arrow indicates the swelling caused by inflammation of the plantar ligament, typical of curb. In severe cases, the swelling may extend proximally to the tuber calcis.

should be clipped from the area and the skin scrubbed with soap and water and prepared with suitable antiseptics. Following tranquilization and local anesthesia, the area of the curb should be injected subcutaneously with a corticoid if no infection is present (Chap. 11, p. 456). This is usually followed by a marked reduction of swelling. In spite of this reduction, some scar tissue may remain after healing has taken place. Treatment includes rest for the affected horse and the application of cold packs, in addition to the anti-inflammatory agents. Ice packs and antiphlogistic pastes are also indicated in acute cases. Chronic cases often are fired or blistered, but the efficacy of these methods of therapy is doubtful. Blistering or firing should not be done for at least ten days after the appearance of an acute curb.

Prognosis

If the horse has good conformation, the prognosis is favorable, providing the initial acute inflammation is controlled with corticoids. Poor conformation, however, serves as a continuing cause, and the prognosis is unfavorable. In most cases, some permanent blemish will remain after recovery, even though most horses will be serviceably sound, if conformation is good.

Capped Hock (see Chap. 5, p. 142)

Weak Flexor Tendons in the Foal

Definition

Some foals are afflicted with very weak flexor tendons at birth. Weak flexors may allow the fetlock to hit the ground, and the toe of the foot will be off the ground (Fig. 6–165). These will usually strengthen in a few days without help, but some do require support (Fig. 6–165).

Etiology

This is a congenital condition, and the true etiology is not known.

Signs

All gradations of the condition will be seen, from mild to severe. When it afflicts the rear legs, the hock conformation also is usually bad (sickle hocks). It is more common for the rear flexors to show weakness than the fore. In some cases, all legs show it.

Treatment

Supporting the foot with a trailer shoe is usually all that is necessary. Since the foal is too small to apply a horse shoe, ordinary triangular hinges 5″ long are used (Fig. 6–165). One is placed on the medial side of the foot and one on the lateral side, and they are either taped or fixed with 2″ plaster of paris bandage to the hoof wall. In just a matter of days, the support can usually be removed. The supports are most satisfactory in the hind foot, because when used on a forefoot the trailer may be stepped on by the hind foot. An ordinary piece of flat steel 2″ wide, 5″ long, and $\frac{3}{16}$″ thick can be substituted for the hinges. The hinges are particularly effective because the area where the pin goes through constitutes a raised heel (Fig. 6–165). Figure 6–165 shows the condition before and immediately after corrective therapy. This indicates the amount of correction that can be achieved by this method.

Prognosis

Prognosis is usually favorable, provided the fetlock joint has not been injured before correction.

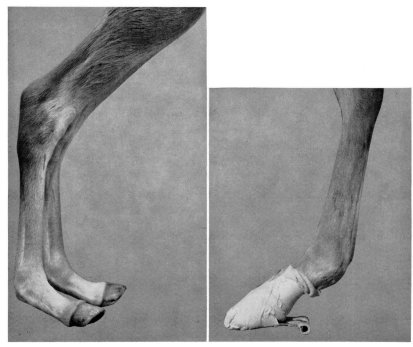

FIG. 6–165. Views of a foal with weak flexor tendons in the rear limbs. The view on the left shows the attitude of the limbs before treatment. The view on the right shows the limbs immediately after placing two 5″ door hinges on the bottom of the foot and taping them to the foot. A piece of steel $\frac{3}{16}$″ thick, 2″ wide, and 5″ long can also be used. Support is necessary for only seven to ten days.

SPECIFIC REFERENCE

MYERS, V. S., and R. L. LUNDVALL. 1966. Corrective trimming for weak flexor tendons. JAVMA 148(12): 1523–1524.

Canker

Definition

Canker is a chronic hypertrophy of the horn-producing tissues of the foot, which may involve any one or all of the feet; it most often is found in the hind feet. It is a rare condition in modern horse practice.

Etiology

The chief etiological agent is presumed to be unhygienic stabling, but exceptions to this may occur. The disease develops in horses that stand in mud or in bedding that is soaked with urine and feces and whose feet do not receive regular attention. The specific cause is believed to be an unidentified infection. Lack of proper frog pressure also may be an etiological factor.

Signs

Lameness usually is not present in early stages of the disease; since neglect of the feet is a contributing cause, the disease may not be detected until well advanced. When the foot is examined, it usually has a fetid odor and the frog, which may appear intact, has a ragged appearance. The horn tissue of the frog loosens easily, and when removed, reveals a foul-smelling, swollen corium covered with a caseous white exudate. The corium shows chronic vegetative growth. The disease may extend to the sole or even to the wall of the foot. It has little, if any, tendency to heal, and the tissues bleed easily.

Diagnosis

Diagnosis can be made by the appearance of the foot and by the offensive odor. It must be differentiated, though, from ordinary thrush.

Treatment

Treatment often is ineffective, and improvement, if it occurs, is slow. All loose horn and affected tissues should be removed and an antiseptic, astringent dressing applied. A 5 percent picric acid solution should be applied under the bandage. Caustic agents, such as a mixture of copper sulfate and zinc sulfate crystals, are sometimes used. Successful treatment of canker with penicillin has been described (Mason, 1962). Penicillin was used at the rate of 3 million units intramuscularly per day until improvement was shown. Then a similar dose was given every second day until the condition was nearly cured, after which treatment was administered every third day. Penicillin ointment was used locally with a foot bandage. Duration of treatment varied from ten days to six weeks. After improvement is noted, an antiseptic powder, such as sulfapyridine powder, or 10 percent sodium sulfapyridine solution can be used. Dressings should be kept on the foot to protect it from further infection, and the horse should be kept in clean surroundings, preferably dry, rocky pastures.

Prognosis

Prognosis is guarded to unfavorable.

SPECIFIC REFERENCES

BANIC, J., and F. SKUSEK. 1960. Experiences in the treatment of canker of the foot. Berl. Munch. Tieraerztl. Wschr. 73: 186.

BJORCK, G., and G. NILSSON. 1971. Chronic progressive pododermatitis in the horse. Eq. Vet. J. 2(3): 65–67.

MASON, J. H. 1962. Penicillin treatment of foot canker. J. S. Afr. Vet. Med. Assoc. 23: 223.

LAMENESSES COMMON TO BOTH LIMBS

Wobbler Syndrome (Ataxia of Foals, Wobbles of Foals, Equine Incoordination)

Definition

The wobbler syndrome of horses is a more or less specific incoordination. The syndrome is recognized universally, but authorities differ as to cause. The condition has been reported in Thoroughbreds, Standardbreds, Arabians, American Saddlebreds, Tennessee Walking Horses, and Quarter Horses. Other breeds undoubtedly are involved.

Rooney (1969) describes three types of wobblers. Type I is rare and of such severity as to cause permanent flexion fixation of the neck, observed by him only three times in 180 wobbler autopsies. Type II is a symmetrical overgrowth of the articular processes that obviously narrows the spinal canal and usually causes clinical signs during the suckling or weaning period. Type III is an asymmetrical overgrowth of one process, usually associated with clinical signs developing during the yearling period. Type II malformations predominate between C3 and C4, while those of type III occur primarily between C4 and C5 and C5 and C6. Several malformations may be present at different levels in the same neck. One is usually more severe than the others. The severity of the clinical signs of ataxia is related to the level at which the malformation and cord damage occurs and not to the severity of the bone malformation itself. As a rule, the closer the lesion to the cervical enlargement, the more severe the clinical signs. He states that malformations of the vertebrae develop during the third month of fetal development.

The vertebral malformation does not automatically cause clinical signs of ataxia. The vertebral malformation is a predisposing lesion that will become clinically apparent only if sufficient arching flexion of the neck occurs. Rooney (1969) estimates that 10 percent of all Thoroughbred horses have predisposing vertebral lesions, and that overflexion of the neck will produce the wobbler syndrome. Horses that have predisposing lesions but do not have a traumatic incident may not develop the condition. This would explain the wide variation in age incidence of the wobbler syndrome.

Etiology

There are several diseases that cause incoordination in horses. Among these are cerebellar hypoplasia, cervical vertebrae fractures, vertebral abscesses, cerebrospinal nematodiasis, rhinopneumonitis virus and ingestion of toxins, such as Sudan grass poisoning. Since true wobbler disease is not due to any of these causes, necropsy of the horse is required to determine the cause of incoordination.

Rooney (1969) believes that 100 percent of the Thoroughbred horses with true wobbler disease show vertebral lesions. He states that there is always a focal area of malacic damage to the white matter (the gray matter is seldom involved), which is related to the most severely malformed vertebral articulation. Single, constant, or repeated subluxation of one vertebra on another occurs because one or both sets of intervertebral articular processes are larger than normal. He believes that this subluxation compresses venous channels, causing stasis, edema, perivenular fibrosis, and myelin destruction. In his opinion, the cause of the articular malformation is not known, but it may be osteochondrosis, possibly due to a defective gene. However, I have seen

cases of wobbler syndrome that had malacic lesions in the cord but no vertebral deformity. Other veterinarians have also had this experience (Dimock, 1950a; Schebitz and Dahme, 1967). Schebitz and Dahme (1967) have used radiography to demonstrate excessive mobility of cervical articulations without observing asymmetry of the cervical vertebrae. This exemplifies the wide variation of opinion on this disease.

A wobbler syndrome also occurs in dogs that is apparently closely related to the disease in horses (DeLahunta, 1972; Wright et al., 1973). Abnormalities of the cervical vertebrae similar to those in horses occur. However, if littermates are separated, cervical vertebral lesions can be produced in those puppies fed high-protein growth ration, which would indicate that not all vertebral abnormalities are necessarily inheritable or produced in the third month of fetal life, as described by Rooney (1969). Many cases of wobbler syndrome in horses occur in foals overfed high-protein growth ration, so that excessive protein and phytic phosphorus are being fed. The phytic acid combines with calcium, making the calcium ion nutritionally nonabsorbable. The high-protein intake stimulates growth, making impossible demands on mineral intake and balance. This combination of factors may lead to uneven development of the cervical vertebrae.

Dimock (1950a) considers wobbler syndrome to be an inheritable disease of horses. In a study of 191 cases of the syndrome, of which 164 were Thoroughbreds, 121 cases had been sired by closely related stallions. Forty-three percent of these cases occurred in one line of Thoroughbreds from one of the foundation lines of the breed. One to 14 percent occurred in other Thoroughbred lines. Dimock believed it is not a simple recessive characteristic, since it was found in more than three times as many males as females. He was unsuccessful in transmitting the disease to healthy horses by blood transfusion or injection of spinal fluid or macerated spinal cord. He did not believe infectious agents are a factor in the condition. Some 85 percent of his cases showed no gross lesions at necropsy. Dimock says that autopsy findings on recently developed cases with typical symptoms reveal cord and bone lesions that could not have developed in a short time. He reports that there is only one case on record of a wobbler sired by a wobbler, so apparently the condition is transmitted by nonwobblers.

Many horse owners associate injury with the production of wobbler syndrome, but in some cases the syndrome has been present in a mild degree before the injury and has gone unnoticed. Following the injury, the horse may appear to become worse due to the actual injury that has occurred. Since the predisposing lesions in the cervical vertebrae may be present in as much as 10 percent of the horse population, a sudden trauma to the neck, especially flexion, may initiate the signs immediately after trauma. In most cases where trauma is blamed for production of the disease, the predisposing lesion was present before the injury.

The etiology probably is best summarized this way: There is a definite possibility that the predisposing cervical lesions of wobbler syndrome are inheritable. While cases actually may occur as a result of traumatic injury to the cervical region, this is not the probable cause of many cases, since it is extremely rare for a horse to show improvement from the wobbler syndrome; if trauma were the only cause, more horses should recover. Still other cases may be due to nutritional imbalances of calcium, phosphorus, vitamin D and/or vitamin A; this has not been proven, and research is required to establish a basis in fact. Nematode invasion of the cord should be considered as a specific condition. Disc protrusion and osteoarthritis of the cervical articular processes may be a cause in some cases, but they are more likely a result of the disease. Toxins are not a probable cause of wobbler syndrome. Cerebellar hypoplasia is a separate entity and should be differentiated.

The cases difficult to explain are those that have cord changes with no demonstrable vertebral changes at necropsy. These may be traumatically induced with no predisposing vertebral lesions, or they may be due to laxity of the intervertebral ligaments, as described by Schebitz and Dahme (1967).

Signs

Signs of the condition may appear at any time from birth to three years of age, but a majority of cases become evident before two years of age.

The disease, which almost always begins as an incoordination of the hind limbs, is always bilateral. In most cases, the forelimbs become involved, to a greater or lesser extent, as the disease progresses. Change is gradual, and any change, whether it be an improvement or worsening of the condition, occurs within the first few weeks. It is rare for any horse to show improvement once the syndrome is evident, but some will improve slightly. Some horses become involved to such a degree that on turning they fall; these may require destruction. Early cases cause dragging of the toes of the hind feet and errors in rate, range, force, and direction of movement. Muscular relaxation in wobbler disease may cause unilateral or bilateral signs of upward fixation of the patella. Upward fixation does not produce signs of incoordination and must be considered secondary to the wobbler syndrome. However, mild cases of wobbler disease may have to be differentiated when bilateral intermittent upward fixation of the patella is present. Although there is muscular relaxation of the hip muscles, there is no atrophy. The tail reflex should be checked, since most wobblers show a weakness of the ventral coccygeus muscles. One of the more typical signs of the wobbler syndrome is the outward swing of the hind limb when the horse is turned in a tight circle (Rooney, 1969). The horse appears healthy in every other way and has normal temperature, appetite, and metabolic functions. Most affected horses tend to reach a certain level of incoordination and remain indefinitely at this point.

Rooney (1963) found significant lesions between C3 and C4 in about 60 percent of the cases, between C2 and C3 and C4 and C5 in about 14 percent each, and least frequently between C5 and C6 and C6 and C7 (5 percent each). Three variations of malformation were observed: (a) Misdirection of articular processes, resulting in fixation, flexion, and anatomical narrowing of the spinal canal; (b) an overgrowth of the ventral medial lip or edge of the articular process encroaching upon the lumen of the spinal canal (this type causes anatomical narrowing of the spinal canal that is exaggerated by flexion); (c) asymmetrical formation of the articular processes, causing them to be of different shapes or size on the right or left articulations (in this form, there is no anatomical narrowing but rather functional narrowing during flexion). In his experience, the last is the most common type of deformity. Other authorities consistently have reported finding pathological changes in the cord from compression by protrusions of cervical discs and from osteoarthritis and enlargement of the articular processes of the cervical vertebrae. Because intervertebral discs in horses are fibrous and contain no central pulp, disc protrusion is not a common cause of cord compression.

Diagnosis

The diagnosis is well defined by the syndrome described above. If recovery from incoordination is shown, it is reasonably certain that the wobbler syndrome was not present. Most other diseases that cause a similar syndrome, e.g., encephalomyelitis, also produce other signs of disease. A horse with incoordination of the hind limbs, or of the fore and hind limbs, but having good health in other respects, should be suspected of having wobbler syndrome.

Rhinopneumonitis virus can cause a similar incoordination. However, most cases of this disease improve with time.

Fractures, tumors, abscesses, cerebellar hypoplasia, nematode invasion of the cord, and other pathological processes involving the brain and spinal cord can cause incoordination. These can usually be differentiated by signs peculiar to the particular condition, or by gross and histological findings at necropsy.

Rooney (1969) suggests that at necropsy the neck be strongly flexed for a few moments before the spinal cord is removed; the lesion site can often be detected and correlated with the articular malformation. Because of the flexion there will be a slight palpable depression at each intervertebral junction. If the moistened finger is run lightly over the ventral surface of the cord (dura removed, eyes closed), one depression will be more obvious than the others.

Treatment

There is no known treatment for this condition, although injection of corticoids has been reported to effect a cure in a few cases. In others, such injections have caused improvement, but the animals suffered a relapse when injections were stopped. Other cases reportedly have responded to some degree to supplemental feeding of minerals and vitamins. In general, it can be stated that no treatment is effective and that after six to eight weeks the horse probably will remain at whatever state of incoordination he is in at that time. Some affected horses can be used for breeding purposes if incoordination is not serious. However, such use has two disadvantages: the likelihood of injury during breeding and the possibility of transmission of the syndrome to the offspring, with the possibility that they may either carry the factor or be affected with the disease.

Prognosis

The prognosis is unfavorable. It is rare for a horse to recover from this disease. In the past, insurance companies have recognized this disease as a legitimate cause for euthanasia.

SPECIFIC REFERENCES

BARDWELL, R. E. 1961. Osteomalacia in horses. JAVMA 138: 158.

DELAHUNTA, A. 1972. Surgical spondylolisthesis in Great Dane dogs—A wobbler syndrome. Slide series produced by A. DeLahunta.

DIMOCK, W. W., and B. J. ERRINGTON. 1939. Incoordination of equidae: "Wobblers." JAVMA 95: 261.

DIMOCK, W. W. 1950a. "Wobbles"—An hereditary disease of horses. J. Hered. 41: 319.

DIMOCK, W. W. 1950b. Wobblers in horses. Ky. Agr. Exp. Sta. Bull. #553.

FRASER, H., and A. C. PALMER. 1967. Equine incoordination and wobbler disease of young horses. Vet. Rec. 80(11): 338–355.

JONES, T. C., E. R. DOLL, and R. BROWN. 1954. *The Pathology of Equine Incoordination*. Proc. Book AVMA, 139–149.

LITTLE, P. B. 1972. Cerebrospinal nematodiasis of equidae. JAVMA 160(10): 1407–1413.

LUNDVALL, R. L. 1969. Ataxia of colts as a result of injuries. Norden News, 6–10 (Summer).

MOYER, W. A. and J. R. ROONEY, 1971. Vertebral fracture in a horse, JAVMA 159(8): 1022–1024.

OLAFSON, P. 1942. Wobblers compared to ataxic lambs. Cornell Vet. 32: 301.

PATTISON, M. 1969. Progressive hind limb weakness in a pony associated with a lesion in the thoracic spinal cord. Vet. Rec. 85(1): 11–12.

ROONEY, J. R. 1963. Equine incoordination. I. Gross morphology. Cornell Vet. 53: 411.

ROONEY, J. R. 1969. Biomechanics of Lameness in Horses. Baltimore: Williams & Wilkins.

SCHEBITZ, H., and E. DAHME. 1967. Spinal ataxia in the horse. Proc. AAEP, 133–148.

SPONSELLER, M. L. 1967. Equine cerebellar hypoplasia and degeneration. Proc. AAEP, 123–126.

STEEL, J. D. et al. 1959. Equine sensory ataxia (wobbles). Aust. Vet. J. 35: 442.

SWANSTROM, O. G. et al. 1969. Spinal nematodosis in a horse. JAVMA 155(5): 748–753.

WRIGHT, F. et al. 1973. Ataxia in the Great Dane caused by stenosis of the cervical vertebral canal: Comparison with similar conditions in the Basset Hound, Doberman Pinscher, Ridgeback and the Thoroughbred horse. Vet. Rec. 92(1): 1–6.

Muscular Dystrophy

Definition

Muscular dystrophy has been observed by the author in two cases. In one case only the semitendinosus muscle was affected, and in the other, the right masseter muscle and the left semitendinosus muscle were affected. Muscular dystrophy differs from simple atrophy in that the muscle completely disappears.

Etiology

The etiology of muscular dystrophy is unknown.

Signs

Complete loss of the muscular tissue is obvious. Signs of lameness have not been observed. In the cases observed by me, the horse affected with dystrophy of the right masseter showed only bone to palpation on the affected side. The semitendinosus on the left hind limb was completely absent. In another case, the semitendinosus on the right hind limb was completely absent. Bilateral dystrophy of both masseter muscles has also been observed. Dystrophy leaves a deformity in the limb and a deep grooving where the muscle was.

Treatment

No treatment is known for muscular dystrophy.

Prognosis

The prognosis is unfavorable, and if dystrophy should involve muscles in other areas, it could cause lameness and permanent disability.

SPECIFIC REFERENCE

CECIL, R. L., and R. F. LOEB. 1963. *A Textbook of Medicine.* 11th ed. Philadelphia: W. B. Saunders. p. 1451.

Traumatic Division of the Digital Extensor Tendons of the Fore and Hind Limb

Definition

Division of the common and/or lateral extensors of the forelimb and the long and/or lateral extensor in the hind limb is relatively common. In the hind limb, the tendon or tendons usually are severed just below the hock joint as a result of wire lacerations. In the forelimb, the common digital extensor or lateral digital extensor often is severed between the fetlock and the carpus, again as a result of wire lacerations. If the laceration is below the middle of the metatarsus in the hind limb, where the lateral and long extensor are combined, only one tendon is cut.

Etiology

Trauma is the etiology in all cases. Wire cuts account for most cases.

Signs

The horse will be unable to extend the toe of the foot. When his foot is put down, the toe may catch and his weight may force the anterior surface of the fetlock to the ground. However, when the limb is set under the horse properly, he can bear his weight normally. The lateral digital extensor may be cut without any accompanying signs in either the fore or the hind limb, because division of the common digital extensor and of the long digital extensor cause most signs. Other signs are contingent upon the extent of the laceration that caused division of the tendons.

Treatment

If the wound is fresh, it should be cleansed, shaved, and sutured. Usually, no attempt is made to bring the tendon edges together with tendon sutures; the extensor tendons have a better chance to rejoin than the flexor tendons, and with time, most horses will regain normal function of the limb. Following suturing of the wound, the limb should be placed in a cast, from hoof wall to above the carpus, with the foot in normal position. Antibiotics can be used locally and/or parenterally, depending upon the severity and contamination of the wound.

The tarsus is difficult to enclose in a cast because of the reciprocal apparatus. The cast should end proximally just below the tarsus in the hind limb. The cast keeps the foot in normal position at all times. The foot and leg should be kept in this cast four to six weeks. The cast should be changed, if necessary, because of breaking of the cast or decreased use of the limb, which might indicate skin necrosis. If a limb is properly padded, though, no necrosis will be encountered.

The foot should be placed in a corrective shoe if the division of the tendon(s) has been present some time when first examined or when the cast has been removed. This shoe has an extended toe of approximately 3″. A metal bar is welded to the toe extension so that it conforms to the shape of the anterior surface of the metatarsus or metacarpus. The front of the limb should be padded and the bar at the front of the limb bound to the leg by adhesive tape, plaster, or elastic bandages. This helps keep the toe in extension. With further improvement, the bar on the anterior surface of the limb may be discontinued, and only the toe extension left on the shoe, until the limb appears to assume nearly normal function. Complete healing usually occurs in about four months, and the horse will again use the extensor tendons normally.

Prognosis

Prognosis is guarded to favorable, depending upon the duration and extent of the wound. The seriousness of the wound itself may be enough to indicate euthanasia. In some cases, wire may cut into the hock joint, making euthanasia advisable, if suppurative arthritis is present. In other cases, the bone may be badly damaged, so the prognosis must be withheld until the case has been evaluated.

Traumatic Division of the Digital Flexor Tendons of the Fore and Hind Limb

Definition

Traumatic division of the digital flexor tendons usually occurs between the carpus and the fetlock or between the tarsus and the fetlock. The greatest difficulty in tendon repair is to re-establish a smooth gliding surface.

Etiology

Trauma is the cause in all cases. Numerous types of accidents may be the cause; they are not all listed here. Injury may occur as a result of backing into or kicking a sharp object or being cut down in a race by a horse coming from behind. In such a case, the hind limb would be involved. A horse may cut his own flexor tendons by overreaching and cutting the tendon area of the forelimb with a toe grab of the shoe on the hind foot of the same side.

Signs

All degrees of laceration have been found. The superficial digital flexor tendon alone may be severed, while in other cases the deep digital flexor also may be severed. In some cases, both flexor tendons and the suspensory ligament may be cut. If the flexors are cut above the middle of the metatarsus or metacarpus, the inferior check ligament also may be severed. If only the superficial flexor tendon is cut, the fetlock joint will drop, but it will not touch the ground. If the superficial and deep flexor tendons are cut, the fetlock will drop and the toe will come up in the air when weight is applied to the affected limb. If both flexors and the suspensory ligament are cut, the fetlock will rest on the ground. When the laceration is below the distal end of the first phalanx, only the deep flexor and the associated digital sheath are cut.

If the wound has been present for some time, there may be infection of the tendon sheath, suppurative tendosynovitis may be present, and varying amounts of swelling in the limb may result. Infection increases the amount of scar tissue formation and decreases the chance of a full recovery. Lameness, which is severe, will vary according to severity and duration of the wound. In some cases, the wounds are greatly lacerated, while in other cases the wound may look as if it were cut with a knife.

Diagnosis

The diagnosis is obvious, but one should determine what structures have been severed by observing the clinical attitude of the foot and by probing of the wound.

Treatment

If the laceration extends through both tendons and the suspensory ligament, treatment may be inadvisable, and euthanasia is sometimes recommended. If the wound is fresh and only the superficial flexor tendon is severed, the wound should be cleaned, shaved, and prepared for surgical correction, and the tendon sheath should be injected with corticoids in combination with antibiotics. The skin edges should be brought into apposition by sutures and the limb placed in a plaster cast from hoof wall to the tarsus (or carpus). This cast should be left in place for approximately four to six weeks and changed as indicated. The cast should be put on with the fetlock slightly flexed so that the tendon will have a better chance to heal. An easy way to cast the lower limb in flexion is to apply a wedge of wood to the bottom of the foot before the cast is applied. The wedge is shaped with the desired amount of thickness at the heel and tapered to the toe. It can be bonded to the hoof wall with an acrylic such as Technovit.* If an effort is made to suture the tendon by surgical procedure, the horse should be confined in lateral recumbency, by using general anesthetic, and the wound extended longitudinally over the posterior aspect of the tendon. The tendon should be sutured with a recommended tendon suture (Boyes, 1964) (see Fig. 6–166). The skin

*Kulzer and Co., Hamburg, West Germany.

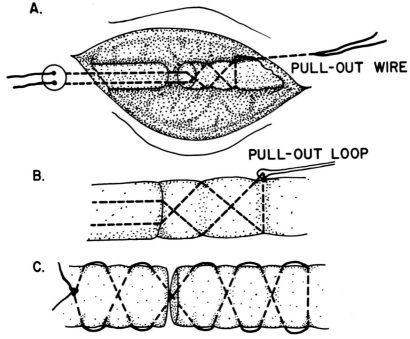

Fig. 6–166. Bunnell's technique for pull-out suture in cut tendons. A, Tendon is sutured with stainless steel wire using a straight needle on each end of the wire. A pull-out wire is placed under the tendon suture, and the loose ends are brought out subcutaneously and through the skin. In the distal fragment of the tendon, the straight needles are passed down through the center of the tendon and subcutaneously for a short distance and out through the skin through a button or other suitable object to prevent pulling on the distal fragment. B, Closeup of technique for suturing the proximal segment of the tendon and placement of the pull-out loop. C, Method of suturing the tendon when no pull-out wire is used. (Redrawn from Boyes, J. H. Bunnell's Surgery of the Hand, 4th Edition, J. B. Lippincott Company, Philadelphia, 1964.)

and subcutaneous tissues should be closed, and the limb, to the carpus or tarsus, placed in a cast so that the fetlock and phalangeal joints are in a flexed position. This should be done to relieve tension on the flexor tendons. Various types of braces may be used with an elevated heel on the shoe. These are satisfactory in some cases, but a strong cast of Zoroc* is usually superior to most types of braces and shoeing. Shoeing and braces of various types are useful when the cast is removed. If the foot is permitted to assume normal position, the sutures almost invariably will tear out. The foot should be kept cast, in this position, for four to six weeks. Change the cast as often as necessary to prevent loosening or skin necrosis. The opposite limb should be kept in a supporting bandage to prevent it from breaking down.

If both flexors are cut, or if both flexors and the inferior check ligament are cut, the horse should be given a general anesthetic, and the wound prepared by shaving and cleansing. The wound should be extended so that the tendons can be seen. They should be sutured with a recommended tendon suture (Boyes, 1964) (Fig. 6–166). One of the most valuable types of tendon sutures is one that can be removed after the wound heals by pulling the sutures out by means of pull wires placed under the sutures during surgery. Sutures in the tendon are less important when the tendon is cut in an area without a sheath (paratenon area). When a tendon is cut within a sheath, the tendon ends are slower to heal (Boyes, 1964). When a tendon pull-out suture is used, the tension is from one end only—the end into which the muscle is attached. The other end is passive. Therefore, the wire suture is spliced into the proximal end and then is passed down through the distal segment and brought out through the skin through

*Johnson & Johnson, New Brunswick, N.J.

a button placed on the skin surface to take the tension. Placing a pull-out wire under the proximal loop makes it possible to remove the suture. Both ends of the pull-out wire are threaded through the skin proximal to the cut ends (Boyes, 1964). After repair of the tendons and closure of the skin, the wound should be protected with sterile petrolatum gauze, and the leg well padded and cast from hoof wall to the tarsus (or carpus), so that the fetlock and phalangeal joints are flexed. This reduces the amount of tension on the flexor tendons, since all sutures will tear out if the foot is allowed to assume a normal position.

After four to six weeks in a cast, the limb should be placed in a supporting bandage and the foot shod with a fetlock-supporting shoe (Fig. 6–167). This enables the fetlock to rest in a leather strap so it will not drop below normal position. This shoe can also be used for division of the superficial flexor tendon only. The shoe should be used for three to six months, depending upon the horse's improvement, and should be reset every four to six weeks. After this, a shoe with 2″ to 3″ trailers on the heels should be used for support until the fetlock regains normal strength. Trailers on front shoes must be shorter to prevent pulling of the shoe by the hind foot.

Antibiotic therapy should be given as indicated with any type of laceration. Whenever an attempt is made to bring the flexor tendons into position by surgical correction, parenteral antibiotic therapy should be continued for at least seven days following the operation.

Prognosis

The prognosis is guarded to unfavorable, depending upon the number of structures that are severed. If both flexors and the suspensory ligament are cut, the prognosis is unfavorable. The presence of

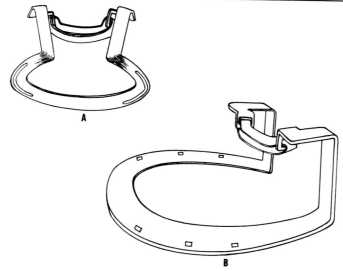

FIG. 6–167. Corrective shoe for traumatic division of the flexor tendons. *A*, Posterior view of the shoe, which has a leather strap to hold up the fetlock joint. *B*, Side view of the shoe showing how the leather strap is inserted to support the fetlock joint. Also note that the heels are about 3″ longer than normal to help support the limb.

suppurative tendonitis makes the prognosis more unfavorable. If the vascular supply is cut, gangrene may result. When a tendon is partially severed or is crushed or bruised from a closed injury, it swells and softens and may rupture from ordinary pull several days to three weeks later (Boyes, 1964).

SPECIFIC REFERENCES

BOYES, J. H. 1964. *Bunnell's Surgery of the Hand.* 4th ed. Philadelphia: J. B. Lippincott Co.
LUNDVALL, R. L. 1969. Tendon injuries of the lower limb. Norden News, 24–28 (Summer).

Windpuffs (Windgalls)
(*see* Chap. 5, p. 146)

Definition

This is distention of a joint capsule, tendon sheath, or bursa, with excess synovia, not accompanied by lameness.

Etiology

Young horses under a heavy training schedule nearly always will develop windpuffs of the fetlock joint capsules, tarsal sheaths, and flexor tendon sheaths. Race horses, rodeo horses, and even gaited horses, subjected to heavy work, will develop windpuffs to some degree as a result of trauma. Once windpuff has started in any area, it usually remains for life. Nutritional deficiency, a possible cause of windpuffs among young horses, should not be overlooked as a possible etiology among those horses not under heavy training. The diet should be closely checked in any young horse to make sure that nutrition is not a factor.

Signs

Firm fluid swelling just above and anterior to the sesamoid bones between the suspensory ligament and the cannon bone indicates articular windpuffs of the fetlock joint capsule. Windpuffs of the flexor tendons occur between the suspensory ligament and the flexor tendons, just above the sesamoid bones. Bursae may swell, and mild distentions of other joint capsules or the tarsal sheath may occur. These are sometimes called windpuffs or windgalls, but the name is usually reserved for conditions below the carpus and tarsus. Long-standing cases may harden as a result of fibrosis of the area. Windpuffs themselves are not a cause of lameness, but when accompanied by arthritis, bursitis, or tendonitis, they should be treated and regarded as a sign of the disease involved.

Treatment

In general, treatment is not effective, nor is it required, if windpuffs or windgalls are not accompanied by lameness. Treatment for serous arthritis and tenosynovitis, described in other sections of this book, should be used when windpuffs are a sign of these diseases. If no lameness is evident, the horse usually is not rested, but the work is decreased for a few days when they first occur. Windpuffs or windgalls usually will remain for the life of the horse. No treatment is recommended, as long as lameness does not occur. If lameness does occur, enforced rest and treatment, as described under arthritis and tenosynovitis, should be employed. Intrasynovial injections of a corticoid usually are the most effective treatment if lameness is present. Injections should be accompanied by adequate rest and supportive wraps of elastic gauze and tape. Swelling will usually diminish if elastic wraps are applied following the injection.

Prognosis

Prognosis is favorable if no lameness is present and guarded if lameness is present. The pathological changes causing the windpuff or windgall should be determined.

Constriction of the Palmar (Volar) or Plantar Annular Ligament

Definition

Annular ligaments are tough, fibrous, thickened parts of the fascial sheath. They are lined with synovia and may act to prevent displacement of the tendon, which would destroy its mechanical efficiency. Tendons lying within annular ligaments suffer great damage when swelling from trauma or infection occurs. Enclosed, they suffer ischemia, then necrosis. The sloughing portion of tendon is replaced by scar tissue that joins the sheath, causing flexing and contracture (Boyes, 1964).

Constriction of the palmar or plantar annular ligament of the fetlock joint occurs as a result of trauma and/or infection. It may occur with a low bowed tendon, or as a result of a wire cut or puncture wound in the area of the palmar or plantar aspect of the fore or hind limb (Wheat, 1968). As the injury or infection heals, there may be a constriction of the annular ligament, which in turn exerts constricting pressure on the superficial flexor tendon and, if severe, pressure necrosis. This causes persistent lameness. The lameness will persist until the ligament is surgically severed to relieve the pressure. Adhesions often form between the superficial flexor tendon and the annular ligament.

Etiology

The inflammation and scar tissue formation that occur with bowed tendon often involve the palmar or plantar annular ligament. In the healing process, the palmar or plantar annular ligament is often incorporated in the fibrous tissue that results from the injury. If this scar tissue contracts, there will be pressure on the superficial flexor tendon. Since annular ligaments are not elastic, swelling of the superficial digital flexor caused by tendosynovitis (bowed tendon) can cause the same signs as constriction of the annular ligament. In some cases, wire cuts or nail punctures occur in the area of the palmar or plantar aspect of the fetlock. As a result, the annular ligament is injured, and in the healing process, it may constrict from scar tissue formation.

Signs

In nearly all cases there will be distention of the tendon sheath of the superficial and deep flexor tendons proximal to the annular ligament. There is often thickening of the superficial flexor tendon, and one may mistakenly assume that the primary problem is low bowed tendon. Viewing the fetlock from the side, one can usually see "notching" at the proximal part of the annular ligament (Fig. 6–168). This notching is caused by constriction of the annular ligament. The lameness is characterized by its persistence; it does not improve with time and usually becomes worse with exercise because of inflammation and increased constriction. Continued pressure produces changes in the superficial digital flexor tendon in the form of inflammation and necrosis. Careful palpation of the area will usually reveal thickening and fibrosis at the junction of the superficial flexor tendon and the annular ligament, leading one to suspect involvement of the ligament.

Diagnosis

Persistent lameness accompanied by a notching at the proximal part of the palmar or plantar annular ligament of the fetlock, combined with palpation of the area that reveals scar tissue formation, is the basis for diagnosis. Most bowed tendons will become sound, at least at the walk and trot, after a few months of rest. In the case of a constriction of the palmar or plantar annular ligament, the lameness

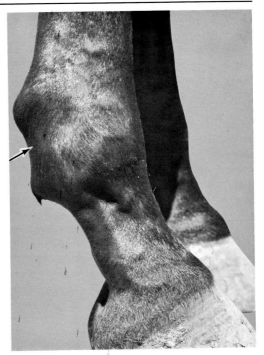

FIG. 6–168. Constriction of the volar annular ligament. Notice the "notched" appearance on the volar aspect of the fetlock above the ergot. The upper swelling is caused by fluid distention of the flexor tendon sheath.

will be persistent. All cases of low bowed tendon should be examined for the possibility of coexistent constriction of the annular ligament, or for enlargement of the tendon sufficient to cause the same signs because of unyielding limitation by the annular ligament.

Treatment

Surgical resection of the palmar or plantar annular ligament is the only effective treatment. Under general anesthesia, and after proper surgical preparation of the area, an incision is made, preferably on the lateral edge of the superficial flexor tendon (Fig. 6–169) behind the digital vessels and nerves. The incision continues through the palmar or plantar annular ligament and through the digital tendon sheath. After inflammation has been pres-

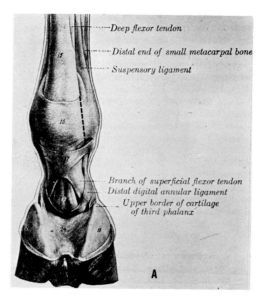

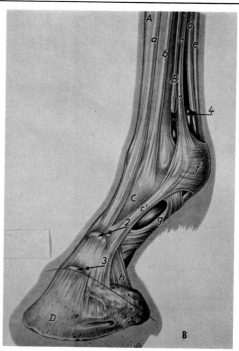

FIG. 6–169. Anatomy specimens showing volar annular ligament. A, 14, Deep digital flexor tendon; 15, superficial digital flexor tendon; 16, volar annular ligament; 17, proximal digital annular ligament; 11, cartilage of third phalanx; 24, digital cushion. [After Ellenberger-Baum, Anat für Kuntler (In Sisson, 1953); courtesy W. B. Saunders Co. and Mrs. J. D. Grossman.] Dotted line indicates line of incision on either medial or lateral edge of the superficial digital flexor tendon. B. A, Third metacarpal bone; B, second metacarpal bone; C, first phalanx; D, third phalanx; a, common digital extensor tendon; b, lateral digital extensor tendon; c, c', suspensory ligament; d, deep flexor tendon; e, superficial flexor tendon; f, volar annular ligament; g, superficial distal sesamoidean ligament; h, ligament to cartilage of third phalanx; i, joint capsule of metacarpophalgeal (fetlock) joint; 2, proximal interphalangeal (pastern) joint; 3, distal interphalangeal (coffin) joint; 4, tendon sheath of superficial and deep digital flexor tendons. (From Topographical Anatomical Diagrams of Injection Technique for Horses. © 1972 National Laboratories. Kansas City, Missouri.)

ent for some time, the ligament and the tendon sheath cannot be separated, and no effort is made to do so. After the palmar or plantar ligament has been resected in its full width, the subcutaneous tissues are sutured with 00 catgut or collagen. The skin is then sutured with a noncapillary, nonabsorbable suture. The horse is put in a snug-fitting support wrap of elastic gauze* and tape† or medicated gauze

bandage.* Exercise is begun in three days, hand-walking the horse and gradually increasing exercise so that adhesions will not unite the incised edges of the annular ligament. Antibiotics are optional, and tetanus antitoxin (or a toxoid booster if the horse has been immunized) should be administered.

*Kling, Johnson & Johnson, New Brunswick, N.J.
†Elasticon, Johnson & Johnson, New Brunswick, N.J.

Prognosis

If the primary involvement is that of constriction of the palmar or plantar annu-

*Medicopaste, Graham Field, Woodside, N.Y.

lar ligament and is not accompanied by extensive changes in the tendon (bowed tendon), the prognosis is favorable. All cases show much improvement, and if tendon changes are not extensive, the horse may be freed of lameness by use of the techniques described above.

SPECIFIC REFERENCES

ADAMS, O. R. 1974. Constriction of the palmar (volar) or plantar annular ligament in horses. VM/SAC, 69 (3): 327.

BOYES, J. H. 1964. Bunnell's Surgery of the Hand, 4th ed. Philadelphia: J. B. Lippincott Co.

WHEAT, J. D. 1968. Personal communication.

Fracture of the First and Second Phalanges

Definition

Fracture of the first and second phalanges is most common among cutting and barrel-racing horses, because such horses often make very sharp turns on one hind leg in their work. These fractures may also occur in the forelegs, but are slightly more common in the hind leg.

Etiology

Trauma is the cause, especially if accompanied by a twisting action. Shoeing with heel calks predisposes to phalangeal fractures. The calks anchor while the weight is on the foot, and the twisting action of a cutting horse or barrel-racing horse causes fracture.

Signs

The bone, or bones, are usually badly comminuted, and crepitation may be obvious. The lameness is severe, and the horse hesitates to put any weight on the affected limb. Swelling will be observable over the pastern area, and, in old cases, bony swelling resembling ringbone will be present. In some cases, only the second phalanx will be fractured, while in others only the first phalanx will be involved (Figs. 6–170 and 6–171). Occasionally, both the first and second phalanges will be

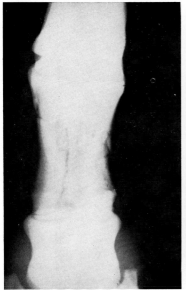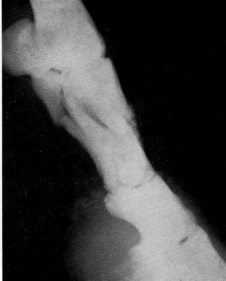

FIG. 6–170. Comminuted fracture of the first phalanx involving both metacarpophalangeal (fetlock) and proximal interphalangeal (pastern) joints. (Carlson, *Veterinary Radiology*, Lea & Febiger.)

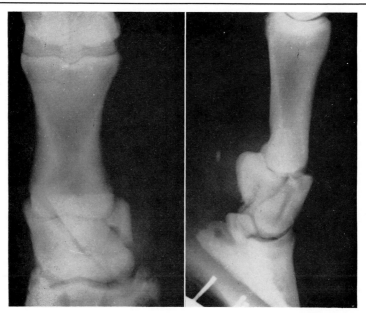

FIG. 6–171. Comminuted fracture of the second phalanx. The prognosis is guarded to unfavorable in this case because it has fractured into the coffin joint. The pastern joint can ankylose with some chance of soundness. (Carlson, *Veterinary Radiology*, Lea & Febiger.)

fractured. Some horses are affected with small chip fractures of these bones, or with single longitudinal fractures, especially of the first phalanx.

Diagnosis

A history of sudden lameness while working, crepitation and signs of inflammation over the phalanges usually are diagnostic. Radiographs are necessary to confirm the damage and to determine which bones are actually broken. Occasionally, luxation of the pastern joint occurs between the first and second phalanx; this causes crepitation similar to that exhibited in fracture. Luxation can be determined by radiographic examination (Fig. 6–172). Crepitation is difficult to produce when there is only one fracture line.

Treatment

Casting the affected limb in plaster is the usual method of therapy. The cast should be applied to the limb with the horse in recumbency. The horse should be surgically anesthetized for repair of first or second phalangeal fracture. A 1,000-lb horse should be given 0.5 mg of promazine per pound body weight, followed by enough 6 percent chloral hydrate IV to make the horse unsteady on his feet. The amount of chloral hydrate will vary from 250 to 500 cc of a 6 percent solution, depending on the tolerance of the individual horse. Following administration of chloral hydrate, 2 gm of 10 percent Surital sodium* are administered rapidly IV. The horse will go down after administration of the Surital, and anesthesia will often last till the cast is dry enough to bear weight; the anesthetic procedure seldom requires more Surital sodium to keep the horse anesthetized for the casting procedure. Pentobarbital may be substituted for Surital if desired. Satisfactory intravenous anesthesia can also be attained with

*Parke, Davis & Co.

5 percent glyceryl guialcolate in 5 percent dextrose with 1 gm thiamylal sodium added per 1,000 cc of solution. It is given to effect—approximately 1 cc of the mixture per pound of body weight. Following anesthesia, the foot is thoroughly cleaned, and any shoes present on either the front or hind feet are removed. If trimming of the hoof wall is required, it is done at this time. The leg is powdered with talcum or boric acid and 3″ stockinette is applied to the limb from the hoof wall to the carpus (or tarsus). Orthopedic felt is applied where the top of the cast will fit.

The limb is positioned so that the fracture ends are in as near normal apposition as possible, and the foot is cast in a slightly flexed position. Start with 4″ or 6″ blue label Johnson & Johnson plaster of paris and put on three rolls before reinforcement is applied. These first layers are not pulled tight, but merely pulled up so that there is no looseness. If resin plaster*

*Zoroc, Johnson & Johnson, New Brunswick, N.J.

is used, fewer rolls are required. One should be very careful to fold the plaster in behind the pastern joint so that it fits snugly for support against the back of the pastern joint. Otherwise, there will be no support in this area for the phalanges. The 6″-wide plaster tends not to support this area sufficiently unless careful attention is paid to this. The plaster of paris goes over the sole and hoof and up to just below the carpus or tarsus. There should be no motion at all in the phalangeal area.

After three rolls of 4″ or 6″ plaster have been rolled on, apply plaster splints ¼″ thick, 15″ long, and 4″ wide to the anterior and posterior surface of the limb, or use a splint 30″ long and bring it across the bottom of the foot. These splints adequately support the cast in the fetlock area. Splints can also be formed from a roll of plaster by merely folding it back and forth to the proper length. These splints should be carefully folded in behind the pastern for support, and then an additional three or four rolls of 4″ or 6″

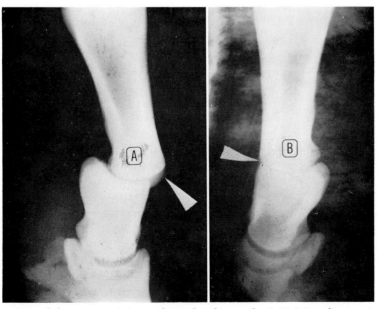

FIG. 6–172. Luxation of the pastern joint on lateral radiograph. *A,* Pointer shows overriding distal end of first phalanx. *B,* The same joint in a plaster cast with the luxation reduced. The pointer shows the decreased joint space, indicating beginning ankylosis as the result of destruction of the articular cartilage.

blue label Johnson & Johnson plaster are rolled on to finish the cast. Green label plaster of paris can be used if faster-setting plaster is required. Application of a walking bar to the cast will aid in immobilization of the joint.

Try to plan the anesthesia so that the horse will stay quiet until the plaster is dry. By the time he tries to get up, the cast should be solid so he can put weight on it without damaging it.

The cast may have to be changed every two to three weeks, depending on the individual case. The whole procedure has to be repeated as described if the cast must be replaced. Repair of a phalangeal fracture may be a long, tedious, and costly affair, but it must be done properly. If the cast shows looseness, it must be changed. It is also changed if ulceration develops at the proximal portion of the cast. It is best to change the cast and be wrong than to leave it and have irreparable damage. At the time the cast is changed, the area can be examined and a corticoid ointment applied to any lesions present. Radiographs could be taken at this time, if necessary. Eight to ten weeks are required for

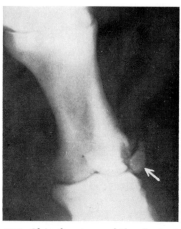

FIG. 6–173. Chip fracture of the first phalanx. Fractures of this type may be repaired, if treated in the early stages, by use of a bone screw. (Carlson, *Veterinary Radiology*, Lea & Febiger.)

a phalangeal fracture to heal. The horse is confined to a stall for at least 30 days after removal of the cast, while strength in the tendons returns. A 3″ trailer shoe is applied to support the tendons for four to six weeks after cast removal.

The pastern joint of the hind leg may become completely ankylosed, as described on page 238, and the horse may still be functional. Ankylosis of the pastern joint in the foreleg causes greater interference with action. The affected horse should not be used for at least six months, and once healing occurs, the foot should be kept properly trimmed and should be shod with a full roller motion shoe. A polo shoe can be substituted for a full roller motion shoe, but in the rest period only.

When only a small chip is broken from the first or second phalanx (Fig. 6–173) or one of these bones is split in a longitudinal direction (Figs. 6–174 and 6–175), it sometimes is beneficial to correct the fracture surgically by applying one or more bone screws transversely through the fragments. When bone screws are used, ASIF* compression technique is preferred (Fackelman, 1973). The limb then should be cast as described above. A walking bar should be applied routinely to the cast in an effort to prevent bending of the screws. Bone screws are beneficial only with minimal fragments. The opposite normal fetlock should be supported by elastic wraps to prevent injury from excess weight-bearing.

When damage to the pastern joint is severe, it is usually best to surgically ankylose the joint, as described on page 238.

Clients should be advised not to shoe cutting horses and barrel-racing horses with calks. Only flat-plate shoes should be used because of the anchoring effect of calks.

*Smith Kline Surgical Specialties, Philadelphia.

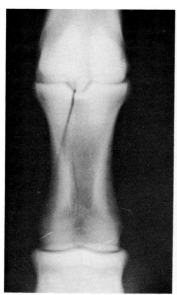
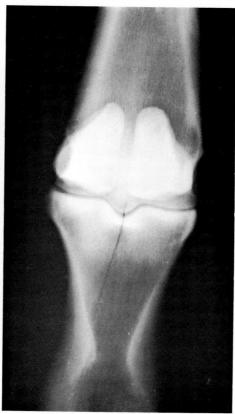

FIG. 6–174. Two examples of longitudinal fractures of the first phalanx. Both would be candidates for compression screws.

Prognosis

If the first phalanx is fractured into the fetlock joint, the prognosis is unfavorable. If the second phalanx is fractured into the coffin joint, the prognosis also is unfavorable. If only the pastern joint is involved, the prognosis is guarded. Some horses can be returned to active use, while others can only be used as brood animals. The normal limb must be protected against excess weight-bearing.

SPECIFIC REFERENCES

FACKELMAN, G. E. 1973. Sagittal fractures of the first phalanx in the horse. VM/SAC. 68(6): 622–636.
VON SALIS, B. 1972. Internal fixation in the horse. AAEP, 193–218.

Rachitic Ringbone
(*see* Chap. 5, p. 127)

Definition

Rachitic ringbone is a fibrous tissue enlargement of the pastern area of young horses. The disease usually develops before the horse reaches two years of age and is most common between six and twelve months of age. Clinically, the fibrous tissue swelling resembles new bone growth caused by true ringbone. In rachitic ringbone there are no bone or joint changes, other than fibrous tissue enlargement, around the pastern joint; therefore, this is not true ringbone or arthritis.

also may be evident (see Chap. 5). Radiographs of the pastern areas will not reveal bony changes but will show soft tissue swelling. On palpation, this swelling may be confused with new bone growth because of its firmness.

Treatment

Determination of the deficient elements in the diet must be made by analysis of the ration and by blood chemistry tests. Once the deficiencies are determined, the diet should be corrected by addition of the deficient elements (see Chap. 5, p. 134). If the diet correction is made early enough, the signs will regress, and as the horse grows older the swellings will not be evident. However, other changes that may accompany rachitic ringbone can permanently disable the horse. Four to six weeks are required after diet correction for favorable changes to be evident.

Prognosis

Prognosis is guarded, but if the diagnosis is established early enough and the diet is corrected, a sound mature condition can be obtained. If changes in the limbs are advanced at the time of the original examination, prognosis is guarded to unfavorable until the effect of the dietary correction can be determined.

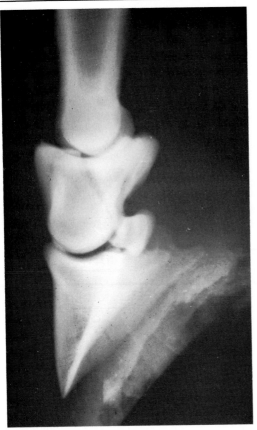

FIG. 6-175. Fracture of the second phalanx. This type of fracture can sometimes be repaired with compression bone screws without arthrodesis of the pastern joint.

Etiology

Rachitic ringbone is due to a deficiency of calcium, phosphorus, vitamin A, vitamin D, or possibly vitamin C, either alone or in combination. Vitamin A, calcium, and phosphorus deficiencies or imbalances are most commonly involved.

Signs

Usually more than one foot is involved. In some foals, both forefeet, both hind feet, or all four feet, are involved. Some lameness usually is exhibited, and joint soreness is evident. Other symptoms, such as enlargement of the carpal joints, bog spavin, and contraction of flexor tendons

Toe Cracks, Quarter Cracks, Heel Cracks (Sand Cracks)

Definition

These are cracks in the wall of the hoof, starting at the bearing surface of the wall and extending to a variable distance up the hoof wall, or cracks originating at the coronary band, as the result of a defect in the band, and extending downward. These cracks, identified as toe, quarter, or heel, depending upon their location in the hoof wall, may occur in either the front or hind feet.

Etiology

Excessive growth of the hoof wall, causing a splitting of the wall, from lack of trimming of the feet, is a common cause. Injury to the coronary band, producing a weak and deformed hoof wall, will lead to cracks originating at the coronary band. Weakening of the wall due to excessive drying or excessively thin walls also causes hoof cracks.

Signs

The presence of the split in the wall will be obvious. Lameness may not be present, but it will become evident if the crack extends into the sensitive tissues, allowing infection to gain access to these structures. An exudate under the cracks or simple inflammation of the laminae may be present, depending upon the size of the opening into the sensitive tissues. The location of the crack will be obvious. Variable lesions will be found above the coronary band in those cases where the crack is due to injury of the band. Lesions may result from lacerated wounds or from other causes, such as overreaching and interfering.

Diagnosis

The diagnosis is based on the presence of the crack, which is easily identified, and is classified according to its location.

Treatment

Treatment will depend upon the location of the crack.

Toe Crack. For toe cracks, the hoof wall on the bearing surface should be lowered about 1″ on either side of the crack. If the crack does not extend into the coronary band, a pattern should be grooved or burned into the crack (as shown in Fig. 6-176) to limit its upward progress. The horse should be shod with a toe clip on either side of the crack to prevent expansion of the wall (Fig. 6-176). Lowering of the wall from the bearing surface of the toe aids in preventing expansion of the crack. The area between the wall and the shoe should be cleaned out daily with a hacksaw blade. The crack should be thoroughly cleaned and tincture of iodine applied if it is determined that infection is present; tetanus antitoxin should be administered if the horse is not on a toxoid program. Toxoid should be given as a

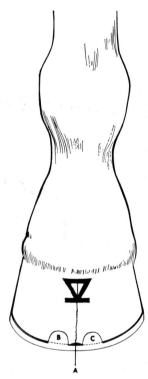

Fig. 6-176. Correction for toe crack. Triangle and bar design below the coronary band is burned or cut in, as shown, to limit the extension of the crack. The hoof wall is trimmed away below the crack so that it will not bear weight on the shoe, as shown by *A*; *B* and *C* are the toe clips used on the shoe to support the wall so that the crack cannot expand under pressure.

booster if the horse has been immunized previously with this product. An alternative method of treatment is to strip out the crack with an electric cast cutter, a hoof groover, a firing iron or a motorized burr. When treated in this manner, the crack is enlarged to about $\frac{1}{4}''$ width and is opened down to, but not into, the sensitive laminae so that it can be filled with epoxy glue or plastic.* A hoof crack amenable to such repair is shown in Figure 6–177. The opening of the crack is made in a triangle shape with the base of the triangle next to the sensitive laminae. This decreases the probabilty of the plastic coming out. In addition, it is very helpful to drill holes in the sides of the crack and thread the

*Technovit, Kulzer and Co., Hamburg, West Germany.

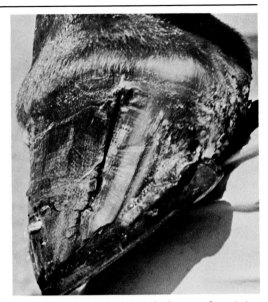

FIG. 6–178. Quarter crack before undermining and drilling. (From Evans et al., 1966; courtesy of Dr. L. H. Evans and JAVMA.)

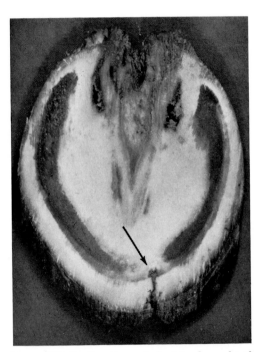

FIG. 6–177. Section through foot to show depth of toe crack into sensitive tissues. Notice walled-off appearance around the defect (arrow). This shows the need to fill some hoof cracks with plastics to protect the sensitive laminae and prevent abscess formation. (Courtesy of Dr. K. J. Peterson.)

holes shoelace fashion with umbilical tape or stainless-steel wire. This adds strength to the repair (Figs. 6–178 through 6–183). Corrective shoeing should be applied as described above. If the horse is not shod but is allowed to go barefoot, the bearing surface of the wall on either side of the crack should be lowered and, whenever possible, a pattern or plastic filling to stop the progress of the crack should be used.

Quarter Crack. For quarter cracks, the bearing surface of the hoof wall should be lowered posteriorly to the crack (as shown in Fig. 6–184). A half-bar shoe should be applied, with the bar on the heel of the affected side (Fig. 6–185). This bar should press against the frog with $\frac{1}{8}''$ to $\frac{1}{4}''$ of pressure when the shoe is applied. This allows the frog to bear the weight that normally would be taken by the hoof wall, which has already been lowered. A pattern should be used at the top of the crack (as shown in Fig. 6–184), if it does not extend into the coronary band. The corrective shoe also may have a quarter

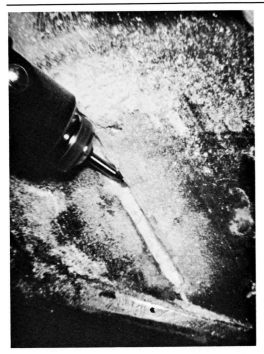

FIG. 6–179. Moto-Tool (Dremel Mfg. Co., Racine, Wis.) in use to undermine quarter crack. (From Evans *et al.*, 1966; courtesy of Dr. L. H. Evans and JAVMA.)

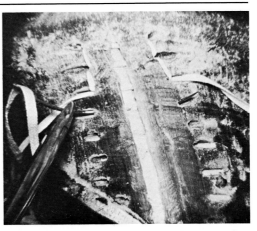

FIG. 6–181. Quarter crack after being undermined and drilled, showing lacing process with a shoemaker's stitch using umbilical tape. (From Evans *et al.*, 1966; courtesy of Dr. L. H. Evans and JAVMA.)

clip on either side of the crack to help prevent expansion of the crack. Quarter cracks may be stripped to $\frac{1}{4}''$ width down to the sensitive laminae, as described for toe crack, and filled with epoxy glue or plastic. The wall may be thinned with a rasp over the area of the crack to make the wall more flexible. Corrective shoeing should be used with rasping of the wall.

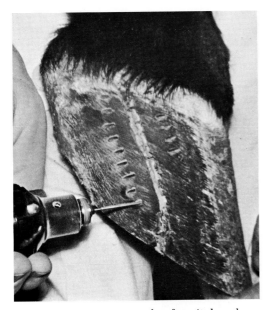

FIG. 6–180. Quarter crack after it has been undermined, showing drill holes for lacing with tape. (From Evans *et al.*, 1966; courtesy of Dr. L. H. Evans and JAVMA.)

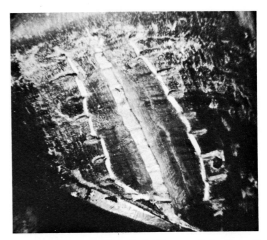

FIG. 6–182. Completed drilling and lacing of quarter crack ready for plastic application. (From Evans *et al.*, 1966; courtesy of Dr. L. H. Evans and JAVMA.)

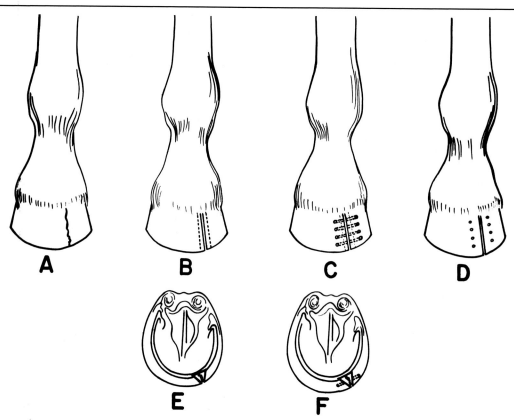

FIG. 6-183. Summary of preparation of hoof crack for repair with plastics. *A*, Hoof crack. *B*, Crack has been undermined in triangular fashion; compare with *E*. *C*, Crack undermined and drilled (dotted lines); compare with *F*. *D*, Crack ready for application of umbilical tape or wire lacing and plastic. *E*, Ground surface view of triangular undermining of crack. *F*, Ground surface view of undermining and drilling (dotted lines).

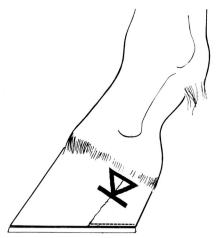

FIG. 6-184. Quarter crack and correction. A triangle and bar design is burned or cut above the crack, as shown. The dotted line indicates the area of hoof wall that should be cut away so it will not bear weight on the shoe.

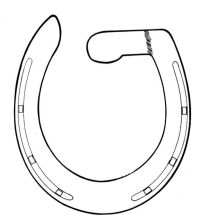

FIG. 6-185. Ground-surface view of a half-bar shoe used in treating quarter crack and heel cracks. The bar is shaped so that it will apply one-eighth to one-fourth inch of pressure against the frog when the shoe is nailed on.

If the horse is not to be shod, the wall should be lowered posterior to the crack, and a pattern should be grooved over the crack to check its spread or the crack should be filled with plastic. Tetanus antitoxin or toxoid if the horse is on a permanent immunization program should be administered if the crack extends into the sensitive tissues.

Heel Crack. Heel cracks should be treated like quarter cracks, except it may not be necessary to apply a half bar to the heel of the shoe. The wall posterior to the crack should be lowered so that it does not touch the shoe or ground.

Whenever the bearing surface of the wall is lowered from the shoe, in any type of crack, the space between the shoe and the wall should be cleaned daily with a hacksaw blade to ensure that dirt does not fill the space and cause pressure. In all cases where it is believed that the crack has permitted infection to enter the sensitive tissues, tetanus antitoxin or toxoid if the horse is on a permanent immunization program should be administered. When there are lacerations of the coronary band that have caused distorted growth of horn, the horn growth should be rasped every two weeks to keep it as nearly normal in shape as possible. Hard, dry areas on the coronary band should be rubbed daily with olive oil to keep them soft.

Any type of hoof crack or hoof defect can be treated by the use of plastics.* Epoxy glues, fiber glass, or special hoof-repair material† can be used. The crack must be thoroughly cleaned and undermined to hold the plastic in place. There are numerous ways to aid binding of the plastic, and one is to enlarge and undermine the crack with a small motor tool burr or Stryker cast cutter, and then traverse the crack with horizontal grooves (Figs. 6–177 through 6–183). Cross drilling and lacing with umbilical tape or wire

prior to applying acrylic have been described above and by Evans *et al.* (1966). The main thing is to give the plastic an anchor to keep it in place. Whatever type of plastic is used, the crack is painted with the catalyst first. The crack is then filled with the glue, fiber glass, or plastic material and allowed to harden. With fiber glass this process can be speeded up by adding more catalyst. After the material is hardened, it can be rasped to conform to the shape of the hoof wall. The best material I have found to date is Technovit.*

Plastics are an excellent way to repair hoof cracks, since they seal the crack and prevent infection of the sensitive tissues. Defects in the hoof wall can also be filled with such plastics (Figs. 6–186 and 6–187). One serious problem with plastic repair is the heat generated by catalysis, which can destroy tissue beneath it, causing abscess formation.

Prognosis

The prognosis is favorable if the crack originates at the bearing surface of the wall and if infection has not entered the foot. The prognosis is guarded if infection is present. In cases where the crack originates in defects of the coronary band, the etiology will be persistent, so corrective shoeing may be necessary for the life of the horse. This makes the prognosis guarded to unfavorable. A considerable period may be necessary for the crack to grow out, because the wall grows approximately $\frac{1}{4}''$ a month.

Infection of cracks may cause foot abscesses that break and drain at the coronary band; this situation is similar to that seen in "gravel."

SPECIFIC REFERENCES

EVANS, L. H., J. J. JENNY, and C. W. RAKER. 1966. The repair of hoof cracks with acrylic. JAVMA 148: 355.

*Technovit, Kulzer and Co., Hamburg, West Germany.
†H. D. Justi Co., Philadelphia.

*Kulzer and Co., Hamburg, West Germany.

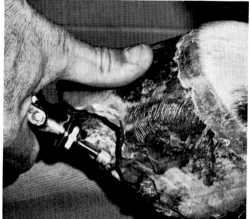

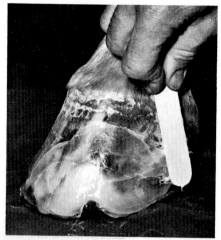

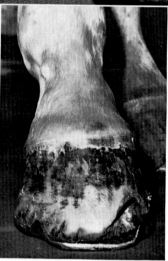

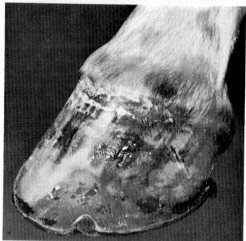

FIG. 6–186. *Top,* Hoof defect being undermined with a motorized burr. *Bottom,* Appearance of defect after it is prepared for plastic application. Note shoe is in place with clips to help hold it. (From Evans *et al.,* courtesy Dr. J. Jenny, Dr. L. Evans, and AAEP.)

FIG. 6–187. *Top,* Applying plastic to foot in Figure 6–114. *Bottom,* Appearance of hoof defect after it is filled with plastic and the hoof has been rasped to normal shape. (From Evans *et al.,* 1966; courtesy Dr. J. Jenny, Dr. L. Evans and AAEP.)

GRAHAM, C. W. 1965. Postoperative results from plastic hoof repair. Proc. 11th Ann. AAEP.

HUTCHINS, D. R. 1969. Acrylics in hoof repair in the horse. Aust. Vet. J., 45: 159–161.

JENNY, J. 1963. Application of plaster cast and plastic repair of the hoof. Proc. 9th Ann. AAEP, 237.

JENNY, J. and L. H. EVANS. 1964. Self-curing acrylic plastics for hoof repair. Pa. Vet. 6: 6.

JENNY, J., L. H. EVANS, and C. W. RAKER. 1965. Hoof repair with plastics. JAVMA 147(12): 1340–1345.

KEOWN, G. 1962. Quarter cracks. Proc. 8th Ann. AAEP, 143.

LUNDVALL, R. L., and J. H. JOHNSON. 1967. Use of plastics in the repair of hooves. Norden News, 9–13 (Fall).

Gravel

Definition

Gravel is a lay term for what supposedly is a migration of a piece of gravel from the white line to the heel area. This does not occur; what does happen is that a crack in the white line permits infection to invade the sensitive structures. Because there is no drainage, inflammation follows the line of least resistance, and drainage occurs at the heel area, as it does with puncture wounds that cannot drain through the sole.

Etiology

A crack in the white line, or in the sole, may occur in feet that are too dry. In addition, chronic laminitis with its associated "seedy toe," causing a poorly defined seal in the toe area of the white line, may cause this condition. The sole and white line should be carefully examined to determine the real cause.

Signs

Lameness usually will appear before drainage at the heel area occurs, but the condition may go undiagnosed until after drainage takes place. Signs of lameness vary according to severity of the infection and location of the entry of infection. The horse will modify his gait, as described in the discussion of puncture wounds of the foot, according to the location of the entry. Careful examination of the white line and sole will reveal black spots, which should be probed to their depth. Examination with a hoof tester will determine the approximate area of penetration. If the black areas are probed to their depth, one will be found that penetrates into the sensitive laminae. After the depth of the crack has been probed, pus often will exude from the wound. When the condition has been present for some time, the heel area will drain at the coronary band. Systemic reaction to the infection varies, but in most cases infection remains localized.

The horse will show a supporting-leg lameness. If routine examination with a hoof tester is made on all lameness cases, some cases can be diagnosed before drainage occurs at the heel.

Diagnosis

Diagnosis is made by careful examination of the foot with a hoof tester. All cases of lameness should have this examination. Most cases can be diagnosed before the heel area breaks and drains, providing the owner seeks help in time. Careful observation of the way the horse sets his foot on the ground will be helpful in localizing the area of penetration.

Treatment

Treatment consists of establishing proper drainage for the infection, as described in puncture wounds of the foot. The foot may be soaked in Epsom salts even if heel drainage has not begun. Applying tincture of iodine to the drainage area in the sole and bandaging the foot until it is healed are necessary. Antiphlogistic pastes can also be used under the bandage. Tetanus antitoxin always should be administered if the horse is not on a toxoid program. Toxoid should be given as a booster if the horse has previously been immunized with this product. After the first week of involvement, bandaging of the foot may be delayed to once every three or four days if it stays dry.

Prognosis

Prognosis is favorable if the condition is diagnosed before drainage at the heel occurs, except in those cases where the foot is subject to recurrence of the condition because of chronic laminitis. The prognosis is guarded if drainage at the heel already has occurred. Careful treatment, though, will permit many of these horses to be returned to complete soundness. If the condition is of long standing, prognosis is unfavorable, because permanent changes already may have occurred.

Thrush

Definition

Thrush, a degenerative condition of the frog involving the central and lateral sulci, is characterized by the presence of a black necrotic material in the affected areas. The infection may penetrate the horny tissues and involve the sensitive structures.

Etiology

The predisposing causes of thrush are unhygienic conditions, (especially when horses are kept in poorly managed stalls or filthy surroundings), dirty, uncleaned feet, and lack of frog pressure resulting from poor shoeing or poor foot trimming. Many organisms probably are involved, but *Spherophorus necrophorus* is the most important of these.

Signs

There is an increased amount of moisture and a black discharge in the sulci of the frog. This discharge, which varies in quantity, has a very offensive odor. When the affected sulci are cleaned, it will be found that they are deeper than normal and may extend into the sensitive tissues of the foot, causing the horse to flinch when they are cleaned. The frog will be undermined, and large areas of it may require removal because of the loss of continuity with the underlying frog. In severe cases that have penetrated into the sensitive structure of the foot, the horse may be lame, and the foot may show the same signs of infection that would be encountered in puncture wound of the foot.

Diagnosis

Diagnosis is based on the odor and physical characteristics of the black discharge in the sulci of the frog.

Treatment

Treatment is cleanliness, removal of the cause, and return of the frog and hoof to normal conformation and condition. The foot should be cleaned daily and the cleft of the frog packed with a proper medication. Medications that may be used include equal parts of phenol and iodine, tincture of iodine, and 10 percent formalin. The best treatment consists of packing the sulci with cotton soaked in 10 to 15 percent sodium sulfapyridine solution. This treatment, which is very effective, should be repeated until the infection is controlled.

The cause can be removed by placing the horse in cleaner surroundings or by daily cleansing of the frog after removal of the debris. Degenerated frog tissues should be removed, and an effort should be made to return the frog to normal by cleaning up all infection. A bar shoe may be applied to exert pressure to the frog until it returns to normal size.

Some veterinarians recommend blistering of the heel areas to stimulate growth of the frog. In some cases it may be necessary to protect the foot with a leather boot to prevent contamination. This is especially true if the sensitive tissues are involved. The hoof wall should be lowered as far as possible to stimulate frog pressure, but normal foot axis should not be changed.

Prognosis

The prognosis is favorable if the disease is diagnosed before the foot has suffered extensive damage. It is guarded if the sensitive structures are involved.

Wounds

Wounds are classified as follows:

Open Wounds

Incised Wounds. These are wounds produced by sharp objects, but where tissue damage is at a minimum. Very little bruising to underlying structures has occurred, and hemorrhage is not severe unless a large vessel has been cut. Separation of wound edges usually is at a minimum, unless the wound is deep, or severs the lines of tension. A minimal amount of pain is present, and the chief danger is damage to underlying vital structures.

Lacerated Wounds. These wounds are usually produced by irregular objects, such as barbed wire, and by horn gores and bites. This type of wound is characterized by extensive damage to underlying tissues, especially to the skin and subcutaneous connective tissue. It may be accompanied by abrasion or contusion. Hemorrhage usually is not profuse, unless large vessels are opened, because the vessels often are torn, and there is a marked constriction of arteries. Pain usually is marked, and the greatest danger is infection, with pockets of pus, tissue necrosis, and gangrene, if tissues are torn away from the blood supply.

Puncture Wounds. These wounds are produced by sharp objects whose length exceeds their diameter, and are characterized by small, superficial punctures with a considerable amount of deep injury. They often are produced by bites, horn gores, nail punctures, and objects such as pitchforks.

Puncture wounds are further classified as:

Penetrating—goes into a body cavity.

Perforating—goes into a body cavity and back out.

Stab—goes into deep tissue only.

Burns. (Burns will not be considered in this discussion.)

Closed Wounds

Closed or subcutaneous wounds are those in which the skin is not broken through all layers. They are caused by external violence that results in tissue damage without loss of continuity of the skin. At a later date, necrosis or sloughing may take place. Closed wounds are classified as:

Wheal. This is a bleb in the skin, usually intradermal; no hemorrhagic extravasation is present.

Abrasions. These are injuries to the superficial surface of the skin or mucous membrane where the epidermis is damaged, but the damage has not extended through all the skin layers or the mucous membrane. These cause oozing of serum and a small amount of hemorrhage. A scab forms over the area of abrasion and constitutes a form of second-intention healing.

Contusions. Contusions are caused by a trauma that causes a rupture of subcutaneous or deep blood vessels. The skin is not broken but subcutaneous hemorrhage occurs. Contusions are classified as follows:

First-Degree Contusion. Here there is some hemorrhage into and under the skin, producing discoloration but very little hematoma.

Second-Degree Contusion. This is a hematoma; if it is small, it will probably be absorbed. If it is large, it may lead to formation of scar tissue and possible blemish. It also may lead to a seroma, after blood cells of the clot are absorbed; the serum remains. This type of contusion most commonly results from kicks over the area of the hip and gluteal region and from rubbing on the brisket region. There is some danger of abscess formation of hematogenous origin.

Third-Degree Contusion. These are so severe that they damage the tissue beyond repair. The skin is not broken from the original blow but thrombosis of the vessels occurs beneath the skin, and sloughing of the superficial areas ensues.

Diagnosis

Diagnosis of a closed wound is usually relatively simple. However, in some cases it may be confused with hernia or abscess, so the swelling always should be tapped, under aseptic procedure, to determine the contents. This is especially important for those hematomas that occur over the abdominal wall and thus must be differentiated from hernia.

The chief danger of all wounds is injury and/or infection to deep structures, especially joint capsules, sensitive portions of the foot, tendon sheaths, blood vessels, and nerves. Lack of free drainage and spread of infection may enhance this danger. Malignant edema and tetanus may be sequelae to wounds, and prophylactic treatment should be used against diseases resulting from wounds that develop anaerobic conditions. Healing of a superficial part of the wound, which traps infection underneath, may lead to an abscess or cellulitis. In other cases, undetected foreign bodies may be left in a wound, later to cause abscessation and sinus tracts.

Conditions Interfering with Healing of Wounds

Interference with Circulation. Circulation in the vicinity of the wound may be hindered by swelling, improper bandaging, laceration, prolonged infection, and exuberant granulation tissue.

Invasive Infection. Infection causing phlegmon or cellulitis will interfere with healing. Drainage should always be established if infection is present. Failure to use aseptic procedures in dressing wounds may be the cause of this type of infection.

Devitalized Tissue. Gapping of wounds leads to drying and will cause tissue to be devitalized. Any tissue that is pulled away from circulation will also be devitalized and will undergo necrosis. A triangular skin flap with the apex of the flap pointed toward the incoming blood supply will usually lose the apex portion of the triangle because of loss of blood supply.

Inadequate Drainage for Collection of Blood and Discharges in the Wound. Inadequate drainage interferes with circulation and forms an ideal medium for growth of bacteria. Hemorrhage should be controlled by ligation, and Penrose* drains should be used to prevent this type of accumulation.

Foreign Bodies. Any foreign body in the wound will interfere with healing and cause a sinus tract drainage.

Continued Trauma to the Wound. This usually results when the horse is not restrained and is allowed to abuse the wound area. Ideally, a wound is immobilized to aid healing. In the lower limb this can be done by means of a plaster cast or a corrective shoe.

Subcutaneous Gases. Subcutaneous gases will produce devitalization of tissue by separating the skin from the underlying structures. Wounds of the axillary space are especially prone to development of subcutaneous air. In some cases subcutaneous gas is due to the type of organism present; e.g., *Clostridium septicum* malignant edema. This is an unfavorable development.

The Effect of Wound Medications. Wound medications often are more detrimental than helpful in the healing of the wound. Irritant antiseptics and drugs should be avoided in all cases. Such drugs as copper sulfate, antimony trichloride (butter of antimony), and alum are irritants. Although these products will destroy superficial exuberant granulation tissue, they irritate the deep tissues so that the end result is a wound with more subcutaneous fibrous tissue than would have resulted if the wound had been treated properly. If exuberant granulation tissue is present, it should be removed surgically by scalpel or cautery. The wound is then kept under a pressure bandage with a corticoid and antibiotic ointment until it is healed. Bandages should be changed frequently enough to avoid irritation. Wet bandages containing wound discharges

*Davol Rubber Co., Providence, R.I.

will delay healing. In most cases, a bandage should not be allowed to stay in place for longer than three days. Contamination should always be avoided when applying a dressing.

Nutrition. Poor nutrition of the horse will delay healing of a wound. Parasitism, bad teeth, and inadequate feeding may contribute to delayed wound healing. All these factors should be considered when poor condition is present.

Treatment of Lacerated and Incised Wounds

The horse, more than other species of animal, must have proper care in treatment of wounds. Mistreatment will result in exuberant granulation, excessive scarring, blemishing, and sometimes unsoundness. Wounds below the carpus and tarsus are especially sensitive, requiring careful treatment to prevent complications. Tetanus antitoxin should always be administered if the horse is not on a toxoid program. Toxoid should be given as a booster when the horse has been immunized previously with this product.

Hemorrhage should be controlled by ligation and/or torsion of the vessels, and the wound should be thoroughly cleansed. After close-clipping an adequate area, hair on the edges of the wound should be shaved for at least $\frac{1}{2}''$ away from the wound edge. Such hair will irritate the wound and may produce enough irritation to cause exuberant granulation tissue. Following shaving, the skin edges should be painted with a skin antiseptic and the wound injected with a local anesthetic such as 2 percent procaine or 2 percent lidocaine hydrochloride. The distal fragment of the wound requires very little local anesthesia because it is torn from the nerve supply. The proximal fragment, though, will be most sensitive. In conjunction with local anesthesia, the horse may be tranquilized to facilitate treatment.

Debridement of all wounds must be done fully and carefully. All dirt, hair, and tissues obviously torn from the blood supply must be removed from the wound. Normal saline solution is recommended for washing wounds. Using sterile gauze sponges and saline, the wound should be thoroughly cleaned so that a healthy surface is present. Wounds may also be thoroughly washed with solutions containing tamed iodine.* These solutions can also be used under pressure (Ingram, 1972) for more thorough cleansing. In all cases, care must be used to avoid increasing contamination of the wound, so rubber gloves are called for. Local antibiotics, such as penicillin-streptomycin mixture used for intramuscular injection, can be placed in a wound or injected into the tissues around a wound. Nitrofurazone† is also an excellent topical antibiotic.

Any fresh incised or lacerated wound that lends itself to suturing should be sutured. This is especially true if the wound is below the carpus or the tarsus. Fresh wounds often will show remarkable healing qualities if properly debrided and sutured. However, this means that the wound must be handled properly. All deep muscular layers should be sutured with catgut, while the skin should be sutured with a nonabsorbable, noncapillary suture. Nonabsorbable sutures should not be buried. In areas of considerable skin tension, the suture lines should be reinforced with the quill-type suture. Skin often tears with triangular-shaped flaps. If the apex of the triangle points toward the blood supply, the tip of the flap is often lost. However, it is worthwhile suturing to minimize skin loss. Local anesthetics containing epinephrine should not be used to anesthetize skin-flap wounds below the carpus and the hock. Circulation to these areas is often borderline, and the use of epinephrine may cause necrosis.

*Betadine, Purdue Fredrick Co., Yonkers, N.Y.
†Furacin, Norwich Pharmacal Co., Norwich, N.J.

If it is obvious that there is going to be pocketing of the wound that will permit the accumulation of discharges, ventral drainage should be established. Whenever there is doubt about adequate drainage, or the possibility of contamination leading to infection and drainage arises, a Penrose* drain should be used. Large wounds requiring suturing in an area difficult to drain can be drained by the use of continued suction.† Some wounds do require this drainage, but the wound still should be sutured and ventral drainage established. If it is not possible to suture a wound because the skin surface has been torn away or because duration or swelling does not permit apposition, debridement and a counterpressure bandage with proper topical medication are recommended. A counterpressure bandage helps keep wound edges in apposition; it should be used until the wound is nearly healed, especially for wounds below the carpus and tarsus. If the pressure is removed, exuberant granulation tissue tends to develop. Bandages should be changed often enough that exudate cannot accumulate and irritate the wound area.

Wounds with large granulating surfaces need a protective covering. This is usually best accomplished by the use of a split-thickness skin graft (Meagher, 1970) or pigskin‡ (Snyder, 1971). When pigskin is used, the bandage and pigskin are replaced at 24- to 48-hour intervals. In some cases, pigskin can be used under a plaster cast for 7 to 10 days. Coverings of this type relieve pain by protecting nerve endings, and they greatly enhance healing.

Ointments containing insulin (10 units of zinc protamine insulin in 1 gm of cream base) have been recommended for smaller granulating areas (Belfield *et al.,* 1970).

Early medication under the bandage should consist of nonirritating ointments containing antibiotics. Mastitis ointments and nitrofurazone are often used. After a granulating surface is present, application of an ointment containing a corticoid is recommended on wounds below the tarsus and carpus. This type of ointment, plus counterpressure bandaging, prevents exuberant granulation tissue. Bandages should become progressively lighter to permit air to reach to the wound.

Wounds that sometimes are impractical to suture, such as those in the upper forearm, where sutures tear out, can be treated very well by shaving and cleansing the wound and by applying daily a soothing wound ointment that contains no irritants.

Wounds below the carpus and the tarsus that are so small that bandaging is not required should be treated daily with agents that tend to retard granulation tissue, such as 2 percent picric acid, 2 percent tannic acid, and triple dye* following shaving and cleansing.

Wounds on the coronary band or the volar aspect of the pastern region are sometimes treated by applying a plaster cast over the sutured wound area. Since immobilizing a wound is one of the fundamentals of wound therapy, a plaster cast does an excellent job of promoting first-intention healing (*see* Chap. 11, p. 433). As long as the sutures remain intact, discharges will be minimal, provided the wound has been properly treated. The cast should be removed in seven to ten days to check on results, and, if necessary, a new one applied.

Wire cuts involving the coronary band require that the wound edges be in close apposition to heal. Otherwise, granulating surfaces that have no tendency to unite will develop. These wounds must either be sutured or be kept under pressure bandage, or both, until healing is nearly com-

---

*Davol Rubber Co., Providence, R.I.
†Snyder Hemovac, Zimmer, Warsaw, Ind.
‡Burn Treatment Skin Bank Inc., Phoenix, Ariz.

*A combination of brilliant green, acriflavine, and gentian violet in an alcohol base.

plete. A plaster cast is the best method of immobilizing the wound. Application of an ointment containing antibiotics under the bandage is recommended. A horseshoe nail may be driven into the toe of the wall to help anchor the gauze bandage so considerable pressure can be applied against the lacerated tissues.

When a joint capsule or a tendon sheath is opened, as the result of a wound, a crystalline penicillin solution should be injected into the joint or tendon sheath. The capsule or sheath and the overlying tissues should be sutured if it is a fresh wound. The leg then should be kept in a snug bandage or a plaster cast, and parenteral antibiotics should be given for four to seven days. Here again, a plaster cast is the best method of immobilization.

Most common mistreatment of open wounds includes permitting wounds below the carpus and the tarsus to heal without counterpressure bandages or sutures, improper cleansing, failing to shave the hair from the wound area, and application of irritant drugs. In no case should caustic or irritant drugs be applied to wounds of horses. Caustic drugs will remove superficial areas of granulation tissue, but at the same time they irritate and stimulate underlying tissue so that this tissue grows back in a short time. Continued irritation may cause a nonhealing wound, exuberant granulation tissue, or excessive fibrosis of the healed wound, causing a permanent blemish. Topical applications of ointments containing a corticoid are much better for this purpose since they relieve inflammation, and, combined with pressure bandages or a plaster cast, are of considerable aid in preventing exuberant granulation tissue. Corticoid ointments are not used if active infection is present. If removal of large amounts of granulation tissue is required, it is best done surgically. Following surgical removal, counterpressure bandaging or plaster cast and application of ointments containing antibiotics are recommended.

Treatment of Puncture Wounds

Puncture wounds are dangerous in horses, since they may lead to malignant edema, cellulitis, or tetanus. Tetanus antitoxin should always be administered unless the horse is on a toxoid program, and parenteral antibiotics are usually recommended. This type of wound may penetrate a tendon sheath or a joint capsule. The wound opening should be properly cleansed and shaved, and the wound flushed daily with antibiotic solutions such as crystalline penicillin.

A puncture wound on the forearm, or above the hock, often causes the distal portion of the leg to become enlarged with edema. This edema may be due to the gravitational effects of the inflammation or to developing cellulitis. If the swelling is due to gravitational effects, counterpressure bandages should be applied. This can be done with elastic gauze and elastic tape or as a modified Robert Jones bandage. Soaking of this type of wound in magnesium sulfate is recommended because of the action of the drug in reducing swelling. The wound opening should be covered with a light bandage, so it is not exposed, and a poultice of Denver Mud* or other satisfactory antiphlogistic paste should be applied under the bandage. Parenteral and local antibiotic medication should be continued until the wound is obviously healing properly. It is sometimes necessary to establish ventral drainage. It is sometimes best to immobilize a lower-limb puncture wound in a plaster cast.

A chronic draining sinus tract in the limbs of horses is very often due to a retained foreign body resulting from a puncture wound. This possibility must be eliminated. Radiographs will not reveal foreign bodies of wood or other soft materials.

*Demco, Inc., Denver, Colorado.

Treatment of Closed Wounds

Minor closed wounds, such as wheals, seldom require treatment. They usually are caused by insect bites or stings, and antihistamines are the usual form of therapy. Abrasions are treated by cleansing of the wounds with normal saline, soap, and brush. A moist antiseptic dressing should be applied, usually in the form of an ointment. These ointments should be continued to keep the scab soft as the lesion heals. If infection develops under the scab, the scab should be removed and antibiotic ointments applied. Abrasions also may be treated with drugs such as triple dye, and acriflavine 1:1000.

Contusions of the second and third degree are those that usually require therapy. For second-degree contusions, cold packs should be applied to stop hemorrhage and limit the extent of the hematoma. Topical application of dimethyl sulfoxide* may be helpful in reducing swelling of seromas and hematomas prior to surgical drainage. After the clot has formed, the serum may be drained in an attempt to obtain union of the skin with the subcutaneous tissue. However, in many cases, union does not occur, so drainage must be established by incision in order to obtain healing. Daily swabbing of the lesion with tincture of iodine should be used to irritate the two surfaces. It is important that the drainage be ventral and that it remain until the wound heals to prevent continual separation of the skin and subcutaneous tissue by serum accumulation. Penrose tube drains are helpful when drainage is required.

In third-degree contusions, a localized area of tissue will usually slough off. All that can be done is to trim out necrotic tissue, keep the wound clean, and prevent infection by local antibiotic ointment.

*Domoso-Syntex Labs., Inc., Palo Alto, Calif.

SPECIFIC REFERENCES

American College of Surgeons. 1960. Care of Soft Tissue Injuries. Philadelphia: W. B. Saunders.

BEEMAN, G. M. 1972. A surgical approach to the repair of equine wounds. Proc. AAEP. 163–171.

BELFIELD, W. O., et al. 1970. The use of insulin in open-wound healing. VM/SAC 65: 455–460.

BOYD, C. L. 1967. Skin autotransplants for wound healing. JAVMA 151(12): 1618–1624.

BRITTON, J. W. 1970. Wound management in horses. JAVMA 157(11): 1585–1589.

BULLARD, J. F. 1967. Adjustable suture for large lacerations. JAVMA 151(6): 718.

DAVIS, L. 1960. Christopher's Textbook of Surgery. 7th ed. Philadelphia: W. B. Saunders Co.

DELAHANTY, D. D., et al. 1968. Wound treatment—Panel discussion. Proc. AAEP, 185–211.

DIXON, R. T., and LARSEN, L. H. 1965. Gamma-ray therapy for granulating wounds. Aust. Vet. J. 41(10): 310–314.

DOUGLAS, D. M. 1963. Wound Healing and Management. Baltimore: Williams & Wilkins.

FORMSTON, C. 1964. Wound management, p. 3. In 3rd Ann. Cong. Brit. Eq. Vet. Assoc.

FRANK, E. R. 1964. Veterinary Surgery. 7th ed. Minneapolis: Burgess Publishing Co.

GUARD, W. F. 1953. Surgical Principles and Techniques. Columbus, Ohio: Published by the author.

HANSELKA, D. V. 1974. Use of autogenous mesh grafts in equine wound management. JAVMA 164(1): 35–41.

INGRAM, J. T. 1972. The pulsating irrigator in the treatment of wounds. Proc. AAEP. 153–166.

JOHNSON, J. H. 1970. Puncture wounds of the foot. VM/SAC 65(2): 147–152.

JOHNSON, J. H. 1972. Septic conditions of the equine foot. JAVMA 161(11): 1276.

KRAEMER, D. C. 1966. Skin autotransplant for granulating wounds. Southwest. Vet. 19(3): 236–237.

MACKAY-SMITH, M. P., and D. MARKS. 1968. Pinch technique for skin grafting. JAVMA 152(11): 1633–1637.

MEAGHER, D. M., and O. R. ADAMS. 1971. Split thickness skin autologous transplantation in horses. JAVMA 159(1): 55–60.

MEAGHER, D. M. 1970. Skin transplantation in horses: Techniques and results. Proc. AAEP, 171–184.

NEAL, P. A. 1971. The treatment of wounds of the lower parts of horses limbs. Vet. Rec. 89(5): 132–134.

ROBERTS, W. D. 1962. Equine wound management. Vet. Med. 57: 773.

ROBERTS, W. D. 1962. Wound management in ranch horses. Proc. 8th Ann. AAEP, 33.

SNYDER, C. 1971. University of Utah Medical School, Salt Lake City. Personal communication.

WALKER, E. R. 1971. The treatment of acute and chronic wounds below the carpal and tarsal areas. Proc. 17th Ann. AAEP, 49–52.

Equine Sarcoid

Definition

Equine sarcoid is a recurring granulation tissue that affects equines. Sarcoid is most common following wounds of the lower part of the limb, but it may involve the head, neck, or prepuce. It is usually characterized by a raw, granulating surface that is somewhat mushroomed-shaped, in that the base of attachment is usually smaller than the granulating surface, or it may appear as a wart-like growth.

Etiology

Etiology has been definitely proven to be a virus (Voss, 1965; Watson, 1973). The lesions have been transmitted from horse to horse, and Olson (1963) has produced similar lesions with bovine wart virus.

Signs

Equine sarcoid is difficult to differentiate from ordinary exuberant granulation tissue. The tendency to recur following surgical removal is indicative of the disease. It often has a mushroom type of growth, with a small base of attachment and a larger raw granulating surface. Sarcoid is common in wounds below the carpus and tarsus. Wounds that occur in areas where motion is present seem especially susceptible to this lesion. It rarely develops when a wound has been treated properly by means of proper nonirritating medications, pressure bandages, suturing, and plaster cast. Sarcoid can occur spontaneously without previous trauma to the skin. Histologically, it is characterized by irregularly arranged fibroblasts with larger than normal nuclei and frequent mitotic figures that tend to form whorls. Proliferation of epithelium with extension and branching of rete pegs into the tumor mass is present. The histology is also similar to exuberant granulation tissue and fibrosarcoma.

Treatment

Equine sarcoid should be surgically removed and the base cauterized by electrocautery when necessary to control hemorrhage or to kill cells that were not removed surgically. It is removed down to below skin level and hemorrhage stopped by means of pressure bandage or thermocautery since hemorrhage is profuse in removal of this type of lesion. If cobalt-60 therapy is available, it should be employed, as it is one of the more successful methods of treatment; 3,000 to 4,000 roentgens of gamma-ray radiation are used after surgical removal. When the lesion is over the carpus, near a carpal bone, the radiation dosage is reduced to 2,000 roentgens because of possible damage to the carpal bones (Gillette, 1966). Whether or not radiation therapy is available, the sarcoid area should be kept clean and all hair kept shaved away from the wound every ten days to two weeks. A corticoid ointment containing antibiotics is applied to the surface of the lesion and a pressure bandage applied using conforming gauze* and elastic tape† until the wound is healed. The bandage is changed at intervals of two to three days and must be used until healing is complete. If the bandage is discontinued before complete healing, the sarcoid may recur. One of the most successful methods of treatment for sarcoid is wide surgical excision. The incision must be wide enough to remove all affected tissue. The wound is then kept

*Kling, Johnson & Johnson.
†Elastikon, Johnson & Johnson.

bandaged, and corticoid ointment* applied when indicated. An excellent wound protection is pigskin.† Split-thickness skin grafting is also helpful in those areas where it is applicable. Plastic surgery techniques using sliding flaps are also very useful when the sarcoid is removed in areas like the head and neck, where such procedures are feasible. The use of a killed vaccine made from the lesions of a horse affected with sarcoid has given variable results. In some cases, vaccines of this type may suppress or inhibit growth of sarcoids.

SPECIFIC REFERENCES

GILLETTE, E. L. 1966. Clinical Radiologist, Colorado State University. Personal communication.

JAMES, V. S. 1968. A family tendency to equine sarcoids. Southwest. Vet. 21: 235–236.

LEWIS, R. E. 1964. Radon implant therapy of squamous cell carcinoma and equine sarcoid. Proc. 10th Ann. AAEP, 217.

METCALF, J. W. 1971. Improved technique in sarcoid removal. Proc. 17th Ann. AAEP, 45–47.

OLSON, C. 1963. *Equine Medicine and Surgery.* Santa Barbara, Calif.: American Veterinary Publications, Inc.

RAGLAND, W. L., et al. 1966. Equine sarcoid epizootic. Nature 210(5043): 1399.

RAGLAND, W. L., G. H. KEOWN, and J. R. SPENCER. 1970. Equine sarcoid. Eq. Vet. J. 2(1): 2–11.

RAGLAND, W. L. 1970. Equine sarcoid. Eq. Vet. J. 2(1): 2.

RAGLAND, W. L., and G. R. SPENCER. 1969. Attempts to relate bovine papilloma virus to the cause of equine sarcoid: Equidae inoculated intradermally with bovine papilloma virus. Amer. J. Vet. Res. 30(5): 743–752.

ROBERTS, W. D. 1970. Experimental treatment of equine sarcoid. VM/SAC 65(1): 67–72.

STRAFUSS, A. C., et al. 1973. Sarcoid in horses. VM/SAC 68(11): 1246.

VOSS, J. L. 1965. Transmission of equine sarcoid. Thesis, Colorado State University.

VOSS, J. L. 1965. Equine sarcoid transmission. Proc. 11th. Ann. AAEP.

WATSON, R. 1973. Personal communication. Department of Pathology, Colorado State University Ft. Collins.

*Kenalog-S, Squibb and Co.

†Burn Treatment Skin Bank, Inc., Phoenix, Ariz.

REFERENCES

Each of the following references describes several types of lameness but was not included in the list of specific references for each section because this would have resulted in needless repetition. References for specific lamenesses can be found at the end of each section.

ADAMS, O. R. 1966. Local anesthesia as an aid in equine lameness diagnosis. Norden News (Jan).

ADAMS, O. R. 1957. *Veterinary Notes on Lameness and Shoeing of Horses.* Published by the author.

ALGER, C. 1904–1905. Clinical study of lameness. Amer. Vet. Rev. 28: 806.

ANNON 1966. Lameness in the horse. Mod. Vet. Pract., 47(5): 51–92.

ARANEZ, J. B., et al. 1962. Preliminary observations on the incidence of leg ailments among race horses in the Philippines. Philippines J. Vet. Med. 1(2): 123–132.

AXE, J. W. 1900. *The Horse in Health and Disease.* London: Gresham Publishing Co. 3 vols.

BAIRD, J. 1933. Lameness and its treatment in the horse. JAVMA 83: 39.

BELL, R. 1899. Shoulder lameness in the horse. Amer. Vet. Rev. 23: 477.

BLOOD, D. C., and HENDERSEN, J. A. 1963. *Veterinary Medicine.* 2nd ed. Baltimore: Williams & Wilkins.

BRENNAN, B. F. 1958. The veterinarian in race track practice. Vet. Scope 3 (summer).

CAMPBELL, D. M. 1934. Shifting lameness in the horse. Vet. Med. 29: 29.

CARLSON, W. D. 1967. *Veterinary Radiology.* 2nd ed. Philadelphia: Lea & Febiger.

CRAWLEY, A. J. 1960. Radiology V. Can. Vet. J. 12: 554.

CHAPMAN, T. 1901. *Lameness in the Horse.* New York: W. R. Jenkins.

CHURCHILL, E. A. 1963. The causes of lameness. Bloodhorse 85: 602.

CHURCHILL, E. A., et al. 1959. Panel on orthopedic surgery. Proc. 5th Ann. AAEP.

CHURCHILL, E. 1968. Care and Training of the Trotter and Pacer. Columbus, Ohio: U.S. Trotting Association.

COCHRAN, D. 1914. Lameness of the hip joint. Amer. Vet. Rev. 44: 491.

COCHRAN, D. 1912–1913. Stifle lameness. Amer. Vet. Rev. 42: 308.

CRAWFORD, H. C. 1932a. Equine lameness: A brief resume. N. Amer. Vet. 12: 29.

CRAWFORD, H. C. 1932b. Radiography: Its limitations as an aid to the diagnostician of lameness. N. Amer. Vet. 13: 39.

DANKS, A. G. 1943. *Williams' Surgical Operations.* Ithaca, N.Y.: Published by the author.

DAUBIGNY, F. T. 1916. Halting or lameness in the horse. JAVMA 19: 648.

DAVIDSON, A. H. 1953. *Lameness, Firing, Etc.* Lexington, Ky.: Third Annual Stud Managers Course.

DAVIDSON, A. H. 1954. *Lameness.* Lexington, Ky.: Fourth Annual Stud Managers Course.

DAVIDSON, A. H. 1965. Equine lameness. MSU Vet. 25(3): 123–131.

DAVIDSON, A. H. 1967. Generalization about equine lameness. Iowa Vet. 38(6): 9–11.

DELAHANTY, D. D., et al. 1958. Orthopedic surgery in the horse—A panel discussion. Proc. 4th Ann. Am. AAEP.

DIXON, R. T. 1963. The nature of injuries causing foot lameness in fast-gaited horses. Aust. Vet. J. 39: 177.

DYKSTRA, R. R. 1927. Anatomical changes in lameness of the horse. JAVMA 71: 425.

Equine Lameness Review. 1961. Vet. Med. 56: 165.

Equine Medicine and Surgery. 1963. (68 authors) Santa Barbara, Calif.: American Veterinary Publishers Inc.

FOWLER, G. R. 1938. Diseases of the foot of the horse. Vet. Med. 33: 216.

FOWLER, W. J. R. 1939. Diagnosis and treatment of lamenesses. Can. J. Comp. Med. 3: 91.

FOWLER, W. J. R. 1940. Diagnosis and treatment of lameness. Can. J. Comp. Med. 4: 249.

FRANK, E. R. 1937. Obscure lameness, N. Amer. Vet. 18: 39.

FRANK, E. R. 1964. *Veterinary Surgery.* 7th ed. Minneapolis: Burgess Publishing Co.

GERTSEN, K. E., and W. O. BRINKER. 1969. Bone plates for fracture repair in ponies. JAVMA 154(8): 900–905.

GIBSON, S. J. 1945. Lameness in horses. Can. J. Comp. Med. 9: 103.

GRAY, T. E. 1961. Foot lameness in the horse. Mod. Vet. Pract. 42: 38.

GRENSIDE, F. C. 1909. Why horses are oftener lame in front than behind. Amer. Vet. Rev. 35: 43.

GUARD, W. F. 1953. *Surgical Principles and Techniques.* Columbus, Ohio: Published by the author.

HANSEN, J. C., et al. 1971. Panel—Chronic lameness. Proc. 17th Ann. AAEP, 279–292.

HANSHEW, E., JR. 1897–1898. Dropped elbow in the horse. Amer. Vet. Rev. 21: 411.

HAYES, I. E. 1947. Shoulder lameness in the horse. Vet. Med. 42: 249.

HICKMAN, J. 1964. Veterinary Orthopaedics. Philadelphia: J. B. Lippincott Co.

HOARE, W. E. 1914. Discussion of ephemeral (transient) lameness. JAVMA 9: 113.

HUME, W. 1913. Neurectomy in foot lameness. JAVMA 8: 115.

JENNY, J. 1963. Hoof repair with plastics. Proc. 9th Ann. AAEP, 137.

JENNY, J. 1961. Management of bone and joint injuries in the horse. Vet. Scope VI.

JENNY, J. 1965. Bone and joint injuries. Mod. Vet. Pract. 46(3): 49–50.

JOHNSON, L. E., et al. 1960. Equine radiology: A panel discussion. 6th Ann. AAEP, 35–64.

JUBB, K. V. F. and P. C. KENNEDY. 1963. Pathology of Domestic Animals, Vol. 1 and 2. New York: Academic Press.

KIERNAN, J. 1894. *Hints on Horseshoeing.* Washington, D.C.: Office of the library of Congress.

LAMBERT, F. W. 1967. Some problems of the hoof in the modern harness horse. VM/SAC 62: 903–906. Sept.

LA CROIX, J. V. 1916. Lameness of the horse. Vet. Pract. Ser. No. 1, Amer. J. Vet. Med.

LIAUTARD, A. 1888. *Lameness of Horses.* New York: W. R. Jenkins Co.

LUNDVALL, R. L. 1961–1962. Lameness of the upper hind leg. Iowa State Univ. Vet. 29: 7.

LUNDVALL, R. L. 1959. Problems in a pony practice. Proc. 5th AAEP.

MACKAY-SMITH, M. P., and C. W. Raker, 1963. Mechanical defects on the equine stifle—Diagnosis and treatment. Sci. Proc. 100th Ann. Meeting, AVMA, 80–85.

MAQSOOD, M. 1944. Thrombosis of the iliac arteries in race horses. Indian Vet. J. 20: 133.

McCUNN, J. 1951. Lameness in the horse, with special reference to surgical shoeing. Vet. Rec. 63: 629.

McDONOUGH, 1913. J. Hock joint lameness. Amer. Vet. Rev. 43: 629.

McDONOUGH, J. 1916. Lameness and its most common cause. JAVMA 49: 653.

McGEE, W. R.: *Veterinary Notebook.* Lexington, Ky. Blood Horse, 1958.

McGEE, W. R. *Veterinary Notes for the Standardbred Breeder.* Columbus, Ohio: U.S. Trotting Association.

McKINNEY, W. J. 1911. Mechanical lameness. Amer. Vet. Rev. 39: 288.

MEGINNIS, P. 1957. Myostitis in race horses. JAVMA 130: 237.

Merck & Co. 1967. *The Merck Veterinary Manual.* 3rd ed. Rahway, N.J.

MILCH, R. A., G. J. BURKE, and I. W. FROCK. 1962. Surgical management of degenerative joint disease in the race horse. JAVMA 141: 1276.

MILNE, F. J., et al. 1964. Panel on lameness. Proc. AAEP, 259.

O'CONNOR, J. J. 1952. *Dollar's Veterinary Surgery.* 4th ed. London: Bailliere, Tindall & Cox.

O'CONNOR, J. T. 1958. Standardbred lameness. Proc. 4th Ann. AAEP.

PAATASAMA, S., et al. 1970. Lameness due to lesions of the radius. Eq. Vet. J., 2(3): 121–124.

PEARSON et al. 1942. *Diseases of the Horse.* Bureau of Animal Industry. Washington, D.C.: U.S. Government Printing Office.

PETERS, J. E. 1940. Lameness incident to training and racing of the thoroughbred. JAVMA 96: 200.

POPE, G. W. 1908. The diagnosis and treatment of lameness. Amer. Vet. Rev. 28: 952.

PRITCHARD, G. C. 1898. Mechanical treatment of lameness. Amer. Vet. Rev. 21: 25.

RAKER, C. W. 1963. Clinico-pathologic conference. JAVMA 143: 1115.

REED, W. O., et al. 1962. Panel on equine lameness. Proc. 8th Ann. AAEP, 191.

REEKS, H. C. 1918. The Horse's Foot. Chicago: Alexander Eger.

ROBERTS, E. J. 1964. Carpal lameness. 3rd Ann. Cong. Brit. Eq. Vet. Assoc., 18.

ROBERTS, E. J. 1966. Some considerations of the problems of equine orthopaedic surgery. Proc. 5th Ann. Conf. Brit. Eq. Vet. Assoc., 37–45.

ROONEY, J. R. 1963. Pathology of equine lameness. Proc. 9th Ann. AAEP, 45.

ROONEY, J. R. 1968. Biomechanics of equine lameness. Cornell Vet. 58 (Suppl. Eq. Bone Joint Dis.): 49–58.

ROONEY, J. R. 1969. Biomechanics of Lameness in Horses. Baltimore: Williams & Wilkins.

ROONEY, J. R. 1966. Congenital contracture of limbs. Cornell Vet. 56(2): 172–187.

SISSON, S. 1953. Anatomy of Domestic Animals. 4th ed. Crossman, J. D., ed. Philadelphia: W. B. Saunders Co.

SMITH, H. A., T. C. JONES, and R. D. HUNT. 1972. Veterinary Pathology. 4th ed. Philadelphia: Lea & Febiger.

SMYTHE, R. H. 1959. Clinical Veterinary Surgery. Vol. 1. London: C. Lockwood & Son.

SMYTHE, R. H. 1960. Clinical Veterinary Surgery. Vol. 2. Springfield, Ill.: Charles C Thomas.

STAHRE, L., and G. TUFFVESSON. 1967. Supracarpal exostoses as causes of lameness. Nord. Vet. Med. 19(7–8): 356–361.

STURGE, E. 1894. Penetrant cauterization in the treatment of lameness from ostitis. Amer. Vet. Rev. 18: 205.

TEIGLAND, M. B., et al. 1960. Orthopedic surgery. 6th Ann. AAEP.

VAUGHAN, J. T. 1965. Analysis of lameness in the pelvic limb and selected cases. Proc. 11th Ann. AAEP.

WALKER, E. R., and PANEL. 1966. Lameness symposium. Proc. AAEP, 329–343.

WHEAT, J. D. 1962. Hypertrophy of synovial membranes. Proc. 8th Ann. AAEP, 208.

WHEAT, J. D. 1963. Trochlear fractures of the tibiotarsal bone. Proc. 9th Ann. AVMA Convention, 86–87.

WHEAT, J. D., and A. RHODE. 1964. Luxation and fracture of the hock of the horse. JAVMA 145: 341.

WHEAT, J. D. 1968–1969. Limb disorders of the racehorse. Victorian Vet. Proc. (Aust.) 27: 29–31.

WHITE, G. R. 1908. Shifting lameness. Amer. Vet. Rev. 34: 482.

WILLIAMS, W. 1891. The Principles and Practice of Veterinary Surgery. New York: W. R. Jenkins.

WRIGHT, J. G., and L. W. HALL. 1961. Veterinary Anesthesia. 5th ed. Baltimore: Williams & Wilkins.

WYMAN, W. E. A. 1898. Diagnosis of Lameness in the Horse. New York: W. R. Jenkins.

Classification of Horseshoes and Horseshoe Nails

HORSESHOES

Horseshoes are classified in several ways, and sizes vary with different types of shoes. Shoes are sometimes classified as iron or aluminum shoes. Plastic shoes are a recent development, and their use to date is limited. Iron shoes denote any type of shoe made of iron or steel and used on a working horse, including a steel racing shoe, which is very light. Aluminum shoes are made primarily for racing horses.

Iron shoes come in different weights: extra extra light, extra light, and light. The extra light shoe is used most commonly. Iron shoes are available in plate shoes, cowboy shoes, pony shoes, keg shoes, mule shoes, and several other types. Iron shoes also can be purchased or made with a variety of heel calks and toe calks or "toe grabs." They can be handmade in any form for corrective shoeing. Cowboy and plate shoes are usually sized from 00 to 8. Sizes 00, 0, and 1 are the sizes most commonly used for saddle horses. Keg shoes are presized and fitted cold, while fitting of most of the others, with the exception of steel and aluminum racing plates and polo shoes, requires heating and cutting of the heels. Keg shoes are available in plates, and with toe and heel calks. Examples of available horseshoes may be seen in Table 7–1.

Polo shoes are iron shoes and come in a separate size pattern, from 00 to No. 3. A polo shoe (Fig. 7–1) has a high inside rim which makes it a full roller motion shoe. Polo shoes should not be used on roping horses because of the tendency of the inside rim to stop the foot when sliding, possibly causing the horse to injure the fetlock area. Aluminum racing plates, also sized in a different manner, vary from size 2 to size 7 (Figs. 7–12 to 7–19). Steel racing plates are sized in the same way, while pony plates range from 00 to No. 4 in pony sizes. In addition to these there are mule shoes, which are shaped to correspond to the shape of the mule's foot. Table 7–2 gives the approximate comparative sizes between manufacturers.

Plastic shoes of various types have been developed and may become popular. Plastic shoes are light, and in the future they may be applied with acrylics rather than nails. Examples of the plastic shoe are the Chyriacos shoe from France for Standardbreds and shoes from the Balanz Racing Plate Corp., New Orleans.

The Nature Plate (Fig. 7–2) acts as a continuation of the hoof wall and concentrates the weight and action of the foot on the outside edge of the wall. In many

383

Table 7–1 Examples of Available Horseshoes[a]

Manufacturer	Type of horseshoe

Diamond Tool and
Horseshoe Co.,
Duluth, Minn.
	Iron
	  Keg-heeled
	  Plain
	  Extra light
	  Uncut heels
	Steel (for racing)
	  Heavy plate
	  Light plate
	  Barrel-racing plate
	Pony shoes

Victory Racing Plate Co., Baltimore, Md	Aluminum racing plates Steel racing plates

Multi-Products Co.,
Lodi, Calif.
	Iron
	  Plain
	  Extra light
	  Uncut heels
	Steel (for racing)
	  Heavy plate
	  Light plate

Regal Racing Ltd.
9729 Lurline Ave.
Chatsworth, Calif.
	Nature plate—Steel
	  Heavy
	  Light (racing)

Hyatt Mfg. Co.,
Sebastopol, Calif.
	Iron
	  Plain—keg
	Plates
	  Heavy plate
	    (roping plate)
	  Light plate

Thoro'Bred Racing
Plate Co.,
Anaheim, Calif.
	Steel racing plate
	  Heavy
	  Light
	Aluminum racing plate
	  Thoroughbred
	  Quarterhorse
	  Standardbred

[a] Not all manufacturers, nor all types of horseshoes, are listed.

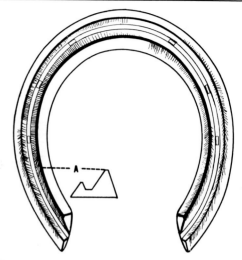

FIG. 7–1. Ground surface view of a polo shoe. This also serves as a full roller motion shoe because of the high inside rim (*A*) on the web. Inset shows a cross section of the web.

Table 7–2 Comparative Horseshoe Sizes

Diamond	Multi- Products	Hyatt	Victory	Thoro'Bred
00	4	4	4	4
0	5	5	5	5
1	6	6	6	6
2	7	7	7	7

ways, it is similar to a full outside rim shoe. It is not a corrective shoe and works best on horses of nearly normal conformation. Application of the shoe is critical and must be done by farriers acquainted with the problems involved. Personal observation leads me to believe this shoe allows more normal use of the foot than does a shoe with a toe-grab. At this time, the shoe is being marketed on a full production scale. The principles of manufacture should allow for a better fit than is available with most shoes.

A shoe may be made with variable amounts of creasing into which the nail heads fit. In some cases no crease is present at all, while in others the crease encircles the shoe which is called a "full swedged shoe." The crease may also be termed "fullering" or "swedging." The branch of a shoe is divided into toe, quarters and heels, and the width of the branch is called the web (Figs. 7–3 and 7–4).

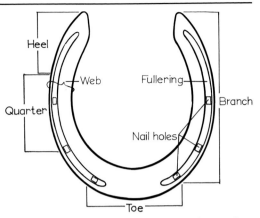

FIG. 7–3. Ground-surface view of a front plate shoe with the parts labeled.

Horseshoe nails also have heads of different shapes. A regular head is larger than the city head, which is small enough to fit into the fullering of the shoe, for shoes such as racing plates. In addition, there are horseshoe nails with frost heads, which are chisel-shaped for increased traction. In shoeing race horses, the Nos. $3\frac{1}{2}$ to $4\frac{1}{2}$ nails with city heads ordinarily are used. For saddle horses, the Nos. 5 and 6 nails commonly are used, with city or

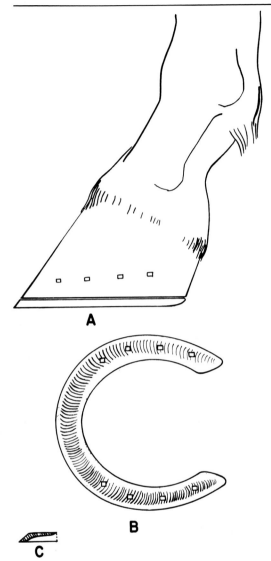

FIG. 7–2. "Nature plate" horseshoe. A, Shows level of shoe matching dorsal hoof wall. B, Ground surface of shoe, showing concavity in the shoe, which places weight-bearing on the outside edge of the shoe. C, Cross section of shoe showing concavity of ground surface. Shaded area represents the shoe; clear portion is removed.

HORSESHOE NAILS

Horseshoe nails usually are sized (from smallest to largest) from $2\frac{1}{2}$ to 12 (Capewell Mfg. Co.) (Fig. 7–5). Capewell No. 3 through No. 6 are used most commonly.

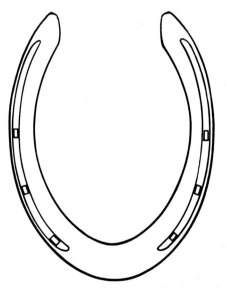

FIG. 7–4. Ground-surface view of a hind plate shoe. Note the pointed appearance of the hind shoe.

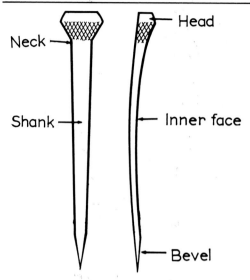

FIG. 7–5. Horseshoe nail with parts labeled.

Table 7–3 Comparative Shoe Nail Sizes

Capewell	Multi-Products Co.
$2\frac{1}{2}$	1
3	
$3\frac{1}{2}$	2
4	
$4\frac{1}{2}$	3
5	4
6	5

regular heads, depending upon the size of the crease in the shoe. The head of the nail, after it is driven in, should project about one-sixteenth of an inch below the ground surface of the shoe.

EFFECTS OF SHOE WEIGHTS

Weights added to the foot alter the gait only at a high speed. Weights are used mostly for gaited horses and trotters. Toe weights, which cause a horse to reach farther, are usually applied as a roller toe weight. Heel weights cause the horse to lift the foot higher in its action. Some trotters may carry as much as 5 to 10 ounces of additional weight on the toe for increased reach.

When weights are added to the branches of the shoe for correction, they may instead aggravate the interference that was to be corrected. When weights are added to the sides, even though on the correct side, increased deviation of the limb may result. Weight reduces speed, decreases agility, and increases fatigue of the limb, so the lightest shoe possible, for the work to be done, should be used.

CORRECTIVE SHOES

A number of descriptive terms are used in discussing corrective shoes:

Roller Toe. There is a rolled toe on the shoe to facilitate easy breakover at the toe (Fig. 7–6B).

Full Roller Motion. The web of the shoe has a high inside rim all the way around the shoe. This can be accomplished in several ways, such as using a polo shoe, which is normally made in this fashion; by welding a quarter-inch round rod around the inside of the web of the shoe, or by grinding off the outside edge of the branch of the shoe all the way around to

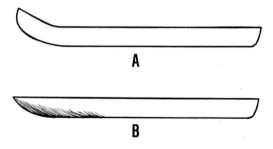

A

B

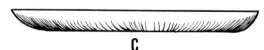

C

FIG. 7–6. *A*, Side view of rocker-toe shoe. The wall must be cut away at the toe to fit the shoe. This permits easy breakover at the toe. *B*, Side view of roller-toe shoe. This shoe also enables the horse to break over more easily at the toe. *C*, Front view of a full-roller-motion shoe, in which the outside of the shoe has been ground off around the entire shoe.

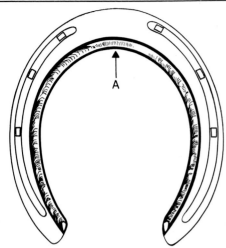

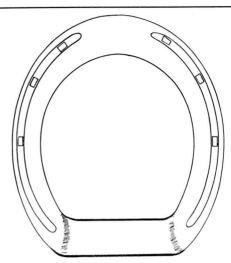

FIG. 7-7. Full-roller-motion shoe made by welding a one-fourth-inch round rod around the inside of the web on the ground surface. A, indicates the rod has gone around the toe as well as the branches of the shoe. This type of shoe enables the horse to break over in any direction more easily.

FIG. 7-8. Ground-surface view of a full-bar shoe. A full-bar shoe can be used to produce or to remove frog pressure.

lower the outside edge (Figs. 7-1, 7-6C, and 7-7).

Bar Shoe. This may be a full bar across the heels or a half bar that extends from one of the branches (Figs. 6-184 and 7-8). Bars on the shoe can be used to increase or decrease frog pressure. A full bar can be used to either increase or decrease frog pressure, while a half bar is usually used to increase frog pressure. To increase frog pressure, the full or half bar must press in against the frog about $\frac{1}{4}$ inch when the shoe is nailed on. The full bar is recessed from the frog if frog pressure is to be lessened.

Rocker Toe (Fig. 7-6A). This is used to increase the ease of breakover on the toe. The hoof wall must be cut to fit the shoe.

Memphis Bar Shoe. There are two bars across the branches, on the ground surface, to cause a roller action (Fig. 7-9).

Trailer Shoe. The shoe has one or both heels extended for corrective purposes (Fig. 7-10 and 9-10, p. 407). Trailers may be used on one or both heels. They should be turned to the outside rather than projecting straight back from the heel of the

shoe. Care should be taken when applying inside heel trailers to a horse that tends to interfere, as the trailer may cut the opposite foot. Care also must be taken in applying trailers to the front foot, as the hind foot may strike them and pull the front shoe. The length of a trailer seldom should exceed $\frac{1}{2}''$. Trailers sometimes work better when applied contrary to rec-

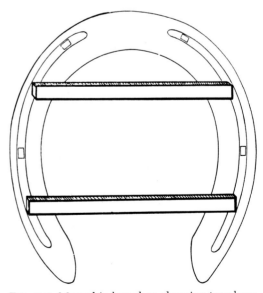

FIG. 7-9. Memphis bar shoe showing two bars welded to the ground surface of the shoe to produce roller action.

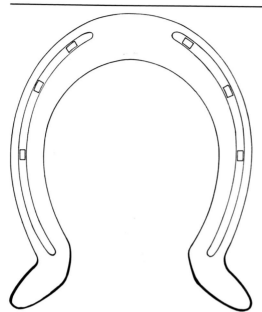

Fig. 7–10. Plate shoe with trailers on both heels. Trailers, which may be put on one or both heels, may be of varying lengths. In general, they should be turned out at a 30° to 45° angle. In addition, calks may be used on one or both heels.

ommended position. Before nailing the shoe tight, the shoes can be reversed to opposite feet and the effect checked.

Rim Shoe (Fig. 7–11 and 7–16). This shoe

has a rim on the outside edge of the web. Such a shoe may be used to increase traction or to correct a condition. The rim may be full or half, depending on need. A full-rim shoe is often used to increase traction of Standardbreds, and its use is increasing in the Thoroughbred (Figs. 7–11 and 7–16).

In many ways, a shoe with a full outside rim is similar in action to the "nature plate" (Fig. 7–2). However, the full-rim shoe has a straight wall, while the "nature plate" has an outside rim that blends with the angle of the hoof wall. Many of the commercially produced full-rim shoes also have a "toe grab" (Fig. 7–16). After close observation of horse tracks on a prepared track, I have concluded that a toe grab is detrimental to the action of the normal foot on well-prepared racing surfaces. Toe grabs, block heels, and sticker heels may have some advantages under adverse track conditions, but they should be used with caution, since the normal action of the horse's foot is well equipped

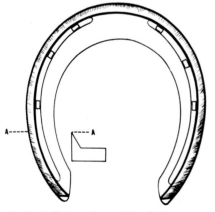

Fig. 7–11. Full-rim shoe. This full rim on the outside edge of the web is used to increase traction, especially among Standardbreds. Inset shows a cross section of the web with rim (A) on the outside.

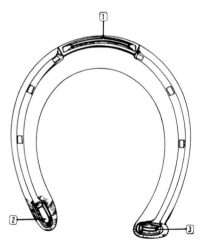

Fig. 7–12. Diagram of aluminum racing plate shoe. 1, Toe grab; 2, block heel; 3, heel sticker. The same forms are available in steel racing plates. Front shoes usually have toe grab only or possibly a heel sticker. Hind shoes often have a toe grab and block heels, or one block heel and one heel sticker for increased traction.

to handle the situation in most cases. Toe grabs, if used, should be low, since they have the effect of blunting the descent of toe into track surface, causing stress to the dorsal aspect of the fetlock and pastern joints and a "scooping" or "climbing" effect when the forefeet leave the ground. The "climbing" effect prevents all but the toe of the foot from being used in the push from the ground, and prevents full useful action of the foot in propelling the horse. Aluminum racing plates are also made with a full inside rim and toe grab. This shoe would be similar in action to a polo shoe, but the toe grab could be detrimental under certain conditions.

Toe Grab. This is a wedge-shaped bar across the toe of the shoe to increase trac-

tion. A toe grab commonly is used on racing plates (Fig. 7–12).

Heel Calks. These are projections of differing shape on the heels; they are called jar calks, heel calks, block heels, or heel stickers, depending upon their shape (Figs. 7–12, and 9–7, p. 406).

Quarter Clips and Toe Clips (Figs. 6–108, p. 279, and 6–176, p. 365). These are used to reinforce the toe or quarter areas in case of hoof cracks. Quarter clips also are used to prevent foot expansion resulting from fracture of the third phalanx.

Figures 7–13 through 7–18 show various corrective aluminum racing plates, and Figure 7–19 shows a shoe for treatment of nail puncture and other conditions that require protection of the sole. Many other

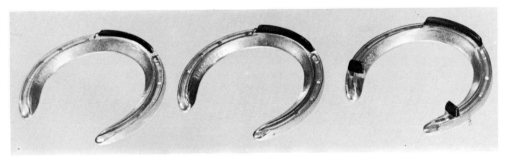

FIG. 7–13. Aluminum racing plates, front shoes. *Left,* low toe; *center,* regular toe. Shoe on right is equipped with jar calks for muddy tracks and turf. (Courtesy of Thoro'Bred Racing Plate Co.)

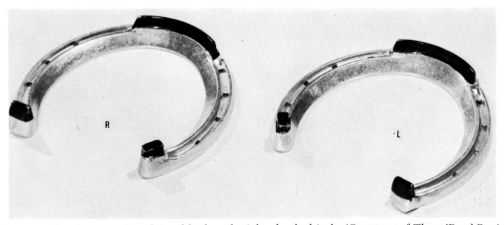

FIG. 7–14. Aluminum racing plates, block and sticker heels, hinds. (Courtesy of Thoro'Bred Racing Plate Co.)

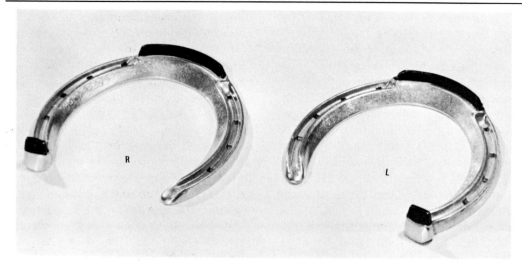

FIG. 7-15. Aluminum racing plates, sticker hinds. (Courtesy of Thoro'Bred Racing Plate Co.)

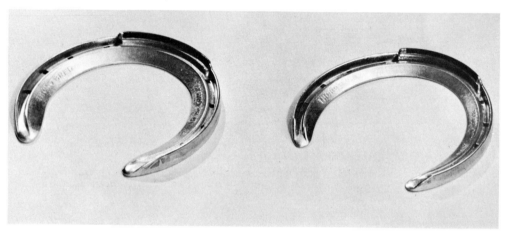

FIG. 7-16. "Level grip" aluminum racing plates, fronts. These are a full-outside-rim shoe with toe-grab. (Courtesy of Thoro'Bred Racing Plate Co.)

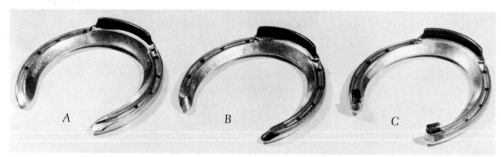

FIG. 7-17. Quarterhorse aluminum racing plates. A, Front; B, plain hind; C, block hind. (Courtesy of Thoro'Bred Racing Plate Co.)

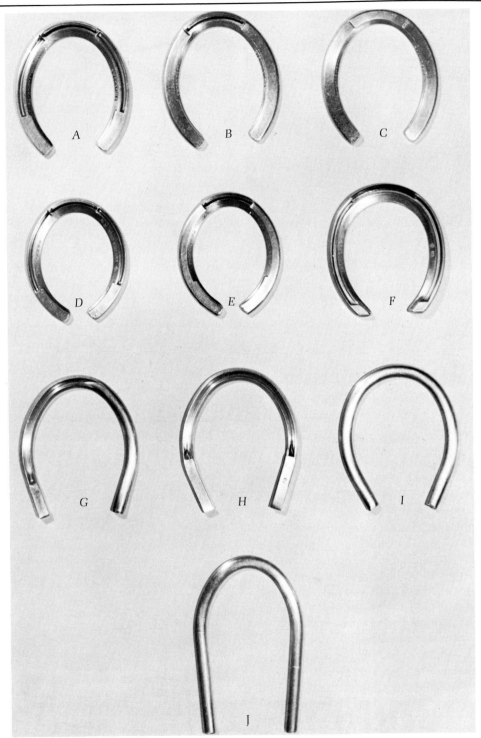

FIG. 7–18. Aluminum racing plates for Standardbreds. *A*, swedge shoe; *B*, standard plate; *C*, standard toeless plate; *D*, No. 5 swedge shoe; *E*, No. 5 standard; *F*, full-rim shoe; *G*, half-round/half-swedge shoe; *H*, full-swedge shoe; *I*, half-round shoe; *J*, half-round bar shoe (bar not completed). (Courtesy of Thoro'Bred Racing Plate Co.)

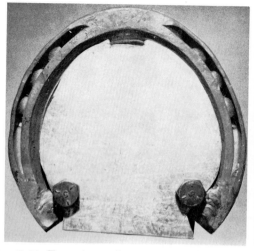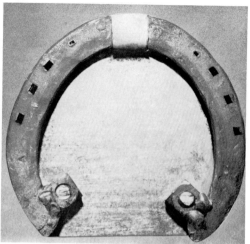

FIG. 7–19. Two views of a treatment shoe that can be used for nail punctures or for protection of the sole when needed for other reasons. The left photo shows the ground surface with two bolts holding a galvanized steel plate to the shoe. Unscrewing these bolts allows the plate to be removed for treating the foot. The right photo shows the shoe as it goes next to the hoof wall. The hoof wall must be lowered at the toe to allow the point of the treatment plate to be inserted between the toe and the shoe.

forms of shoes are available, but it is impractical to try to describe them here.

SHOE PADS

The basic reason for using a pad is to protect the foot. Shoe pads are made of leather, plastic, or rubber. They are used to decrease concussion to the bottom of the foot, especially to the sole. Pads can be classified as full pads or rim pads. A full pad covers the entire sole of the foot, and a rim pad is a full pad with the center section cut completely away after nailing, so that it is only the width of the shoe all the way around. Soft rubber pads may be made from silicone rubber,* which can be mixed immediately prior to use, or from tire retreading rubber, which can be form-fitted to the bottom of the foot. Both silicone rubber and retread rubber must be covered with an additional pad of leather or plastic. The soft rubber pads are best described as cushioning material

*Hoof Cushion, Miller Harness Co., New York.

with a pad over them. Solid rubber pads approximately $\frac{1}{8}''$ thick are also available for use alone. Plastic pads made of Neolite or polyvinyl are quite rigid and tough. Leather pads are more susceptible to damage from moisture.

REFERENCES

ASMUS, R. A. 1946. *Horseshoes of Interest to Veterinarians.* Plant City, Fla.: Ken Kimbel Book Company.

AXE, J. W. [1900.] *The Horse in Health and Disease.* London: Gresham Publishing Co. *Vol. III.*

HOLMES, C. M. 1949. *The Principles and Practice of Horse Shoeing.* Leeds: The Farriers Journal Publishing Co., Ltd.

RICHARDSON, C. 1950. *Practical Farriery.* London: Pitman Publishing Co.

SIMPSON, J. F. 1968. The theory of shoeing and balancing, p. 293. *In* Care and Training of the Trotter and Pacer. Columbus, Ohio: U.S. Trotting Association.

SPARKS, J. 1971. New horseshoe approximates the unshod equine foot. VM/SAC 66: 110.

SPARKS, J. 1969: Personal communication.

War Department. 1941. The Horseshoer. Tech. Man. TM 2-220. Washington, D.C.

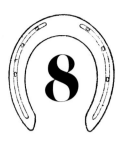

8

Trimming and Shoeing the Normal Foot

Trimming should be done every four to six weeks on horses that are used barefoot, and shoes should be reset every four to six weeks on horses that are shod. Shoeing is done at two- to four-week intervals on race horses. The object of proper trimming is to make the shape of the foot, the angle of the foot axis, and foot level (Fig. 8–1) as nearly normal as possible (see Chap. 1). However, over-enthusiastic trimming aimed at creating a "perfect" foot axis is unwise, because each horse has its own normal axis of pastern and hoof, and any radical alterations may produce pathological changes.

The foot should be trimmed so that pastern and hoof axis form an unbroken line (Figs. 1–32 and 1–35, p. 22 and 24).

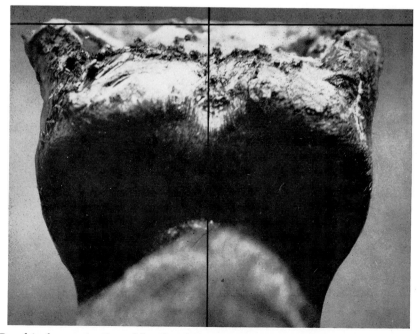

FIG. 8–1. Graphic demonstration of foot level. An imaginary line bisecting the limb longitudinally and a transverse line across the heels should give two 90° angles at their intersection. If the transverse line is tilted either way, the foot is off level.

Even if a horse does not have a normal foot axis, drastic changes should not be made if the pastern axis and hoof axis are of the same angle. The horse should be observed at rest and in motion to better determine the angles of the feet best suited to that particular horse. Following observation, the foot should be cleaned of all debris with a hoof pick. Dead portions of the sole and frog should be cut away with a hoof knife. Only shallow cutting is done, because normal frog and protective layers of the sole should not be removed. Keeping in mind the proper angles for this particular horse, the wall should be trimmed with hoof nippers (Fig. 8–2). One usually begins at the heel and trims to the opposite heel, or trims from the heel toward the toe (Fig. 8–3). If the wall is trimmed near the sole, all around, the wall will be concave at the quarters; thus, more wall should be left projecting below the sole at the quarters than at the heel or toe. The wall usually should be trimmed approximately to the level of the frog, but never past the sole. One should watch the angle of the hoof nippers carefully and avoid creating irregularities in the bearing surface of the wall (Fig. 8–4). The bars

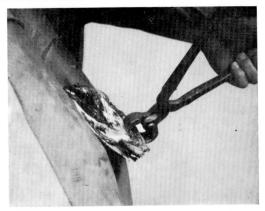

FIG. 8–3. Trimming the foot. This view shows one side which has been trimmed from heel to toe; this should be followed by trimming of the other side.

should only be trimmed to the level of the wall at the heels and not removed.

A tang rasp (Fig. 8–2) should be used to smooth the foot and level it following proper trimming. The rasp should be held flat and level so that one wall is not made lower than the other (Fig. 8–5). "Opening the heels" or cutting away the wide part of the frog, between the bar and the frog,

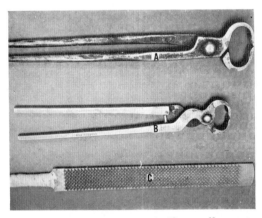

FIG. 8–2. Foot instruments. A, Shoe puller; note the deep throat on this instrument as compared with B. B, Hoof nipper; The cutting edges of the hoof nipper have a long taper to facilitate cutting of the hoof wall. C, Tang rasp used to rasp the foot.

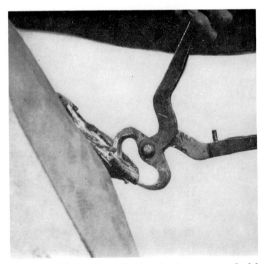

FIG. 8–4. Note that the hoof nippers are held so that the bearing surface of the hoof wall will be flat after trimming. One must be careful not to trim the wall to a taper from inside out.

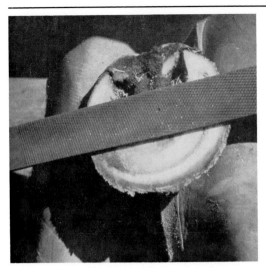

FIG. 8–5. This shows the final preparation of the foot for shoeing with a tang rasp. The rasp must be held so that one side of the wall is not cut below the other.

a caliper, measuring the center of the toe of the hoof wall from the coronary band to the point where the toe touches the ground. This distance is then measured on a ruler and will aid in keeping the length of the toe the same on opposite front or hind feet. In some breeds, such as Standardbreds, the length of toe may be critical, but at the same time, the proper angle must be kept (Simpson, 1968).

SHOEING THE NORMAL FOOT

Shoeing, accurately described as a "necessary evil," should be done only when required for traction, when the use to which the horse is put causes excessive wear of the feet or when necessary to complement or correct the gait. Horses are

should *not* be done, as this weakens the heel area and may cause contraction.

If the horse is to go barefoot, about a quarter of an inch of wall should project below the sole at the heel and toe. Sharp outside edges of the wall should be smoothed to reduce the chance of splitting or cracking of the hoof wall. If the horse is to be shod, the wall should be trimmed level with the sole at the toe, and as low as necessary at the quarter and heel to establish the proper foot axis.

One of the most common shoeing errors is cutting down the heels of the wall so that the angle of the hoof wall in front will be within ideal "normal" limits. This causes a break in the hoof and pastern axes, as shown in Figure 8–6. The hoof and pastern axes should be left as a continuous line even though the horse is too upright in the pasterns. Changing this angle as described will increase pressure between the deep flexor tendon and the navicular bone, thereby increasing the chances of navicular disease.

Careful attention should also be paid to the length of the hoof wall (Fig. 8–7). The length of the toe can be measured with

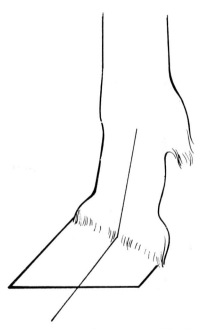

FIG. 8–6. A long upright pastern with a broken foot and pastern axis caused by lowering of the heels in an attempt to produce normal angulation of the hoof wall. This puts even greater stress on the navicular bursa by forcing the deep flexor tighter against the navicular bone, and is a common example of improper trimming in an attempt to force normal angulation of the pastern.

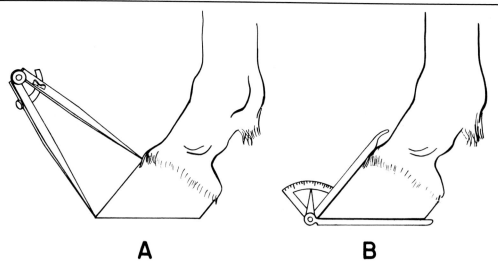

Fig. 8–7. *A*, A method of measuring and comparing length of the dorsal portion of the hoof wall. *B*, Use of foot protractor to measure hoof angle.

usually shod on the basis of tradition and not on the basis of scientific study. This is probably the reason that improvement in shoeing has been slow. Normal feet should have shoes reset every four to six weeks. After the foot is properly trimmed and leveled, as described above (Fig. 8–8), the desired shoe of the correct size should be selected. To be the correct size, the

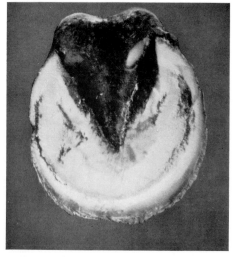

Fig. 8–8. A foot that has been trimmed and rasped and is ready for application of a shoe.

shoe should follow the contour of the hoof wall, and the heel of the shoe should be about $\frac{1}{4}''$ longer than the heel of the hoof. The shoe definitely should be fitted to the foot rather than the foot fitted to the shoe (Fig. 8–9). The branches of the shoe should extend beyond the wall about $\frac{1}{16}''$ at the heel and quarter to allow for foot expansion. The size of the shoe also is determined by the last nail hole of the shoe. This nail hole should not be past the bend of the quarter of the hoof wall, or two thirds of the length of the foot measured from the toe. Expansion of the foot is limited if nails extend beyond the bend of the quarter of the wall.

The shoe should be accurately centered on the foot (Fig. 8–9). For those horses with normal feet, the shoe can be centered by using the point of the frog as a guide. For horses that toe-in or toe-out, the frog usually points off center, so the shoe cannot be centered by this method.

Shoes may be applied hot or cold, but the hot method is preferred because more accurate shaping can be done with a hot shoe. However, the shoe still must be fitted to the foot, rather than being burned into place to save time. Final shaping of

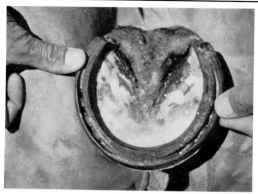

FIG. 8–9. A shoe of proper size for the foot. The shoe is centered by using the frog for a pointer, if the foot is normal. The shoe is wider than the wall at the quarters by about $\frac{1}{16}''$.

machine-made shoes usually can be done by hammering the cold shoe into form. For most pleasure horses, a plate shoe, such as a flat plate, is preferable to a shoe with heel calks. Heel-calk shoes are not recommended for horses used for general-purpose riding, since they distort the correct foot axis. If heel calks are used, a toe grab of the same height must be used to maintain proper foot axis. Such a combination relieves the frog of pressure, except in very rough terrain. Heel calks should not be used on horses whose work consists of many quick turns. Cutting cattle, barrel racing, pole bending, and reining are in this category. In these events, the horse often twists with the entire body weight on one foot, especially a hind foot. If the heel calks anchor the foot, the first or second phalanx may fracture.

If the foot is worn excessively on one side as a result of poor conformation, it may not be possible to level the foot properly by trimming. In this case, the branch of the shoe on the low side should be shimmed with leather or Neolite so that the foot is level when the shoe is in place.

Once the shoe is fitted to the foot, the nails should be driven in. A nail should

be selected with a head that protrudes about $\frac{1}{16}''$ above the ground surface of the shoe after it is driven in. If the head is too small, it fits too deeply in the crease, and the shoe becomes loose. The nail holes should be over the wall, starting at the outer aspect of the white line (Fig. 8–10). Authorities differ on which nail should be driven in first; some claim that the right heel nail should be driven in first, while others say that the right toe nail should be first. Location of the nail to be driven in first does not matter greatly, as long as the shoe is balanced so that it does not sit too far to the medial or lateral side and is not out of position in relation to the toe after the driving of the first nail. The shoeing hammer should be used to tap the shoe into position after driving the first nail. If the heel nails are driven first, the toe nails should be next and if the toe nails are driven first, the heel nails should be next; and the remaining nails should follow.

The beveled side of the nail point should be toward the inside so that it is directed outward when driven in. The beveled side can be identified by the rough spot on the head, since they are both on the same side of the nail (Fig. 7–5). The nail should be held straight and its

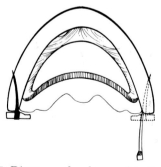

FIG. 8–10. Diagram of a shoe nail in the proper place. The nail should enter at the white line and come out approximately $\frac{3}{4}''$ above the junction of the shoe and hoof wall, or about one third of the length of the hoof wall from the coronary band to the ground surface.

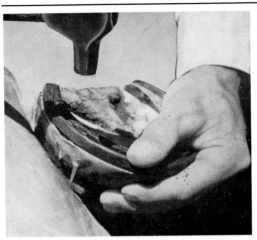

FIG. 8-11. Exit of nail following driving. As nearly as possible the nails should come out in an even line.

course appraised for its approximate exit on the hoof wall (Figs. 8-10 and 8-11). In general, the nail should come out approximately $\frac{3}{4}''$ above the junction of the shoe and hoof wall, or at about one third of the way up the wall. If the nail comes out too low or too high, it should be pulled and redriven.

If the horse flinches noticeably during the driving of the nail, the sensitive laminae may have been punctured. In such case, tincture of iodine should be applied to the nail opening and the nail should be pulled and left out, or a new nail should be driven in at the proper spot. Tetanus antitoxin should be administered and the horse should be watched closely for signs of foot infection.

The path of a horseshoe nail, upon entering the horn structure of the wall, should be parallel with the horn fibers so that the nail does not cut or sever these fibers. The point of the nail will follow a path parallel with the horn fibers if light blows of the driving hammer are used. To force the nail through the outer surface of the wall at the desired point, the shoer should use light blows until the nail is driven two thirds of the required height,

then he should strike a sharp, hard blow on the head of the nail to force the point through the surface of the wall at the desired height. The bevel on the point of the nail causes the nail to angle outward. The bevel is most effective when the nail is being driven rapidly through the horn. Nails driven to a uniform height add to the good appearance of the work; however, if the nail comes out the wall at a point near the desired position, it is advisable to allow it to remain, provided the horn is sound. If it is removed to make a better appearance, the second perforation may weaken the wall and cause a loose shoe.

Under ordinary circumstances, three nails on either side are enough, but most machine-made shoes have four nail holes per side. All four holes need not be filled. As soon as each nail is driven, it should be bent over so the point will not injure the shoer if the horse jerks the foot away (Fig. 8-12). The nail can be bent by using the claw of the hammer. After all nails are driven in and bent over, they should be clinched by placing a small block of steel on the bent edge of the nail and hitting the head of the nail with the hammer (Fig. 8-13). Nails should be clinched firmly, but not so tightly that the horse will be "nail bound." Following clinching, the nails should be cut so about $\frac{1}{8}''$ of nail protrudes (Fig. 8-14). Then, using the rasp, a small

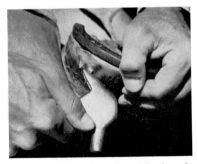

FIG. 8-12. Bending of nails with the claws of the shoeing hammer so that they will not injure the shoer if the horse pulls the foot away.

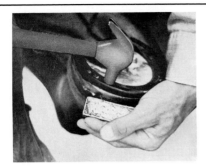

FIG. 8–13. Clinching the nails by the use of a clinching block and hammer. The clinching block is held under the bent edge of the nail and the head is struck with the hammer to clinch the nail firmly.

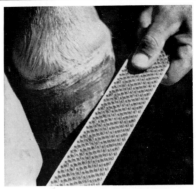

FIG. 8–15. The rasp should be used to cut a small groove under each nail so that the nail can be clinched into the groove with a tong.

groove should be cut under each nail where it emerges from the wall (Fig. 8–15). Clinching tongs then should be used to clinch the nail into the groove. The clinched end should be rasped lightly and the hoof wall smoothed at its junction with the shoe (Fig. 8–16). Only a minimum amount of rasping should be done or the hoof will be deprived of its protective outer covering. The shoe should fit well enough to the wall that no rasping has to be done to fit the toe to the shoe. After shoeing, the horse should be observed at rest and in motion to see if the shoes fit properly.

REMOVING HORSESHOES

Shoes should be removed by cutting the clinched nail ends on the hoof wall with a clinch cutter, or by filing off the clinches with a tang rasp (Figs. 8–17, 8–18, and 8–19). The foot then should be picked up and placed between the knees so that pulling pinchers can be used (Fig. 8–20). The pinchers should be placed under the shoe, starting at the heel, the handles closed and pushed away from the person pulling the shoes, and slightly toward the median line of the foot (Fig. 8–21). After one heel is loosened, the opposite heel

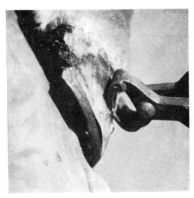

FIG. 8–14. The nails are cut so that approximately $\frac{1}{8}''$ of the nail protrudes above the hoof wall.

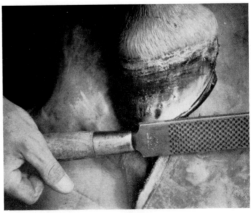

FIG. 8–16. Final light rasping of the nails and rasping of the line between the shoe and the hoof wall.

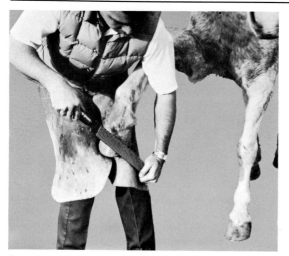 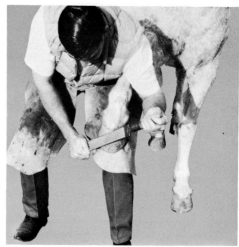

FIG. 8–17. Removing inside (left) and outside (right) nail clinches with a hoof rasp. (Courtesy of Dr. Mike Kirk.)

should be loosened. The pinchers should not be twisted, and the foot of the horse should be braced with one hand under the toe so that no injury will be done to the fetlock joint. The procedure should be continued by moving down each of the branches as the shoe is loosened (Fig. 8–22). The pulling should be gentle enough that undue pain is not caused and no sprain occurs. After the shoe has been removed, any pieces of nail left in the hoof wall should be pulled and the foot trimmed, as previously described.

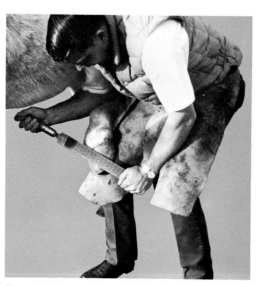 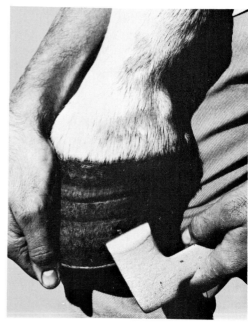

FIG. 8–18. Removing nail clinches on hind shoe with a hoof rasp. (Courtesy of Dr. Mike Kirk.)

FIG. 8–19. Cutting nail clinches with clinch cutter.

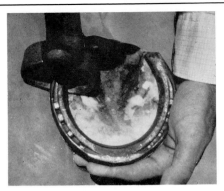

FIG. 8–20. Application of a shoe puller under the heel of one side of the shoe.

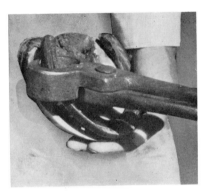

FIG. 8–21. Pushing the shoe pullers away from the operator and toward the midline.

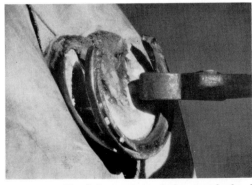

FIG. 8–22. Final loosening of the inside heel after loosening of the outside heel. The pullers should be reapplied on the shoe until it works free of the foot.

REFERENCES

ARMISTEAD, W. W., and C. M. PATTERSON. 1957. *Care of Horses' Feet.* Texas Agr. Exp. Sta. Bull. MP-198.

AXE, J. W. [1900.] *The Horse in Health and Disease.* London: Gresham Publishing Co. *Vol. III.*

BERNS, G. H. 1918–1919. Lameness of obscure origin and some of its causes. JAVMA 54: 217.

BUTZOW, R. F. 1961. Anatomy and care of the equine foot. Ill. Vet. 4(4): 98.

CANFIELD, D. M. 1971. Rebel with a cause. Thoroughbred Mid-America, 12–14 (March–April).

CHAPMAN, G. T. 1901. *Lameness in the Horse.* New York: W. R. Jenkins.

CHURCHILL, F. G. 1912. Practical and Scientific Horseshoeing. Wheaton, Ill.: Kjellberg and Sons.

DOLLAR, J. A. 1898. *Handbook of Horse Shoeing.* New York: W. R. Jenkins.

FRANK, E. R. 1964. *Veterinary Surgery.* 7th ed. Minneapolis: Burgess Publishing Co.

GRAHAM, C. W. 1965. Care of the horse's foot. Vet. Med. 60(3): 255.

HOLMES, C. M. 1949. *The Principles and Practice of Horseshoeing.* Leeds: The Farriers Journal Publishing Co., Ltd.

KIERNAN, J. 1894. *Hints on Horseshoeing.* Washington, D.C.: Office of Library of Congress.

LAYTON, E. W. 1965. Care of the horse's foot. Vet. Med. 60(3): 248.

LUNGWITZ, A., and J. W. ADAMS. 1897. *A Textbook of Horseshoeing.* 11th ed. Philadelphia: J. B. Lippincott Co.

McDONOUGH, J. 1916. Lameness and its most common cause. JAVMA 49: 653.

PEARSON et al. 1942. *Diseases of the Horse.* Bureau of Animal Industry. Washington, D.C.: U.S. Government Printing Office.

Phoenix Manufacturing Co. 1943. *How to Care for the Feet of Horses and Mules.* Joliet, Ill.

PROCTOR, D. L. 1953. *Anatomy, Care and Trimming of Feet.* Lexington, Ky.: Third Annual Stud Managers Course.

RICHARDSON, C. 1950. *Practical Farriery.* London: Pitman Publishing Co.

RUSSELL, W. 1907. *Scientific Horseshoeing.* Cincinnati: C. J. Krehbiel and Co.

SIMPSON, J. F. 1965. The theory of shoeing and balancing, p. 293. *In* Care and Training of the Trotter and Pacer. Columbus, Ohio: U.S. Trotting Association.

SPARKS, J. M. 1970. Prevention of Lameness in horses. Proc. AAEP, 67–81.

SPRINGHALL, J. A. 1964. Elements of Horseshoeing. Brisbane: University of Queensland Press.

War Department. 1941. *The Horseshoer.* Tech. Man. TM 2-220. Washington, D.C.

Corrective Trimming and Shoeing

FUNDAMENTALS OF CORRECTING FAULTS IN GAITS

If a horse is to maintain a normal gait, his feet must be balanced and in alignment with the body at the moment the feet leave the ground. Faults in the gaits of a horse may occur if the rider is unskilled or the horse's equipment is not properly adjusted. The horseshoer obviously has no control over these matters, but a skillful horseshoer can control the position of the foot in rest and in flight. However, the shoer must understand the structure of the foot and leg of the horse and the action of leg and foot in flight before he can successful apply corrective measures. Each horse must be considered individually in order to select the type of shoe that will correct a faulty gait. Even though two or more horses have the same fault in gait, each may require a separate method of shoeing for correction.

Also, shoeing alone will not always completely correct a faulty gait, though it will often reduce the harmful effects of such a fault. Some horses, though, do not follow the usual pattern when affected by malformations. For example, a horse that toes out may land on the inside toe and wall or on the outside wall, depending on whether he is base-wide or base-narrow. Therefore, it is essential that careful observation be made to determine the animal's way of going so that proper correction can be made. The effect of shoeing should be studied, and if necessary, more than one method of shoeing should be tried to see which is most effective.

The veterinarian, through his knowledge of anatomy and physiology of the limb, is well qualified to recommend corrective shoes, even though he may not be a skilled horseshoer. Study of the basic principles of shoeing, plus the application of physical laws, will usually indicate an effective method of correction of most faulty gaits.

Although the art of making horseshoes has been lost in most communities, corrective shoes can be fashioned from ordinary plate shoes by using some welding and ingenuity. Many types of corrective shoes can be made by simply welding metal to a common shoe. The shoe should be fitted to the horse and then taken to a welder for the proper additions. For example, extension-toe shoes can be made of round steel rod welded on the shoe to form a lateral extension. Bars, both half and full, can be welded on and shaped by the welder. Quarter clips and toe clips of $\frac{1}{8}''$ thick steel can be added (Figs. 6–108, p. 279, and 6–176, p. 365).

Even though all of the methods of correction may be recommended for a particular condition, often several methods of correction are attempted before the

402

best method is found for that individual. *As a general rule it is best to use the least severe corrective measure that will produce a functional gait.* Radical changes may produce pathological changes in the limb. Corrective shoeing follows physical laws, and keen observation of the gait and way of travel of a horse will give the necessary clues to correcting the problem. Some defects, however, are so bad that they cannot be corrected. Corrective measures should start with corrective trimming in the young horse, when possible. Faulty gaits in mature animals cannot be corrected; they can only be modified and improved.

In general, for corrective shoeing, one must remember that the horse will perform best when he is trimmed and shod with his own angulation of hoof wall and toe length, keeping the pastern and hoof axes unbroken (see p. 22). This will vary from horse to horse, and each individual must be given consideration, even when he varies from what are considered to be normal ranges. Occasionally, a horse will show a type of gait interference such as overreaching or scalping that will require change in angulation for correction. Angle changes not greater than 2° can be made in an attempt to correct the problem. Angle changes not greater than 2° will lessen the likelihood of damage to the limb. At subsequent shoeings, additional changes of angle not exceeding 2° can be made.

CORRECTIVE TRIMMING

In corrective trimming it is sometimes not necessary to trim the worn hoof away but is necessary only to pare down those areas that have grown too long as a result of poor conformation. The object of corrective trimming is to trim the foot until it is level and has normal foot and pastern axis for the horse (Figs. 1–32 and 1–33, p. 22).

Some writers recommend trimming a horse's foot until it lands flat. They mistakenly call this "landing level." A horse that is trimmed to land flat often does not have a level foot (see Fig. 8–1). The theory behind trimming a horse so that he wears his foot or shoe evenly is to reduce uneven concussion to the foot. For example, a horse that is base-narrow, toe-in lands on the outside of the foot. If the outside wall is trimmed off until the foot lands flat, the foot is considerably off level (low on the outside wall) and increased stresses have been placed on the lateral aspect of the fetlock joint. The lateral collateral ligament of the joint will also be stressed, and the angulation of the joint surfaces will be changed so that there is likelihood of damage (compression of the medial aspect of the joint). In general, stresses producing lameness will be less if the foot is trimmed level and not so that it will land flat.

The feet should be observed in flight from both front and rear to determine where the foot lands. The wall on which the foot lands will be low, and the opposite wall is trimmed to level the foot (Figs. 8–1 and 9–1). The hoof should be trimmed so that there is no break in the foot and pastern axes (see Chap. 1).

If a horse is base-narrow and toes in, or is base-narrow and toes out, the outside wall and heel are usually worn too low, and a compensating portion must be removed from the inside wall from toe to heel to level the foot. If the horse is base-wide and toes out, the inside wall and heel may be worn down, and the outside wall must be trimmed to bring the foot near a normal foot level. It is important to observe the gait of the horse carefully and to watch where the foot lands from both front and rear before deciding where to correctively trim the foot. Squaring the toe and leveling the foot of young horses helps them break over the center of the toe. If a horse is shown at halter, squaring

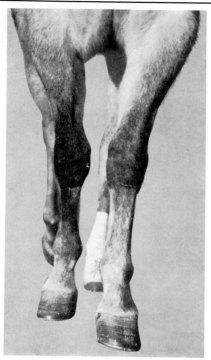

FIG. 9-1. Base-narrow, toe-wide horse landing on the outside wall. Notice how the right forelimb is in a toe-out position while the left forelimb is landing on the outside wall. With the foot landing in this way, the outside wall will be lower than the inside wall if corrective trimming is not used at each shoeing.

the toe may cause a judge to mark the horse down. By watching the horse walk, one can determine how the foot lands. If the foot is put down unevenly, that area of the wall that takes most of the weight when the foot lands will be low, while other areas of the wall will be high and, therefore, must be lowered (Fig. 9-1). Any portion of the wall that has begun to flare outward as the result of poor conformation must be rasped down on the outside of the wall and trimmed to the proper level (Fig. 9-2). Rasping the ground surface of the flare-out wall so that the wall does not bear weight may also aid the hoof wall in growing straight. If the wall is rasped on the outside and ground surface consistently, the hoof wall tends to regain a more normal shape.

CONDITIONS THAT REQUIRE CORRECTIVE SHOEING

All corrective shoes listed here should be applied to a level foot; the foot may also be shimmed with leather under one of the shoe branches. In either case, the foot is level when the shoe is applied.

Base-Wide, Toe-Out in Front (Splay-Footed, Toe-Wide)
(Fig. 1-11, p. 8)

In a base-wide toe-out conformation, the foot is not level because the horse wears off the inside wall from toe to heel. The foot breaks over the inside toe and lands on the inside toe and wall. This condition should be corrected, if possible, by trimming the outside wall from toe to heel to level the foot. Even if no shoe is to be used, this method should be followed. The feet of young foals can be rasped periodically in this manner, and some correction will take place as the foals grow. Once the foot is leveled, numerous methods of correction can be applied. If the foot is excessively off level, a leather shim can be used under the low wall to raise the branch of the shoe on that side.

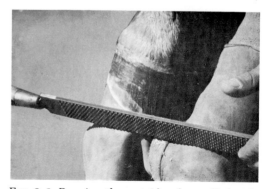

FIG. 9-2. Rasping the outside of a wall that is flared outward. In time a foot may be changed to a more normal shape by proper trimming and rasping of the flared portions.

A. *Half-Rim Shoe*
(Figs. 9–3 and 9–4)

This type of shoe has a rim on the outside edge of the inside branch from the heel to approximately the first nail hole. This shoe raises the inside of the foot when it is placed on the ground and interferes with breakover, except at the center of the toe. A $\frac{1}{4}''$ rod welded to the outside edge of the inside branch will accomplish the same purpose (Fig. 9–4).

B. *High Inside Rims and Open Toe*
(Fig. 9–5)

In this type of correction, a $\frac{1}{4}''$ rod is welded to the inside of the branches of the shoe from the heel to the first nail hole of both branches. This helps the horse break over the center of the toe. The same thing can be accomplished by welding the rod on the outside of the branches and leaving the toe open, but this makes breakover somewhat more difficult (Fig. 9–6).

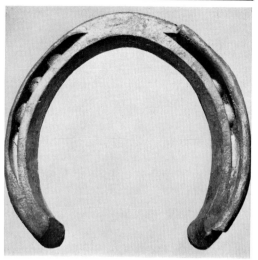

FIG. 9–4. Half-rim shoe using $\frac{1}{4}''$ round steel rod welded on the outside edge of the branch of the shoe from the first nail hole to heel. This type of shoe is used with the rod on the outside branch for base-narrow, toe-out or toe-in and on the inside branch for base-wide, toe-out horses.

C. *Calks* (Fig. 9–7)

A calk is set at each of the heels, and then one in the area of the first nail hole on each side. This accomplishes the same purpose as the quarter-inch rod mentioned in B, by forcing the horse to break over the center of the toe.

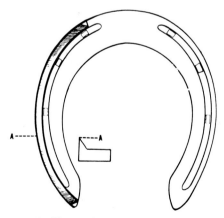

FIG. 9–3. Half-rim shoe. This shoe can be used for either a toe-in or toe-out condition to help raise the side of the foot that is low and to aid in causing breakover at the center of the toe. Inset shows cross section of web with rim (A) on outside.

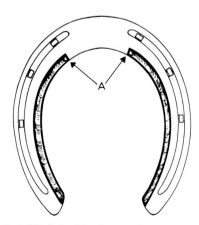

FIG. 9–5. High inside rims with open toe. This shoe aids breakover at the center of the toe (A) for toe-in or toe-out. Breakover is made easy because of the high inside rim.

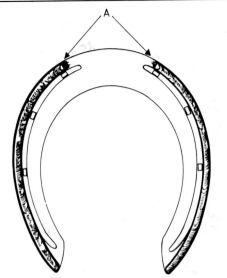

FIG. 9-6. High outside rims with open toe. The high outside rim is made of $\frac{1}{4}''$ round steel rod welded to the outside of the web. This aids in forcing the foot to break over the center of the toe (A), but more leverage is applied than when a high inside rim is used.

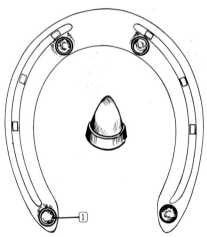

FIG. 9-7. The use of calks (1) to force breakover at the center of the toe for toe-in or toe-out condition. These calks are approximately $\frac{1}{2}''$ high and are pointed at the ground surface. Inset shows close-up view.

D. Steel Bar across the Area of Breakover (Fig. 9-8)

In this case a piece of steel approximately $\frac{1}{4}''$ to $\frac{3}{8}''$ square and $1\frac{1}{2}''$ long is

welded to the toe of the shoe at the area where the foot is breaking over. The bar interferes with breakover at that point and forces the foot to break over the center of the toe.

E. Square-Toe Shoe (Fig. 9-9)

This shoe will aid many mild cases of toe-out. As the foot starts to break over, the square toe forces the foot to break over the center of the toe. The shoe should be fitted so that the square portion of the toe is even with the toe of the hoof wall. A square toe can be combined with shoes A and F.

F. Short Inside Trailer (Fig. 9-10)

This is of value in forcing the foot to land straight. As the foot lands, the trailer catches the ground and turns the foot in. The trailer should be turned out at a 30° to 45° angle and should not exceed $\frac{1}{2}''$ in length. If a horse wings-in badly, caution must be exercised, or the trailer may lac-

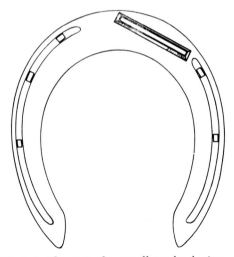

FIG. 9-8. The use of a small wedged piece of steel across the area of breakover to force the foot over the center of the toe. This bar should be placed over the area where the foot breaks over.

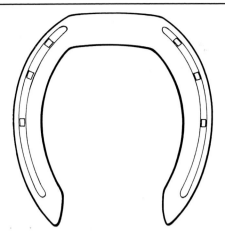

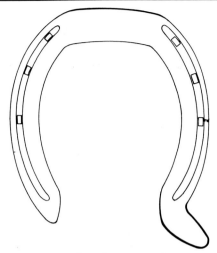

FIG. 9–9. Ground surface view of a square-toe shoe. The square-toe shoe is a useful shoe for toe-in or toe-out condition of either the front or hind feet. If the square portion of the shoe is fitted flush with the edge of the toe, the squared edges aid in forcing the foot to break over the center of the toe as the foot leaves the ground.

FIG. 9–10. Ground surface view of a square-toe shoe with trailer. If the square-toe shoe, shown in Figure 9–9, is not sufficient, a trailer may be added. The trailer is added to the inside heel for base-wide toe-out horses, and to the outside heel for base-narrow toe-in or toe-out horses.

erate the opposite limb. A short calk on the trailer may be of additional aid. A trailer can be used with *A, B, D, E, G,* and *I* corrective shoes listed here.

G. *Toe Extension* (Fig. 9–11)

An extension from the shoe, or a welded extension, projects from the inside toe, helping to force the horse to break over the center of the toe. A toe extension interferes with breakover on the inside toe. The extension should blend with the shoe and extend to the second nail hole. This can be dangerous on a splay-footed horse, since most such animals tend to wing inside, and the extension may cause trauma to the opposite forelimb.

H. *Half Shoe* (Fig. 9–12)

One half of a plate shoe or steel racing plate is used on the inside half of the foot where the wall is wearing excessively. This aids in leveling the foot and delaying

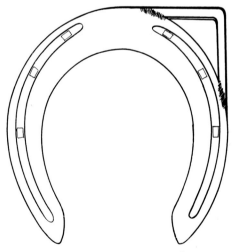

FIG. 9–11. Ground-surface view of toe-extension shoe. The toe extension is added to aid in forcing the foot to break over the center of the toe. The toe extension is used on the inside of the toe for base-wide toe-out horses and on the outside of the toe for base-narrow toe-in and toe-out horses.

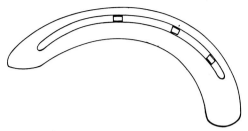

FIG. 9–12. Ground-surface view of a half shoe. A half shoe may be applied to the area of the foot wall that shows the greatest wear in toe-in or toe-out conformation. In base-wide toe-out conformation, the half shoe should be added to the inside of the hoof; for base-narrow toe-out and base-narrow toe-in conformation, it should be added to the outside wall. The toe end is beveled to blend into the wall.

wear on the inside wall. The ends are beveled to blend with the wall.

I. *Plate Shoe with Thinned Outside Branch* (Fig. 9–13)

This shoe is thinned from the first nail hole on the inside branch to the heel of

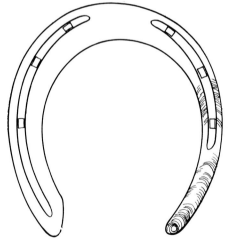

FIG. 9–13. Ground surface view of plate shoe with thinned branch. The thinned branch is placed on the outside wall in horses with base-wide toe-out conformation and on the inside wall in horses with base-narrow toe-in or toe-out conformation. This type of shoe sometimes works better when applied in reverse to these directions.

the outside branch. The thickness of the inside branch, plus the thinned outside branch, tends to turn the toe forward and cause the foot to break over the center of the toe. This shoe may also work with the thinned branch on the inside wall.

Base-Narrow, Toe-Out, Landing on Outside Wall in the Forefeet
(Fig. 1–6, p. 6)

This is a bad conformation and is aggravated by shoeing methods ordinarily used for base-wide, toe-out conformation. The outside of the wall is low because the weight of the horse falls on this area (Fig. 9–1). The foot breaks over the outside toe, wings to the inside and lands on the outside wall. The feet are leveled by lowering the inside wall and toe. Any of the methods of shoeing for base-wide, toe-out conformation can be used by reversing the correction; however, the following methods of shoeing seem to be the most successful.

A. *Half-Rim Shoe*
(Figs. 9–3 and 9–4)

This type of shoe has a rim on the outside edge of the outside branch of the shoe from the heel to the first nail hole. This shoe raises the outside of the foot when it is placed on the ground and interferes with breakover except at the center of the toe. A $\frac{1}{4}''$ round steel rod welded to the outside edge of the outside branch will accomplish the same purpose (Fig. 9–4). This is one of the most successful methods of shoeing base-narrow, toe-out conformation.

B. *High Outside Rims and Open Toe*
(Fig. 9–6)

In this type of correction, a $\frac{1}{4}''$ steel rod is welded to the outside edge of both branches of the shoe from the heel to the first nail hole. This helps the horse break over the center of the toe.

C. *Square-Toe Shoe* (Fig. 9–9)

This shoe will aid many mild cases of toe-out. As the foot starts to break over, the square toe forces the foot to break over the center of the foot. The shoe should be fitted so that the square portion of the toe is even with the toe of the hoof wall. A square-toe shoe can be combined with shoe *A* or *D*.

D. *Short Outside Trailer* (Fig. 9–10)

This trailer is of value in forcing the foot to land straight. As the foot lands, the trailer catches the ground and turns the foot in. The trailer should be turned out at a 30° to 40° angle, and its length should not exceed approximately $\frac{1}{2}''$ to prevent interference. A short block heel on the trailer may be of value. A trailer of this type can be used with shoes *A* and *C*. Occasionally, this trailer works best on the inside heel with this conformation; this alternative should be considered.

E. *Half Shoe* (Fig. 9–12)

One half of a plate shoe or steel racing plate can be used on the outside half of the foot where the wall is wearing excessively. This aids in leveling the foot and delays wear on the outside wall. The end is beveled to blend with the wall.

F. *Toe Extension* (Fig. 9–11)

Extension from the shoe, or a welded extension, projects from the outside toe, helping to force the horse to break over the center of the toe. A toe extension interferes with breakover on the outside toe. Extension should blend with the shoe and extend to the second nail hole. It can be combined with shoe *D*.

Base-Narrow, Toe-In (Pigeon-Toed) (Toe Narrow) (Fig. 1–7, p. 7).

With toe-in conformation, the feet usually are off-level. In this case, the horse tends to wear down the outside toe and wall, since breakover occurs on the outside toe, and the foot lands on the outside wall. Corrective trimming is done by paring down the inside wall until the foot is as level as possible. If the foot is excessively off-level, a leather shim is placed under the outside branch of the shoe to bring the foot to normal level. In correcting toe-in conformation, many of the same methods used to correct base-narrow, toe-out can be used.

A. *Half-Rim Shoe*

The half rim can be a $\frac{1}{4}''$ rod welded on the outside of the branch of the shoe beginning at the heel and ending about the first nail hole on the outside of the branch. This helps to force the foot to break over the center of the toe (Figs. 9–3 and 9–4).

B. *One-Fourth-Inch Rod on the Outside of Both Branches*

The rod, which extends from the heel to the first nail hole, aids the horse in breaking over at the center of the toe (Fig. 9–6).

C. *Calks*

Two heel calks and a calk at the area of the first nail hole on the outside of each branch of the shoe will help the foot break over at the center of the toe (Fig. 9–7).

D. *One-Fourth-Inch to Three-Eighth-Inch Square Steel Bar One and One Half Inches Long*

If such a bar is welded over the point of breakover on the outside toe, it interferes with breakover at this point and causes the foot to break more nearly toward the center of the toe (Fig. 9-8).

E. *Short Trailer on the Outside Heel* (Fig. 9-10)

This is sometimes of value in catching the foot as it lands and turning it straight, preventing the horse from landing in a toe-in position. A small block heel may be added to the bottom of this extension. Such a trailer can be used in conjunction with *A, B, D, F, G,* and *I* corrective shoes listed here.

F. *Square-Toe Shoe* (Fig. 9-9)

This accomplishes the same purpose as for toe-out: It forces the foot to break over the center of the toe. It is one of the best and mildest methods of correction. The square toe should fit the outside edge of the toe of the wall.

G. *Toe Extension* (Fig. 9-11)

This is added to the outside of the toe area and should extend as far as the second nail hole. It forces the foot to break over the center of the toe. There is little danger of interfering with toe-in conformation, since in nearly all cases the foot tends to break in an outside arc.

H. *Half Shoe* (Fig. 9-12)

One half of a plate shoe or steel racing plate is added to the outside half of the wall. This aids in leveling the foot and delaying wear to the outside wall. The edges of the shoe should be beveled to blend with the wall.

I. *Plate Shoe with a Thinned Inside Branch* (Fig. 9-13)

The shoe is thinned from the first nail hole on the outside branch to the heel of the inside branch. The normal thickness of the outside branch, plus the thinned inside branch, tends to turn the toe forward, causing the foot to break over the center of the toe. This shoe also may work with the thinned branch on the outside wall.

Base-Wide, Toe-In, Landing on the Inside Wall of the Forefeet

This is bad conformation, and it is aggravated by some shoeing methods ordinarily used for base-narrow, toe-in conformation. The inside wall is low because the weight of the horse lands on this area. The feet should be leveled and shod so that the inside toe and wall are slightly raised. To raise the inside wall, a piece of $\frac{1}{4}''$ steel rod should be welded to the outside edge of the inside branch of the shoe from the heel to the first nail hole (Figs. 9-3 and 9-4). Leather shims under the inside branch can be used if necessary. This tends to level the action of the foot and to force the foot to break over the center of the toe. It is difficult to correct this type of defect.

Contracted Heels

Treatment of contraction of the foot is based on producing frog pressure. This must be accomplished in order to reestablish normal foot function; but above all, the primary cause of contraction must be corrected. In other words, an accurate diagnosis must be established before treatment. In addition to disease, dryness of the wall will contribute to contraction. Proper moisture in the hoof can be aided by the daily application of animal- or vegetable-base oils in hoof dressings. To help prevent dehydration, the periople should not be removed when shoeing the horse.

If the work of the horse does not require shoeing, proper trimming to allow frog pressure may promote foot expansion, provided the trimming is done often enough. If the horse requires shoeing but does not do heavy work, a tip shoe can be used (Fig. 9–14). Other shoes, such as a half-bar shoe, full-bar shoe, T shoe, slipper shoe of Broué, and slipper and bar clip shoe of Einsiedel, may be used (Figs. 6–185, 7–8, 9–15 and 9–16). When a half-bar or full-bar shoe is used, the half or full bar must press inward about $\frac{1}{4}''$ against the frog when the shoe is set. More complicated methods of treatment, such as the Smith expansion shoe, a Chadwick spring (Fig. 9–17), and Deffay's vise can be used, but these are not necessary in most cases. The front of the toe area on the hoof wall can be rasped in conjunction with the use of a Chadwick spring. This will make the toe area more flexible and the action of the spring more effective. Care should be taken not to attempt too rapid expansion of the heels, or lameness may result.

In addition to shoeing, other procedures sometimes used to aid expansion of the quarters include thinning the region of the quarters with an ordinary farriers' rasp. Be careful not to rasp a $\frac{1}{2}''$ wide portion of the wall immediately below the coronary band. The greatest thinning should start $\frac{1}{2}''$ below the coronary band and at the

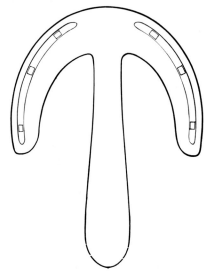

FIG. 9–15. Ground-surface view of a T shoe. This shoe is used for contraction of the foot. The center bar exerts pressure on the frog to promote foot expansion. The heel areas of the hoof wall are unshod to aid frog pressure. The wall of the toe area may be cut more deeply to receive the tip portion of the shoe.

heels. Thinning should decrease gradually for $2\frac{1}{2}''$ to 3″ forward and downward, until at the ground surface of the wall the normal thickness is left (Fig. 9–18C). The foot should be shod with a pressure-bar shoe

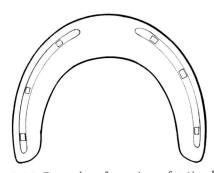

FIG. 9–14. Ground-surface view of a tip shoe. This shoe may be used in contraction of the foot to protect the toe from wear yet leave the heels unshod for frog pressure. The ends of the shoe are tapered to blend into the wall, or the wall of the toe is cut more deeply to receive the shoe.

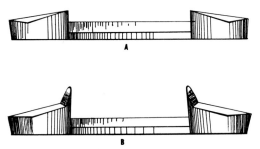

FIG. 9–16. A, Posterior view of slipper shoe of Broué. This shoe permits the heels to slide outward when the foot is put down to promote expansion of the heel. B, Posterior view of a slipper and bar clip shoe of Einsiedel. The inside clips prevent the heels from coming together, and the taper of the walls aids in causing the heels to go outward when the foot is set down.

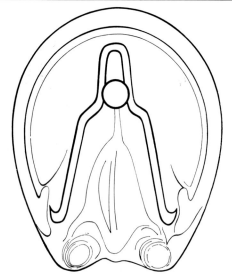

FIG. 9–17. Chadwick spring in place in a foot. The Chadwick spring is forced outward by a round pin in the center, as shown. The pin can be hammered outward if more pressure is needed against the heels. The heels are under constant pressure from the spring.

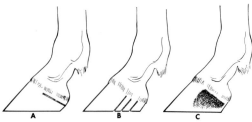

FIG. 9–18. Methods of increasing hoof wall flexibility and expansion. A, Groove $\frac{1}{4}''$ wide $\frac{1}{2}$–$\frac{3}{4}''$ below the coronary band to aid in heel expansion. The groove does not penetrate the sensitive laminae, or the blood supply. B, Three vertical grooves along the quarters of the hoof wall to promote hoof expansion. These grooves do not penetrate the sensitive laminae or the blood supply. C, Rasping away the quarters of the hoof, with the deepest areas of rasping $\frac{1}{2}''$ below the coronary band and the thinnest at the bearing surface of the hoof wall. The rasping extends from the heel of the wall 3″ forward. All these methods aid in expansion of the quarters of the foot. They are used in hoof contraction, sidebones, and sometimes for laminitis. A foot with chronic laminitis may be grooved at the toe and across the sole instead of at the quarters.

and the foot treated daily with a hoof compound to prevent the wall from cracking.

Another method of promoting expansion of the wall is to groove the wall over the quarters and heels with a series of vertical lines, or simply by one groove paralleling the coronary band $\frac{3}{4}''$ below it (Fig. 9–18A,B). This groove should extend from the heel forward for 3″ to 4″. Following either method of grooving the wall, a pressure-bar shoe should be applied. The grooves, which aid in expansion of the heel areas of the hoof, may be placed in the hoof wall with a Stryker cast cutter, a hoof groover, or a firing iron. Such grooving methods give the hoof wall a chance to expand. When a single groove parallel to the coronary band is used, the proximal portion of the hoof wall may actually expand and overlap the hoof wall below it in the process of growing out.

Ringbone

This condition is discussed in Chapter 6. Corrective shoeing consists of shortening the toe and applying a full-roller-motion shoe to transfer the action from the pastern and coffin joints to the shoe area. If the horse has good conformation, the toe alone can be rolled; if not, a full-roller-motion shoe should be applied.

Sidebones

This condition is discussed in Chapter 6. Corrective shoeing is usually intended to roll the foot or shoe on the affected side. The affected side of the shoe is given a roller motion by grinding off the outside edge of the branch of the shoe. Full-roller-motion shoes also may be used (Figs. 7–1, 7–6, and 7–7).

A shoe with swedged-up heels and rolled toe may be used on horses that work on soft ground where a full-roller-motion shoe may lose its effectiveness upon sinking into soft dirt (Fig. 9–19).

Navicular Disease

This condition is discussed in Chapter 6. Corrective shoeing may delay or eliminate the necessity of a posterior digital neurectomy in a horse that is not used in such strenuous work as racing. A roller toe, swedged-up heel (Fig. 9–19), full bar, and slippered heels are used (Fig. 7–8 and 9–16). The raised heels and rolled toe make it easier for the horse to break over and land in a way that decreases concussion of the deep flexor against the navicular bone. The raised heels also reduce frog pressure, and the full bar across the center third of the frog eliminates trauma to this area and prevents the painful reaction that occurs. The slippered heels tend to cause the wall to slide outward and thereby help to overcome both contraction that is already present and that which would be induced by the raised heel and bar. In addition, it is wise to thin or groove the quarters (Fig. 9–18) to aid wall expansion that is stimulated by the slippered heels. It is also sometimes helpful to apply retread rubber or silicone rubber to the bottom of the foot and cover it with a pad, in addition to the above corrective shoeing.

Cow Hocks

Roping horses having this condition slide wide when stopping. This is corrected by use of a small heel calk on the inside heel of the shoe of the hind feet. When the horse slides, the calk tends to force the hind feet to slide straight. Cow-hocked horses used for other purposes can be shod with a small inside trailer on the hind shoes, and, in some cases, with the addition of a heel calk to the trailer. As the foot lands, the heel calk tends to hold the foot inward, forcing it to break over straight. If the horse tends to interfere, the trailer may hit the opposite limb. A trailer is sometimes effective on the outside branch, except for use with roping

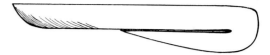

FIG. 9–19. Side view of shoe with swedged-up heels and rolled toe. This type of shoe causes a quicker breakover of either the front or hind foot. It has been used in navicular disease to protect the frog from pressure, and it is sometimes used for bone spavin in Standardbreds.

horses. Before the shoes are set completely, this outside trailer can be checked by reversing the shoes. A square toe on the shoe will help the foot break over the center of the toe, and an inside trailer with a calk may be used, if necessary (Fig. 9–10).

Bone Spavin

When corrective shoeing is used for bone spavin, the heels should be raised with calks and a short outside trailer should be used. In speed horses, calks may slow the horse, and the heels of the shoe can be turned back on themselves to make a smooth calk that will slide (Fig. 9–19). In trotters and pacers, a Memphis bar shoe (Fig. 7–9, p. 387) or an oval bar across the heels is sometimes used. A second method is to use a $\frac{1}{4}''$ steel rod on the inside of the branches, leaving the inside toe open (Fig. 9–20). This tends to force the horse to break over the inside toe, which is the object of most corrective shoeing for spavin. This action tends to relieve pressure in the spavin area. Shoeing, though, often is not helpful, and this condition can best be treated surgically, as described in Chapter 6.

Cross-firing

Cross-firing is a condition in which the inside of the toe, or inside of the wall of the hind foot, strikes the inner quarter or under surface of the inner branch of the shoe of the opposite forefoot. It is most

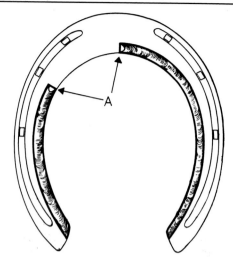

FIG. 9–20. Ground-surface view of a shoe that causes a tendency to break over the inside of the foot (A) in bone spavin. The raised areas are of $\frac{1}{4}''$ round steel rod welded to the inside branches, while the inside of the toe is left open. This shoe is for the left hind foot.

likely to occur in pacers, especially those that toe out in front and toe in behind. With this conformation, the flight of the fore feet is forward and inward during the first half of a stride, and the flight of the hind feet is forward and inward during the last half of the stride. This causes foot contact. Corrective shoeing is used to force the front and hind feet to move forward in a manner that will approximate a straight line, correcting the deviations in flight. If the foot can be forced to point straight ahead on landing and can be forced to break over near the center of the toe again on takeoff, straight-line flight is more nearly accomplished. Corrective shoeing to widen the flight of the hind foot is also used.

Shoeing the Front Feet

1. Since most cross-firing horses toe out in front, corrective shoeing for toe out is used. Shoeing methods A, B, E, and G in the discussion of correcting base-wide,

toe-out (p. 404) may be used. In addition, the edge of the ground surface of the inside branch of the shoe should be rounded, so that if striking does occur, it will not break the skin.

2. The inside branch can be fitted with a $\frac{1}{4}''$ to $\frac{3}{4}''$ trailer on any of the shoes listed above, so that it will strike the ground just before the lateral branch, thereby rotating the toe inward.

3. A cross-firing horse should always wear quarter boots for protection.

4. A square toe shoe is often used on trotters and pacers to straighten break-over.

Shoeing the Hind Feet

1. Short trailer on outside branch.

2. The inner branch is cut short and is thinned progressively from the toe to the heel.

3. Bevel or round the ground surface edge of the inside branch. This is used in trotters and pacers and is called a half-round shoe on the inside and a half-swedge shoe on the outside. The swedged portion is used on the outside branch to widen the gait in pacers, and on the inside branch to narrow the gait in trotters.

Other methods of corrective shoeing, discussed under toe-out, may be used in front. Other types of shoeing the hind feet are discussed under toe-in (p. 409).

Forging and Overreaching

Forging is a defect of the trotting gait in which the toe of the hind foot overtakes and strikes the bottom of the front foot of the same side at the moment the front foot is starting flight (Fig. 4–3). The front foot is too slow in breaking over and leaving the ground to avoid the forward extension of the advancing hind foot.

Overreaching is similar to forging except the hind foot comes up more quickly than it does in forging. This means that the hind foot steps on the heel of the front foot on the same side before the forefoot can leave the ground or just as it is leaving the ground (Fig. 4–3). In this case, the shoe of the front foot is often pulled because the toe of the hind foot steps on the heels of the shoe on the front foot.

Forging and overreaching may be due to faulty conformation, leg weariness, improper adjustment of the saddle, improper riding, or improper shoeing. Faults in conformation that tend to cause forging include a short body with relatively long legs; front or hind feet set too far under the body; short front legs and long hind legs. Leg weariness causing forging and overreaching may result from debility or overexertion. Improper preparation of the feet, or improper shoeing, may slow the breakover of the front feet, decreasing the height of their action, and cause forging. Young horses with good conformation and properly balanced feet often are subject to forging while being trained and developed. In this case, forging is caused by fatigue of underdeveloped muscles.

Corrective Shoeing for Forging and Overreaching

The method of correction should be governed by the cause of the forging and the nature of the work the horse performs. The horse should be ridden at a walk and a trot to determine the rate of speed at which forging and overreaching are most pronounced. One should watch for lack of coordination between the front and hind feet during flight. Look for conditions that would aggravate an unbalanced gait. Determine if the conformation is good or faulty, if the feet are balanced laterally from toe to heel, and if the shoes are correctly fitted and are of suitable weight. Three fundamentals are essential in correcting forging or overreaching:

1. The front foot must leave the ground more quickly to avoid being struck by the oncoming hind foot.

2. The hind foot must take a slightly shorter stride so it will not hit the front foot.

3. The heel of the front shoe and the toe of the hind shoe must be shortened to avoid contact.

Methods of Shoeing

1. Prepare and balance the front feet and shoe with light-weight rocker or rolled-toe shoes of equal weight. Prepare and balance the hind feet, but leave the hoof a little longer than normal, and shoe the horse with light-weight shoes. Fit the hind shoe fully to the point of the toe, and extend the heels back about $\frac{1}{2}''$ to $\frac{3}{4}''$ beyond the buttresses. The heels of the shoe should be turned slightly outward.

This increases the rapidity of breaking over of the front feet and decreases the rapidity of breaking over of the hind feet. The extended heels tend to stop the hind foot as it is being put down.

2. Prepare and balance the front feet, and shoe with rocker or rolled-toe shoes equal in weight. Prepare and balance the hind feet and shoe with heel calks $\frac{1}{2}''$ long, $\frac{1}{4}''$ deep, and $\frac{1}{8}''$ wide and a rocker toe.

This method of shoeing induces greater hock action in the elevation of the hind feet in flight but decreases forward extension. Therefore, there is more clearance between the front and hind feet in action. The calks tend to stop the hind foot before it hits the front foot.

3. Prepare and balance the front feet, and shoe with rocker or rolled-toe shoes of equal weight. Prepare and balance the hind feet, leaving the hoof a little longer than normal; shoe with a square-toe shoe; extend the heels of the shoe back about $\frac{1}{2}''$ to $\frac{3}{4}''$ beyond the buttresses; turn the heels of the shoe out slightly. The straight section of the shoe at the toe should be set back about $\frac{1}{4}''$ from the outline of the wall at the toe. The wall that projects beyond the shoe at the toe should not be removed.

This method of shoeing increases the

rapidity of breaking over the front feet and causes higher action. The preparation of the hind feet, plus the greater length of shoes, delays the breakover of the hind feet, thus allowing more time for the front feet to be carried to sufficient elevation to allow clearance. By setting the shoe back from the point of the toe you prevent the clicking noise when the hind foot strikes the front shoe. The extended heels on the rear shoes stop the hind feet more quickly and thereby aid in avoiding contact with the front feet.

4. Prepare and balance the front feet, and shoe with rocker or rolled-toe shoes of equal weight. Prepare and balance the hind feet, keeping the toe short; shoe with square-toe shoe. This allows the hind foot to break over quickly, causing it to go higher and allowing the front foot to get out of the way.

A full-roller-motion shoe (Chapter 7, Figs. 7–1, 7–6 and 7–7, pp. 384 and 386) can be substituted for a rolled toe or rocker toe in corrections of the forefeet. A polo shoe acts as a full-roller-motion shoe if no other type is available or if such a shoe

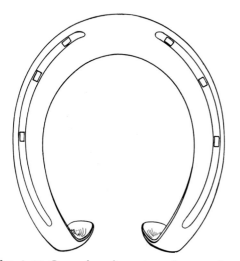

FIG. 9–21. Ground-surface view of spoon shoe. The spoons extend upward and cover the heels of the foot. They must fit closely at the heels; they prevent the horse from pulling a shoe if he overreaches.

cannot be made. The high inside rim facilitates breakover in any direction.

If one is unable to stop forging or overreaching, a spoon on the heels of the front shoes may be applied so the shoe cannot be pulled. A spoon closely fits the heels of the front foot and covers the bulbs of the heel, thereby giving the hind shoe no area in which to pull the front shoe (Fig. 9–21). This type of shoe must be changed often, or it may cause corns.

Elbow Hitting

When a horse is hitting his elbow during motion, he is breaking over quickly and the carpus is flexing easily as the foot leaves the ground. There are two obvious ways of decreasing this flexion: (1) The heel may be lowered, thus changing the angle and slightly delaying the breakover. The angle should not be decreased more than 2° to avoid any great changes in the pastern and foot axes. If the length of the toe is not a primary consideration, the lengthening of the toe will also aid in delaying breakover. (2) Since the condition is usually present in trotters, it may be that half-round shoes acting as full-roller-motion shoes allow the foot to leave the ground easily and quickly; this may be the cause of elbow hitting. Sometimes, merely changing to a flat shoe will delay the foot enough to stop elbow hitting. In addition to the flat shoe, a standard swedge shoe may be used to slightly delay the breakover. A full-swedge shoe may be used if desired.

If the gait is considered nearly perfect and the elbow hitting is mild, using elbow boots for protection of this area is an obvious answer.

Interfering

Interfering is a fault of the gait that causes the horse to strike any part of the inside of one leg with the inside of the foot or shoe of the opposite foot. The injury may be at any spot, from the coronary band to the carpus of the front legs. Injuries are more common to the front legs, and the fetlock joint and second metacarpal bone are most commonly injured. Temporary causes of interfering include fatigue, faulty preparation of feet, and improper shoeing. Faulty conformation may be a permanent cause. Such horses are either base-wide or base-narrow with toe-out conformation (see Chap. 1). They often are narrow-chested or, in the case of the hind limbs, cow-hocked.

Corrective Shoeing for Interfering

For extrinsic causes, correct any obvious faults in shoeing or trimming. Be sure that the shoes are of proper weight and proper fit.

For conformational causes, the methods of correction vary, depending upon whether the horse is mature or still growing. If correction is begun early with a foal, corrective trimming may prevent interference by gradually straightening the feet (p. 403). Before application of corrective shoes, the horse should be observed at the walk and trot to determine the degree of severity of interference. If interference cannot be seen, chalk may be put on the hoof wall and shoe to determine where interference is occurring and whether one or both feet are involved.

In the forelimbs, most of the shoeing methods used to correct base-narrow or base-wide, toe-out horses also will aid in preventing interference (p. 404, 408). In the hind limbs, most of the shoeing methods used to correct cow hocks will also aid in correcting interference (p. 413).

1. If the horse strikes the inside portion of the fetlock of the forelegs, prepare and balance the feet, and shoe with a square-toe shoe. The straight section of the shoe should come to the point of the toe, level with the outline of the wall, and should extend laterally slightly beyond the wall on both sides of the toe of the hoof. The inside branch of the shoe should be rasped and smoothed on the outside edge of the ground surface for the entire length of the branch, so that if it does strike, it will not injure the tissues.

2. The base-wide, toe-out horse can be shod with a medial (inside) extension of the toe of the shoe as described under base-wide, toe-out conformation (p. 404). This is often a good shoe for those horses that definitely deviate from the fetlock to the foot. These shoes are fitted even with the wall at the point of the toe. The outline of the shoe extends $\frac{1}{4}''$ beyond the outline of the wall at the junction of the oval and straight sections. Graduate the fullness to zero at a point just to the rear of the second nail hole of the shoe. From this point to, and including, the heel, the shoe should be closely fitted to the wall. The outside portion of the toe should be closely fitted, but full from the bend of the outside quarter to the heel (slightly fuller than for normal shoeing). The edge of the ground surface of the inside branch of the shoe should be rasped and smoothed.

The medial toe extension forces the foot to break straight over the toe, and this tends to reduce the inward swing during flight. The fullness of the shoe at the natural breaking-over point of the foot on the inside toe acts as a lever to turn the foot to a straight forward position while the heels are being raised. Handmade shoes are preferable to factory shoes.

3. The base-narrow, toe-wide horse can be shod with a half-rim shoe on the outside branch from the first nail hole to the heel (Figs. 9–3 and 9–4). A short inside trailer can also be used. The foot should always be leveled before applying this type of shoe. In some cases, this means that the outside wall must be shimmed with leather. Other methods of corrective shoeing are described under base-narrow, toe-out conformation (p. 408).

4. If the horse is striking the inside por-

tion of the hoof at the coronary band, and if the cause is a narrow chest and front legs that are too close together, the feet should be balanced, prepared, and shod with rocker-toe shoes made of extra light shoes. The inside branch of the shoe should be closely fitted, and the outside edge of this branch should be rasped and smoothed. It is advisable to use interference boots for this condition if the horse is to be used for long rides; leg weariness tends to aggravate the condition.

5. If the horse is striking the inside portion of the fetlock joints in the hind legs, and the cause is faulty leg conformation because the horse is bow-legged (see Chap. 1), such a horse is base-narrow. The feet should be prepared, leveled, and shod with extra light shoes with square toes and a trailer on the outside branch (Fig. 9–10). The trailer should not exceed $\frac{3}{4}''$ in length, with a turned heel calk about $\frac{3}{8}''$ high. If the heel calk is not turned on the shoe, it may be welded to the ground surface. The inside branch of the shoe should be closely fitted, following the outline of the wall from the quarter to the buttress and rasped and finished smoothly. No heel calk should be put on the inside branch of the shoe. Such a shoe, when properly adjusted, will balance the foot and reduce the inward swing of the foot in flight.

6. If the horse is striking the inside portion of the fetlock joints on the hind legs, and the cause is faulty leg conformation because the horse is cow-hocked and the feet are in toe-out position, the feet should be prepared, leveled, and shod with inside extension-toe shoes with trailers on the inside branches, but with no calks (Fig. 9–11). The trailer should be about $\frac{1}{2}''$ long and should be turned out at a 30° to 45° angle. The inside branch of the shoe should be closely fitted and rasped and smoothed. This type of shoe tends to force the foot to break over the center of the toe and reduces inward swing of the foot

in flight. A square-toe shoe with an inside trailer may be substituted for a shoe with inside toe extension. The square toe should be fitted to the front edge of the toe wall.

7. Most trotters and pacers interfere in front and usually hit the knee. Horses that will not hit on a mile track may contact on a half-mile track. Every effort is made to use a correction that will not slow down the feet. A shoe with longitudinal calks is sometimes used. These calks are 2″ to 3″ long, $\frac{1}{8}''$ wide, and $\frac{1}{4}''$ deep. They are set inside of the nail holes on the branches beginning at the first nail hole.

Corns

These are discussed in the section on corns in Chapter 6.

Toe and Quarter Crack

Corrective shoeing for toe and quarter cracks is discussed under these conditions in Chapter 6.

Wire Cuts in the Coronary Band

A bar shoe—either half or full—is used to place pressure on the frog. The hoof wall is shortened on the affected side beneath the wire cut area. The wall is trimmed so it will not bear weight, and the weight that would be borne on this portion of the wall is transferred to the frog by use of the bar. This reduces movement in the area of the cut and aids healing (Fig. 9–22).

Flexor Tendonitis or Suspensory Ligament Injury

In this case, the heels are raised with blunt heel calks to remove some of the pressure from the flexor tendons. Trimming of the toe alone may be of value. Proper levels and angles are observed, but

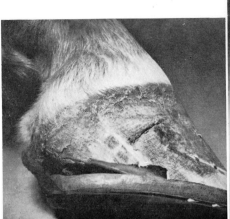 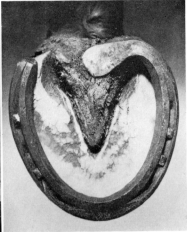

FIG. 9–22. Use of half-bar shoe to correct hoof wall or quarter crack defect. *Left,* Hoof wall lowered to prevent weight bearing from the wall defect to the heel. *Right,* Ground-surface view of half-bar shoe shows how the weight is taken on the frog rather than over the hoof defect area.

the heel is raised by the shoe. Care must be taken so that the tendons do not contract when the heels are raised for long periods of time.

Flat Feet

In trimming of the foot, the sole should not be trimmed excessively and the frog should not be trimmed at all. The wall should be trimmed, but only enough to smooth it for application of a shoe.

The shoe should be seated moderately on the sole. If seating is excessive and bearing is allowed only on the wall, there is a tendency for the wall to push outward and the sole to drop still farther. Conversely, if the web of the shoe is too wide and too much bearing is given to the sole, there will be excessive pressure on the sole, and sole bruising, with lameness, will result. The shoe should cover the whole of the wall and the whole of the white line but should just touch upon the sole. The heels of the shoe should be of full length to avoid causing a corn. In addition, shoe pads of leather or Neolite may be necessary.

Dropped Sole or "Pumiced Foot"
(Fig. 6–81, p. 252)

In less severe forms, corrective shoeing similar to that discussed for flat feet may be of value. A broad-webbed shoe that will give wall pressure, plus protection to the white line to prevent further dropping of the sole, is indicated. Avoid creating sole pressure if possible; pads of leather or Neolite may be necessary. In many cases, the white line is very wide. In some cases, seedy toe is present as a result of the separation of the sensitive and insensitive laminae, and rotation of the third phalanx may be present. Further corrective measures are discussed in the section on chronic laminitis (Chap. 6).

REFERENCES

ADAMS, O. R. 1965. Corrective shoeing for common defects of the forelimb. Proc. 11th Ann. AAEP.

ARMISTEAD, W. W., and C. M. PATTERSON. 1957. *Care of Horses' Feet.* Texas Agr. Exp. Sta. Misc. Publ. MP-198.

ASMUS, R. A. 1946. *Horseshoes of Interest to Veterinarians.* Plant City, Fla.: Ken Kimbel Book Company.

Britt, O. K. 1959. Corrective shoeing. Southeastern Vet. 2: 49.

Churchill, E. A. 1968. Care and Training of the Trotter and Pacer. Columbus, Ohio: U.S. Trotting Association.

Churchill, F. G. 1912. Practical and Scientific Horseshoeing. Wheaton, Ill.: Kjellberg and Sons. (Facsimile reprint, 1964.)

Dollar, J. A. 1898. Handbook of Horseshoeing, New York: W. R. Jenkins.

Graham, C. W. 1965. Care of the horse's foot. VM/SAC 60: 255–261.

Holmes, C. M. 1949. The Principles and Practice of Horseshoeing. Leeds: The Farriers Journal Publishing Co., Ltd.

La Croix, J. V. 1916. Lameness of the Horse. Vet. Pract. Ser. No. 1, Am. J. Vet. Med.

Lambert, F., Jr. 1966. The role of moisture in the physiology of the hoof of the harness horse. VM/SAC 61: 342–347.

Lambert, F., Jr. 1968. An experiment demonstrating rapid contraction of a standardbred horse hoof from moisture loss during flooring. VM/SAC. 63: 878–881.

Lungwitz, A., and J. W. Adams. 1897. A Textbook of Horseshoeing. 11th ed Philadelphia: J. B. Lippincott Co.

Marks, D., et al. 1971. Use of an elastomer to reduce concussion to horses' feet. JAVMA 158(8): 1361–1365.

McCunn, J. 1951. Lameness in the horse, with special reference to surgical shoeing. Vet. Rec. 63: 629.

Norberg, O. K. 1968. Silicone rubber hoof pad. Proc. AAEP, 336–337.

Owen, D., et al. 1970. Farrier science for the general practitioner. Proc. AAEP, 43–52.

Reeks, H. C. 1918. Diseases of the Horse's Foot. Chicago: Alexander Eger.

Richardson, C. 1950. Practical Farriery. London: Pitman and Sons.

Russell, W. 1907. Scientific Horseshoeing. Cincinnati: C. J. Krehbiel and Co.

Simpson, J. F. 1968. Care and Training of the Trotter and Pacer. Columbus, Ohio: U.S. Trotting Association.

U.S. Department of Agriculture. 1942. Diseases of the Horse. Bureau of Animal Industry. Washington, D.C.: U.S. Government Printing Office.

War Department. 1941. The Horseshoer. Tech. Man. TM 2-220. Washington, D.C.

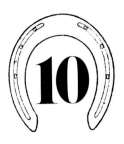

Natural and Artificial Gaits

Natural gaits of the horse are the walk, trot, and gallop. The running walk, amble, rack (broken amble or singlefoot), and pace may be either natural or artificial gaits. The canter is a restrained or collected gallop.

A three-gaited horse is required to show at walk, trot, and canter. Five-gaited horses, in addition to the three gaits mentioned, must also show a "slow-gait" (fox trot or amble) and a fast rack. Tennessee Walking Horses (Plantation Walkers) must show the flatfoot walk, running walk, and the canter.

For descriptive purposes, the terms "near" and "off" are used to describe the feet in motion. The "near" side of a horse is the left side, while the "off" side is the right.

The terms "step" and "stride" are used as descriptive terms in determining distance covered by the feet. A step is the distance between the footprints of the two forelimbs or between the two hind limbs. It is not the distance between the forelimb and the hind limb. The distance between footprints of the right and left forelimb or between footprints of right and left hindlimb would be measured. The stride is the distance between successive imprints of the same foot or feet. A stride is therefore longer than a step.

The Walk (Fig. 10–1)

This is a four-beat gait. Walking can be of various forms, but regardless of the form, it must be an even four-beat gait. When a regular sequence identified by four hoof beats at precise intervals, is lost, the horse is no longer walking. The walking sequence is lateral because both feet of one side hit the ground before the two feet of the opposite side strike. Propulsion results primarily from the hind limbs, and the forelimbs simply follow. The length of stride in the walk will usually vary between $5\frac{1}{2}'$ and 6′. This distance is measured between successive imprints of the same foot. The step will vary between 33″ and 39″ and is the measurement made between the imprints made by a pair of forefeet or the imprints made by a pair of hind feet. The sequence of hoof beats can be described according to this pattern: (1) near-hind, (2) near-fore, (3) off-hind, (4) off-fore (Fig. 10–1). This gait is sometimes described as beginning with a forelimb as: (1) off-fore, (2) near-hind, (3) near-fore, and (4) off-hind. This description is not proper according to the way the horse starts, but it is proper after he is in motion.

In the walk there is never a moment at which fewer than two feet are in contact with the ground. There is no period of suspension and no moment when only one foot is in contact with the ground.

The Flat-Foot Walk

The flat-foot walk is the natural walk of the Tennessee Walking Horse. The feet land in the same sequence as described above, but, because of the normal loose action of the horse, this gait propels the horse forward very rapidly.

The Running Walk

This is the fast walk of the Tennessee Walking Horse. It is a four-beat gait intermediate between a walk and a rack. In this gait, the hind foot oversteps the foot print of the front foot from a few inches

to as much as 18″, giving the horse a gliding motion. The gait is characterized by a bobbing and nodding of the head, a flopping of the ears, and a snapping of the teeth, in rhythm with the movement of the legs. It is easy on both horse and rider. Upon close observation, the gait resembles a pace with the hind foot hitting ground before the fore foot of the same side.

The Trot (Fig. 10–2)

The trot is a two-beat gait in which opposite fore and hind feet hit the ground together. The left forelimb and right hind limb move together, as do the right forelimb and left hind limb. A trot can be of various forms, but to be a true trot it must be in two-beat time. An "impure" trot is

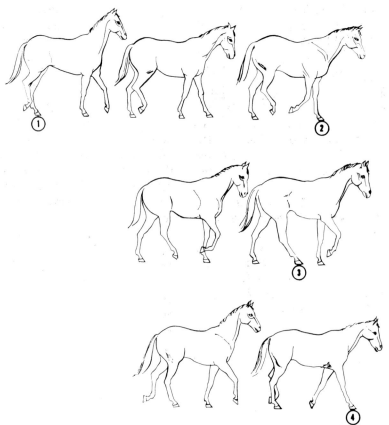

FIG. 10–1. The walk. Numbers indicate the foot sequence in the four-beat gait.

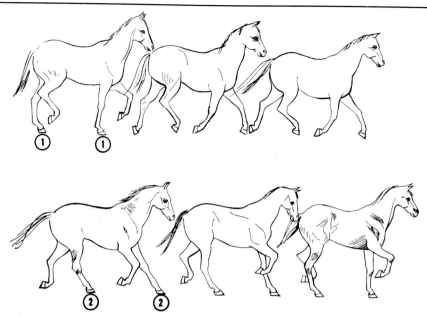

FIG. 10–2. The trot. Opposite fore and hind limbs pair to make this a two-beat gait. Numbers 1 and 2 show the pairing of the limbs.

one in which the forelimb hits the ground before the diagonal hind limb or vice versa. When the hind limb is in advance of the correct tempo, forging may be evident in feet on the same side. The length of stride in a trot will vary from slightly over 9′ in an ordinary horse to 17′ or more in a racing trotting horse.

The trot is sometimes classified as ordinary trot, collected trot, and extended trot. A Standardbred horse characterizes the extended trot with length and rapidity of individual strides. Standardbreds are also referred to as being "line-gaited trotters" when the front and hind feet on the same side are seen to travel on a direct line with each other, when viewed from front or behind. They are said to be "passing-gaited trotters" when the hind feet land outside the front feet (Simpson, 1968). The Hackney characterizes the collected trot with extreme flexion of knees and hocks. In the trot, there is a diagonal base of support, but there may be a moment of suspension during the interval at which one pair of limbs is moving toward

the ground and the other pair is leaving the ground.

The Gallop or Run (Fig. 10–3)

In a straightaway gallop, the horse normally changes leads periodically to relieve fatigue. As a horse turns to the left, he should lead with the left forelimb and right hind limb, and as he turns to the right, he should lead with right forelimb and left hind limb. When a horse is in the left (near) fore lead, the right (off) hind limb is said to be the lead hind limb, but when a horse is in the right (off) forelimb lead, the left (near) hind limb is said to be the lead hind limb. A horse should change leads, both in front and in back, at the same time during the period of suspension when the lead forelimb leaves the ground (Fig. 10–4). However, some horses change lead in front without changing in back immediately; this makes the gallop rough and difficult for the rider. When this happens, the horse is off-lead behind and runs like some dogs, landing on the

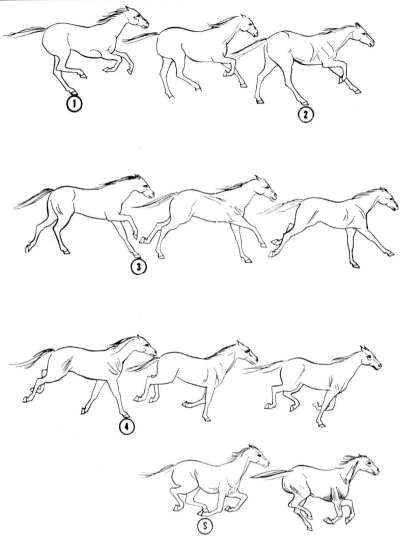

FIG. 10–3. The gallop. The gallop is a four-beat gait with a front and opposite hind limb leading and the other fore and hind limbs paired. This illustration shows a right forelimb and left hind limb lead with the sequence of foot beats indicated by numbers. A period of suspension exists, as shown by S, after the lead forefoot leaves the ground.

lateral hind leg on the same side as the leading forefoot instead of the opposite hind foot. The gallop is a fully extended gait in which the head is stretched forward and the strides reach their maximum length. The three-time beat of the canter is not possible at this speed, so the gallop becomes a gait of four beats. The length of stride in a gallop will vary between 15′ and 22′. Some horses can stride in excess of 22′. The difference is essentially in the spring of the leg in the leading forefoot.

Using as example a horse with the right, or off-fore, leading, the gallop sequence is as follows: (1) near-hind, (2) off-hind, (3) near-fore, and (4) off-fore (followed by a period of suspension) (Fig. 10–3). The gait is very similar to the canter, with the exception that the paired, nonleading diagonal limbs do not land together. The non-leading hind limb lands slightly before the nonleading forelimb. The forelimb with which the horse leads and its diagonal hind limb bear more weight and are subject to more fatigue than are the opposite diagonals. The propulsion is chiefly from the hind limbs, while the forelimbs are subject to great concussion.

In a left or near-fore lead, the beat is as follows: (1) off-hind, (2) near-hind, (3) off-fore, and (4) near-fore (followed by a short period of suspension). Another way of describing the same beat, beginning with the lead limb in an off-fore (right)

lead would be: (1) off-fore (suspension) (2) near-hind, (3) off-hind, (4) near-fore. In a near-fore (left) lead, the beat is as follows: (1) near-fore (suspension), (2) off-hind, (3) near-hind, (4) off-fore.

The Canter (Fig. 10–5)

The canter is a restrained gallop, which, like the gallop, imposes greater wear on the leading forefoot and its diagonal leading hind foot. It is a three-beat gait in which two diagonal legs are paired. The single beat of the paired legs falls between successive beats of the two unpaired legs.

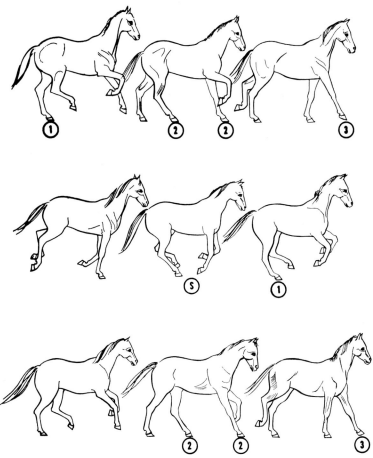

FIG. 10–4. This shows the correct change of leads in a canter. In the first sequence the horse is in a right (off) forelimb lead with a left (near) hind-limb lead. At S the horse is in a period of suspension and properly changes leads at this time, coming down with right (off) hind-limb lead and a left (near) forelimb lead, as shown by the second sequence of foot beats.

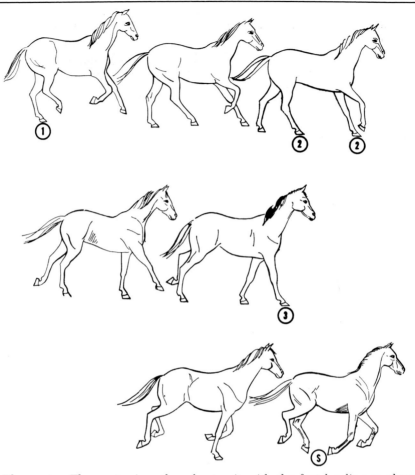

FIG. 10–5. The canter. The canter is a three-beat gait with the feet landing as shown by the numbers, followed by a period of suspension (S). The nonleading fore and hind limbs are paired to cause one beat of the three beats.

The unpaired legs act independently and are the lead limbs. The forelimb with which the horse leads and its diagonal leading hindlimb bear the most weight and are subject to more fatigue than are the paired limbs. This is the reason leads should be changed frequently. The length of stride in the canter will vary between 9'8" and 11'8". The distance between steps will usually vary between 37" and 43". In a right or off forelimb lead, the beat is as follows: (1) near-hind, (2) diagonal off-hind and near-fore together, (3) off-fore (followed by a short period of suspension) (Fig. 10–5). Another way of describing the same beat, beginning with the lead limb in an off-fore (right) lead would be: (1) off-fore (suspension) (2) near-hind, (3) diagonal off-hind and near-fore together. In a near-fore (left) lead, the beat is as follows: (1) nearfore (suspension), (2) off-hind, (3) near-hind and off-fore together.

If the canter is exceptionally animated (collected), a four-beat gait may result, similar to the four-beat gait of the gallop. When the gait becomes a four-beat cadence, the paired fore and opposite hind limb do not land together; the hind limb lands just before the forelimb, or the fore-limb lands shortly before the hind limb. When the horse changes leads in a canter, both the fore and hind limbs should change leads at the same time, or a dis-agreeable gait will result. When the horse changes stride in front but not in back, the hind limb on the same side as the leading forefoot lands before the hind limb oppo-site the lead forefoot.

The Pace (Fig. 10–6)

The pace is a fast two-beat gait in which the lateral fore and hindfeet strike the ground simultaneously. It is a faster gait than the trot, but is not as rapid as the gallop. Such a gait is not suited to mud or snow. Because the gait causes a rolling motion, the horse is said to be a body or leg pacer, depending upon the amount of rolling of the body during movement. The base of support is always on the two lat-eral limbs and there is a brief moment of suspension as two limbs leave the ground and the other two strike it. The length of stride in the pace is 12′ to 14′.

The "Slow Gaits" (Running Walk, Fox Trot, or Amble)

The five-gaited horse must show one of the slow gaits and a rack, in addition to the walk, trot, and canter.

The Fox Trot

This is a slow, short, broken trot in which the head usually nods during movement. The horse brings each hind-foot to the ground an instant before the diagonal forefoot strikes.

The Rack or Singlefoot (Broken Amble)

This is an artificial gait, in most cases. An exaggerated walk of four beats, it is a fast, flashy gait in which each foot meets the ground separately at equal intervals. Originally known as the singlefoot, the rack is easy on the rider but difficult on the horse. It should not be confused with the pace, which it resembles because the hind foot lands just before the forefoot of

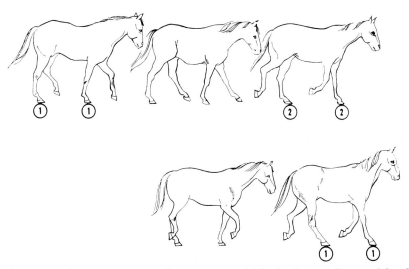

FIG. 10–6. The pace. The pace is a two-beat gait in which the lateral fore and hind limbs are paired, with the feet landing as shown.

the same side. The rack differs from the running walk in that there is more up and down motion of the limbs, and the hind foot does not overreach the forefoot as much as in a running walk.

The Amble

The amble is a pace of walking speed and is classified as a "slow gait." Some authorities have said the amble is not a pace because the hind foot lands slightly before the forefoot. There is no period of suspension, since one foot is always on the ground. The legs work in lateral pairs, but the forefoot of one lateral pair remains on the ground until the hind foot of the opposite lateral pair touches the ground. Therefore, it is not a true pace.

Backing

This is done at the two-beat diagonal gait of the trot. Both left-hind and right-fore and the right-hind and left-fore move in unison when the horse is backing with any speed.

REFERENCES

Axe, J. W. [1900.] *The Horse in Health and Disease.* London: Gresham Publishing Co. *Vols. 1 and 3.*

Hildebrand, M. 1959. Motion of the running cheetah and horse. J. Mammal., 40(4): 481.

Hildebrand, M. 1960. How animals run. Sci. Amer. 202(5): 148.

Hildebrand, M. 1965. Symmetrical gaits of horses. Science 150: 701.

Self, M. 1946. *The Horseman's Encyclopedia.* New York: A. S. Barnes & Co.

Simpson, J. F. 1968. The theory of shoeing and balancing, p. 293. *In* Care and Training of the Trotter and Pacer. Columbus, Ohio: U.S. Trotting Association.

Smith, F. 1921. *A Manual of Veterinary Physiology.* 5th ed. Chicago: Alexander Eger.

Taylor, B. M., C. M. Tipton, M. Adrian, and P. V. Karpobith. 1966. Action of certain joints in the leg of the horse recorded electrogoniometrically. Amer. J. Vet. Res. 27: 85.

Wynmalen, H., and M. Lyne. 1954. *The Horse in Action.* New York: A. S. Barnes & Co.

Methods of Therapy

PHYSICAL THERAPY

The aim of physical therapy is the restoration of function and promotion of tissue healing by assisting normal physiological processes. Methods of physical therapy are cold, heat, massage, exercise, light, electricity, manipulation, and mechanical devices. Not all of these methods are applicable to horses. The physiological response to physical therapy is its effect on the vascular supply; this in turn reproduces similar changes in deeper tissues.

Cold

The application of cold is used in treatment of acute and hyperacute inflammatory processes. It aids in relief of pain and is used to prevent edema and tissue swelling. There is a decrease in tissue metabolism and possibly some anesthesia. Cold is best combined with compression bandage and rest to further limit swelling. Cold can be applied through a bandage and is used during the first twenty-four to forty-eight hours after trauma has occurred. After this time, it is of no value. It is applied for 20- to 40-minute applications, and at least one hour should elapse before it is reapplied.

Cold application can be made by running cold water through a hose on the part or by using a tub or canvas bag to cover the limb. This type of moist therapy should not be used if there is an open wound. Ice bags or ice contained in plastic is very helpful in acute noninfectious inflammatory processes. This type of therapy limits swelling from the acute injury and will shorten the recovery period. Swelling is limited by vasoconstriction. If cold is applied too long, there may be a reflex vasodilation, and there is also the possibility of vasodilation after the cold is removed. These are additional reasons for using compression bandage in conjunction with cold application. Alternating heat and cold are often used on acute noninfectious inflammatory conditions (such as sprain) after an interval of 24 hours following the injury. Cold is used for injury of muscles, tendons, ligaments, and joints and for burns.

Heat (Thermotherapy)

Heat can be applied as radiant heat, conductive heat, and conversive heat (Hickman, 1964). Physiological effects of the three methods are basically the same. Radiant heat is applied by infrared light, and conductive heat by hot water bottle, electric heating pad, hot fomentations, and poultices. Conversive heat is developed in tissues by resistance to high-frequency electrical energy (diathermy) or sound waves (ultrasound).

Heat is used in an attempt to cause resorption of swelling caused by blood or serum. Heat causes vasodilation and in-

429

creases the number of phagocytes in the area, as well as increasing oxygen supply to the part. There is increased metabolism in local cells, increased lymph flow and a rise in local temperature caused by the vasodilation. Vessel permeability is also increased, and this must be considered when using heat because increased vessel permeability can lead to increased absorption of toxins or occurrence of tissue edema following its use. Heat is usually not used alone, but is combined with active or passive action, either manually or by exercise. Heat can spread bacteria and toxic products deeper into surrounding tissues and should not be applied if infection is present. Heat should not be used until infection is under control by antibiotics. Heat should not be used on any injury until 24 to 48 hours have passed.

Superficial Heat

Some methods of applying heat cause only superficial inflammation that does not extend far beneath the skin. Hot water poultices, heating pads, turbulator (whirlpool), and ultraviolet light are used for this purpose. Hot water poultices and turbulator are application of moist heat, and drugs may be added to facilitate penetration. For this purpose, magnesium sulfate or mild liniment solutions are commonly used. Magnesium sulfate also acts as an agent to draw swelling from the tissue, because of the higher osmotic tension in the magnesium sulfate solution. Magnesium sulfate should be added at the rate of approximately two cups per gallon of water for this purpose. A turbulator can be used to give passive massage to the part during the application of hot water heat. A turbulator is a motorized device that agitates the water around the part by pump action. These are expensive and carry some risk of electrical shock. An inexpensive turbulator can be made by reversing a vacuum cleaner hose so that the air blows from the machine instead of sucking air. With the vacuum hose deep in the water that is around the limb, the machine blows air through the hose and turbulates water around the part. Superficial heat of this type is often combined with massage, and following application of heat by one of the above methods, the part may be massaged using alcohol or other mild rubefacient solutions. These solutions do not have any particular therapeutic value, but they aid the massage and cause a superficial erythema. Often the liniment may be credited with improvement of a part, when improvement was actually the result of the heat and massage.

For deeper penetration, infrared light, both luminous and nonluminous, is used. The luminous type of infrared is used mostly for atmospheric heating for young pigs and calves. It also can be used for frostbite or to aid in pointing abscesses. There is a danger of a thermal burn caused by infrared light, and the source should be at least 18″ away from the part being treated. There is no pain initially, and evidence of thermal burn appears later. It can be applied for 20- to 40-minute applications and repeated at hourly intervals if necessary. The nonluminous type of infrared light heats a metal coil and this coil radiates the infrared light. This form is usually the best type to use since there is no danger of bulb breakage.

Deep Heat

Diathermy. Diathermy will penetrate to a depth of approximately 2″. There is a problem of arcing and electrical shorting in treating animals. Ultrashort-wave diathermy units are available in which the current oscillates several million cycles per second. The tissue heats because of resistance to this energy and it is unable to expel the heat produced. Diathermy treatment can be used twice daily if necessary.

Heating by high-frequency electrical energy is obtained by including the tissues in the circuit. The high-frequency electrical energy passes from one electrode through the tissues to the other electrode. Resistance in the tissues produces a variable rise in tissue temperature due to a variation in the degree of impedance to the electrical energy. Therefore, all tissues will not be heated to the same degree. The greater the fluid content of the tissue, the higher the temperature recorded. Fatty tissues are the most resistant and may be damaged earlier than other tissues. Bone and tendon have lower water content and do not heat as much as the surrounding moist tissues. Diathermy is a relatively impractical way of treating horses. The difficulty in getting the coils to adapt to the part, the possibility of the horse moving and damaging equipment, plus the danger of possible short-circuit shocking of the horse, make this method of therapy cumbersome, and it is not commonly used. If bone screws or pins are present in the bone, they may heat to a high enough temperature to cause bone necrosis.

Ultrasound. Ultrasound consists of ultra-high-frequency sound waves produced by conversion of high-frequency electrical energy waves to sound waves by the crystal in the head of the instrument. A mechanical vibration is produced by the sound waves. This crystal converts electricity to sound, which is measured in watts of output per square centimeter of head surface. Use of ultrasound involves the passage of these high-frequency sound waves (above 20,000 cycles per sec) through tissues. The resistance of the tissues to these waves produces heat. This heat will penetrate to the bony structures of a joint or limb. Ultrasound is best used for deep heat penetration of muscles (myositis), nerve damage, tendon injury, trauma, bursitis, and scars in contracted tissue. In some cases, it may be better than corticoids for these conditions, and it can

be used in combination with them. Ultrasound restores function by the relief of pain by the production of heat. It is not of value in bone damage, and if enough is used, bone destruction may occur because of the heat produced. It has been said by some that the bone chips from sesamoids and other small bones can be removed by use of this agent. However, this is undesirable since healthy bone may be demineralized as a result of inflammation caused by this treatment.

Ultrasound penetrates deeper (approximately 3″ to 5″) than does diathermy or other forms of heat application described, and it also causes a micromassage of tissue. The chassis of the machine should always be grounded to prevent accidental shock to the horse.

For tendons or superficial tissue, 0.5 watts per square centimeter of head surface is used. For deeper penetration, 1 to 2 watts per square centimeter of head surface is used. Duration of application varies between five and ten minutes, and the head should be kept in motion and in contact with the skin. Ultrasound waves do not pass through the air or through hair on the surface of the body. The part should be clipped and shaved, and a coupling agent, such as mineral oil, must be used to establish contact between the head and tissue. High doses of ultrasound will cause a rise in tissue heat to as high as 106° (Burdick Corporation, 1961). The temperature rise can cause bone or tissue damage, and care should be taken not to use too high a dosage for too long a time. The head should be kept in motion to prevent heat from accumulating in the tissues underneath the head surface.

Ultrasound should not be used for 48 to 72 hours after injury since it can cause hematoma and seroma if used before this. It can disseminate cancer cells, and so should not be used if cancer is present or suspected. It should not be used over an area of local anesthesia because the horse cannot feel it and thus will not object to levels of heat high enough to cause discomfort. Ultrasound can be used more safely than diathermy in the presence of bone pins, screws, and other metallic objects.

Ultrasound can be used up to ten days prior to radiation therapy, but it is not used for at least two months after radiation therapy has been administered because radiation therapy causes a prolonged inflammatory reaction (Dixon, 1965). Ultrasound is of most use when there are no bone changes and when only soft tissues are damaged.

Massage

Massage is used in subacute and chronic swelling and can be combined with the use of liniments, although the main benefit is from massage. The lubrication quality of the liniment usually aids in the massaging. Many liniments receive credit for being good therapeutic agents, when it is actually the massage that reduces edematous swelling and aids in relieving pain of an injured tendon or joint. The effect is transitory, and treatment must be repeated several times a day to be of most value. Massage aids in reducing tissue edema and also in freeing scar tissue adhesions of the skin to underlying tissues.

Treatment with Faradic Current

Treatment using faradic current has been described by Strong (1967). Faradic current is an intermittent alternating electrical current from a secondary winding of an induction coil. This electric current stimulates contraction of muscle and can be varied in intensity and timing so that muscles are contracted and relaxed, thereby preventing atrophy and promoting mobilization of joints. It is said to prevent adhesions and help disperse inflammatory fluids and hematoma. The instrument is called Transeva and is manufactured by the Trans-S.E.V.A. Limited

Electrahouse, Weyhill, Haslemere, Surrey, England. It is said to be tolerated by 99 percent of horses, even those that are high-strung. The instrument is operated by battery to eliminate the possibility of electrocution. This type of therapy is indicated primarily in sprain injury of joints and strain injury of muscles. It probably hastens recovery from this type of injury and helps to alleviate muscular soreness.

Exercise

Depending on the condition, exercise is frequently used to aid in rehabilitation. It is primarily used in subacute and chronic conditions and is used to remove swelling, especially in puncture wounds of the limb, midline incisions, and castrations. Whenever possible, it is combined with massage and the use of liniments. It may also be used to rehabilitate and strengthen the limb after injury to tendon or ligaments. In any case, it must be used with judgment, since the horse will often tend to overdo when allowed free access to a corral or pasture. Exercise on a hand lead is usually best when the horse is beginning exercise after surgery for fractured carpus, sesamoid fracture, and similar conditions. After the initial excitement has worn off, after several days of hand leading, the horse can be turned into a small lot and from there into a pasture as the limb strengthens.

When facilities are available, swimming is an excellent way to rehabilitate and condition the musculature of a horse without concussion to the limbs. It should be used whenever possible to strengthen the limbs after surgery before regular training procedures are reinstituted.

OTHER METHODS OF THERAPY

Immobilization of the Part

Immobilization is one of the most beneficial methods of therapy for acute inflammatory conditions, but it can be difficult to employ in horses because they may resist the restraint. Immobilization of the part will aid in preventing the spread of inflammation and will reduce swelling as it reduces movement. It also permits the tissues to heal with minimal scar formation. Immobilization will also support damaged structures to aid their healing, which is especially valuable in healing of tendons. Immobilization is best done by the use of a plaster cast. When this is not possible or feasible, compression bandages such as Ace bandages, cotton bandages, or nylon bandages may be of help. Compression bandages should not be used in acute infectious inflammatory conditions until the infection is under control by the use of antibiotics. Unless the infection is controlled by antibiotics, the compression might tend to force bacteria and associated toxic products deeper into the tissues. In no case should a compression bandage be left on longer than three days without changing. Skin loss from necrosis can occur if this rule is not observed. Strong liniments should not be used under bandages because they can cause blistering.

At this point, it might be well to mention the fact that ordinary gauze is extremely inelastic and, when left in place for longer than 24 hours, may cause loss of skin. When gauze is used under a compression bandage, it is usually best to use the type known as "Kling"* or "conforming" gauze, which is much more elastic and does not rigidly oppose the tissue. The same is true of ordinary adhesive tape, and preferably only elastic adhesive tape is used.†

Application of a Cast

A cast is applied to allow healing of bone and tendon, to immobilize a wound,

*Johnson & Johnson Co.
†Elasticon, Johnson & Johnson Co.

and to offer support to a limb to prevent contraction of tendons or overstress. In this discussion the use of a cast for fracture of long bones is not described.

The following are examples of plaster of paris and plaster-resin products available for use. The products from Vetco Div., Johnson & Johnson Co., New Brunswick, N.J., are used for examples.

1. Blue label "specialist" plaster of paris, fast-setting, five to eight minutes. Available in 2″ to 6″ widths. This product is satisfactory for ordinary splinting.

2. Extra-fast-setting, green label "specialist" bandages. Available in 2″ to 6″ widths. Setting time two to four minutes.

3. Zoroc resin-plaster bandages. Zoroc combines plaster, resin, and catalyst in one product. It is applied in the same way as other plaster bandages but is stronger and shows more resistance to the effects of moisture. It is available in 3″ to 6″ widths. Setting time five to eight minutes. Zoroc bandages are more than twice as expensive as the blue and green label plaster bandages, but fewer of them are used. Zoroc is destroyed upon exposure to air, and if the roll feels granular it should not be used. If care is taken either to paint the bottom of the cast with quick-drying enamel or to cover it with rubber inner tubing to prevent moisture from seeping through and destroying the bottom portion of the cast, a water-resistant cast material is usually not necessary.

4. Plaster of paris splints. These are available in the blue and green label products, the blue label with a setting time of five to eight minutes and the green label with a setting time of two to four minutes. The following sizes are available: 3″ × 15″, 4″ × 15″, and 5″ × 30″. A splint of this type can also be made by rolling an ordinary plaster bandage back and forth on itself until the proper length and thickness are attained.

5. Orthopedic stockinette. This is available in 2″ to 10″ widths and can be cut to length.

6. Orthopedic felt. For protecting the skin at the top of the cast and for padding around prominences.

Application of Cast for Lacerations in the Lower Limb (Lower Metacarpal or Metatarsal Region to the Coronary Band). Lacerations of this region often involve tendon(s) and/or tendon sheath. Application of a cast to lower limb lacerations often proves to be one of the best methods of therapy. It immobilizes the tissues while they heal and causes union of lacerated surfaces where it might not normally occur with just a pressure bandage. This is especially true in lacerations in the region of the coronary band.

The wound is clipped, shaved and cleansed. Debridement of the wound is done and sutures are placed if practical or indicated. The wound is dressed with sterile bandages and the limb covered with stockinette. A cast may be put on in the standing position under tranquilization if the horse is of good disposition. Otherwise, it is best to administer tranquilization, 6 percent chloral hydrate until incoordination exists, and then put the horse down with 1 gram of thiamylal sodium.* An additional gram of thiamylal sodium can be given a 1,000-pound horse to keep him immobilized during the casting procedure. Glyceryl guaiacolate† (5 percent) containing 1-2 gm thiamylal sodium per liter of solution can be substituted as a restraining anesthetic if desired. After the limb is covered with stockinette, three rolls of 4″ or 6″ blue label Johnson & Johnson plaster of paris are applied, enclosing the foot wall and extending to just below the carpus or tarsus. Optionally, $\frac{1}{4}$″ × 3″ orthopedic felt can be placed under the top of the cast in a ring formation around the limb. Orthopedic felt can also be placed around the coronary band to prevent chafing, but this is not necessary when the foot is completely immobilized by the cast. After three rolls of

plaster have been applied, plaster splints (4″ × 15″ or 5″ × 30″) are used on the dorsal and volar surfaces of the limb. A $\frac{1}{4}$″ thickness of plaster splints is used on each surface. The splint should go over the bottom of the sole of the foot and conform closely to the pastern and fetlock areas. The first rolls of plaster are put on with very little tension. They are merely laid over the limb and smoothed without pulling them tight. After the plaster splints are applied, an additional three or four rolls of 4″ or 6″ plaster are used to reinforce the cast. More tension can be put on these latter rolls because the first rolls of plaster and the plaster splints are beginning to dry and will resist pressure. This does not mean that one can put great pressures on the plaster but it should be pulled up reasonably snug. The cast is allowed to dry; the horse should not be permitted to bear weight on the cast until it has dried.

When the cast is applied while the horse is standing, the reinforcing splints are applied first (Fig. 11–1). A plaster splint 4″ or 5″ wide, 30″ long, and $\frac{3}{8}$″ thick is applied down the front of the limb, under the foot and up the caudal aspect of the limb. This is applied over a stockinette bandage. Orthopedic felt $\frac{1}{4}$″ thick is placed around the leg just under the tarsus or carpus. Approximately three rolls of 4″ or 6″ plaster bandage are applied snugly over these splints. More pressure must be put on the plaster bandage when applying it in the standing position, because the plaster splint has been applied first. If these rolls are not applied tight enough, especially over the orthopedic felt, the cast will be loose. After these rolls of plaster and the plaster splint have hardened to the extent that they will hold the foot in position, the foot is picked up and the cast is moistened and finished with an additional three rolls of plaster. These last rolls cover the foot and reinforce the fetlock area. In this way, the normal foot position can be maintained, whereas the normal position cannot be

---

*Surital, Parke, Davis & Co.
†Summit Hill Laboratories.

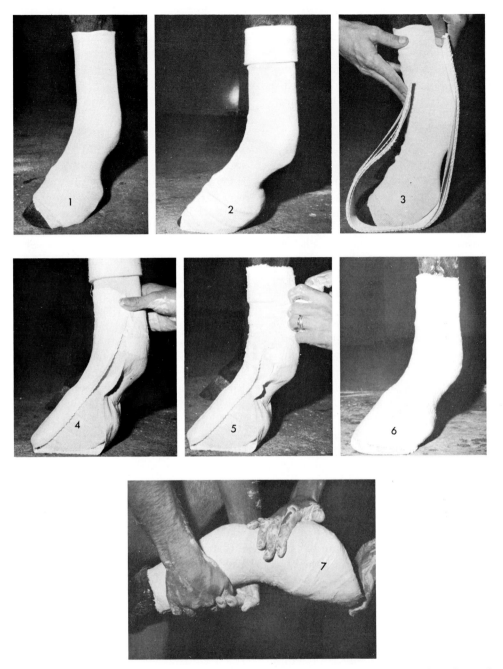

FIG. 11–1. Application of a standing plaster cast. *1*, After the leg is cleaned, dried, and powdered, a double layer of stockinette is applied. *2*, A piece of $\frac{1}{4}''$ orthopedic felt is applied just below the carpus or tarsus. *3*, A plaster splint is applied. *4*, The plaster splint is moistened and contoured to the limb. *5*, Four-inch plaster of paris rolls are then applied firmly over the plaster splint. Extra pressure must be applied over the orthopedic felt at the top to keep the cast from being loose at this point. The plaster is applied more snugly than when the cast is applied in the recumbent position, because the plaster splint is applied later in a recumbent cast. *6*, The horse is allowed to stand a few minutes to allow forming of the cast without complete drying. The cast is then moistened and the limb is picked up and the cast is finished with the limb in the flexed position. *7*, The limb has been picked up and the cast finished in this position. If the plaster is moistened beforehand, the layers will form a firm bond. This allows complete normal positioning of the foot.

maintained if the cast is put on the limb with the foot picked up from the floor from the beginning. The standing cast is most helpful in wounds of the lower limb. It is not sufficiently snug for fractures of the phalanges.

When applying a cast over a wound, it is usually necessary to remove the cast in approximately eight days and apply a new one because of discharges that occur. When the cast is removed, strong odors may be present, but these are not necessarily indicative of destructive changes and are usually due to putrefaction of discharges from the wound. The wound is thoroughly cleansed and a new cast applied in a similar fashion to the first one. After removal of the second cast, in another eight days, the wound is usually healed sufficiently that a cast is no longer necessary if a tendon is not cut, and the wound can be treated by a pressure bandage and topical medication.

Cast Following Removal of Sesamoid Fractures, for Fractures of the First and Second Phalanges, and for Other Orthopedic Procedures in the Lower Limb. The horse is ordinarily under surgical anesthesia for an orthopedic procedure and the cast is put on in the recumbent position. If an incisional area is present, it is bandaged with sterile gauze and elastic tape. The limb is then covered with stockinette, and the proximal portion of the cast just below the carpus or tarsus is covered by $\frac{1}{4}'' \times 3''$ orthopedic felt. Three rolls of 4″ or 6″ blue label Johnson & Johnson plaster of paris are applied to the limb, including the hoof and sole. These rolls are applied without tension. Special emphasis is placed on supporting the posterior aspect of the pastern. After the three rolls of plaster are applied, plaster splints (4″ wide, 15″ long) are placed on the dorsal and volar surfaces of the limb. These splints also cover the bottom of the foot. The splints are molded carefully to the limb, and an additional three rolls of 4″ or 6″ plaster are used to reinforce the

cast. These latter rolls may be pulled fairly snugly because the original rolls of plaster and splints will act as protection against getting the cast too tight. In addition to uses already mentioned, this cast can be used following surgery to promote ankylosis of the proximal interphalangeal joint, following removal of fractures of the extensor process of the third phalanx, and following removal of chip fractures of the first phalanx into the metacarpophalangeal joint. It also can be used for longitudinal articular fractures of the third metacarpal bone that have no separation of fragments (see Chap. 6, p. 359). The foot of the cast is protected from moisture by spraying with quick-drying enamel or applying a piece of rubber over the bottom of the cast.

The addition of a walking bar to the cast is very helpful when treating fractures of the first and second phalanx. This addition of the bar will distribute weight-bearing to the sides of the cast and help prevent movement of the fracture fragments.

Cast for Protection of the Carpus Following Carpal Surgery. The cast is applied with the horse in a recumbent position as soon as the skin incision is closed with sutures. Orthopedic felt is used to pad the limb in the region of the accessory carpal bone and lateral and medial malleoli of the radius. Orthopedic felt is placed over these areas to make the adjacent limb the same circumference as these points (Fig. 11-2). This distributes pressure more evenly and aids in preventing skin necrosis over these prominences. The limb is then covered with stockinette after the incision is bandaged. Orthopedic felt $\frac{1}{4}'' \times 3''$ is placed just above the fetlock joint and at the proximal portion of the cast just below the elbow joint. Four rolls of 6″ plaster are then placed on the limb between the elbow joint and the proximal aspect of the metacarpophalangeal joint. Following this, plaster splints 4″ wide, 30″ long, and $\frac{1}{4}''$ thick are placed over the

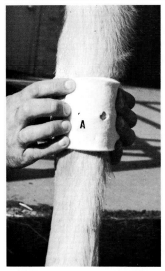
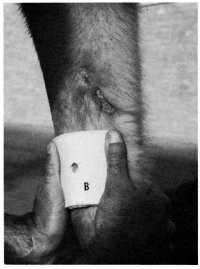
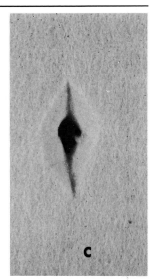

FIG. 11-2. A method of protecting the skin over the accessory carpal bone (A) and the medial malleolus of the radius (B), when bandaging or casting the carpus. An elliptical hole is cut in the orthopedic felt (C), and the felt is contoured over the prominence.

dorsal and volar surfaces of the limb. The first rolls of plaster are only laid upon the limb and not pulled up snugly. After the application of the plaster splints, three to four more rolls of 6″ plaster of paris is put on the cast to reinforce it. These latter rolls can be pulled more tightly than the first ones because of the resistance of the original plaster in the drying process. All casts should be rubbed thoroughly to cause blending of the layers. This cast is removed six to eight days after carpal surgery. The cast acts as protection against injury to the carpus while the horse is recovering from anesthesia, and is an excellent pressure bandage during the period. It is followed up with elastic pressure bandages for an additional thirty days.

Casting Procedure for Immobilization of the Hock. Casting of the hock joint must be done carefully or necrosis over the tuber calcis or the malleoli of the tibia may occur. Casting this area is frequently indicated for wounds on the anterior surface of the tarsal joint. Other indications are fractures, tendon lacerations, luxation of the tarsal joint, and rupture of the gas-

trocnemius muscle. In most cases, it is best for the cast to include the hoof. The tremendous muscular power of the hind limb is somewhat restrained by including the hoof rather than stopping the cast at the fetlock joint.

A 1,000-lb horse is restrained with 0.5 mg/lb promazine,* enough 6 percent chloral hydrate to make him unsteady on his feet (250 to 500 cc) and 2 gm of thiamylal sodium† given intravenously. This will ordinarily give enough anesthesia to allow application of a cast and time enough for it to dry before the horse attempts to get up. Glyceryl guaiacolate‡ (5 percent) containing 1–2 gm thiamylal sodium per liter of solution can be substituted as a restraining anesthetic if desired. The wound is cleaned and dressed, if one is present, and the limb is covered with stockinette. Orthopedic felt $\frac{1}{4}″ \times 3″$ is applied in the region of the malleoli of the tibia so that the adjacent limb is built out to the level of these prominences. It is best

* Promazine, Ft. Dodge Laboratories; Sparine, Wyeth Laboratories.
† Surital, Parke, Davis & Co.
‡ Summit Hill Laboratories.

to do it in this fashion rather than try to pad the prominence itself. The limb is covered with stockinette and several rolls of 6″ blue label Johnson & Johnson plaster bandage are applied. In most cases, four to five rolls are applied before applying plaster splints. These initial rolls are not pulled down tightly but laid on to conform to the limb without putting on pressure. At this time, blue label Johnson & Johnson plaster splints 5″ × 30″ and $\frac{3}{8}$″ thick are applied to the plantar and dorsal surfaces of the limb. These splints are centered over the point at the hock. One strip on the plantar surface and one strip on the dorsal surface are used. This will reinforce the cast in the area of greatest stress. An additional four or five rolls of plaster are then applied to the limb. The cast is carried up close to the stifle joint and down to and including the hoof wall. If desired, plaster splints may also be applied in the region of the fetlock joint, including the foot. If tendon injury has occurred, it is best to apply splints in this area as described for the forelimb extending proximally to just below the tarsal joint.

In order to avoid skin necrosis over the point of the hock, the hock must be restrained so that no motion occurs. The cast is removed in six to eight days if it is being used for a wound. If being used for a fracture, it is removed and changed as it loosens. Six to eight weeks in a cast are required for severed flexor tendons or ruptured gastrocnemius tendon.

Cast material other than plaster of paris and resin-impregnated plaster of paris is available. This cast material is fiber glass applied in two different ways. In one instance, the 4″ × 10′ fiber glass cloth rolls are dipped into a polyester-resin-catalyst mixture and applied over a light plaster of paris cast (Hanselka et al., 1972). Three to five thicknesses are usually adequate. One-half to one hour is required to set the material into solid cast. This time can be shortened by adding more catalyst or

using a heat lamp. The resin mixture is very irritating to hands, and rubber gloves should be worn for application. The cast is cut off with a cast cutter. The materials* are available through most marine supply dealers.

Another form of fiber glass used for cast material is "Lightcast".† In this case, the material is set with an ultraviolet light. The procedure is as follows (Alexander, 1971): Lightcast stockinette is applied to the limb, and beveled orthopedic felt‡ is used for padding. Four-inch Lightcast tape is then applied starting at the hoof. Successive wraps are made by overlapping one-half width of the tape, and at the top the edges are exactly aligned to gain strength. Three to five layers are usually adequate. The cast is cured with an ultraviolet light that is used after the first wrapping and again after the second and third. Time varies from 90 seconds on the first wrap to three minutes for the final wrap. When the cast is too long for the light to cover it, the curing is done in two stages by exposing the distal and proximal parts to the Lightcast light separately. The chief disadvantage to this method of cast application is the cost of the material and ultraviolet light.

Application of Counterirritation

Counterirritation is used to stimulate a subacute or chronic inflammatory process to a more acute process in the hope that resolution will occur when the acute inflammation heals. Counterirritants may be classified by strength:

Rubefacient Drugs

These produce redness and mild heat by increasing circulation. They are commonly present in various braces and liniments. Many terms are applied to

*Pettit Paint Co. Inc., San Leandro, Calif.
†Solar Laboratories Inc., Torrance, Calif.
‡Quaker Felt & Gasket Co., Philadelphia.

products used for rubefacient effect. The terms "liniment," "tightener," "brace," and "sweat" are often used. In reality there is very little difference among them.

A *liniment* is any combination of drugs used for rubefacient effect; examples are as follows: A preparation of camphor and cottonseed oil; camphor and soap liniment —a preparation of hard soap, camphor, rosemary oil, and alcohol; chloroform liniment—a preparation of chloroform with camphor and soap base.

A liniment usually contains one or more of the essential (volatile) oils. Their use on the legs of a horse can result in considerable edema and skin soreness. If the reaction is severe or neglected, scars and denuded areas can result. A horse should not be ridden while skin soreness or edema are present. The blistering effect of a liniment is increased when a bandage is used to cover the area where liniment was applied.

A *tightener* is a term applied to various drug mixtures that appear to aid removal of edema or filling of a joint capsule or tendon sheath. The so-called tightener effect comes about from removal of edema or synovia so that the tendons and suspensory ligament are more palpable. In most cases, this effect is not due to the drug but to the massage with which the drug is applied and to the compression bandage that is applied over the area after the tightener has been rubbed in. An example of a tightener is as follows: tincture of belladonna—4 oz. (not used in preparations prescribed at race tracks); tannic acid powder—2 oz.; menthol crystals—2 oz.; camphor crystals—1 oz.; alcohol—q.s. 1 qt. There should be no skin soreness when a product of this type is used. It is applied daily and covered with a cotton and roll bandage for five days.

A *sweat* is a product that causes some moisture accumulation on the skin following its use. Most products including alcohol will do this. The skin of a horse can actually exude serum from its surface

in the presence of inflammation. A plastic wrapping, oiled silk, or waxed paper is usually applied around the limb after the use of this type of drug mixture. These wrappings themselves can cause the skin to "sweat." In addition to alcohol alone, equal parts of alcohol and glycerin are also used for this action. Many other proprietary remedies are available. Plastic sheeting can be wrapped over the drugs applied and bandaged over to increase the "sweat" effect.

A *brace* is a mixture of drugs that is used routinely following workouts. The limbs of the horse are rubbed down prior to putting on leg wraps each night. In most cases the massage used in applying the mixture is of much more benefit than the mixture itself, but the drugs are given credit for action such as prevention of tendon sheath and joint capsule filling. Massage, plus the compression bandage, would accomplish the same purpose in most cases. Alcohol (ethyl or isopropyl) will serve this purpose satisfactorily. A proprietary remedy* made of wormwood (oil of chenopodium), thymol, chloroxylenol, menthol, and acetone is also very popular. This latter mix is also sometimes used as a "tightener" and a "sweat."

There is great overlapping of the above compounds, and in many cases, "secret formulas" are only variations of common drugs like camphor, ammonia, alcohol, oil of wintergreen (methyl salicylate), turpentine, glycerin, acetone, menthol, and thymol. Depending on concentrations of various products incorporated in them, they may or may not produce a severe irritation when enclosed under a bandage. Some types of leg paints are used that contain iodine, which will produce blistering if applied several days in a row under wraps. A mixture of 120 cc 7 percent tincture of iodine, 30 cc turpentine, and 30 cc glycerin is an example of a type

*Absorbine Jr., W. F. Young Inc., Springfield, Mass.

of leg paint that can produce this effect. If this type of product is used, it is better not to apply a bandage over it, because a severe skin irritation can result.

In summary, one would have to say that most of these products are not really effective, but the massage and bandaging that go with them probably are. As long as the product does not cause pain to the horse and irritation to the skin, no harm is done. The rubefacient effect is very temporary and must be repeated once or twice daily for any beneficial effect at all. An area of muscular soreness or joint soreness that is massaged will show pain relief following application of this type of drug. However, in just a short time the effect is gone. Plastic sheeting applied to the limb after application of these drugs enhances their effect. However, it also increases the irritant effect and could damage tissues.

Blisters or Vesicants

These agents produce blistering and inflammation of the skin down to the subcutaneous tissue. Red iodide of mercury and cantharides (Spanish fly) are examples.

General rules for application of blisters:
1. Clip area.
2. Apply blister with a piece of cork or stick. Do not use hand.
3. Rub in for about five minutes.
4. Remove according to directions on blister as early as six to eight hours later and as late as twenty-four hours later.
5. Apply petroleum jelly on outer ring where blister was applied so that if it runs, it will not disturb adjacent tissues.

Precautions in applying blisters:
1. The horse must be cross-tied while the blister is in effect, because if he is able to lick or chew the area, considerable damage to the tongue and mouth may result. A neck cradle may be necessary after the blister is removed.
2. Do not use red iodide of mercury on very young horses because of severe irritation that may occur.
3. When a blistering agent such as red iodide of mercury has been used, it may interfere with interpretation of radiographs because of deposits of iodine on the skin. The limb should be thoroughly scrubbed before x-ray films are taken.
4. Always give tetanus antitoxin or have the horse on a tetanus toxoid program before using a blister.

Conditions for which blistering agents are used (subacute or chronic inflammation):
1. Chronic inflammations of joints (hock, stifle, fetlock, carpus)
2. Chronic bone conditions (ringbone, bog spavin, exostosis, sidebones)
3. Tendonitis
4. Tendosynovitis
5. Synovitis
6. Curb
7. Pointing abscesses

Contraindications are:
1. Acute and hyperacute inflammatory conditions
2. Open wounds
3. Flexor surfaces except the fetlock
4. Near mucous membranes
5. Weak or emaciated animals
6. Recent injection of corticoids in the area (within thirty days)

Results of blistering:
1. Blistering and scurfing of the skin—its effectiveness is questionable, especially in bony conditions. In general, it can be said that blistering is an ineffective and painful method of therapy. Results obtained are due to the enforced rest of the horse.

Therapeutic Cautery (Firing)

Purpose. To produce an acute inflammatory process in a chronic or subacute inflammation in hope that it will undergo resolution.

Indications. It is one of the most misused therapeutic agents in veterinary therapy. It is often used on normal tissue and for conditions for which it is contraindicated.

Conditions for which therapeutic cautery is used are listed below (*Caution— Always radiograph a joint before using any type of therapy*):

(a) Soft tissue damage, especially around joints, ligaments, and tendons.

(b) Carpitis (popped knee). In this condition it is of most value when no periosteal new bone growth is present.

(c) Chronic arthritis.

(d) Osselets. Osselets is one of the conditions for which firing may be of definite value. By creating an acute inflammation, resolution of the chronic serous arthritis may occur as healing takes place. This also usually makes it easier to obtain the proper rest for the horse. Four to six months' rest should follow firing of osselets. It is of little value after periosteal new bone growth involves the joint.

(e) Tendosynovitis and tendinitis. Although firing is commonly used on these conditions, there is little indication to do so. There is already too much inflammation and scar tissue present.

(f) Sesamoiditis. Firing is of doubtful value in this condition. It is commonly used but seldom effects a cure.

(g) Bone spavin. Bone spavin is commonly fired in an effort to aid ankylosis of the distal intertarsal and tarsometatarsal joints. These joints may ankylose regardless of whether firing is done. Surgical arthrodesis is of more value.

(h) Splints. Splints are commonly fired even though they will heal without any therapy. Rest must be enforced to obtain healing of the splint and firing usually will aid in forcing this rest.

Contraindications for Therapeutic Cautery

(a) Near open wounds.

(b) Areas of dermatitis or infection.

(c) Acute inflammation. Any area that is fired should be rested until the acute inflammation has subsided.

(d) Flexor surface of a joint, especially the flexor side of the carpus where skin folds upon itself.

(e) Healthy tissue. In some areas it is a common procedure to fire horses prior to training in the mistaken belief that it will strengthen the parts. Scar tissue is not as strong as normal tissue, and it is poor practice to fire in this fashion.

(f) Very young horses.

(g) Weak and emaciated animals.

(h) New bone growth in an active stage. Firing may cause a flare-up of the bone activity and the new bone growth may be greater than it would have been otherwise.

(i) Areas where corticoids have recently been used (within thirty days).

Instruments for Firing

(a) Ether firing iron. This instrument makes objectionable noise, and when the flame goes out, it makes a loud report that disturbs the horse.

(b) Hand-made irons. Hand-made irons are constructed so that the point is backed up by a large portion of iron. The heat in the iron will keep the point hot so that four or five points can be made in the skin before it requires reheating. This type of iron is usually heated by a blowtorch.

(c) Crude apparatus such as hot nails has been used in the past.

(d) Electric cautery. This is by far the best instrument for therapeutic cautery. Different-sized points are available, as well as instruments for cauterizing and removal of granulation tissues (see Fig. 11–3). These instruments are silent and portable. A selection of point size decreases danger of puncturing a joint capsule. A smaller point should be used for firing fetlocks than for carpal joints.

(e) Line-firing instruments. Line firing is not recommended and does not cause any more irritation than blistering. A flat instrument, $\frac{1}{8}''$ wide, is ordinarily used, and the skin must not be penetrated with the instrument. Lines should not be closer than $\frac{1}{2}''$ apart. Various lines and chevron patterns are made but these are strictly up to the artistic ability of the operator. Point firing is more effective than line firing.

Point Firing. If at all possible, the horse should be fired in a standing position. A tranquilizer can be given for sedation of nervous horses. Many horses that are docile become alarmed when they smell burning skin. In some cases, two or three penetrations of the skin are all that can be made before the horse moves. By making only two or three firing holes and then stopping before the smoke reaches the horse's nostrils, this can be overcome. A horse that is fired in a recumbent position invariably has an irregular firing pattern.

The technique used is outlined below:

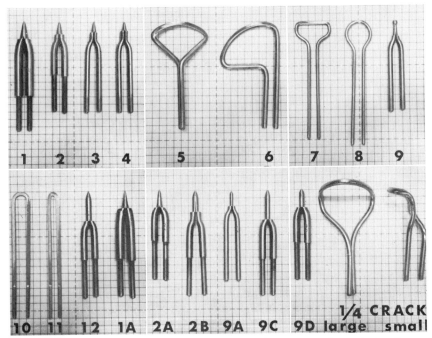

Fig. 11–3. An illustration of accessories for an electric firing iron. Instruments for point firing, line firing, cautery and removal of granulation tissue are shown. (Courtesy Nicholson Manufacturing Company, Chicago, Ill.)

1. The area to be fired is clipped with a No. 40 clipper blade.
2. The skin surface is then scrubbed with soap and water and a skin antiseptic applied. All scurf must be removed.
3. Induction of local anesthesia:
   a. Carpus. The carpus can be blocked in two ways. The author prefers to infiltrate the anterior surface of the carpus subcutaneously with 1 percent procaine. A line block is put across the top of the carpus, and then, by injecting down the sides of the carpus and under the skin of the dorsal surface, a pad of 1 percent procaine is formed under the entire skin area. This type of block produces good anesthesia and protects the joint capsule as well, by cooling the firing point.

   The carpus can be anesthetized by blocking the median, ulnar, and musculocutaneous nerves. This block is effective for anesthesia but does not give as much protection to the joint capsule. Protection of the joint capsule is advisable in case a horse jumps suddenly into the firing iron. When a procaine pad has been used, the firing point will rarely penetrate the capsule because of the cooling effect of the procaine. The capsule can be inadvertently punctured if there is no protective pad.

   b. Fetlock. Modern anesthetics make it possible to completely anesthetize the fetlock, using a ring block approximately 3″ above the metacarpophalangeal joint. The volar nerves are located between the suspensory ligament and the deep flexor tendon (Fig. 4–12). Both medial and lateral volar nerves are blocked at this point, and then a subcutaneous block is used to complete a ring block around the limb (see Chap. 4, p. 109). Special attention should be given to blocking a small nerve that runs between the second and third and third and fourth metacarpal bones. It lies in the groove at the junction of these bones, and a 25-gauge needle is used to carry local anesthetic to the bone at these points. At all other points around the limb, it is satisfactory to use subcutaneous block. With a drug like 2 percent lidocaine hydrochloride* the block can be completed with approximately 12 cc of the local anesthetic.

   c. Other areas such as a bone spavin or splint can be blocked by subcutaneous infiltration of the local anesthetic over the part.

A point-firing pattern can be set up in a block pattern or diagonal pattern (Fig. 11–4). When applying the point, it is better to make the pattern first; then if the points are not deep enough, they can be retraced until the firing point has reached proper depth. Holes in the pattern should not be closer than $\frac{3}{8}''$ to $\frac{1}{2}''$ to each other.

There are several factors to consider in point-firing:

1. Heat of firing iron. A cherry-red heat is the correct heat for firing. If it is hotter than this, it will burn tissue excessively.
2. Length of time firing point is in the skin. It is better to touch a firing hole twice quickly than to hold the iron in place too long. Leaving the firing point too long in the skin or making the holes too close will cause necrotic areas that can coalesce and cause sloughing of skin.

*Xylocaine, Astra Laboratories.

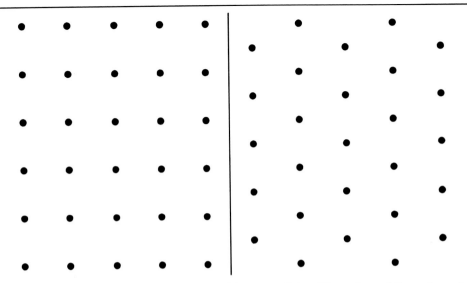

Fig. 11-4. Rectangular and diagonal pattern used for point-firing. The points of the pattern should not be closer than $\frac{3}{8}''$ to $\frac{1}{2}''$ apart.

3. Excessive pressure. It may cause penetration of a synovial structure or penetrate bone. Bone penetration causes risk of osteomyelitis or local bone necrosis and is done only over splints or bone spavin.
4. Sudden movements of the horse. One arm resting on the horse can often give the operator an indication that movement is about to occur.
5. Penetration of artery or vein. When firing the fetlock joint, care should be taken not to penetrate the digital artery or vein on the abaxial surface of the sesamoid bone. Although this is usually not serious, it is unsightly and can be avoided by not allowing the firing point to penetrate beneath the skin in this area.

Line Firing. Line firing is ordinarily used along the volar surface of tendons or over the long axis of the stifle joint. It is done under local anesthetic and the edge of the instrument should not be greater than $\frac{1}{8}''$ wide. I feel that line firing is so ineffective that it does not deserve consideration. It causes no more inflammation than an ordinary blister.

Aftercare of Firing. I discourage the use of a blistering agent after firing. Some veterinarians have recommended the use of mercuric iodide blisters following firing. If the firing points are as deep as they should be, the blister may cause severe sloughing of skin by causing subcutaneous tissue necrosis. This sloughing is serious, unsightly, and requires a long healing period. A leg paint, in my opinion, is preferable to a blistering agent. A leg paint that is effective in producing prolonged irritation as well as having some anesthetic qualities is compounded as follows: 2 parts 7 percent tincture of iodine, 1 part glycerine, and 1 part liquid phenol. Although it can be argued that the alcohol in the tincture of iodine will neutralize the phenol, this does not seem to be entirely true. Enough of the phenol is neutralized that it does not cause necrosis, and the presence of some phenol seems to have an anesthetic effect. It is rare to have a horse that will chew at a bandage when this type of leg paint is used. The leg paint is applied daily for 21 days, using a brush to apply the paint into the wounds. The limb is then wrapped for protection with 14″ × 16″ combine pads* and muslin wraps. Leg paint acts as a local anesthetic and a germicidal agent, and it prolongs irritation. In approximately ten days, a scaling will occur that shows that the superficial layers of skin are sloughing as a result of the leg paint. This is not serious and does not go deeper than the very superficial layers of the skin. After 21 days the leg paint is stopped, but the limb is kept in wraps for a variable period of time. The horse should be rested six months following firing.

Unfortunate sequelae of firing:
  Sloughing of skin
  Tetanus
  Wound infection and septicemia
  Laminitis (from the inflammation produced by firing)
  Suppurative arthritis and synovitis (from penetrating a synovial membrane with a firing iron)

General Considerations for Firing. Radiographs are essential to proper evaluation of the bones and to a well-founded decision on whether firing should be used. This procedure will help prevent missing chip fractures and other conditions that contraindicate firing. Firing is most favorable for chronic and subacute conditions of soft tissue but it is also used where periosteal new bone growth has occurred but is not in the active stages. Firing is of no value if periosteal new bone growth involves the articular surface of a joint.

Other Methods of Producing Counterirritation

Methods of producing irritation with caustic agents have been used, but they are not recommended. The application of acid to a perforated piece of plastic to allow the acid to cause necrosis of skin

*Johnson & Johnson Co.

at selected points approximately $\frac{1}{2}''$ apart has been described, but it is not as effective as therapeutic cautery.

Injection of irritants to produce counterinflammation has been described (Milne, 1960). This technique has been shown to be more effective in producing inflammation than either firing or blistering. Injection of Lugol's iodine diluted from 1:2 to 1:20 has been used, as well as 5 percent aqueous iodine solution. These irritating products are injected along tendons in 1- to 1.5-cc amounts, approximately 1″ apart. A total of 10 to 15 cc of the irritating product is used. This is followed by bandaging. Light work is instituted five to six weeks after injection. Unfortunately, in most tendonitis cases, there is already too much scar tissue and inflammation. This type of treatment may aid resolution of tendosynovitis by increasing blood supply, as is claimed for Asheim's operation (see Tendosynovitis, Chap. 6). Such injections must be done following careful preparation of the skin by clipping, scrubbing, and application of skin antiseptic to prevent possible infection and sloughing.

Radiation Therapy

Radiation therapy is another way of producing deep inflammation. Contrary to some reports that would indicate that it has an anti-inflammatory effect, it actually produces an inflammatory reaction that can last for approximately six weeks (Dixon, 1965). The phenomenon of immediate improvement from lameness does occasionally occur, but this may be the result of damage to nerve endings. A minimum of 90 days' rest must be allowed following radiation therapy for best results. Long-term improvement is probably due to smoothing by osteophytes.

Radiation therapy can be applied in a number of ways. The most satisfactory methods have employed the therapeutic x-ray machine or gamma radiation using cobalt-60 needles. Cobalt-60 needles have proven to be the most easily handled and the most satisfactory method of radiation therapy. Radium has also been used, but in case of an accidental breakage of a radium container, the radium powder can contaminate an area for several years. This makes it undesirable to use around horses. Cobalt-60 is prepared in wires and if the outer container should break, the wire is easily found with a counter. Radon gas enclosed in glass or beads has also been used and has the advantage of having a very short half-life, but it is expensive, since it can be used only once. The same radiation safety procedures must be used with radon as with any other radioactive source. Unfortunately, radon and radium presently are available in some states without license. In some cases, practitioners are endangering themselves because they do not fully appreciate the dangers involved in radiation therapy.

Cobalt-60 needles can be placed in packs and taped directly over the area to be irradiated. This is a distinct advantage over a therapeutic x-ray machine, with which the slightest movement of the horse will change the intensity of the beam on the area to be irradiated. In all cases, radiation therapy should be administered by a person specially trained in the use of this therapy and not done without proper precautions both for the horse and for persons in contact with the horse. It is usually best not to follow radiation therapy with a treatment like ultrasound, which also produces deep inflammation. The long-lasting inflammation already present from radiation therapy could be aggravated enough by ultrasound to produce damage to bone or soft tissue.

The rate of the therapy and the energy of the source must be computed carefully or results will vary. When cobalt-60 packs are used, the strength of the pack should be sufficient to administer the therapy at the rate of 12 to 20 roentgens per hour. Experimental work has shown that in-flammation following this type of therapy lasts six weeks or more and that actual decrease in bone density occurs (Dixon, 1965). This decreased bone density is the result of inflammation and does correct itself after approximately 40 days. Decrased bone density could, in theory, lead to a fracture if the horse is not properly rested.

Before radiation treatment, the affected joint must be radiographed. This will ensure that the cause of lameness is not a small chip fracture or other conditions best handled surgically. If articular cartilage is destroyed, radiation therapy has been recognized as palliative only. Therefore, if joint narrowing, sclerosis, or cyst formation are noted radiographically, results will not be as favorable.

The following conditions are treated with radiation therapy: chronic traumatic arthritis and osteoarthritis of the carpal joint, chronic traumatic arthritis and osteoarthritis of the metacarpophalangeal joint, periosteal new bone growth of the carpal bones, and other conditions where a deep prolonged inflammatory reaction is indicated. Generally, the type of arthritic lesion that seems to respond most satisfactorily to radiation therapy is one in which the changes are periarticular only. These changes may be soft tissue changes only or may have progressed to new bone growth. The dosage for the above conditions is usually 750 to 1,000 roentgens.

Radiation therapy is also effective on some cases of equine sarcoid, equine fibrosarcoma, and equine squamous cell carcinoma. When radiation therapy is used on these conditions, a dose that is strong enough to kill superficial and deep cells is used. The dosage for treating equine sarcoid, fibrosarcoma, and squamous cell carcinoma will range from 4,500 to 6,000 roentgens. Two thousand roentgens are used to treat sarcoid over the carpus because of proximity to the carpal bones, leading to possible demineralization.

Poultices or Cataplasms

These agents work through high osmotic tension to draw fluid from the part toward the surface. Examples of such agents are Denver Mud,* magnesium sulfate, fuller's earth (impure aluminum silicate), boric acid paste, kaolin poultice (combination of kaolin, glycerin, water, and aconite), and Unna's paste. Poultices tend to limit infectious or noninfectious inflammatory processes. They are very good over puncture wounds. Some of these agents are not applied directly to the skin, for they might cause excessive moistening of the skin. An agent like Denver Mud can be applied directly on the skin with little detrimental effect. A bandage is placed over the poultice, and it is usually left in position for 12 to 48 hours. A poultice may be reapplied at intervals several times. Covering the poultice with plastic sheeting increases its efficiency.

These agents are very useful after surgery if there is a tendency for more than average swelling to occur. They can be applied over the surgical wound and around the rest of the limb and can be kept under bandage. Applications are changed periodically according to the type of agent used.

Unna's paste is popular in other countries as an antiphlogistic poultice (Irwin and Hofmeyr, 1961). It is also used for supporting bandages. It is made by mixing the following ingredients: zinc oxide, 150 gm; gelatin, 150 gm; glycerine, 350 ml; and water, 350 ml. The solid ingredients are mixed and the liquids are added, and the mass is stirred and heated in a double boiler. When the material acquires the consistency of heavy paint, it is ready for use. When cold, the paste assumes the springy consistency of foam rubber. Unused paste is reheated in the double boiler and used as required. The paste is applied to a conforming gauze bandage using a 2″

*Demco Corp., Denver, Colo.

brush. The paint is liberally applied to the part to be bandaged and to the gauze as it is rolled on. Adequate paste should be painted onto the gauze to ensure that each layer of bandage adheres to its predecessor. No knots, pins, or other fastening devices are necessary. The horse is kept away from dust and bedding for 20 minutes, giving the paste time to set. The bandage is firm but flexible and can stay in place for several days. Removal is readily effected by cutting the bandage longitudinally, and peeling it off. This type of bandage is used in a horse for support for flexor tendons, as a pressure bandage to aid resorption of excess synovia, to prevent swelling in the legs of a horse confined to stable, and as pressure bandaging of a wound in an effort to prevent excessive granulation tissue. This paste can also be used instead of pine tar and oakum in cases of punctured sole in the convalescent stage.

There are commercially available medicated gauze bandages* that accomplish the same purpose as the paste bandage described above. They serve as support bandages as well as poultice bandages. They are often used after surgery as support bandages when a plaster cast is not required.

The Use of Anti-inflammatory Agents

The use of anti-inflammatory agents is now well established in veterinary medicine. The products used are corticoids and phenylbutazone (Butazolidin, Jensen-Salsbery Laboratories) oxyphenylbutazone (Tandearil, Geigy) and methylated, fluorinated Prednisolone-Dexamethasone (Azium, Schering). Depending on the individual product, these drugs can be given in a variety of ways. New additions to the field are claimed to be more effective

*Gelocast, Duke Laboratories South Norwalk, Conn.; Medicopaste, Graham Field Laboratories, Woodside, N.J.

than older ones that were formerly popular. The main use of these products has been for anti-inflammatory action in lamenesses, especially arthritic involvements. It has been found that they also can be used with judgment to aid in relief of postsurgical pain and swelling. When used in this manner, they must be used with discretion and be covered by the use of parenteral antibiotics. Although phenylbutazone and oxyphenylbutazone are effective for these purposes, they can apparently lower the resistance of the wound to infection, just as the corticoids do. The routine use of these drugs after joint surgery will occasionally be accompanied by postsurgical infection and destruction of the operated joint. The corticoids also are used by injection locally into tendosynovitis, splints, and other local inflammatory conditions. Tendosynovitis can also be treated parenterally with corticoids while the lesion heals in a cast. Intra-articular use of corticoids is popular and beneficial in many cases. However, in many cases it is used to alleviate symptoms of lameness without allowing sufficient rest for healing of the part. In this case, additional damage is done to the joint while the horse goes on with racing workouts. This eventually leads to a complete degeneration of the joint. The same can be true of parenteral injection of corticoids and phenylbutazone derivatives.

One should not use a counterirritation method after the use of an anti-inflammatory drug. In some cases, a joint is injected and a blister or point firing is used over the joint. This is completely contraindicated, since it amounts to using two exactly opposite methods of therapy. When a horse has received intra-articular injections for a lameness, e.g., carpal fracture or sesamoid fracture, it is advisable to wait a while before performing surgery for removal of the chip fracture. The prognosis is poor, since the chip fracture should be removed as soon as possible

after it occurs. The intra-articular injection or parenteral use of corticoids and/or phenylbutazone derivatives allows the horse to use the joint and causes degenerative changes as a result of the fracture. In addition, corticoid injections may lower the tissue resistance of the part, making it more likely that infection will result from surgery. This type of therapy should be discouraged, and before a surgical procedure is done on a joint, inquiry should be made as to how many times it has been treated with a corticoid, or how long the horse has been on parenteral or oral therapy with corticoids or phenylbutazone derivatives.

Intra-articular Injection

Controlled research by Meagher (1970) has shown that the use of corticoids in the carpal joints is detrimental and contraindicated when fractures are present and when the horse is worked after the corticoid injections. Under these circumstances, injection of a long-acting corticoid caused demineralization of the fragment and cartilage erosion. Dehiscence and infection of operative wounds occurred when the fractures were removed. This may be the result of the synovial membrane rapidly taking up the corticoid from the joint, from which it is slowly eliminated (Uvarov, 1963). These changes were not present in carpal joints that had fractures but no corticoid injections. Meagher's conclusion was that corticoids should not be used in cases of carpal fractures and that any injection of a corticoid into a joint should be followed by at least 30 days of rest.

Corticoids are being grossly misused at present. No joint should be injected with a corticoid without prior radiologic examination. Intra-articular injections of corticoids will permit a horse to use a joint that has extensive pathologic changes, thereby causing further degenerative changes. If a fracture is present, the joint should not be injected if any long-term working future is expected for the horse. The ill-advised injection of a corticosteroid during the time of degenerative arthritis or reparable fractures frequently causes a more rapid destruction of the joint with the production of extensive degenerative lesions that cannot be corrected by surgery. This causes many hopeless cases to be presented for surgery when the corticosteroids are no longer effective, whereas if they had been operated upon early, a successful result could have been anticipated (Meagher, 1970). Surgery for joint fractures following corticoid injections is often disastrous. Only if the racing future of the horse is considered extremely short should corticoid injections be considered. In addition, there is good evidence that repeated injections of corticoids into a joint can cause joint destruction by degeneration of joint cartilage (Meagher, 1970). This can occur even though aseptic technique is used. The addition of hyaluronic acid to a corticoid may improve results by contributing to joint lubrication, possibly lessening the likelihood of cartilage damage (Rydell et al., 1970).

The site of action of corticoids, following intra-articular injection, appears to be the synovial membrane. These drugs cause a suppression of inflammation that allows recovery of cellular function. Synovial fluid volume is reduced, and its viscosity is increased to normal. To obtain optimal results, the hormone should be injected directly into the synovial space; however, it also has been established that injection of the drugs into tissues that are inflamed from noninfectious causes is of considerable therapeutic aid. Such noninfectious conditions include acute bowed tendon, splints, and bucked shins (see Chap. 6). One should remember that the long-acting steroids often cause calcification if injected into soft tissue (Fig. 11–5). Long-acting steroids are for use within the joint only.

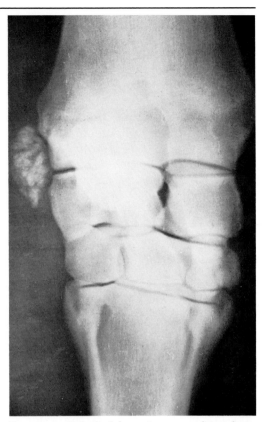

FIG. 11–5. Calcified hematoma resulting from injection of the carpus with a corticoid. When passing the needle into a joint there is a danger of hitting blood vessels. In some cases the resulting hemorrhage will calcify as shown. A small needle, and an attempt to miss all skin vessels when passing the needle, will help in preventing such a complication. Calcification is sometimes caused by the long-acting corticoids when injected into soft tissue, presumably by the chemicals used to delay absorption.

The exact mode of anti-inflammatory action of the corticoids is unknown; however, some investigators believe the hormone acts as a buffer or shield between irritants and susceptible cells. Other authorities claim that the activity of the injured cell is altered so that it is less effective in producing some of the specific factors responsible for inflammation. The inflammatory responses to irritants are decreased and fibrosis is prevented because mesenchymal cell (fibrocyte) proliferation is inhibited. Corticoids delay healing by inhibiting hyaluronadase activity and inhibiting fibrocyte proliferation. In addition, the capacity of tissues to wall off infectious agents is reduced. However, the steroids seem to increase the "insult threshold" of the cell, allowing the restoration of cell function in what would otherwise be a disabling environment. Whatever the mode of action, the value of corticoids in the treatment of joint inflammation is quite firmly established in veterinary practice. Adequate rest must accompany the use of corticoids, for they merely decrease inflammation while healing occurs. Too often, the corticoids are used to mask symptoms, and the horse is allowed to further damage the part.

General Technique. Before any joint cavity is invaded, it is of utmost importance that the skin area be clipped, shaved, and washed thoroughly. A surgical preparation of the injection area should be done. Introduction of bacteria into the joint cavity from the exterior greatly lessens the chances of satisfactory recovery and may even lead to a condition more serious than the one already present. Aseptic precautions also should be observed when using these drugs subcutaneously around local inflammatory conditions such as splints.

A 20-gauge needle should be of sufficient size for most injections; the length of the needle is determined by the area to be injected. In sensitive or nervous animals, infiltration with local anesthetic agent prior to the injection may be necessary; a 25-gauge needle should be used for this purpose. The needle should be pushed into the area quickly without the syringe attached; this avoids the breakage of a needle under the skin if the horse moves quickly.

Entrance into the joint cavity can be confirmed by withdrawing synovial fluid into the syringe. All fluid that can be withdrawn easily should be removed before injection. In some cases, the fluid will run freely through the needle so no syringe is necessary to aspirate the fluid. The end of the needle will move freely when properly positioned in the joint capsule or tendon sheath. If the needle is in the proper place, the injection of fluid will be accomplished easily and without undue pressure from tissue resistance. In some cases, it may be extremely difficult to withdraw any volume of fluid. The cause for this is not always apparent, but it may be that villae plug the lumen of the needle. In such a case, the injection should be continued without prolonged efforts to withdraw fluid.

The amount of corticoid to be injected depends on the size of the joint and the degree of inflammation. The following doses are approximate and vary with the size of the joint:

Hydrocortisone Acetate.—50 to 100 mg in a joint. More can be used in large joints and for subcutaneous injection over an inflammatory process. This product is one of the earliest of the steroid group and is now seldom used since there are other products that are longer-lasting and more effective and have fewer side effects.

Prednisolone (Sterane, Pfizer; Meticorten, Schering). 50 to 100 mg, depending on the size of the joint. More can be used for large joints or for subcutaneous injection over an inflammatory process.

Prednisolone Tertiary—Butylacetate (Hydeltrone—T.B.A., Merck & Co.). 50 to 100 mg, depending on the size of the joint. More may be used in large joints or for subcutaneous injection over an inflammatory process.

9-Fluoroprednisolone Acetate (Predef 2X, Upjohn).—5 to 20 mg, depending on the size of the joint. More can be used in large joints or for subcutaneous injection over an inflammatory process.

Triamcinolone Acetonide—Synthetic Corticosteroid (Kenalog I.M., Squibb).—5 to 15 mg, depending on the size of the joint. More may be used in a large joint or for subcutaneous injection over an inflammatory process.

Methylprednisolone (Depo Medrol, Upjohn).—40 to 80 mg in large joints. This long-acting corticoid is quite effective intra-articularly.

9-Alpha-Difluoro,16-AlphaMethylprednisolone-Flumethasone (Flucort, Syntex).—The dose in horses is 1.5 to 2.5 mg intramuscularly or intra-articularly. It is similar to dexamethasone but can be given intra-articularly, while dexamethasone cannot. This is a long-acting steroid.

Prednisolone Sodium Succinate (Solu-Delta Cortef, Upjohn).—This product is primarily for intravenous use to establish a quick level of steroid effectiveness.

Betamethasone Acetate and Betamethasone Disodium Phosphate (Celestone Soluspan, Schering).—This is a repositol steroid that can be given intra-articularly and intramuscularly. The dose is 1 to 2 cc for large joints, and the concentration is 6 mg per cc. This is a long-acting steroid.

All the above corticoids are contraindicated in the presence of infection without supporting antibiotics. The above list is not complete, but it gives a representative sample of products available. No product should ever be used intra-articularly if it is not specifically manufactured for this purpose.

The interval between injections is dependent upon the severity of the condition and the degree of response to the previous injection. Some severe inflammatory conditions should be injected every two or three days, while less severely affected areas will respond with less frequent injections. After the injection of a corticoid into a joint or tendon sheath, the area should be wrapped to establish counterpressure and to promote absorption of excess fluid.

In some cases, a bandage can be used around the joint, leaving a diamond-shaped opening to aid in forcing fluid from the needle after the joint is punctured. Elastic material such as a rubber-impregnated bandage is of most value in producing this effect.

Some products cause joint swelling after administration. This swelling usually disappears in 24 to 72 hours, and the effect of the drug can then be determined. Products that consistently cause swelling soon after injection should be discontinued. (Cortisone should never be used in joints, since it must be converted by the liver into hydrocortisone in order to produce results.) All the above products may be used intramuscularly for supportive therapy following intra-articular injection. The same doses are used intramuscularly.

After injection, the joint may be manipulated to aid the mixing of synovial fluid and the corticoid suspension. For routine work, it is sometimes advisable to include some antibiotic agent with the corticoid to combat any bacterial organism that might be present without obvious clinical evidence. Crystalline penicillin or crystalline chloromycetin are used for this purpose. Adrenocorticotropic hormone (ACTH) is used intramuscularly to stimulate the adrenal cortex to secrete hydrocortisone as follow-up therapy to injections of corticoids. The usual dose is 200 to 400 units repeated at three- to seven-day intervals.

Specific Injection Sites for the Horse

DISTAL INTERPHALANGEAL (COFFIN) JOINT (Figs. 11–6 and 11–7).—This should be injected from either the medial or lateral side of the midline on the anterior aspect of the foot. The needle should be held in a vertical position and pushed into the joint from just above the coronary band. Fluids injected into the coffin joint may be able to pass into the navicular bursa and the digital flexor tendon sheath by osmosis.

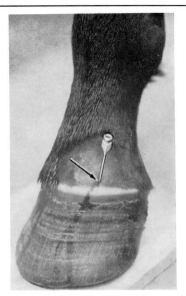

FIG. 11-6. Twenty-gauge, 2″ needle in place to inject the coffin joint. Arrow shows area penetrated by the needle.

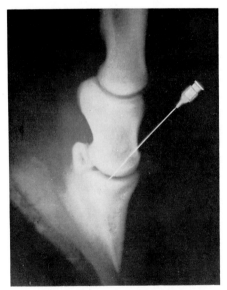

FIG. 11-7. Radiograph showing needle in place to inject the coffin joint. This is the same foot and needle shown in Figure 11-6.

NAVICULAR BURSA (Figs. 11-8 through 11-11).—The navicular bursa should be injected from the posterior aspect of the foot, the needle being directed parallel to or slightly below the angle of the coronary

band. A complete description of the procedure is found under Navicular Disease (Chap. 6, p. 260).

METACARPOPHALANGEAL (FETLOCK) JOINT (Figs. 11-12 and 11-13).—The volar

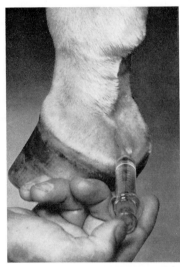

FIG. 11-8. Infiltrating the heel area with a local anesthetic using a 25-gauge $\frac{1}{2}$″ needle in preparation for injection of the navicular bursa. (Reprinted from *Veterinary Scope*, 7(1): 3, 1962; courtesy of Upjohn Company.)

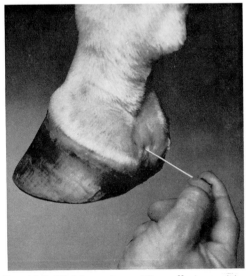

FIG. 11-9. Eighteen-gauge 2″ needle in position where the area has been anesthetized in Figure 11-8.

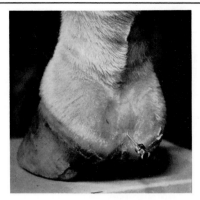

FIG. 11-10. Eighteen-gauge 2″ needle in place in the navicular bursa.

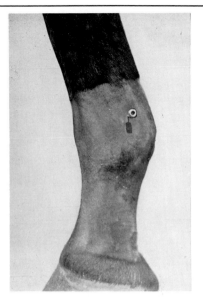

FIG. 11-12. Location of injection into the volar pouch of the fetlock joint. The needle should be positioned just anterior to the sesamoid bone, between the palmar aspect of the cannon bone and the suspensory ligament.

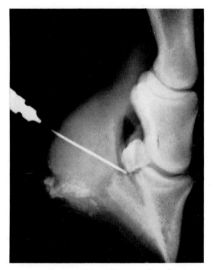

FIG. 11-11. Lateral radiograph showing 18-gauge, 2″ needle in place in the navicular bursa. The dark area above the navicular bone is air that has been injected through the needle to better outline the bursa for radiographic purposes.

pouches of the fetlock joint should be injected from either the medial or lateral side of the leg. The pouches lie between the caudal side of the cannon bone and the suspensory ligament.

CARPAL JOINT.—Injection into the radiocarpal or intercarpal joint is usually easiest with the carpus in a flexed position. When the joint capsule is distended, it is a simple matter to inject the most promi-

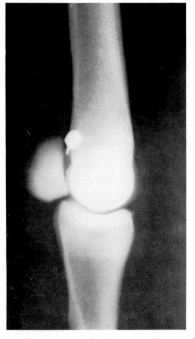

FIG. 11-13. Radiograph showing the needle in position for injection of the volar pouch of the fetlock joint capsule.

nent portion of the swelling with the horse standing. However, if the joint capsule is not distended, it is best to flex the joint to pass the needle (Figs. 11–14, 11–15, 11–16). Injection should be made from the anterior aspect into the joint desired. In many horses there is no communication between the radiocarpal and intercarpal joints. Therefore, the injection should be made into the exact area desired. The

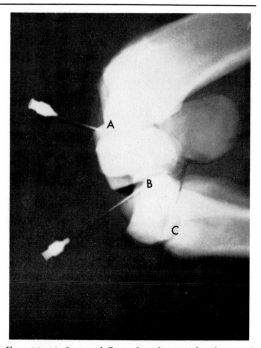

FIG. 11–16. Lateral flexed radiograph of carpal joint with needles in the radiocarpal joint (*A*) and intercarpal joint (*B*). (*C*) shows the carpometacarpal joint, which does not open. The fluid of the radiocarpal joint is separate from that of the intercarpal and carpometacarpal joints in most cases. The joint fluid of the intercarpal and carpometacarpal joints is confluent. (Courtesy of Norden Laboratories.)

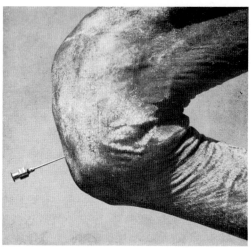

FIG. 11–14. Injection of the intercarpal joint on a flexed carpus.

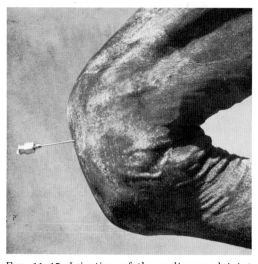

FIG. 11–15. Injection of the radiocarpal joint on a flexed carpus.

intercarpal and carpometacarpal joints communicate (see Chap. 4, p. 100).

HUMERORADIAL (ELBOW) JOINT.—The elbow joint is somewhat difficult to palpate for injection. The joint is flexed repeatedly until the articulation can be distinguished. The needle can be passed from either the anterior side or the posterior aspect into the joint (Fig. 11–17).

SCAPULOHUMERAL (SHOULDER) JOINT.— The shoulder joint is injected in a notch between the two parts of the lateral tuberosity of the humerus (Fig. 11–18). In most cases, this tuberosity can be palpated and the needle carefully passed into the joint.

TIBIOTARSAL (HOCK) JOINT (Fig. 2–14, p. 46; Figs. 11–19 and 11–20).—Injection of

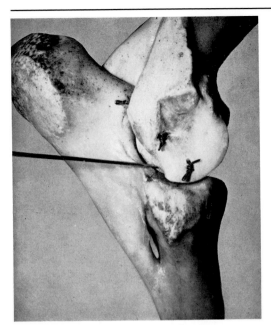

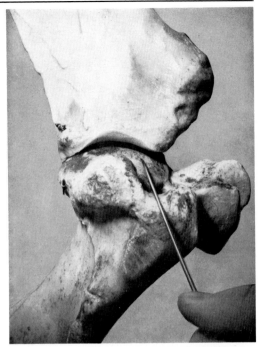

FIG. 11-17. Injection of the humeroradial (elbow) joint. This joint is more difficult than others to inject. The joint is flexed repeatedly until the articulation is determined. The needle can be passed posteriorly as shown or from the anterior aspect.

FIG. 11-18. Injection of the scapulohumeral (shoulder) joint. The needle is passed in the notch between the two processes of the lateral tuberosity of the humerus. The most posterior portion of the lateral tuberosity can usually be palpated, and the needle is passed in front of it.

the tibiotarsal joint should be at the anteromedial aspect of the hock over the most prominent portion of the joint capsule. Care should be taken to avoid the saphenous vein where it crosses the joint.

FEMOROTIBIAL (STIFLE) JOINT.—Injection of the stifle joint can be made into the joint capsule between the medial patellar ligament and the medial collateral ligament of the stifle joint. The femoropatellar pouch can be injected between the middle and medial patellar ligaments or between the middle and lateral patellar ligaments (Fig. 11-21). The femoropatellar pouch communicates through a slit-like opening with the medial portion of the femorotibial joint capsule. This means that the femoropatellar pouch can be injected, and in most cases the injected material will reach the medial portion of the femorotibial joint capsule. The lateral portion of the femorotibial joint capsule

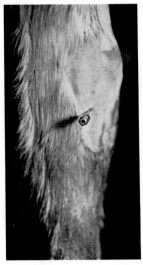

FIG. 11-19. Anterior view of injection of the right tibiotarsal joint. The needle is to the lateral side of the saphenous vein.

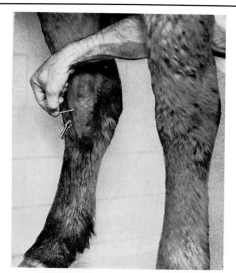

FIG. 11-20. Area of penetration for injection of the tibiotarsal joint for bog spavin. The needle should be forced through the joint capsule, either on the outside or the inside of the saphenous vein, indicated by the arrow.

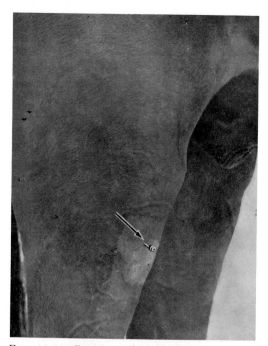

FIG. 11-21. Position of eighteen-gauge, two-inch needle for injecting the femoropatellar pouch, between the lateral and middle patellar ligaments. Arrow indicates the skin area the needle has penetrated.

communicates with the femoropatellar pouch in a small percentage of cases, and if it is desired to have the injected material reach this area, the femorotibial joint capsule should be injected directly between the lateral patellar ligament and the lateral collateral ligament or between the medial patellar ligament and the medial collateral ligament of the femorotibial joint (see Chap. 4, Fig. 4-22).

COXOFEMORAL (HIP) JOINT.—The hip joint is injected through the notch that lies just anterior to the trochanter major of the femur. The trochanter major is followed down on the anterior edge, and the needle passed through the notch in front of it into the joint, as shown in Figure 11-22.

Subcutaneous Injection of Corticoids

When a corticoid is to be injected into subcutaneous tissues, as in the case of bowed tendon or splints, the area should be closely clipped, scrubbed, and prepared with a good skin antiseptic. If the injection is not made under aseptic circumstances, it may cause a suppurative process. Corticoids may be used subcutaneously in most acute, noninfectious inflammatory processes. Corticoids are sometimes used parenterally or locally and followed by the use of a blister. This type of therapy is contraindicated. The corticoids act as an anti-inflammatory agent and the blisters act as an inflammatory agent. There should be at least thirty days between the use of these two methods of therapy. Long-acting corticoids may cause calcification of soft tissues.

Anti-inflammatory Agents with Action Similar to Corticoids

1. *Butazolidin** (phenylbutazone).— Butazolidin is used intravenously and

*Jensen-Salsbery Laboratories.

orally for pain relief in arthritis, but there is no form for intra-articular use. This drug produces an anti-inflammatory action similar to the corticoids. Full doses of a corticoid and phenylbutazone simultaneously are contraindicated. One or the other may be used for anti-inflammatory activity but not full doses of both at the same time. Smaller doses of each are commonly used together. Full doses of each are not used simultaneously because adverse effects caused by these drugs are more likely to occur. The intravenous dose of Butazolidin is 1 to 2 gm per 1,000 pounds of body weight, with a limit of five successive days. The oral dose is 2 to 4 gm daily per 1,000 pounds of body weight. The intravenous form of phenylbutazone should not be given intramuscularly, because in some cases it causes abscess formation. Therapy should be discontinued upon signs of gastrointestinal upset, icterus, or blood dyscrasia. Administration of pain-relieving drugs like corticoids and phenylbutazone should *not* be used as a substitute for accurate diagnosis.

2. *Tandearil* (Oxyphenylbutazone, Geigy).—Tandearil seems to be quite an effective anti-inflammatory agent. It can be used following invasion of a joint for chip fracture for preventing postsurgical pain and swelling. The horse is not kept on the product for longer than ten days, and during its administration its use is covered by antibiotics. The usual initial daily dosage is 2 to 5 gm orally, with gradual reduction of the dose after four days.

Nonsteroidal Anti-inflammatory Drugs for Use in Lameness of Osteoarthritic Origin

A number of drugs are being used clinically and experimentally for relief of lameness. At present, no definitive conclusions can be drawn about their use. A brief description of a few of these products follows. Similar drugs are undergoing

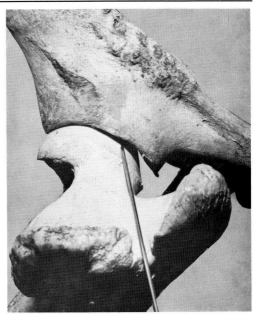

FIG. 11–22. Injection of the coxofemoral (hip) joint. The needle is shown passing through the notch on the anterior side of the trochanter major. Once the needle passes through this notch, it can be pushed gently into the joint capsule. Synovial fluid can often be aspirated.

investigation, but are not approved for use.

1. Meclofenamic acid [N-(2,6-dichloro-m-tolyl) anthranilic acid].* A study was done on this drug by four investigators (Riley *et al.*, 1971) in a variety of lameness. The drug was given orally at a dosage rate of 1 mg/lb for 7 days and for 21 days. There was no toxic effect, and they believed that there was improvement in a significant number of cases. Other research (Voss, 1973) showed it to be effective for relief of pain in pedal osteitis and laminitis and ineffective in osteoarthritis. It has not yet been approved by FDA.

2. Palosein† (orgotein). This is described as a metalloprotein congener isolated from bovine liver. It contains copper and zinc and when administered parenterally is said to be distributed rapidly

*Parke, Davis & Co.
†Diagnostic Data Inc., Mountain View, Calif.

throughout the body. It is claimed that in addition to its anti-inflammatory effect, orgotein protects against shock reactions produced by antigenic challenge after prior sensitization. This might make it useful in various diseases with allergic manifestations, as well as help to ensure that repeated injections of the material would not cause allergic reaction (Cushing et al., 1972). The recommended dosage is 5 mg of Palosein intramuscularly every other day for two weeks and twice a week thereafter for a 4–5 week period, or a total of 15–17 doses. Clinical tests sponsored by the manufacturer claimed good results in a wide variety of bone, joint, and soft tissue problems. Time and use will help to determine its true value. The cost of the drug is a limitation to its use at the present time.

3. Adenolin Forte (Adenosine-5-Monophosphate). This drug is claimed to be an effective nonsteroid anti-inflammatory agent that is useful in treating acute arthritis, bursitis, tendinitis, and other collagen diseases. The drug is said to aid in proper restoration of muscle function and to furnish coenzyme replacement of adenosine-5-monophosphate. Opinion on the use of the drug in horses is variable. Any analgesic effects seem to be temporary.

4. Indocin* (indomethacin MSD). Indocin is a nonsteroidal drug with anti-inflammatory, antipyretic, and analgesic properties. Its mode of action, like others of this group, it not known. It seems to be most indicated in arthritic conditions, but its use in horses is not well documented. The manufacturer stresses that it is not a simple analgesic and that it should be used with caution, since it may be accompanied by serious side effects.

Dimethyl Sulfoxide (DMSO)†

Dimethyl sulfoxide is an oxidation product of dimethyl sulfide and is a by-product of kraft paper processing. It was, and still is, used as a preservative for various cells and tissues. It is a solvent and mixes with many other common solvents and with water. It is extremely hygroscopic and will absorb 70 percent of its weight from air under the right temperature and humidity conditions. This hygroscopic property makes sealing the bottle after use mandatory. Its penetration of the skin reaches a maximum when it is mixed with 10 percent water.

The mechanism of penetration has not been fully explained (Diamond Labs, 1972), but it may be combination with intracellular water. A number of products, such as steroids, seem to be absorbed from the skin when combined with DMSO.

Various claims have been made for the drug, but most claims have not been substantiated by adequate research. In the hands of the author, the drug was only mediocre in value. It apparently has its greatest use in reducing acute swelling of noninfectious origin. Seromas, hematomas, and edema from trauma, when the skin is not broken, apparently respond quite well to application of this drug. However, in most other types of treatment, the drug seems to be of little value. It is contraindicated on raw wound surfaces. DMSO apparently can carry drugs through the skin, and various claims have been made for remedies utilizing this quality. Treatment of ringworm with thiabendazole to increase the penetrability of the fungicide has been tried and claimed to be of value. DMSO will carry irritating drugs into tissue, and one should be very cautious before using it on an area to which any type of blistering material containing iodine, turpentine, camphor, or similar substances has been applied previously, because it may cause severe reaction due to deep penetration by these agents. Corticoids have been mixed with DMSO with the hope that they would be carried to deeper tissues; as yet, however, no experimental evidence has proven this

*Merck Sharp and Dohme, West Point, Pa.
†DOMSO, Syntex Laboratories, Palo Alto, Calif.

to be valid. Frequently, the topical application of DMSO causes a transient irritation in the skin that may cause the horse to bite at the area treated. The drug should not be applied with bare hands, and the maximum daily dose is 100 cc divided equally in two or three applications (Diamond Labs, 1972).

REFERENCES

ALEXANDER, J. T. 1971. The application of a fiberglass cast to the equine forelimb. Proc. 17th Ann. AAEP, 269–278.

BRACKEN, F. 1965. Physical therapy in veterinary medicine. Ann. Conf. Vet. Colorado State University.

BRONEMARK, P. I. 1967. Observation on the action of intra-articularly administered prednisolone, tertiary butyl acetate (Codelcortone) and methyl prednisolone acetate (Depomedrove) in the normal rabbit knee joint. Acta Orthopoed. Scand. 38(2): 247.

BUNN, C. E. E., and J. E. BURCH. 1955. Hydrocortisone in the treatment of traumatic arthritis in thoroughbreds. N. Amer. Vet. 36: 458.

BUNIM, J. J. (ed.). 1959. A decade of anti-inflammatory steroids, from cortisone to dexamethasone. Ann. N.Y. Acad. Sci. 82: 797.

BURDICK CORPORATION. 1961. Ultrasonic Therapy Abstracts from Current Literature. Milton, Wisc.

BUSCHKE, F. 1958. Progress in Radiation Therapy. New York: Grune & Stratton. pp. 16, 17, 20.

CARLSON, W. D. 1967. Veterinary Radiology. 2nd ed. Philadelphia: Lea & Febiger.

CHARYLULU, K. K. N. 1964. Recent advances in radiation therapy. J. Vet. Rad. Soc. 5: 70.

CLAPP, N. K., W. D. CARLSON, and J. P. MORGAN. 1963. Radiation therapy for lameness in horses. JAVMA 143(3): 277.

CUSHING, L. S., et al. 1972. Treatment of Orthopedic Disorders in Horses by Palosein. Mountain View, Calif.: Diagnostic Data Inc.

DAVIDSON, A. H., and W. C. FRANK. 1966. Anti-inflammatory agents in equine surgery. Mod. Vet. Pract. 47: 46–49.

DENNY, B. 1959. Short wave radiotherapy in veterinary practice. Brit. Vet. J. 115: 341–350.

Diamond Labs Inc. 1972. Questions and Answers DOMSO. Des Moines, Iowa.

DILLON, R. 1956. Corticosteroids in the treatment of certain equine lamenesses. Vet. Med. 51: 191.

DIXON, R. T.: 1965. Some effects of cobalt 60 gamma irradiation of the equine carpus. Thesis, Colorado State University.

DUNN, P. S. 1972. A clinician's views on the use and misuse of phenylbutazone. Eq. Vet. J. 4(2): 63–65.

EBERT, E. F. 1962. Clinical use of phenylbutazone in large animals. Vet. Med. 57: 33–35.

FARQUHARSON, B. 1966. Lameness symposium. Proc. AAEP, 329.

FRANK, E. R. 1964. Veterinary Surgery. 7th ed. Minneapolis: Burgess Publishing Co.

FRASER, A. C. 1961. The treatment of lameness by faradism. Vet. Rec. 73(5): 94.

GARNER, H. E., L. E. ST. CLAIR, and H. J. HARDENBROOK. 1969. Clinical and radiographic studies of the distal portion of the radius in race horses. JAVMA 149(12): 1536–1540.

GARMER, L. 1965a. Corticosteroid injection for treatment of leg injuries. Nord. Vet. Med. 17(10): 516–529.

GARMER, L. 1965b. Osseous metaplasia, a complication of local corticosteroid treatment in the horse. Nord. Vet. Med. 17(10): 529.

GAUNT, R., et al. 1958. The adrenal cortex. Ann. N.Y. Acad. Sci. 50: 509.

GILLETTE, E. L. 1965. Radiation therapy. Ann. Conf. Vet. Colorado State University.

GILLETTE, E. L., and W. D. CARLSON. 1964. An evaluation of radiation therapy in veterinary medicine. J. Amer. Vet. Rad. Soc. 5: 58.

GORMAN, H. A., et al. 1968. The effect of oxyphenylbutazone on surgical wounds. JAVMA. 152(5): 487–491.

GUARD, W. F. 1953. Surgical Principles and Techniques. 2nd ed. Ann Arbor, Mich.: Edwards Brothers, Inc.

HAYES, I. E. 1954. Treatment of equine coxitis with intra-articular hydrocortisone. N. Amer. Vet. 35: 673.

HANSELKA, D. V., et al. 1972. External fixation of a large animal fracture with a resin-bonded fiberglass cast. VM/SAC 67: 519–525.

HICKMAN, J. 1964. Veterinary Orthopaedics. Philadelphia: J. B. Lippincott.

HOLLANDER, J. E. (ed.): Arthritis. 8th ed. Philadelphia: Lea & Febiger.

HOPES, R. 1972. Uses and misuses of anti-inflammatory drugs in race horses—I. Eq. Vet. 4(2): 66–68.

HOUDESHELL, J. W. 1970. The effect of a corticosteroid on blood and synovial fluid in horses. VM/SAC 65: 963–966.

HUNT, M. D. 1963. The role of corticosteroids in equine practice. 2nd Ann. Cong. Brit. Eq. Vet. Assoc. 25–28.

IRWIN, D. H. G., and C. F. V. HOFMEYR. 1961. Unna's sticky paste as a practical aid to bandaging. J. S. Afr. Vet. Med. Assoc. 32(3): 431.

JACOB, S. 1964. Dimethyl sulfoxide. Paper presented at Washington State Veterinary Conference.

JOHNSON, L. E., et al. 1960. Panel on equine radiology. Proc. 6th Ann. AAEP, 35.

KATTMAN, J., and J. KRUL, 1960. Intra-articular injection of penicillin and streptomycin. Veterinarni Medicina 5: 55.

LEWIS, R. E. 1965. Radiation therapy of sarcoids and carcinomas. Mod. Vet. Pract. 46(1): 37.

MacKay, A. G. 1967. Articular cartilage erosion. Can. Vet. J. 8(6): 134–135.

Mankin, H. J., and K. A. Conger. 1966. The acute effects of intra-articular hydrocortisone on articular cartilage in rabbits. J. Bone Joint Surg. 43: 1383.

McGinnis, P. J., and E. F. Lutterbeck. 1951. Roentgen therapy of inflammatory conditions affecting the legs of thoroughbred horses. N. Amer. Vet. 32: 540.

McGinnis, P. J., 1954. Further clinical experience with radiation therapy in race horses. N. Amer. Vet. 35: 431.

Meagher, D. M. 1970. The effects of intra-articular corticosteroids and continued training on carpal chip fractures of horses. Proc. AAEP, 405.

Merck & Co. 1967. Merck Veterinary Manual. 3rd ed., Rahway, N.J.

Milne, F. J. 1960. Subcutaneously induced counter-irritation. Proc. 6th Ann. AAEP, 25.

Miner, R. W., G. Pinius et al. (ed.). 1955. Hydrocortisone, its newer analogs and aldosterone as therapeutic agents. Ann. N.Y. Acad. Sci. 61: 281.

Morgan, J. P. 1964. Personal communication.

Moss, M. S. 1972. Uses and misuses of anti-inflammatory drugs in race horses—II. Eq. Vet. J. 4(2): 69–73.

Murray, D. M. 1967. Current concepts on intra-articular infections of corticosteroids. 28th Ann. Con. for Vet., Colorado State University.

Nordensson, L. G. 1965. Intermittent ultrasonic treatment of certain forms of lameness in horses. Svensk. Vet. 17: 165–168.

O'Connor, J. T. 1969. Avoiding and treating the untoward effects of the corticosteroids. Proc. 15th Ann. AAEP, 75–83.

Ohme, F. W. 1962. Phenylbutazone in the treatment of soft tissue reactions of large animals. Vet Med. 57: 229–231.

Owen, D. 1971. Arthrocentesis techniques in treating equine joint disease. Proc. 17th Ann. AAEP, 263–267.

Panel Report, 1963. Use of firing. Mod. Vet. Pract. 44(3): 54.

Panel Report, 1967. Corticosteroid therapy. Mod Vet. Pract. 48(8): 54–67.

Quinlan, J. 1959. Intra-articular and intra-thecal prednisolone in the treatment of traumatic inflammation of synovial structures in equines. J. S. Afr. Vet. Med. Assoc. 30(3): 235.

Raker, C. W. 1962. Injection and radiography of movable joints. Norden News 37(4): 6–8.

Riley, W. F., Jr. 1956. Corticosteroids in the treatment of certain equine lamenesses. Vet. Med. 51: 191.

Riley, W. F., et al. 1971. Preliminary report on a new non-steroidal anti-inflammatory agent in the horse. Proc. 17th Ann. AAEP, 293–308.

Rydell, N. W. et al. 1970. Hyaluronic acid in synovial fluid. Acta. Vet. Scand. 11(F2): 139–155.

Silver, I. A., and D. B. Cater. 1964. Radiotherapy and chemotherapy for domestic animals: I. Treatment of malignant tumors and benign conditions in horses. Acta Radiol. (Ther) 2: 226.

Simkin, B. 1964. Corticosteroids in clinical practice. Eye Ear Nose Throat Mon. 43: 47–54.

Sisson, S. 1953. Anatomy of Domestic Animals. 4th ed. J. D. Crossman, ed. Philadelphia: W. B. Saunders Co.

Stevenson, A. C. et al. 1972. Chromosome findings in horses treated with phenylbutazone. Eq. Vet. J. 4(4): 214–216.

Stihl, H. G., and A. Leuthold. 1964. Subcutaneous iodine therapy of chronic tendonitis in the horse. Schweiz. Arch. Tierheilk. 106: 218.

Strong, C. L. 1967. Horses' Injuries. London: Faber and Faber.

Temple, J. L. 1960. Fluoprednisolone in race horse practice. JAVMA 137: 136.

Thom, M. 1950. Some indications for x-ray and radium therapy in large animal practice. Proc. 87th Ann. Meeting, AVMA, 63.

Thom, M. 1955. Radiation therapy, using x-ray. N. Amer. Vet. 36: 111.

Thom, M. 1963. Equine Medicine and Surgery. Santa Barbara, Calif.: American Veterinary Publishers Inc. p. 513.

Thom, M. 1966. Radiation therapy of joint and tendon lesions. Proc. AAEP, 325–327.

Thom, M., et al. 1960. Panel on equine radiology. Proc. 6th Ann. AAEP, 35.

Tiegland, M. B., and V. R. Saurino. 1968. Clinical evaluation of dimethyl sulfoxide. Ann. N.Y. Acad. Sci. 141(1): 471.

Trussell, W. E. 1965a. Clinical response to intra-synovial injection of flumethasone in a horse. Vet. Med. 60: 60.

Trussell, W. E. 1965b. Intrasynovial injection of flumethazone. VM/SAC 60: 610–615.

Uvarov, O. 1963. Corticosteroids in equine practice. 2nd Ann. Cong. Brit. Eq. Vet. Assoc., 29–35.

Van Kruiningen, H. J. 1963. Practical techniques for making injections into joints and bursae of the horse. JAVMA 143(10): 1079–1083.

Van Pelt, R. W. 1960a. Arthrocentesis of the equine carpus. Vet. Med. 55: 30.

Van Pelt, R. W. 1960b. The role of intra-articular adrenocortical steroids. Mich. State Univ. Vet. 20: 68.

Van Pelt, R. W. 1961. Equine intra-articular injections. Mich. State Univ. Vet. 21: 54.

Van Pelt, R. W. 1962a. Intra-articular injection of the equine carpus and fetlock. JAVMA 140(11): 1181.

Van Pelt, R. W. 1962b. Properties of equine synovial fluid. JAVMA 141(9): 1951.

Van Pelt, R. W. 1963. Clinical and synovial fluid response to intrasynovial injection of 6a-methylprednisolone acetate into horses and cattle. JAVMA 143(7): 738.

VAN PELT, R. W. 1966. Arthrocentesis and injection of the tarsus. JAVMA 148(4): 367–377.

VAN PELT, R. W. 1967a. Characteristics of tarsal synovial fluid. Can. J. Comp. Med. Vet. Sci. 31(12): 342–347.

VAN PELT, R. W., 1967b. Intra-articular corticosteroid therapy in bog spavin. JAVMA 151(9): 1159–1171.

VAN PELT, R. W. 1968. Changes in blood and synovia in bog spavin. Amer. J. Vet. Res. 29(3): 369–579.

VAN PELT, R. W. et al. 1970. Intra-articular betamethasone in arthritis. JAVMA 156(11): 1589–1599.

VAN PELT, R. W., et al. 1971. Effects of intra-articular injection of flumethasone suspension in joint diseases of horses. JAVMA 159(6): 739–753.

VAN PELT, R. W. and W. F. RILEY. 1967. Prednisolone therapy for bog spavin. JAVMA 151(3): 328–338.

VIGUE, R. F. 1960. Clinical evaluation of prednisolone trimethylacetate in arthritis and general inflammatory conditions of horses. Southwestern Vet. 13: 103.

VM/SAC Staff Report. 1970. Dimethyl sulfoxide (DMSO). VM/SAC 65: 1051.

Voss, J. 1973. Personal communication. Colorado State University, Ft. Collins.

WHEAT, J. D. 1955. The use of hydrocortisone in the treatment of joint and tendon disorders in large animals. JAVMA, 27: 64.

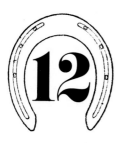

Radiology

Joe P. Morgan, D.V.M., Vet. med. dr.

The importance of diagnostic radiology in the diagnosis of lameness in horses cannot be overestimated. A radiographic study permits visualization of bone or joint lesions suspected on the basis of a physical examination and, frequently, diagnosis of diseases that would otherwise not be suspected. Often, radiographs provide additional information helpful in making a prognosis, e.g., identification of the extension of a fracture line into a joint space, observation of a small chip fracture associated with overextension of a joint, or the finding of a secondary periosteal change indicative of a chronic disease process. One of the greatest values of a diagnostic radiographic study is often overlooked—utilization of the study as a permanent record for later reference at the time of follow-up studies. The current status of a bone lesion is more easily determined when follow-up radiographic studies are available for comparison. The significance of diagnostic radiology in postoperative studies should be obvious.

Radiology can be misused as an aid in diagnosis and treatment of equine lameness. It is easy in a busy practice to make the radiographic examination before the physical examination. This places the physical examination in the secondary role of confirming the radiographic findings. This is a serious error and one that leads to erroneous diagnoses. The clinician should perform his physical examination carefully and select the several possible diagnoses. This places the radio-graphic examination in the proper role of confirming or rejecting each of the preselected diagnoses. Only in this way can the clinician avoid being overimpressed by positive radiographic findings that may have clinical importance but may *not* represent the cause of the lameness. An example would be the radiographic finding of minimal periarticular new bone growth indicating old injury to a joint, while the more important puncture wound in the sole, which does not cause as prominent a radiographic finding, is the cause of the acute lameness.

It is important to understand that definite requirements must be met before a radiographic study can be considered diagnostic. A satisfactory number of views of good technical quality must be made, with the central beam directed correctly. Meeting these demands necessitates using an adequate x-ray machine properly and requires correct processing of the radiographs. A diagnostic radiograph requires use of costly equipment and valuable time. Therefore, the wise practitioner will learn the operation, capabilities, and limitations of his x-ray equipment to assure that the studies will be of diagnostic quality.

Radiographs are the property of the veterinary clinic or practitioner. Fees charged for examinations entitle the client to a complete report of the study. The client should be allowed an opportunity to examine the radiographs with the veterinarian. All radiographs should be

462

properly identified and should be retained by the veterinarian for possible comparison with follow-up studies. It is not desirable to "lend" radiographs to clients. Problems are created by an owner or trainer having possession of radiographs without the knowledge necessary to make a correct interpretation. If consultation is desired, radiographs should be forwarded to another veterinarian for his examination, requesting that they be returned when they are of no further value.

Equipment and techniques that may be used to obtain diagnostic radiographs helpful in interpreting lameness in horses are described in this chapter. The construction and theory of operating x-ray machines may be found elsewhere (Carlson, 1967; van der Platts, 1961; Douglas and Williamson, 1972). Excellent textbooks on radiation physics are also available (Johns and Cunningham, 1969; Goodwin et al., 1970; Christensen et al., 1972).

RADIOGRAPHY

A number of separate items must be considered, in terms of cost and contribution, in production of a diagnostic radiographic study. The most expensive item is the x-ray machine. However, the quality of diagnostic radiographs cannot be guaranteed just because one has purchased an expensive and highly rated machine. The correct use of accessory items such as film holders, beam collimators, positioning aids, and film processing facilities contributes heavily to the final results.

X-Ray Machine

Many practitioners are concerned only with the minimum requirements of an x-ray machine that can produce diagnostic radiographic studies. Limitation of this type is a mistake. Larger, more powerful units permit radiographic examinations to be performed more easily, in less time, with fewer views repeated, which enables one to arrive at a diagnosis more easily. Thus, the purchase of a machine that meets only minimum standards is false economy. The final selection of a diagnostic radiographic machine is based on many factors.

Milliamperage

Milliamperage (ma) is a major factor in determining the quantity of x-rays produced and is, therefore, a good indication of the type of examination that can be performed with a machine. Many small x-ray machines have constant ma with no provision for alteration. Other small units have variable settings in the range of 10 to 30 ma. Larger, more expensive equipment has maximum ma values ranging from 50 up to 1,600, usually in 100- or 200-ma increments, and relatively simple controls for adjustment.

The relationship between ma and time is a direct one. Therefore, a higher ma setting allows for a corresponding decrease in required exposure time. A second advantage of a high-ma setting is that the greater amount of radiation produced permits examination of thicker portions of the horse.

Radiographs obtained with a setting of 0.1 sec and 100 ma are identical to those obtained with a setting of 1.0 sec and 10 ma, assuming that all other factors remain constant. The product of milliamperage and time is called milliamperseconds (mas); equal mas settings will produce radiographs of equal density or contrast. This relationship can be seen in two examples:

1. $0.1 \text{ sec} \times 100 \text{ ma} = 10 \text{ mas}$
   $1.0 \text{ sec} \times 10 \text{ ma} = 10 \text{ mas}$

2. $0.05 \text{ sec} \times 30 \text{ ma} = 1.5 \text{ mas}$
   $0.1 \text{ sec} \times 15 \text{ ma} = 1.5 \text{ mas}$
   $0.15 \text{ sec} \times 10 \text{ ma} = 1.5 \text{ mas}$
   $0.3 \text{ sec} \times 5 \text{ ma} = 1.5 \text{ mas}$

Exposure Time

Exposure time is one of the most important considerations in determining whether an x-ray machine is adequate for large-animal examinations. Exposure times of 0.1 sec or less generally ensure that the problem of motion during the exposure will be minimal. If the exposure times are longer than 0.1 sec, there will frequently be motion of the horse, film holder, or tube. The range of available exposure times is great, and some units have minimum settings of 0.003 and 0.001 sec.

Reviewing the relationship between ma and exposure time, it is obvious that a short exposure time can be obtained only in association with the utilization of a high milliamperage. Conversely, a machine with a low milliamperage (15–30 ma) must utilize exposure times of rather long duration (0.1–0.5 sec).

Kilovoltage

The kilovoltage potential (kVp) determines the quality of the x-ray beam and thus its ability to penetrate tissue. Higher kVp settings produce more penetrating beams, with a higher percentage of radiation reaching the film. Some units do not have a control for changing kVp and employ what is referred to as a "constant kVp" setting.

A kVp setting of 75 to 85 is adequate for penetrating most distal portions of a mature horse's leg. Lower kVp settings can be of value when radiographing immature horses and for soft-tissue techniques. A higher kVp setting allows for use of a lower mas setting. This would generally mean a short time of exposure. The inverse relationship between kVp and mas can be seen in the following settings, all of which will produce comparable radiographs if other factors are unchanged.

60 kVp and 4.0 mas (10 ma × 0.4 sec)
70 kVp and 2.0 mas (10 ma × 0.2 sec)
80 kVp and 1.0 mas (10 ma × 0.1 sec)
90 kVp and 0.5 mas (5 ma × 0.1 sec)

In the range of kVp settings normally used, adding 10 kVp and dividing the mas in half will produce a comparable radiograph. Conversely, subtracting 10 kVp and doubling the mas maintains radiographic density at a similar level.

Mobility

The degree of mobility required in an x-ray unit is generally determined by the type of practice and how the machine is to be used. If most examinations are to be conducted in a central clinic, a larger machine is recommended. Such a machine might be one of the heavier portable units (Fig. 12-1), a lighter portable unit (Fig. 12-2), or a stationary transformer and control unit with a ceiling-suspended tube (Fig. 12-3). If survey examinations are to be made in the field, an easily transportable unit is needed. Many compact portable units are adequate for survey radiography of equine limbs in the field (Fig. 12-4).

A high-powered x-ray machine may be rendered useless by limitations in movement of the tube head. Examination of the extremities of the horse requires that the tube be easily positioned and the direction of the x-ray beam be quickly and easily altered. The tube head must reach to near ground level to permit lateral views of the foot and digit. It is also essential that the tube head be easily moved to avoid accidental damage by the horse. The continual development of new x-ray equipment has made it possible to suspend the tube from the ceiling (Fig. 12-3). Such an installation facilitates positioning as well as maintenance of the area, and the factor of increased safety to the tube is a definite advantage. Regardless of configuration, the machine and/or tube

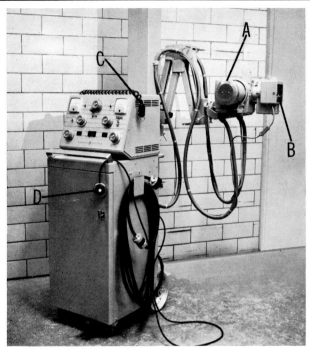

FIG. 12–1. A 300-ma mobile x-ray machine that has an easily positioned tube head (A). The machine is equipped with an adjustable lead shutter diaphragm (B), hand switch (C), and foot switch (D).

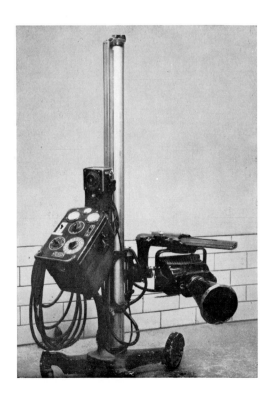

FIG. 12–2. A 15-ma mobile x-ray machine that is adequate for most examinations of the extremities of horses.

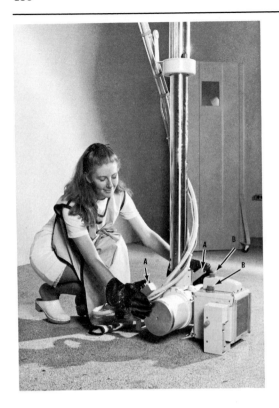

FIG. 12–3. Ceiling-suspended x-ray tube with stationary generator (not shown). Tube housing is equipped with handles (A), making tube movement easy; controls (B) to alter size of illuminated field; and controls on the handles for exposure. Note that the tube drops to the level of the floor.

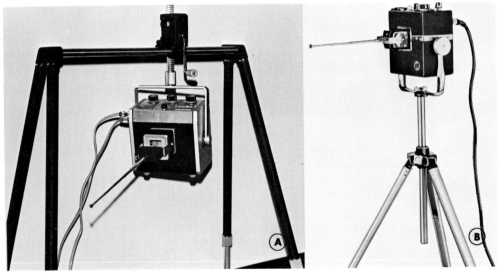

FIG. 12–4. This lightweight portable machine is adequate for radiographing the distal extremities of horses. The machine can be used suspended (A), supported on a tripod (B), or can be hand-held or rested on a block for support.

should move as quietly as possible, and locks should not create excessive noise.

Other Factors To Consider in Evaluation of an X-Ray Machine

Other controls that may be present on an x-ray machine include those for measuring and regulating voltage on the incoming line. This determination is important, since other settings on the machine are dependent on the value of the incoming voltage. An unnoticed drop or rise in incoming voltage produces a less or more highly penetrating beam than expected, resulting in improperly exposed film. The more commonly experienced problem is a drop in line voltage and subsequent unexpected loss in radiographic density. This may happen if rural electrical lines with varying voltage are used; use of a long extension cord or the simultaneous use of heavy motors (such as air conditioners) on the same circuit may also cause such a drop. Large x-ray units may automatically compensate for changes in line voltage.

A low noise level is important during radiography of a horse, since too much machine noise can increase the difficulty of handling a nervous animal. Machines utilizing a rotating anode tube may be objectionally loud, and this should be evaluated before purchase. Operation of the timer should also be quiet, to ensure that the horse will remain calm at the exact moment of exposure. A foot switch to activate the exposure is desirable (Fig. 12-1), as it frees a pair of hands to assist in restraining the horse. A foot switch can usually be wired to the timer at little extra cost. Locating the exposure switch on the tube housing makes repositioning of the tube possible up to the time of the exposure (Fig. 12-3).

Ideal X-Ray Machine

An ideal x-ray machine for use in examining the extremities of horses must have most of the following characteristics:

A high degree of mobility of both the unit and the tube head

Timer, ma selector, and kVp control that permits a sufficiently penetrating exposure in a short time, preferably 0.1 sec or less, at a focal-film distance of 36–40″ (90–100 cm)

A method of monitoring and controlling the incoming line voltage

A foot switch

Minimal machine noise

Safety from electrical and radiation hazards

Accessory Equipment

Accessory items are frequently as important as the x-ray machine itself. Included are positioning aids, cassette holders, beam-collimation devices, beam filters, and grids. Most items are available commercially, but some may be produced locally to better satisfy needs created by a specific machine or situation.

Aids in Positioning

Positioning aids are perhaps the most important of the accessory equipment items. These devices are usually wooden blocks placed to ensure that the foot or digit and cassette are held in the same position on successive studies with little risk of motion.

The type of blocks required depends entirely on the specific x-ray machine and the type of radiographic examination desired. If the x-ray tube cannot be lowered to floor level, it is necessary to elevate the foot to allow true lateral projections. Examples of positioning aids are presented in the discussion on specific radiographic positionings (p. 494–550).

Cassette Holder

Cassette holders are essential as radiation protection devices. Although an operator wears protective lead gloves and a lead apron, it is an unacceptable practice to position the hands or any part of the body within the primary x-ray beam. A slot may be cut in a wooden positioning device and serve to hold the cassette. The cassette holder may be fashioned of metal or wood with a handle that permits the assistant to remain outside the primary beam (Fig. 12–5).

Beam-Collimation Devices

X rays radiate from the target in the tube in straight lines in all directions. The rays that escape from the tube form the primary beam. It is important that x-ray machines be equipped with a method of controlling the size of the primary beam as it leaves the tube. Control of the beam size means that a smaller area on the patient is exposed to radiation, and exposure to the primary beam of persons assisting with the examination is more easily avoided. By limiting the area of tissue exposed to the primary beam, the amount of secondary or "scatter" radiation is also lowered. Scatter radiation is "soft," less penetrating radiation that is produced when the primary beam strikes an object. It travels in all directions and, in sufficient amounts, can cause generalized graying of the film.

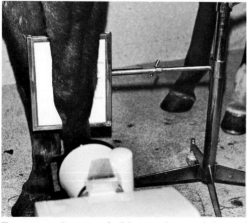

FIG. 12–5. Cassette holder with capability of altering height of cassette and length of arm.

Many different types of cones, cylinders, lead apertures, and lead-shutter diaphragms are available for controlling the size of the primary beam (Fig. 12–6). These items range from simple, inexpensive lead apertures to costly lead-shutter diaphragms. Frequently, the field of primary radiation is illuminated by a light so that the irradiated area is more easily determined. When used with an adjustable lead-shutter diaphragm, an illuminated field permits exposure of the smallest area compatible with a diagnostic study (Fig. 12–7).

Aluminum Filter

Insertion of a thin aluminum filter within the primary x-ray beam removes a large percentage of the "soft," less penetrating portion of the primary beam, which has little effect in creating a latent image on the film. Exposure dose to the skin of the patient is decreased by approximately 50 percent when 1.0-mm aluminum is used as the filter. Exposure dose to the skin is cut by 80 percent when 3.0-mm aluminum is used as the filter (Trout *et al.,* 1952). The filter may be taped against the tube housing or fastened to the base of the cone, or it may be an integral part of the tube housing assembly. Since the filter also removes some of the more penetrating rays, the thickness of the filter that can be used depends somewhat on the maximum capability of the x-ray machine. Use of a thick filter with a low-power generator would require higher kVp settings or longer exposure times that would be unsatisfactory. The x-ray beam from a large generator could be heavily filtered and compensatory increases easily made in either kVp or ma settings. Exposure times for radiographs of comparable density made at 60 kVp using 1.0-mm aluminum filtration need only be increased approximately 20 percent. Selection of a 1.0-mm aluminum filter represents a compromise that provides good absorption of the less energetic portion of the primary

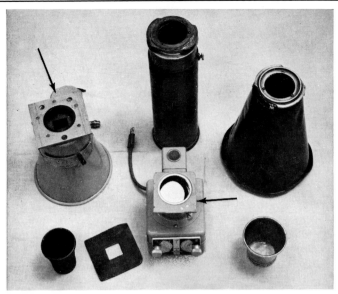

FIG. 12–6. Various methods of controlling the size of the primary beam. More desirable types can change the size of the radiation field and illuminate the area that is irradiated (arrows).

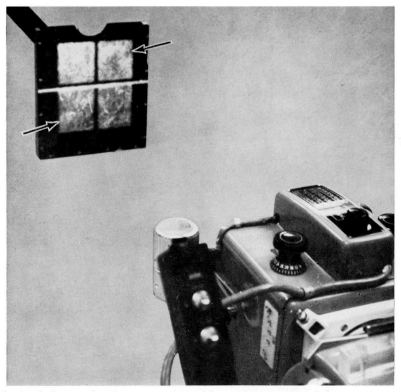

FIG. 12–7. The lead-shutter diaphragm is adjustable, and exact size of the opening can be determined by the area illuminated on the cassette holder (arrows). This ensures that the size of the exposed area is as small as possible. (Photo furnished through the courtesy of the Department of Clinical Radiology, Royal Veterinary College, Stockholm, and Elema-Schönander AB, Stockholm.)

x-ray beam without requiring an increase in exposure factors (ma or time) that will lead to problems in motion during exposure.

Wedge filters are blocks of aluminum that diminish greatly in thickness from one side of the radiation field to the other; they are used deliberately to cause uneven radiation exposure to the part being radiographed. They are useful in examinations of the horse's leg in areas of unequal tissue thickness such as the posterior-anterior projection of the stifle joint. A greater number of x rays are available to penetrate the thick distal femur than the less dense tibia.

Grids

A grid is a thin wafer with alternating lead and radiolucent strips. Grids are used to decrease the amount of secondary radiation reaching the film, which produces "fogging" and a gray film lacking in contrast. The more distal areas of the horse's limbs (less than 12 cm thickness) can be adequately examined without using a grid. A grid is needed when the thickness of a radiographed part exceeds 12 cm.

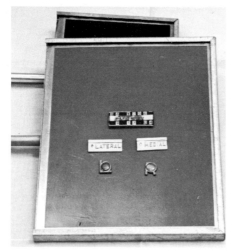

FIG. 12-8. Lead markers that identify the radiograph and indicate left or right leg and lateral or medial side.

Thus, it is used in examinations of the stifle joint, pelvis, shoulder joint, and elbow joint. The quality of special views of the navicular bone can often be improved by the use of the grid. A grid focused at 40″ (100 cm) with an 8:1 ratio and 60–80 lines per inch (25–30 lines per cm) is recommended.

Distance from Tube to Film

Since change in the tube–film distance requires compensatory change in kVp or mas settings, a standard distance is usually recommended. Alteration of this distance affects the definition of the radiographic image, the better radiographic definition being obtained at the greater distances. The distance depends on the quality of the x-ray generator. A high-powered unit could be used at 40″ (100 cm) or greater, but a less powerful unit could be used as close as 20″ to 25″ (50 to 60 cm) to permit a shorter exposure time. The loss in detail due to the short tube–film distance would be more than compensated for by the improvement in detail resulting from the elimination of movement in the brief exposure time. Shortening of the tube–film distance from 40″ (100 cm) to 30″ (75 cm) would permit a 50 percent decrease in ma or time.

Film Markers

All radiographs should be clearly identified with the name of the veterinarian or his clinic, the date on which the radiographs were made, and a number or name to identify the patient. One type of film marking is the use of lead numbers and letters either placed in a holder or taped directly to the face of the film holder when the exposure is made (Fig. 12-8).

A second type of marker utilizes a disposable, lead-impregnated tape that is placed on the outer surface of the cassette. This is used with a permanent plate containing the name and address of the vet-

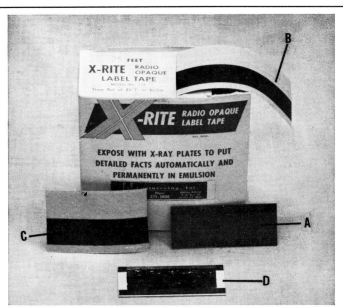

FIG. 12-9. Type of radiograph marker. A plate contains the name and address of the veterinarian or clinic (*A*). Lead-impregnated tape is available in a roll (*B*) from which a small piece is cut (*C*) and additional information written with pen or pencil. This tape is then placed on the plate (*D*) and the marker placed on the cassette.

erinarian in lead letters. Date, name or number of the case, and other information can be easily written or typed on the tape (Fig. 12-9).

A third type of marker requires that a lead block be built into the cassette or placed on its surface. The block shields a corner of the film from exposure by the x-ray beam. The film is removed from the cassette in the dark room and a typed card with appropriate information is placed next to the unexposed corner. A light is then flashed through the card onto the film, and the typed or written letters create unexposed shadows on the film (Fig. 12-10).

A fourth method of identification is to write on the film with a pencil or other pointed device before it is developed. It is also possible to scratch the softened gelatin easily while the film is in the wash water.

Additional markers that are needed include those used to identify fore and hind, right and left, and medial and lateral as-

pects (Fig. 12-8). A marker in the shape of an arrow is useful to indicate a soft-tissue lesion or an area of severe pain. When viewing the radiograph, attention is immediately directed to this particular

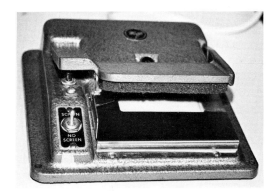

FIG. 12-10. Type of radiograph marker. An unexposed corner on the exposed radiographic film is "flashed" by an ordinary incandescent light through a typed (or handwritten) card with necessary identifying information. This records the information on film before processing.

area. A useful film marker is available that assists in recording the direction of the primary beam (Reid, 1962, 1965).

Types of Film and Film Holders

Two basic types of film and film holders are of importance in equine radiography. Screen-type film is placed in rigid cassettes with intensifying screens. Non-screen-type film is placed in a nonrigid, lightproof holder.

Screen Technique

The most useful combination in radiographic examinations of the horse is the screen-type film placed in a rigid cassette with intensifying screens. The cassette protects and supports the intensifying screens and films. Both the film and screens are available in several speeds, determined primarily by crystal size. Larger crystals and thicker layers in either film or screen permit a reduction in the amount of radiation required for an exposure, unfortunately at the expense of minimal loss of radiographic detail or definition. Generally speaking, the faster films and screens are still recommended; the improvement in detail due to elimination of motion of the horse more than compensates for the minimal loss of detail caused by the increase in crystal size or number of crystals in either the screens or film. The various screen speeds produced by two companies are shown in Table 12–1.

Since speed of both films and screens varies, it is advisable to use only one combination so that only one technique chart is needed. Cassettes are available in varying sizes. An 8″ × 10″ (20 × 25 cm) cassette is most convenient for use on horses. Larger cassettes may be divided so that two or more exposures can be made on the same film (Fig. 12–11). A 7″ × 17″ (18 × 43 cm) cassette is of great value in recording the degree of deformity of long

bones, such as might be present in congenital and nutritional diseases in foals.

Dirt or chemical staining of the intensifying screens are the cause of many film artifacts (Eastman Kodak Co., 1968), which appear as white, unexposed areas corresponding to the shape and size of the foreign material. Screens should therefore be cleaned frequently, before the dirt becomes imbedded in the surface of the screen. Cleaning is done by using either a soft brush or cotton to carefully wipe the surface. Drops of processing solution must be removed as soon as possible by absorbing them with a damp piece of cotton to avoid permanent staining. If dust cannot be removed or if chemical stains are present, it is necessary to use either soap and water or a commercial cleanser. Organic solvents such as ether, alcohol, and acetone attack the screens and are not suitable. Screens become discolored and less efficient with age and should be replaced when they are seen to be a yellow-gray color on visual examination. Similar exposures made with new and old screen pairs will produce different-quality radiographs even though the screen pairs were the same speed originally. It is important therefore not only to have the screens of the same speed but to ensure that they are of comparable age. Use of damaged or old screens is the cause of a large percentage of artifacts that compromise the film quality in equine radiology to the point of rendering the examination unsatisfactory.

The outside of the cassette should also be kept clean to prevent the admittance of dust onto the screens when the cassette is opened. If cassettes must be used in dusty or dirty locations, a plastic bag or similar device should be used as a protecting cover.

Nonscreen Technique

There is no intensification of the x-ray beam when a cardboard holder or com-

Table 12-1　Types of Intensifying Screens

Manufacturer	Screen	Speed	MAS factor
Dupont	Cronex Xtra Fine Detail	Very slow	4.0
	Cronex Xtra Fine Fast Detail	Slow	2.0
	Cronex Xtra Fine Par Speed	Par	1.0
	Cronex Xtra Fine High Speed	Fast	0.87
	Cronex Xtra Fine Hi Plus Screen	Very fast	0.5
Radelin (U.S. Radium Corp.)	UD (Ultrafine detail)		4.0
	T-2 (General purpose)		1.0
	TF-2 (High speed)		0.5
	STF-2 (Super high speed)		0.35

parable lightproof device is used to support nonscreen film. Therefore, an exposure time three to five times longer than that required for screen-type film is needed. Nonscreen holders are, therefore, suitable only for specific examinations. Nonscreen film is available with different speeds. The faster type should be used. Nonscreen film is available prepackaged in cardboard holders that are discarded in the darkroom before the film is developed. This type of holder is desirable if the area to be examined is soiled with blood or other debris since the holder will be quickly disposed of.

Nonscreen film is used only with a cardboard holder, not with a screened cassette. The nonscreen-film technique is much less expensive because there is no need for cassettes, and, in addition, it

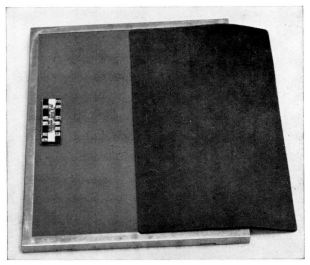

FIG. 12-11. A lead-impregnated rubber sheet used to divide a cassette. Two or more exposures can then be made on the same film. The identification marker uses lead letters.

produces a radiograph with excellent detail. However, these advantages are offset by the much greater exposure time or ma required to obtain comparable film density. The opportunities for use of non-screen technique in diagnosing lameness in horses are definitely limited.

Developing a Technique Chart

Individual exposure guides, based on the capabilities of a given machine and the particular wishes of the veterinarian, can be readily prepared. These charts prevent unnecessary waste of time and film due to incorrect exposure factors (Fig. 12–12). The same combination of ma, time, and kVp settings for a particular view when used on different x-ray machines will not produce identical radiographs because of differences in speed of intensifying screens, age of intensifying screens, speed of film, tube–film distance, amount of beam filtration, temperature and time of developing film, and inherent differences in the settings of x-ray machines.

The value of a chart is appreciated mainly after one has acquired confidence in its listed values and is assured that radiographs of diagnostic quality will be obtained with the best combinations of ma, kVp, and time.

As many factors as possible must be standardized before formulating a chart. The value of incoming line voltage should be determined, if possible, and controlled. Tube–film distance must be standardized for satisfactory beam intensity without distortion. The aluminum filter and beam collimator to be used must be in place. The type of intensifying screens and film speed have an important bearing on exposure factors and should be determined. The chart is usually made for use without a grid, since most studies can be made this way.

After these factors are known, trial exposures may be made of, for instance, the fetlock of an average-sized adult horse. The film may be divided by rubberized-lead sheets, or a separate film may be used for each trial exposure. Past experience with the machine will be of help in deter-

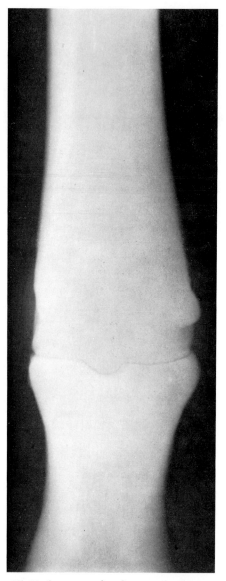

FIG. 12–12. An example of exposure factors so incorrect that the film is worthless. In this underexposed radiograph of the fetlock joint, it is impossible to evaluate the joint space or the condition of the proximal sesamoid bones. This is a common fault and should be corrected.

mining the technique for trial exposures. The exposure time should be as short as possible and the mas setting probably as high as possible. The kVp should be selected last. An exposure of 70 to 80 kVp and 1.5 to 2.0 mas should be approximately correct for most machines. After the first exposure is made, additional exposures should be made, with the time doubled and then redoubled. The radiographs should then be processed and examined. Developing time should be a full 5 minutes, and the temperature of developing solutions should be carefully controlled at 68°F (20°C). The tube–film distance must be constant for each exposure. Of the resultant radiographs, one should be dark (overexposed), one light (underexposed), and one of diagnostic quality (correctly exposed) (Fig. 12–13).

If all of the radiographs are overexposed, as indicated by dark films, the kVp should be reduced by 10 or the mas by half. Three additional exposures should then be made at varying exposure times, as in the first trial. If none of the original exposures is satisfactory because of underexposure (a light film), an increase in exposure factors will be required. If possible, the kVp should be increased by 10, and, again, the three trial exposures should be repeated. If it is not possible to increase the kVp, then the exposure time or the ma must be doubled. This technique of increasing or decreasing factors is continued until a satisfactory radiograph is obtained. The acceptable radiograph is the one that appeals to the individual and that best permits evaluation of both bone and soft tissue. Examples of corrections to be made for over- or underexposure in the trial series are given below:

Original trial exposures
1. 70 kVp and 1.5 mas
   (15 ma and 0.1 sec)
2. 70 kVp and 3.0 mas
   (15 ma and 0.2 sec)

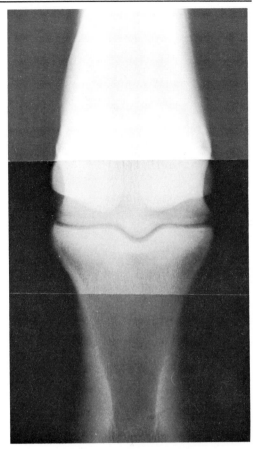

FIG. 12–13. Three radiographs that demonstrate the difference expected in "trial" exposures preparatory to development of a technique chart.

3. 70 kVp and 6.0 mas
   (15 ma and 0.4 sec)

If all exposures are dark (overexposed), decrease the settings to:
1. 60 kVp and 1.5 mas
   (15 ma and 0.1 sec)
2. 60 kVp and 3.0 mas
   (15 ma and 0.2 sec)
3. 60 kVp and 6.0 mas
   (15 ma and 0.4 sec)
or
1. 70 kVp and 0.75 mas
   (15 ma and 0.05 sec)
2. 70 kVp and 1.5 mas
   (15 ma and 0.1 sec)

3. 70 kVp and 3.0 mas
   (15 ma and 0.2 sec)

If all exposures are light (underexposed), increase the settings to:
1. 80 kVp and 1.5 mas
   (15 ma and 0.1 sec)
2. 80 kVp and 3.0 mas
   (15 ma and 0.2 sec)
3. 80 kVp and 6.0 mas
   (15 ma and 0.4 sec)

or

1. 70 kVp and 3.0 mas
   (15 ma and 0.2 sec)
2. 70 kVp and 6.0 mas
   (15 ma and 0.4 sec)
3. 70 kVp and 12.0 mas
   (15 ma and 0.8 sec)

If the procedure is performed exactly as described, some exposures will be duplicated. However, by following each step, the ideal technique can be achieved. This *standard technique* can be used for most examinations of the foot, digit, metatarsus, and metacarpus.

The technique for radiography of the carpus and tarsus, and for other special studies, must utilize higher kVp and/or mas. The *darker technique* is achieved either by increasing the kVp of the standard technique by 10 or by doubling the time of exposure or the ma of the standard technique. All other factors remain constant.

Special views, such as that of the third phalanx with the horse standing on the cassette, require a *lighter technique*, formulated by lowering the kVp of the standard technique by 10 or by halving the time or ma of the standard technique. All other factors remain constant.

If the *standard technique* is 80 kVp and 3.3 mas [100 ma and 0.033 (1/30) sec], then the *darker technique* will be

90 kVp and 3.33 mas
   [100 ma and 0.033 (1/30) sec], or
80 kVp and 6.66 mas
   [200 ma and 0.033 (1/20) sec], or

80 kVp and 6.66 mas
   [100 ma and 0.066 (1/15) sec],

and the *lighter technique* will be
70 kVp and 3.33 mas
   [100 ma and 0.033 (1/30) sec], or
80 kVp and 1.67 mas
   [50 ma and 0.033 (1/30) sec], or
80 kVp and 1.67 mas
   [100 ma and 0.017 (1/60) sec]

The above procedure establishes three basic techniques: a standard technique applicable for most of the common views; a darker technique useful for thicker parts of the horse's leg; and a lighter technique for specialized areas. The values obtained remain constant for a particular x-ray machine. It will be obvious that the techniques used in examination of the foot of a draft horse must be increased, just as the techniques used for a foal or pony can be decreased by one-half. Thus, the practitioner most usually deals with only three different sets of exposure factors. One of these three techniques will produce satisfactory radiographs for most problems encountered in routine examinations.

Preparation of the Horse

Before radiographic examination of an extremity is attempted, the leg should be examined and all dirt and debris brushed away. As will be explained later, this is especially necessary in studies of the third phalanx and the navicular bone (Figs. 12–14 and 12–15). It may be necessary to scrub the hoof with a brush and water to clean the sole. Any radiopaque substance, such as iodine solution, blister, or scurf on the skin, will create increased density and "white" shadows on the radiograph (Figs. 12–15 through 12–18). If possible, any bandages should be removed to eliminate confusing lines on the radiograph (Fig. 12–18).

The presence of a shoe on the horse's foot during radiography compromises the amount of information that can be ob-

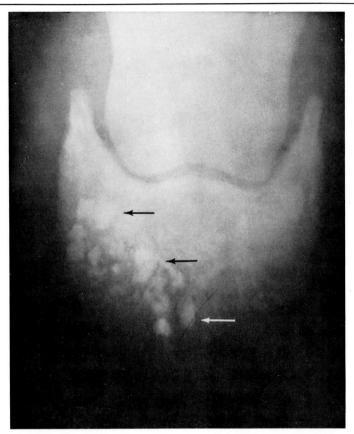

FIG. 12-14. The sole had not been thoroughly cleaned before radiographic examination. The multiple radiopaque areas (arrows) are due to dirt and gravel. A study of this quality should not be considered satisfactory.

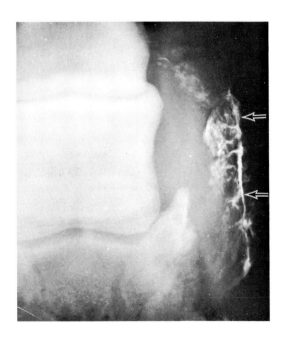

FIG. 12-15. Radiopaque shadow (arrows) caused by a heavy granulation tissue due to severe laceration of the lateral aspect of the heel and frequent administration of iodine products.

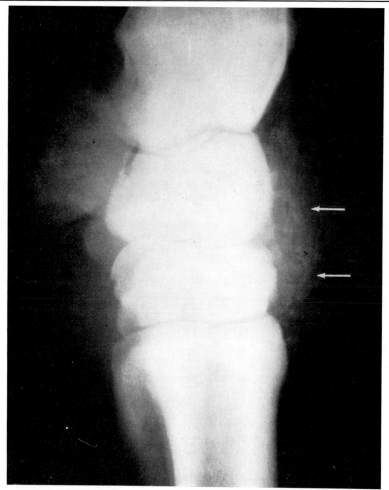

FIG. 12–16. It is impossible to fully interpret the condition of the anterior aspect of the carpal bones (arrows) on this radiograph because of the use of blistering compounds containing radiopaque iodine.

tained from the radiograph. It is possible that a fracture or other pathological change may be hidden by the shadow created by the shoe.

Film Processing

The most common errors made in radiography of horses are related to the processing of exposed radiographic film. The area used as a darkroom must be clean, lightproof, and uncluttered. If undeveloped film should accidentally come into contact with spilled processing chemicals, specific artifacts will appear on the radio-

graph. Pressure, creasing, buckling, or static electricity can also cause artifacts, dictating care in the handling of film. Because of the number of different errors possible in the darkroom and the frequency of these errors, it is not difficult to explain the trend toward purchase of automatic processors. These are costly if purchased new, and the cost of maintenance and replenishing of solution is high. Still, in the practice using radiography frequently during the day, the automatic processor will save time by decreasing the number of repeat examinations necessitated by technical problems.

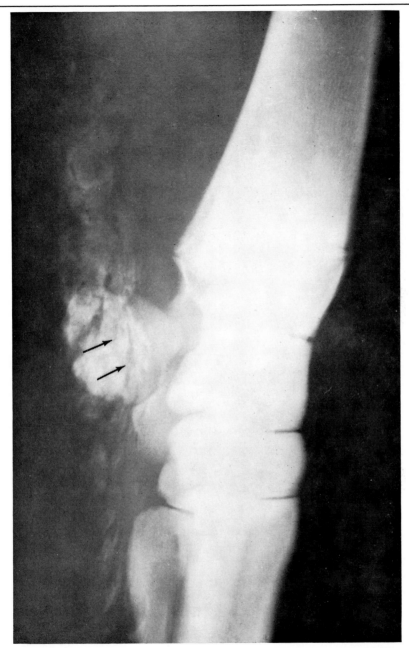

FIG. 12-17. The presence of dirt on the hair and skin can make accurate radiographic interpretation impossible. Note the false "fracture" lines (arrows) through the accessory carpal bone.

Developing

Technique charts should be based on a full five-minute developing time. Since many radiographs will be made with portable units with which it is difficult to establish exact settings, a certain amount of sight developing must be tolerated. The film should be visually inspected using a red darkroom light after approximately one minute of developing time to determine whether it will be greatly overexposed or underexposed. If the film is removed from the developer at one min-

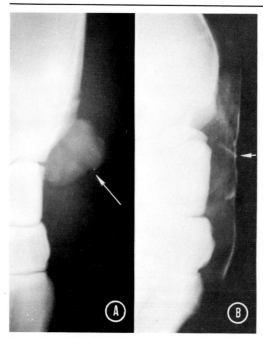

Fig. 12-18. Radiographs of the carpus. (A) A soft-tissue scar on the skin creates a dense shadow anterior to the distal radius (arrow). (B) A heavy bandage casts linear shadows anterior to the carpus (arrow).

ute or less and shows *correct* finished film density (darkness), then the film has been *greatly overexposed.* The processed radiograph will be gray and lacking in contrast.

Five-minute developing time is recommended because it permits a reduction of exposure factors. This could permit a shorter exposure time. In use of a technique chart based on five-minute developing time, the actual length of the developing time is not as critical as it would be with three-minute developing. The film may be removed from the solution at four to six minutes with little difference in film density. The advantage of this greater freedom in time of developing is obvious.

Fixing

If film is not washed before it is placed in the fixer solution, the pH of the fixer will be altered by the residual developer, necessitating earlier replacement. Films must remain within the fixing solution for approximately one minute before any light is allowed to reach the radiograph. Total time within the fixer should be twice the clearing time. Clearing time is the length of time required for the radiograph to lose the milky appearance it has when first placed in the fixer. Clearing time is approximately one minute but will lengthen proportionally with the age of the fixer solution. Film can safely remain in the fixer for as long as 10 to 20 minutes. Longer times in the fixer necessitate slightly longer washing times in clear water to avoid streaking on the dry film.

Washing

It is usually stated that films should be washed for 20 minutes. This length of time is dependent on whether water is constantly flowing through the tank and on the number of films that have been processed in the same water. The greater the intensity of water circulation, the shorter the washing time can be.

Processing Temperatures

The optimal temperature for all processing solutions is 68°F (20°C); the range should not be allowed to exceed 60° to 75°F (15° to 24°C). The temperature of the developing solution influences the time required for complete development as well as the resulting quality of the film. Charts are available to determine changes in the length of developing time for given changes in solution temperature. Generally, warmer solutions cause more rapid development, while colder solutions slow the chemical reaction and require longer developing times.

Processing Solutions

Processing solutions can be prepared from powders or from concentrated solutions. The latter are easier to work with and eliminate the problem of powder settling on counter tops. How often processing solution must be replaced is determined by the number of films processed and the care given to processing solutions. A green or brown developer solution and prolonged clearing time in the fixer solution signify an unsatisfactory condition and the need to replace solutions. In many areas, it is possible to contract for replacement of processing solutions on a regular basis.

Processing in Trays

Radiographs may be processed in flat trays of plastic, hard rubber, or enamel. Bottled solutions can be poured into the trays and then back into bottles after use. The film must be constantly agitated during processing to prevent the appearance of lines where the film rested on the bottom of the tray. This type of film processing can be performed within a light-tight black bag with openings for admitting the hands. This may be a technique required for studies made away from the clinic, but it should not be considered an acceptable way of processing radiographs made regularly in the clinic.

Drying and Filing

The film can be dried in a cabinet with heat and fan, or it can be hung for room air drying. Once it has dried, the corners should be clipped and the films placed in an envelope suitably identified for filing.

Technical Errors

Various technical errors are encountered in radiography, and they often destroy the diagnostic qualities of the radiograph. The failures arise from not following correct radiographic procedures and processing, causing incorrect

handling and processing. Table 12-2 lists most common technical errors, their appearance on the radiograph, their cause, and method of correction.

RADIOGRAPHIC INTERPRETATION

Every effort should be made to read the radiograph objectively and to evaluate soft tissues and each joint space carefully. Many obvious lesions have been overlooked when studies are performed only to confirm a clinically suspected lesion. In other cases, lesions are overlooked because radiographs were not studied to a greater extent after a first pathologic change was observed.

The radiograph should not be read when wet. A wet film should be examined only to see if the exposure is correct, the desired anatomical areas have been included on the film, the positioning is adequate, and radiographic detail is sharp. A final conclusion concerning the radiographic study should be made only from a dry radiograph.

A definite pattern must be established in reading a radiograph. It is important that this pattern be repeated in evaluating each radiograph so that no part is overlooked. It is essential to use a viewbox, not the nearest desk lamp or the sunlight. It is most important to have access to a high-intensity light for use in evaluating cortical surfaces and soft tissues (Fig. 12-19). Most small chip fractures and minimal areas of periosteal new bone growth will be missed completely without use of a "bright" light.

Tissue Density

Difference in tissue density is the factor that permits radiographic diagnosis. The tissue with greatest density is bone, which appears radiographically as a white shadow. Soft-tissue structures with high water content, such as muscle, tendons,

Table 12–2 Technical Errors

Appearance on the Radiograph	Cause	Correction
Image dark (background dark)	Film overexposed because of incorrect machine settings	Lower kVp, ma, or time setting
	Film overdeveloped because of too long a time in the developer	Correct length of time in developer solution (5 min)
	Film overdeveloped because of high temperature of processing solution	Correct temperature to 68°F (20°C)
	Film overexposed because of too short tube–film distance	Correct tube–film distance
	Film overexposed because beam filter not in position	Replace filter
	Film exposed to light or other source of radiation	Throw film away and start again
Image gray with no contrast, "fogged" (background dark)	Film exposed to light fog	Correct defective safety light
	Film exposed to light fog	Correct light leaks in darkroom
	Film exposed to light fog	Do not view films until they are completely fixed
	Film exposed to chemical fog due to high temperature	Correct developing temperature to 68°F (20°C)
	Film exposed to radiation during examination	Remove loaded cassettes from room during examination
	Film exposed to chemical fog	Discard old processing solutions
	Film exposed to scatter radiation	Use grid on tissue thickness greater than 11 cm
	Films exposed to backscatter radiation	Use lead-backed cassettes
	Film overexposed and underdeveloped	Correct exposure factors and develop film for 5 minutes
	Film old	Discard film
Image light (background light)	Film underexposed because of incorrect exposure	Increase kVp, ma, or time setting
	Film underdeveloped because of too short time in developer	Correct length of time in developer solution (5 min)
	Film underdeveloped because of low temperature of processing solutions	Correct temperature of processing solutions to 68°F (20°C)
	Film underexposed because of too long tube–film distance	Correct object–film distance
Black marks (not generalized)	Linear scratches on film	Handle film carefully
	Crescent marks due to bending film after exposure	Handle film carefully
	Static electricity (linear dots or "tree" pattern)	Handle film without causing friction
	Developer solution on film (fingerprints, blotches)	Clean bench surface in darkroom and dry hands before loading film
	Black areas on two films processed together caused by film sticking together in fix and not clearing properly	Gently agitate film in fix
	Black areas on film due to light exposure	Correct light leaks
White artifacts	Fingerprints or blotches due to fixer on film prior to processing	Clean bench surface in darkroom and clean hands before handling film
	Bubbles due to nonagitation of film	Agitate film briefly after placing in developer

Table 12-2   (Continued)

Appearance on the Radiograph	Cause	Correction
	"Hair" marks or irregular marks due to dirt or debris on intensifying screen	Clean or replace intensifying screens
	Crescent marks due to bending film before exposure	Handle film more carefully
	White areas on two films processed together because films stuck together in developer	Gently agitate films in the developer
	Linear streaks where emulsion has been scratched away	Handle film carefully
	Irregular white marks due to dirt or medicaments containing iodine on skin	Clean leg prior to radiography
	White streaks near edge of film due to cracks in screens	Replace screens
Yellow radiograph	Irregular yellowing of radiograph with age due to improper fixation of the film	Replace exhausted fixer or fix film for correct length of time
Yellow patches	Film sticking together (or to edge of tank) during fixing	Agitate film gently during fixation, avoid crowding films in fix tank
	Improper timing	Rinse correct length of time
Distorted, magnified, or blurred radiographic image	Object motion	Try again
	Tube motion	Check tube locks or method of stabilizing the tube
	Film (cassette) motion	Use sturdy cassette holders
	Object–film (cassette) distance too great	Position film (cassette) closer to organ of interest
	Image distorted because central beam not perpendicular to film (cassette)	Reposition film (cassette) so central beam perpendicular to cassette
	Image distorted because central beam not directed to center of film	Reposition tube so central beam hits center of film (cassette)
Heavy lines across radiograph	Grid lines due to use of tube–film distance outside range of grid focus	Use correct tube–film distance as determined by individual grid
	Grid lines heavy on one side of film and more normal on other side of film because grid not perpendicular to central beam	Reposition grid perpendicular to central beam
	Grid lines heavy on one side of film and more normal on other because central beam not centered on midline of grid	Reposition so central beam perpendicular to midline of grid
	Grid lines heavy on both edges of film because grid used upside down	Turn grid over so primary beam hits side indicated
	Grid lines randomly heavy and distorted because of grid damage	Replace grid
Edges of film black (exposed)	Light leak because of improperly fitting cassette back	Replace felt or repair damaged cassette
Edge(s) of film white (underexposed)	Cone cut because of incorrect centering	Reposition so central beam hits center of cassette

Table 12–2   (Continued)

Appearance on the Radiograph	Cause	Correction
Clear spots on films	Water spots causing multiple artifacts on film	Use detergent to lower surface tension to hasten drying without spots, and do not splash water on films when drying
Film cloudy and streaky (crusty when dry)	Streaky with sticky feeling because of failure to fix long enough	Fix longer or replace exhausted fixer solution
	Film sticky and cloudy because of failure to rinse adequately	Rinse adequately
Reticulation pattern	Emulsion "slips" because rinse is too hot	Lower temperature of rinse water

and skin, are of next higher density, appearing gray on a properly exposed radiograph. It is necessary to use a bright light to evaluate soft tissue areas (Fig. 12–20). Deposits of fat are less dense and provide contrast around tendons and muscle bellies. Cartilage is much less dense than bone and causes the radiolucent appearance of joint spaces. Air is the least dense, but it is not normally found in the equine leg. When air is present, following intra-articular injection or a break in the continuity of the skin, it appears as a black shadow on the radiograph. Radiopaque

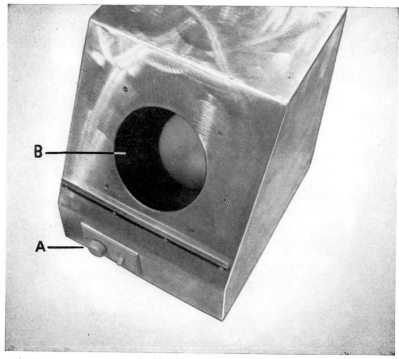

FIG. 12–19. A high-intensity viewer is essential for study of the bone margins and soft tissues. This viewer has a rheostat (A) with which to control the amount of light. It also has a heat-absorbing glass (B) to prevent damage to the radiograph.

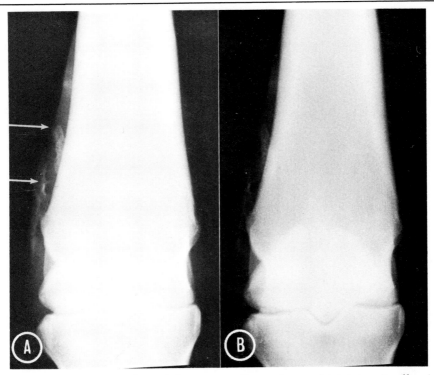

FIG. 12–20. Two photographs taken of the same radiograph on a high-intensity illuminator (*A*) and regular view box (*B*), demonstrating how a "bright" light is necessary in order to visualize soft-tissue calcific densities (arrows) that would otherwise have been overlooked.

foreign bodies such as glass, metal, gravel, dirt, or iodine solutions create white shadows of various shades, depending on size, density, and quantity of the material. (Figs. 12–15 through 12–18).

Views

Terms used in discussing the various radiographic projections describe the manner in which the x-ray beam passes through the animal. In an anterior-posterior (AP) view, the x-ray beam enters the leg anteriorly and exits posteriorly before striking the film. The posterior-anterior (PA) view is seldom used except in a PA view of the stifle joint or shoulder joint. The lateral view is made with the beam directed either lateral-medial or medial-lateral. Usually it is more convenient to make the exposure with the x-ray machine lateral and the cassette medial.

An exception is a lateral view of the elbow with the cassette held lateral to the elbow joint and the central beam directed just cranial to the pectoral muscles. Oblique views are most conveniently referred to by the same terminology. An anterior-lateral/posterior-medial oblique is made with the x-ray tube anterior and lateral and the film held posterior and medial. This view is also referred to as an anterior-posterior medial oblique view.

It is absolutely imperative to make more than one projection of an anatomical area to be radiographed (Fig. 12–21). Since a radiograph is only a representation of two dimensions, the second study made at right angles to the first permits evaluation of the third dimension. Additional oblique views are of value in radiographic examinations of the fetlock joint, proximal sesamoid bones, carpus, and tarsus.

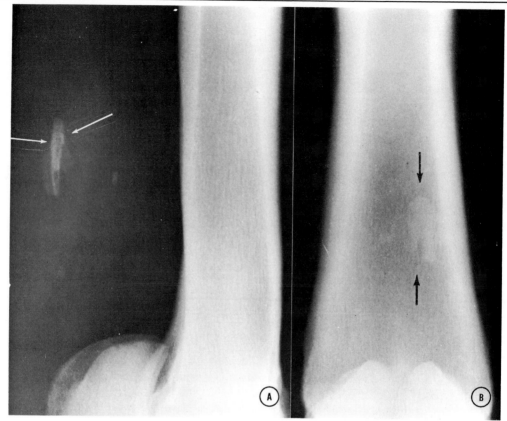

FIG. 12–21. Calcific densities (arrows) that are easily noted on the lateral projection (A) but more difficult to identify on the AP (B) projection because of the superimposed metacarpal bone. This is one example of the importance of including two views in each radiographic examination.

Flexed lateral-medial studies of the carpus and fetlock joint permit better evaluation of the joint surfaces. Small chip fractures adjacent to the joint margins are often shifted in position between the extended and flexed lateral projections, making interpretation of the radiographic study more accurate.

Dorsoventrally directed x-ray beams are used to provide tangential projections of the carpus, stifle, and navicular bone. The tangential view of the carpus projects the anterior portions of the distal radius and carpal bones for better evaluation (p. 525). The patella and the way it fits into the patellar groove are better evaluated with a similar projection directed along the anterior aspect of the distal femur (p.

545). The navicular bone can be projected between the angles of the third phalanx with a vertically directed beam posterior and parallel to the axis of the phalanges (p. 513). Table 12–3 lists the recommended projections for various anatomical areas of the horse.

Examination of Immature Animals

When a radiographic examination is to be made of the limbs of a horse in which epiphyseal closure has not occurred, it is important that the opposite leg also be radiographed. This simple precaution will help to prevent an erroneous diagnosis of "lesions" related to this growth area of the

Table 12–3   Recommended Views for Radiographic Examination of the Horse

Anatomical area	Recommended view
Foot	1. AP 2. Lateral
Third phalanx	1. AP (60°) 2. AP (Standing on film) 3. Lateral
Navicular	1. AP (60°) 2. AP (30°) 3. Lateral 4. Tangential view (Proximal-distal)
Fetlock joint (Proximal sesamoids)	1. AP 2. Lateral, extended 3. Lateral, flexed 4. Medial oblique 5. Lateral oblique
Metacarpals (Metatarsals)	1. AP 2. Lateral 3. Medial oblique 4. Lateral oblique
Carpus	1. AP 2. Lateral, extended 3. Lateral, flexed 4. Medial oblique 5. Lateral oblique 6. Tangential view—distal radius 7. Tangential view—proximal row carpal bones 8. Tangential view—distal row carpal bones
Elbow	1. AP 2. Lateral (leg extended cranially)
Shoulder	1. PA (obliques) 2. Lateral (through chest)
Hock	1. AP 2. Lateral 3. Medial oblique 4. Lateral oblique
Stifle	1. PA (technique for proximal tibia) 2. PA (technique for distal femur) 3. Lateral 4. Tangential view (patella)
Hip	1. VD, frog-leg 2. VD of each hip joint

bone. Normal closure times for each of the various cartilaginous growth plates are known to vary with different breeds and lines of horses, and probably with nutritional levels and with certain systemic diseases. A summary of the findings of both published and unpublished studies, based primarily on Quarter Horses and Thoroughbreds, is given (Table 12–4). The times generally do not agree with those published in anatomy texts because closure has been determined radiographically instead of by gross examination of the specimen.

SPECIAL DIAGNOSTIC PROCEDURES

One of the few special procedures available for aiding in the radiographic diagnosis of lameness of horses is the injection of a radiopaque contrast medium to outline a sinus or fistulous tract. There is frequent opportunity for use of this technique. A second procedure, arthrography, has not received the attention that it deserves in aiding the diagnosis of lameness. Arthrography in its several forms can provide definite, additional information concerning the condition of the joint capsule, synovial membrane, and articular cartilage.

Injection of Sinus Tract or Fistula

Injection of a radiopaque contrast medium to outline sinus tracts or fistulae is easy to perform and is not painful to the horse. The information gained may be of great help in surgical treatment of the problem.

By definition, a sinus is a tract leading from the skin or mucous membrane to a deep-seated focus of suppuration, vestigial structure, or an aberrant secreting tissue. A fistula is an abnormal tract leading from a mucous membrane to another mucous surface or to the skin. These abnor-

Table 12–4 Age of Epiphyseal Closure in the Horse

Age of Horse

Epiphyseal Line	6 months	9 months	12 months	18 months	2 years	2½ years	3 years
Front Leg							
First phalanx (proximal)	▭						
Second phalanx (proximal)	▭						
Third metacarpal bone (distal)	▭▭						
Radius (distal)					▭		
Radius (proximal)				▭			
Ulna (proximal)					▭▭▭		
Ulna (distal to distal radial epiphysis)	▭						
Humerus (distal)				▭			
Humerus (proximal)				▭▭▭			
Humerus (lateral tuberosity)					▭▭▭		
Humerus (medial epicondyle to distal epiphysis of humerus)	▭▭▭						
Hind Leg							
First phalanx (proximal)	▭						
Second phalanx (proximal)	▭						
Third metatarsal bone (distal)		▭▭					
Tibia (distal)				▭			
Tibia (proximal)					▭		
Tibial crest							
united with proximal tibia		▭▭					
united with tibial shaft							▭
Fibula (distal with tibia)					▭		
Femur (distal)					▭		
Os calcis	▭						

Age of epiphyseal closure based on Quarter Horse and Thoroughbred breeds, both male and female. The age of epiphyseal closure given here is based on radiographic determination, which will be earlier than actual closure determined histologically.

▭▭▭▭▭▭ Age during which closure usually takes place.

mal tracts may constantly drain pus, necrotic tissue, or the contents of the gastrointestinal or urinary tract.

Three techniques have been successfully utilized for radiographic exploration of these tracts. Regardless of the technique used, radiographs must be made in at least two projections, preferably AP and lateral.

The first technique involves occluding the orifice of the tract with a blunt, conical rubber nozzle placed on a syringe. Several 4″ × 4″ gauze pads or comparable material can be wrapped around the opening to seal the tract. The contrast material is then injected into the tract in an attempt to force contrast material throughout the sinus tract or fistula while occluding the orifice (Fig. 12–22).

The second technique, used with larger tracts, involves injection of a contrast medium through a rubber catheter placed in the tract. As with the first technique, the secret of obtaining good visualization lies in occluding the orifice of the wound.

In the third technique, which is the most rewarding, the extent of the sinus tract is probed gently by advancing a thin polyethylene catheter as far as it will penetrate prior to injection of the contrast medium. The catheter may become lodged in a blind socket, making it necessary to move the catheter in several different directions to find additional tracts. Because the focus of suppuration or the primary site is often distant from the orifice of the fistula or sinus tract, it is important to introduce the catheter as far as possible prior to injection. Multiple tracts occasionally have a common orifice and it is necessary to outline all the tracts with the contrast if possible.

Iodine is used as the radiopaque substance in most of the contrast media available for injection. Water-soluble solutions are more easily injected but tend to drain out more quickly. Care must be taken to wipe the areas around the orifice, since any radiopaque medium that may

have drained onto the skin will create a shadow on the radiograph.

Viscous products are somewhat more difficult to inject to the depth of the tract but may provide more satisfactory coating of the wall and do not drain out as quickly.

Even though the tract may be infected, injections should be made by aseptic technique. The unlikely possibility of iodine sensitivity should be considered after the injection of an iodine containing contrast medium.

If a large cavity is entered, visualization is aided by injection of both contrast material and air (Fig. 12–23) and making radiographs in various positions to give a double-contrast demonstration of the contours of the cavity. Occasionally, injection of either negative or positive contrast directly into a suspect fluid-filled pocket provides additional information about its etiology (Fig. 12–24).

Arthrography

Additional information concerning the condition of the synovial membrane, joint capsule, and articular cartilage is gained by radiography of the joint following injection of either air or positive-contrast medium into the joint space. A local anesthetic is used prior to placing a needle into the joint space to be studied, using the same care as when performing an aseptic joint tap. As much joint fluid as possible should be removed before injection of 5 to 10 cc of either air or 50 percent diatrizoate sodium.* The needle is then removed and the joint is massaged lightly to assure distribution of the contrast media. Radiographic studies are then made as quickly as possible, using routine positioning.

One of the main purposes of the technique is to outline the width of the articular cartilage and demonstrate minimal

*Hypaque, Winthrop.

changes in thickness that would otherwise be much less obvious. Distension and possible rupture of the joint capsule is another change noted with this technique. Severe changes in the synovium are easily demonstrated, but minimal changes may be difficult to interpret. Recent findings concerning the pathogenesis of degenerative joint disease suggest that periarticular osteophytes may not play as significant a role in the diagnosis of this condition as was once thought (Marshall, 1969). If this observation is proven to be true, changes in the articular cartilage and synovium

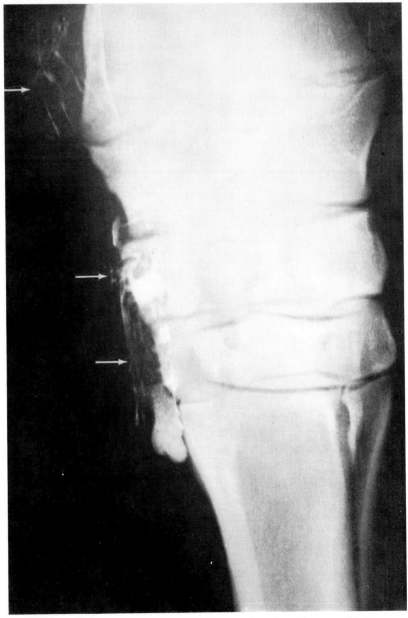

FIG. 12-22. The origin of clear fluid draining just proximal to the radiocarpal joint was not known. By injecting contrast medium into the fistulous tract, it could be determined that there was a direct communication with the tendon sheath of the common digital extensor muscle (arrows).

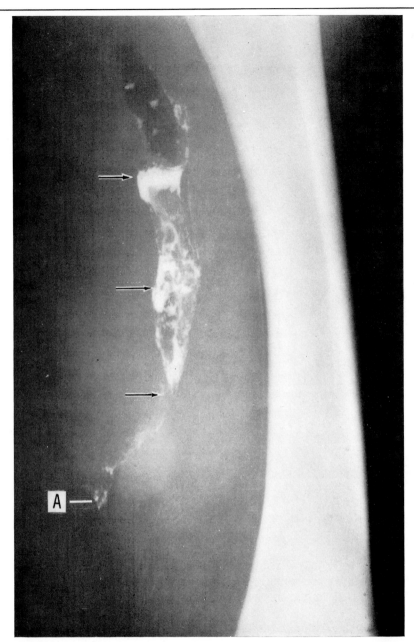

FIG. 12-23. Injection of a sinus tract with opaque contrast medium and a small amount of air outline the extent of the tract. The point of drainage just proximal to the carpus (A) is seen, as is the total length of the tract (arrows). The cause of the lesion was a wood splinter, not positively identified.

must be evaluated by some method other than the simple determination of the presence of periarticular osteophytes on the radiograph. Arthrography may provide this special technique.

RADIATION SAFETY

Any of the body tissues may be injured by overexposure to x-rays, with the skin, gonads, and blood-forming organs being

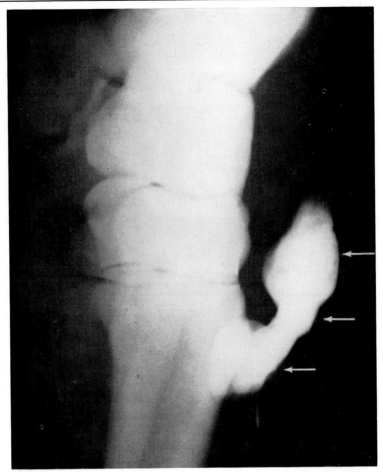

FIG. 12–24. By use of contrast medium, more is learned about a fluctuating soft-tissue swelling anterior to the carpus. The extent of the fluid-filled cavity (arrows) and its failure to communicate with the joint cavities is noted.

especially sensitive. Ionizing radiation can cause both somatic and genetic damage; it also has short-term, long-term, and cumulative effects.

There are three basic rules of radiation safety: (a) Place something between yourself and the radiation (e.g., lead apron). (b) Keep exposure time as brief as possible (i.e., use fast-intensifying screens so the exposure time can be cut). (c) Increase the distance between you and the radiation, remembering the inverse-square law.

Rules for radiation safety are given below:

1. Remove personnel from the room who are not involved in the procedure. Use restraining devices so that the examination can be done with as few people as possible.

2. Always wear protective aprons when assisting in positioning an animal for diagnostic study. Aprons should be evaluated for tears or cracks periodically. This can be done by placing them on a cassette and making routine exposures (Fig. 12–25). Lead aprons should be 0.5-mm lead-equivalent at 85 kVp.

3. Always wear protective gloves if hands are placed near the primary beam. Check gloves for breaks or tears, espe-

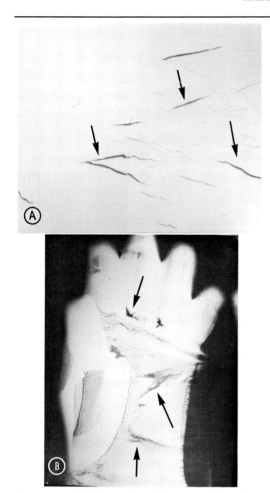

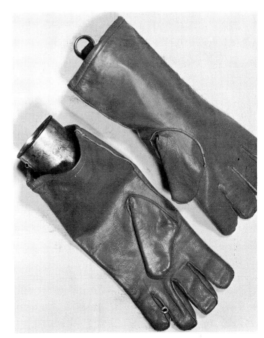

FIG. 12–25. Radiographs of the central portions of a damaged lead apron (A) and lead glove (B) demonstrate the value in checking both of these protective devices for cracks or breaks (arrows).

your body is behind the cassette. Do not position your feet so that they are beneath the cassette with a vertical beam.

7. Use collimation so that there is an unexposed border on each film that proves that the primary beam did not exceed the size of the cassette. This precaution (a) restricts primary beam to a minimum area; (b) exposes as little tissue as possible to the primary beam for patient safety; and (c) decreases the amount of scatter radiation.

8. When possible, use fast film, fast-intensifying screens, and high-kVp technique to cut exposure factors.

9. Use a 2.0-mm aluminum filter installed at the tube housing part to remove softer x-rays. This decreases production of scatter radiation and reduces patient exposure.

FIG. 12–26. Useful life of lead gloves can be prolonged by using devices such as hooks to hang gloves or an open-ended cylinder (can with ends cut away) to prevent the gloves from being stored before they have dried. The moisture on the inside of the gloves hastens deterioration of the lead.

cially since the gloves are often used to handle intractable animals (Fig. 12–25). Lead gloves should be 0.5-mm lead-equivalent at 85 kVp.

4. Give proper care to protective gloves and aprons so that they do not crack because of being folded while moist (Fig. 12–26).

5. Never permit any part of the body to be within the primary beam, whether gloved or not. Use cassette holders.

6. Never position yourself when using a horizontal x-ray beam so that a part of

10. When people are working in the room during exposure, keep the distance from the primary beam as great as possible. (Remember the inverse-square law.)

11. All personnel should wear monitoring film badges outside their aprons. Film rings can be worn on hands if desirable. Film badges are dental-size film inserted in a badge that incorporates metal filters so that amount and type of radiation can be estimated.

12. Never permit anyone under the age of 18 in the room during a diagnostic procedure. Never permit pregnant women in the room during a diagnostic procedure.

13. If possible, rotate personnel who assist with radiographic examinations.

14. Do not direct the x-ray beam into an adjacent room that is regularly occupied.

15. Plan your radiographic procedure carefully and avoid unnecessary retakes.

RADIOGRAPHIC POSITIONING AND NORMAL RADIOGRAPHIC APPEARANCE

For the discussion of positioning, the extremities of the horse have been arbitrarily divided into convenient anatomical divisions. Structures seen on commonly used views are generally discussed together. Methods of positioning are described and illustrated, and examples of normal radiographs are shown. Epiphyseal closure as determined radiographically is discussed. Pertinent comments are included to aid in the recognition of normal structures and in the avoidance of erroneous diagnoses.

The definition of terms frequently used in describing positioning will make the following discussion more meaningful. The useful x-rays are referred to as the *primary beam*, the geometric center of which is the *central ray* or *central beam*. The central beam is perpendicular to the tube axis, and its direction is used in describing tube position and angle. The central beam should always be directed to the midpoint of the area under study. It also should be perpendicular to the long axis of the leg and to the surface of the cassette.

Radiographic techniques for all of the more commonly used views are described in terms of the *standard, darker,* or *lighter* technique. More than one method of obtaining a particular view may be described. It is important that the method finally selected be used repeatedly and that it be one that can easily be duplicated with your equipment. This is important so that familiarity with the appearance of the anatomical structures on the resulting radiograph can be established. Mistaken diagnoses often occur when radiographs of the same anatomical area are made in slightly different positions.

Digit

The phalanges and interphalangeal joints are adequately visualized on a single film, and generally only the anterior-posterior and lateral views are required for a routine radiographic study of the digit. Oblique views may be necessary to gain full appreciation of some lesions.

Views

The anterior-posterior view is made with the leg extended slightly forward (Fig. 12–27). The hoof is elevated on a block to allow the cassette to be positioned posteriorly and "below" the hoof. The central beam is directed at the pastern joint or at the specific area thought to be clinically unsound (Fig. 12–28). It is important that a marker be placed on the cassette so that medial or lateral sides of the foot can be easily identified.

The lateral view usually requires that the foot be elevated so that the central beam can be directed at the point of interest (Figs. 12–29 and 12–30). It is also important to have the foot straight and not deviated medially or, more commonly,

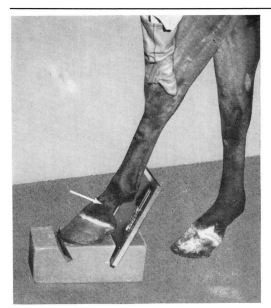

FIG. 12–27. Radiographic technique for the AP view of the digit. By using a block of this type, the cassette can be placed "below" the hoof. Better visualization of the coffin joint is obtained in this way. No part of the helper need be in the primary beam (arrow).

laterally, because of the resulting difficulty in directing the central beam perpendicular to the long axis of the foot. If the horse has any conformational problem, care must be taken to ensure that the central beam is perpendicular to the long axis of the foot at the point of greatest interest.

Special views of the digit are not ordinarily required, but oblique views may be desired to locate a foreign body more positively or to determine the origin of a small chip fracture. Oblique views are made in a manner similar to that used for oblique views of the proximal sesamoid bones (see p. 502). All views of the digit can be made with the *standard* technique.

Diagnosis

Improper positioning of the foot or tube may result in the appearance of asymmetrical joint spaces, leading to a false diagnosis of primary or secondary joint disease. If positioning is extremely poor, minimal joint changes will not be detected radiographically.

In an AP projection of a properly positioned foot, the fetlock, pastern, and coffin joints can be visualized. The fetlock joint is normally narrower than the other two joints, and the pastern joint is narrower than the coffin joint as seen on this pro-

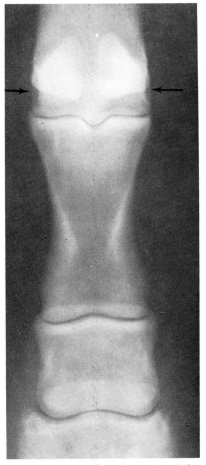

FIG. 12–28. Normal AP radiograph of the digit of a mature horse. In the AP projection, the fetlock joint appears narrower than the other two joints and the pastern joint appears narrower than the coffin joint. The collateral ligaments of the fetlock joint attach on small concave depressions on the lateral and medial aspects of the distal end of the cannon bone (arrows).

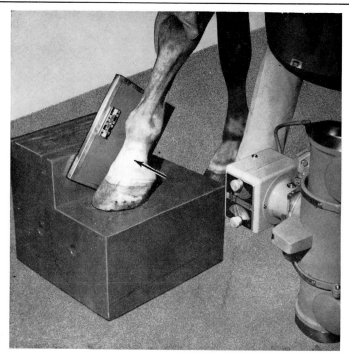

FIG. 12–29. Radiographic technique for the lateral view of the digit. Since the tube will not lower to the floor, the foot has been elevated. The cassette is positioned in a slot so no part of the helper is within the primary beam. The central beam is marked (arrow).

jection. Evaluation of the width of the joint spaces is important since it permits early determination of secondary joint disease. The subchondral bone in the proximal end of the first and second phalanges is normally denser and appears as a sclerotic transverse band. The marrow cavity of the first phalanx narrows markedly at the junction of the middle and distal thirds and then widens in the distal third. The shadow of the navicular bone is cast over the distal portion of the second phalanx and the coffin joint. The proximal border of the navicular bone can be evaluated. The standard exposure is often too light to permit evaluation of the proximal sesamoid bones, and lesions involving these small sesamoid bones can easily be overlooked on this study.

The ergot casts a radiopaque shadow on the midportion of the first phalanx on an AP projection. Examination of the radio-graph made in the lateral projection with a high-intensity light demonstrates this structure to be posterior to the proximal portion of the first phalanx. Shadows caused by uneven thicknesses of tissue in the sole and frog may simulate fracture lines in the navicular bone.

The middle distal sesamoidean ligament attaches distally on the posterior aspect of the first phalanx. On the lateral view, this attachment is often seen to be roughened, and the cortex is always thicker. This commonly noted change has little clinical significance. Calcification in this ligament is occasionally noted, indicating past trauma to this area. The superficial distal sesamoidean ligament attaches on the posterior aspect of the proximal end of the second phalanx. With age, this joint of attachment frequently roughens without clinical significance.

The lateral view frequently shows a

roughened area on the anterior aspect of the distal end of the second phalanx, which is more obvious if the view is slightly oblique. This roughened appearance is due to the fossae for attachment of the collateral ligaments in this area and attachment of the common or long digital extensor tendon. Pathological changes can occur in this area, but the minimal changes described are not thought to be of clinical significance.

Studies of the digit on the hind leg are performed in essentially the same manner. The AP view is somewhat more difficult to make because the tube must be located just behind the elbow. If the hock is rotated inward, it is much easier to position the tube for the AP view.

Epiphyseal Closure

Three epiphyseal plates are normally seen on views of the digit of a newborn foal. They are located in the distal metacarpal and metatarsal bones, in the proximal first phalanx, and in the proximal second phalanx. The epiphyseal plate in the distal metacarpal or metatarsal bone begins to close at five months, appears partially closed at nine months, and is completely closed at one year. In the proximal portion of the first phalanx, closure occurs between four and nine months. The epiphyseal plate in the proximal portion of the second phalanx also begins to close at four months and closure is complete at nine months (see Table 12–4). Union begins in the central portion of these bones and gradually expands to the periphery of the bone. The distal metacarpal (tarsal) metaphysis widens at the time of closure of the distal epiphyseal plate. This widening and apparent sclerotic appearance persists for several months until bony remodeling restores a more normal radiographic appearance. Care must be used to avoid erroneously interpreting this widened sclerotic bone as pathologic change associated with

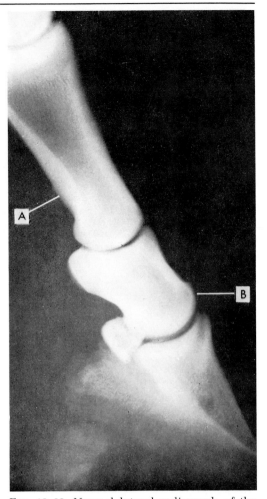

Fig. 12–30. Normal lateral radiograph of the digit of a mature horse. The pastern joint is well seen because the central beam was directed at this point. The area of attachment of the middle distal sesamoidian ligament is slightly roughened (*A*). Changes more extensive than seen here are still within the range of normal. A roughened appearance on the anterior aspect of the second phalanx may be normal. This can be due to the areas of attachment of collateral ligaments (*B*) or the common/long digital extensor tendons.

epiphysitis or metabolic imbalance. In all three of these growth plates, closure in the hind leg seems to occur slightly later than in the comparable plate in the front leg (Fig. 12–31).

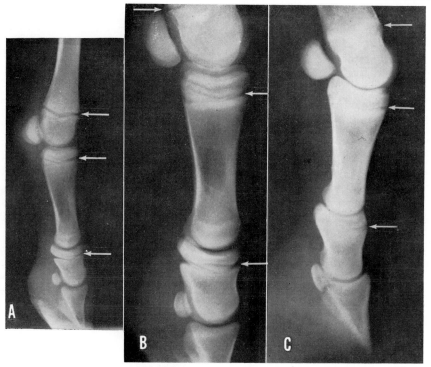

FIG. 12–31. Stages of epiphyseal closure as seen on the lateral view of the digit. The studies are typical of a newborn foal (A), five weeks of age (B), and six months of age (C). The degree of closure of the epiphyseal lines (arrows) can be seen. Note the much wider joint spaces seen on the radiographs taken at birth.

Proximal Sesamoid Bones and Fetlock Joint

Routine radiographic examination of the proximal sesamoid bones and fetlock joint consists of an anterior-posterior view, a lateral view, two oblique views, and a flexed lateral projection.

Views

The AP view is made in the same way as the AP view of the digit, except that both cassette and central beam are elevated (Fig. 12–32). It is recommended that the central beam be angled downward instead of being parallel with the floor. By thus angling the beam, the proximal sesamoid bones are seen superimposed through the distal end of the third metacarpal or metatarsal bone. If a horizontal beam is utilized on the AP view, the proximal sesamoid bones will be superimposed over the fetlock joint space, and diagnosis of lesions in the proximal sesamoid bones is more difficult. Care must be taken in positioning both leg and tube to produce a symmetry of the bones on the radiograph. Medial or lateral markers must be used.

If the fetlock joint is of primary interest, the *standard* technique is adequate. To demonstrate the proximal sesamoid bones, it is imperative to use the *darker* technique (Fig. 12–33). It is often advantageous to compare radiographs made with both techniques.

The lateral view usually requires that the foot be elevated in such a way that the central beam is parallel with the floor and perpendicular to the leg and cassette.

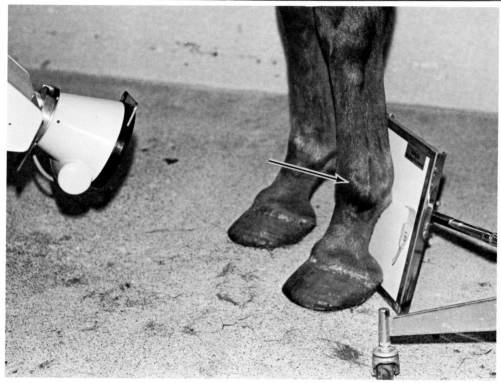

FIG. 12–32. Radiographic technique for the AP view of the proximal sesamoid bones and fetlock joint. The central beam is marked (arrow).

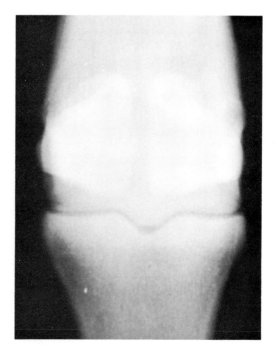

FIG. 12–33. Normal AP radiograph of the proximal sesamoid bones and the fetlock joint of a mature horse.

The view is made in a manner similar to that described for the lateral view of the digit, except that the cassette and central beam are elevated (Fig. 12–34). *Standard* technique is adequate for the lateral view (Fig. 12–35).

There is a high incidence of chip fractures originating from the anterior aspect of the proximal end of the first phalanx and from the proximal sesamoid bones. These small bone fragments are best seen on the oblique views, which would, therefore, be considered a part of the routine examination of this area. The tube is positioned anterior-lateral and the cassette posterior-medial to demonstrate either the lateral proximal sesamoid bone or the anterior-medial aspect of the fetlock joint (Fig. 12–36). The opposite oblique view will project the medial proximal sesamoid or the anterior-lateral aspect of the fetlock joint. Oblique views are made at approximately 45° angles. *Standard* technique is used for the oblique views (Fig. 12–37). The flexed lateral projection is of great value in evaluation of the articular surface of the proximal sesamoid bones or posterior aspect of the distal end of the metacarpal (metatarsal) bone (Fig. 12–38). Examination of the fetlock area of the hind leg is done essentially in the same manner as a study of the fore fetlock.

Diagnosis

In examining the edges of the proximal sesamoid bones, care must be taken to recognize the difference between the normal fine vascular grooves and small fracture lines. Sesamoiditis causes rarefaction of the bones, and the vascular channels become more prominent. If changes are not recognized a horse may continue in training and be predisposed to later fracture. New bone production on the abaxial aspect may result from tearing of the suspensory ligament; new bone production

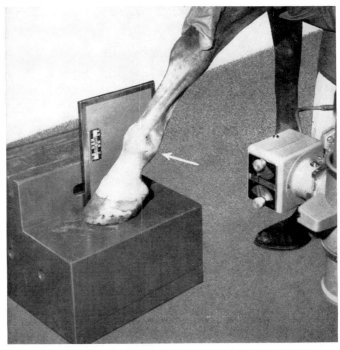

FIG. 12–34. Radiographic technique for the lateral view of the proximal sesamoid bones. Usually the foot must be elevated to obtain a true lateral projection. The central beam is marked (arrow).

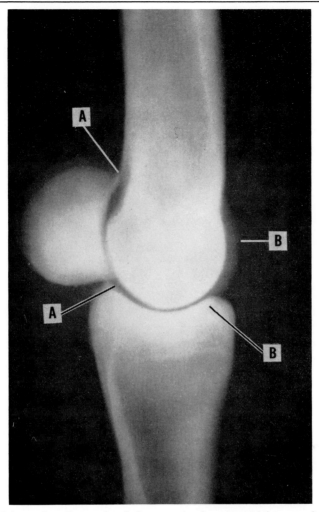

FIG. 12–35. Normal lateral radiograph of the proximal sesamoid bones of a mature horse. If positioning is correct, the fetlock joint can be easily studied. The posterior portion of the sagittal condylar ridge (A) may resemble a fracture fragment. The anterior portion of this ridge (B) extends below the proximal end of the first phalanx.

originating at the base of the proximal sesamoid bones is usually due to tearing of the distal sesamoidean ligaments.

On the true lateral view, a radiopaque shadow resembling new bone production or a chip fracture is frequently seen posterior to the distal end of the cannon bone. This shadow represents the posterior portion of the sagittal condylar ridge. If the lateral view is slightly oblique, one of the joint surfaces of the first phalanx may be superimposed over the distal end of the

proximal sesamoid bone, causing a shadow that resembles a chip fracture from the sesamoid bone.

Small concave depressions on the lateral and medial aspect of the distal end of the cannon bone are seen on the AP view and are the site of attachment of the collateral ligaments for the fetlock point. If the AP view is slightly obliqued, one area of attachment is not seen and the other appears much more obvious. Such a difference in appearance can errone-

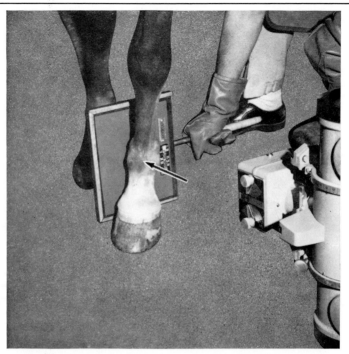

FIG. 12–36. Radiographic technique for the oblique view of the proximal sesamoid bones. This position will demonstrate the lateral proximal sesamoid bone to good advantage. The central beam is marked (arrow). This technique may be used for oblique views of the digit by using a lower focus with the beam. It is a valuable view when examining for position of a small bone chip in the fetlock joint. In this case, the medial oblique view should also be taken.

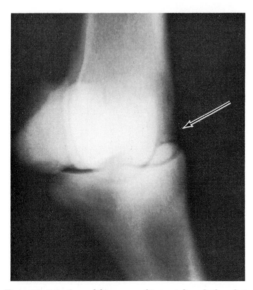

FIG. 12–37. An oblique radiograph of the fetlock joint, demonstrating the value of such a study in diagnosis of small chip fractures (arrow) that originate from the anterior lip on the first phalanx.

ously suggest pathologic change. Periosteal new bone can be present on the lateral and medial aspects of the distal extremity of the metacarpal (metatarsal) bone as a result of an old sprain at the attachment of the collateral ligaments.

Epiphyseal Closure

Normally, there are no epiphyseal plates in the proximal sesamoid bones. Epiphyseal closure in the metacarpal bone and first phalanx is illustrated in Figures 12–39 and 12–40. Closure times for the epiphyseal plates in the distal metacarpal or metatarsal bones and the proximal portion of the first phalanx has been discussed earlier (p. 497 and Table 12–4). Bipartite sesamoid bones that radiographically resemble fractures have been reported. These bipartite sesamoid bones form from two ossification centers rather

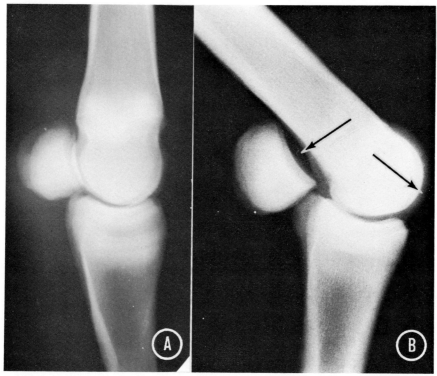

FIG. 12-38. Lateral radiograph of the fetlock joint extended (A) and flexed (B), demonstrating the ease with which the articular surface of the distal cannon bone (arrow) and the articular surfaces of the proximal sesamoid bones (arrow) can be evaluated on the flexed lateral study.

than one, and union does not occur. Since the two centers do not fuse, the radiolucent plate does not represent a true epiphyseal plate. This abnormality is usually bilateral and is often present in both front and hind legs.

Third Phalanx

Radiographic examination of the third phalanx requires considerable preparation. All dirt and debris must be removed from the hoof wall and sole to prevent the appearance of multiple artifacts on the radiograph. The shoe must be pulled if the radiographic study is to be of maximum value. A routine examination consists of two AP views and a lateral view. Oblique studies are utilized to gain additional information about the angles of the third phalanx. Medial or lateral markers must be used with the AP and oblique projec-

tions. Studies are performed in essentially the same manner for the fore and hind legs.

Views

Because of the unique shape of the third phalanx, it is impossible to evaluate the entire bone and adjacent coffin joint on a single AP view, and two AP views should be made. The first is made in the manner described for radiography of the digit (p. 494). The cassette must be positioned "below" the bulbs of the heels. The central beam is directed at 45° and centered at the coronary band. The beam is then perpendicular to the long axis of the foot. This view permits good evaluation of the coffin joint and adjacent bones. *Standard* technique is used for this study.

A second AP view is made with the foot placed directly on the film holder (Fig.

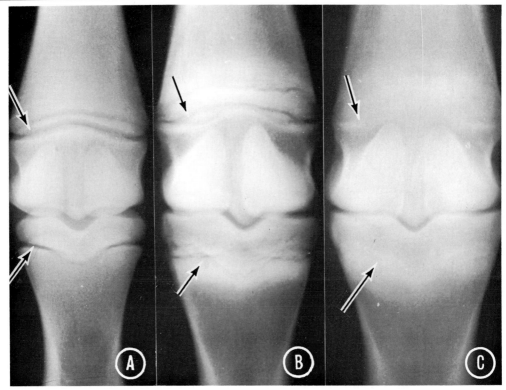

FIG. 12–39. States of epiphyseal closure as seen on the AP view of the fetlock joint. The studies are typical of a newborn foal (A), four months of age (B), and nine months of age (C). The change in appearance of epiphyseal plates can be seen (arrows).

12–41), permitting study of the cancellous bone that comprises most of the third phalanx (Fig. 12–42). Cassettes can be placed directly on the floor or slightly elevated on a block. Elevating the feet may help to prevent the horse from placing its full weight on the cassette. The cassette can be placed in a protective "tunnel" to prevent damage while the foot is in position (Fig. 12–41). If a screened cassette is used without any protective device, the leg should be extended slightly forward. The helper should then place his knee behind and slightly under the carpus to support part of the weight of the leg and prevent the horse from stepping forward on the cassette. The central beam is directed toward the floor, perpendicular to the hoof wall and centered just distal to the coronary band. If screened cassettes are used, the *lighter* technique is adequate. Even though the hoof wall appears to be thicker in this view, the density of the hoof and the third phalanx is less. With the horse standing on the film, the problem of motion is minimized and a nonscreen technique with the film placed in a cardboard holder can be used. With nonscreen film, the mas should be increased 4 to 5 times over the mas used with the *lighter* technique.

Oblique views of the third phalanx are frequently necessary and are taken with the film holder on the floor and the hoof placed on the film holder. The tube is moved 45° medially or laterally, and the central beam is centered just below the coronary band (Fig. 12–43). Such views allow good visualization of one of the angles of the third phalanx and better

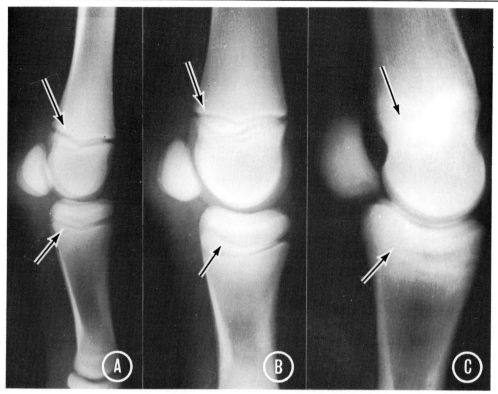

FIG. 12-40. States of epiphyseal closure as seen on the lateral view of the fetlock joint. The studies are typical of a newborn (A), four months of age (B), and nine months of age (C). The change in appearance of epiphyseal plates can be seen (arrows).

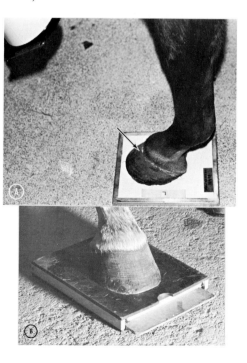

FIG. 12-41. Radiographic technique for the AP view of the third phalanx. A, The central beam is marked (arrow). B, Use of a tunnel in radiography of the third phalanx that provides protection to the cassette.

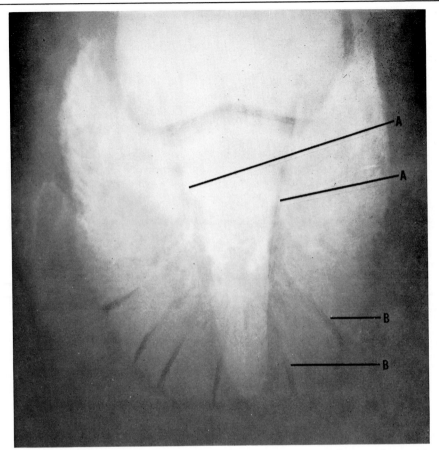

FIG. 12–42. Normal AP radiograph of the third phalanx of a mature horse taken with the hoof resting on the cassette. Lateral sulci of the frog (A) and vascular channels in the bone (B) present problems in diagnosis.

demonstration of fractures in these areas (Fig. 12–44). *Lighter* technique is used for this view if a screened cassette is used.

The deep sulci of the frog cast prominent shadows on the AP views of the third phalanx. These lines interfere with diagnosis but have been tolerated in the past. It is now strongly recommended that the sole be packed with an easily molded material of similar density to occlude the shadows. Substances that have been utilized as packing materials include green surgical soap paste* and Play-Doh.†

*Malone Oil Co. Ltd., Scarborough, Ont.
†Rainbow Crafts, Cincinnati, Ohio.

A technique has been described recently in which a water bath especially designed to fit over a cassette is placed on a focus-type grid. Water has the same density as soft tissues and eliminates the shadows cast by the sulci of the frog since it completely fills the frog without artifact (Fig. 12–45). It is necessary to use a grid since the water causes an increase in the amount of secondary radiation produced. The exposure factors would have to be increased an appropriate amount depending on the grid ratio.

A lateral view of the third phalanx usually requires that the foot be elevated so that the central beam is parallel with the

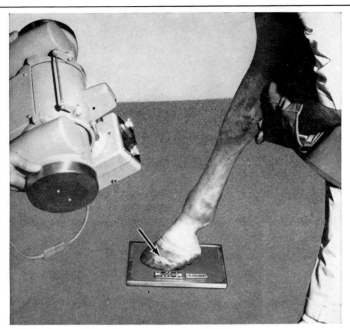

FIG. 12–43. Radiographic technique for the oblique view of the third phalanx. The technique shown does not require use of any block but places the cassette directly on the floor. The central beam is marked (arrow).

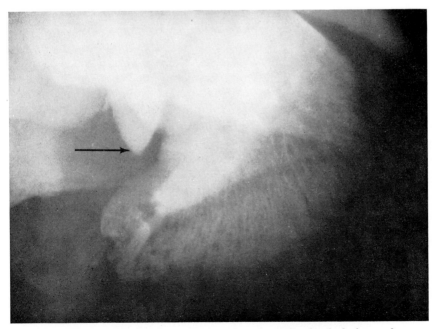

FIG. 12–44. Normal oblique radiograph of the lateral angle of the third phalanx of a mature horse. The angle of the navicular bone can also be studied on this view (arrow).

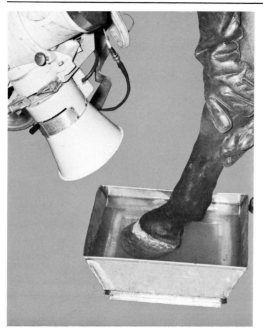

FIG. 12–45. Water bath in use with x-ray grid and cassette underneath. Radiograph being taken. (Courtesy of Dr. J. Lebel.)

floor and perpendicular to the third phalanx (Figs. 12–46 and 12–47). The amount of elevation required is determined by the equipment available. As with all lateral views, the leg must be straight if a joint space is to be visualized. The central beam is centered on or just below the coronary band in the midportion of the hoof. This view is made with the *standard* technique.

Diagnosis

Both AP views are required for evaluation of both the distal interphalangeal (coffin) joint and the entire third phalanx. It is important to be able to evaluate the coffin joint for primary or secondary joint disease or to determine if a fracture line enters the joint space. These changes often cannot be seen on the weight-bearing study. Conversely, a fracture in the distal portion of the third phalanx cannot be judged solely on the AP view, which better demonstrates the coffin joint.

Radiographic study of the third phalanx presents specific problems in diagnosis. The presence of artifacts caused by improper cleaning of the sole and frog indicate that the examination should be repeated.

Radiolucent shadows in the third phalanx are caused by numerous grooves for vessels and may resemble radiolucent fracture lines. The pattern of these normal grooves is symmetrical, whereas a fracture line presents an unsymmetrical appearance. In addition, most vascular grooves radiate from the semilunar canal, making their direction different from that of the typical fracture of the third phalanx.

A notch called the "toe stay" is often present in the distal tip of the third phalanx and should not be confused with bone lysis secondary to osteomyelitis secondary to a sole abscess.

The cartilages of the third phalanx may be seen in various stages of ossification (sidebones). This degenerative process usually begins just proximal to the angles of the third phalanx and progresses away from the bone (Fig. 12–48). However, it is not uncommon for the process to begin in the portion of the cartilage farthest from the third phalanx and to progress toward the third phalanx (Fig. 12–49). At the point where the two areas of ossification approach each other, the radiolucent line resembles a fracture.

The extensor process of the third phalanx on the lateral radiograph commonly presents a sharp appearance, a finding that is usually not of clinical significance. Pedal osteitis is a condition often overlooked as a cause of lameness. The main changes seen with this condition are

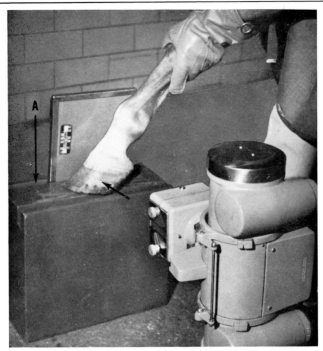

FIG. 12-46. Radiographic technique for the lateral view of the third phalanx. This type of block allows the cassette to be positioned below the level of the sole (*A*). This places the third phalanx in better position on the film. The central beam is marked (arrow).

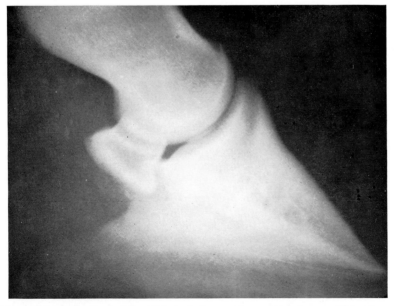

FIG. 12-47. Normal lateral view of the third phalanx of a mature horse. This view is primarily of value in diagnosing fractures of the extensor process and rotation of the third phalanx. Other fractures of the third phalanx are frequently not seen on this view.

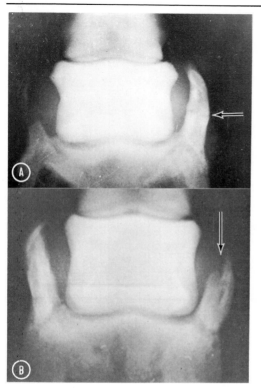

FIG. 12–48. AP radiographs showing the pattern of ossification within the lateral cartilages of the third phalanx. *A*, The degree of ossification is asymmetrical, with a suggestion of a fracture line (arrow). This may be a fracture, or it may be a point of fusion between two separate areas of ossification. *B*, The degree of ossification is asymmetrical but more nearly the same. The "double" hook (arrow) is not uncommon.

roughening of the outline of the third phalanx. It is usually best seen at the angle of the third phalanx on the AP projection. However, the lateral view may often demonstrate the changes. In severe cases, there is marked decalcification at the edge of the bone and small spicules of well-defined bone. Often the margin of the bone is not distinct and appears blurred. A study by von Salis (1961) warned of over diagnosis of the irregular appearance of the borders of the third phalanx.

Epiphyseal Closure

No epiphyseal plates are normally seen on radiographs of the third phalanx. Radiolucent lines are sometimes identified extending across the tip of the angles of the third phalanx on the oblique views, separating a small fragment of bone that resembles a fracture fragment. If clinical signs are localized to this area, a view of the same area of the opposite foot or another angle of the same foot may be used for comparative evaluation.

Navicular Bone

Diagnostic studies of the navicular bone are difficult to obtain and require specific positioning of both tube and foot. Medial or lateral markers must be used on both AP and oblique views.

Views

Oxspring (1935) described the "upright pedal route" as a method of obtaining an AP view. A specially constructed stand

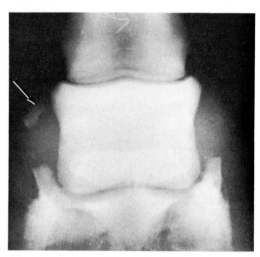

FIG. 12–49. AP radiograph of the pattern of ossification within the lateral cartilage of the third phalanx that demonstrates an abnormal but not uncommon pattern, with the tip of the lateral cartilage (arrow) ossified unilaterally.

held the wall of the toe perpendicular to the ground, and the cassette was placed vertically, posterior to the heels. The central beam was directed parallel with the ground, centered at the coronary band. This technique has been modified so that the anterior wall of the hoof is not quite perpendicular but is tipped forward slightly. The central beam is still parallel with the ground and centered at the coronary band (Fig. 12–50).

Another technique advocated for use in obtaining the AP view is referred to as the "high coronary route." This view is taken with the foot resting on the cassette, with the central beam angled at approximately 60° to the ground and centered at the coronary band. In a variation of the "high coronary route," the toe is placed on a small wooden block to overextend the foot (Fig. 12–51).

The purpose of these special positions for the AP view is to cause an apparent elevation of the navicular bone on the radiograph, permitting the navicular bone to be seen projected through the second phalanx (Fig. 12–52). Special blocks must be fabricated to permit exact duplication of positioning for each examination.

The AP view, regardless of the technique used, is made through a great amount of tissue. Use of a grid will eliminate scatter radiation and produce a study of better diagnostic quality. The *darker* technique is used on the various AP views, since the navicular bone must be seen projected through the second phalanx. Additional compensation must be made for the grid if it is used. The sole should be "packed" on the AP studies to eliminate superimposed shadows. The "water-bath" technique is also beneficial

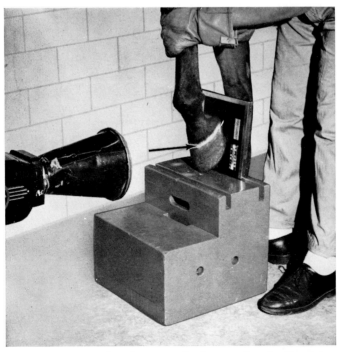

FIG. 12–50. Radiographic technique for the navicular bone using the "upright pedal route." The central beam is marked (arrow). This picture was posed to show one of the most common radiation hazards. The assistant has positioned his leg directly behind the horse's foot within the primary beam.

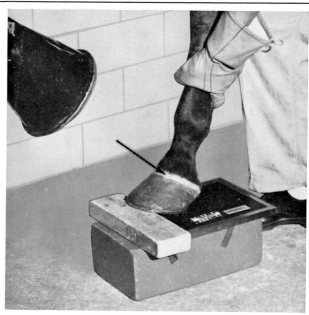

Fig. 12–51. Radiographic technique for the navicular bone using the "high coronary route." The cassette has been placed on a block to prevent the horse from putting his full weight on it. The small block is used to produce further extension of the foot. The angle of the central beam is approximately 60°. The central beam is marked (arrow).

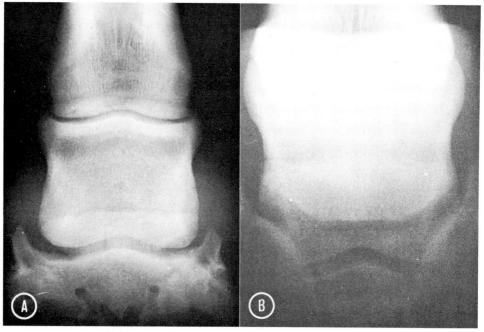

Fig. 12–52. AP radiographs of the navicular bone made by use of the two normal positions of the navicular bone. (A) on the routine AP view and projections demonstrating the elevation of the navicular bone and (B) by use of a central beam directed as in the "high coronary route." Note the better evaluation of the navicular bone in B.

in evaluation of the navicular bone (*see* Chap. 6, p. 267). Changes not easily identified on the more routine studies can be seen more clearly.

The lateral view is made in essentially the same manner as the lateral view of the third phalanx (Fig. 12–46). The central beam is directed posteriorly and proximally so that it is centered on the navicular bone. To obtain true lateral views, the foot must usually be elevated on a block.

The navicular bone may also be studied in a dorsoventral (DV) view, as described by Morgan (1972), projecting a portion of the bone free of other osseous structures. The DV study is made with the horse standing on the cassette. The tube is positioned posterior to the cannon bone and angled anteriorly 10–20° from the perpendicular. The central beam is directed between the bulbs of the heels (Fig. 12–53). The *lighter* technique is used for this study. This study provides an opportunity to view a portion of the navicular bone without superimposition of other bones. The posterior cortex (ligamentous sur-

face) is well identified and is evaluated as to thickness. The medullary cavity can be studied for the presence of lucent zones representing the cystic areas and increased prominence of the vascular channels noted on the AP views (Fig. 12–54).

Oblique studies of the navicular bone, to demonstrate the tips of the bone, are made in the same manner as the oblique view of the third phalanx (Fig. 12–43). The *lighter* technique is used for the oblique study.

Diagnosis

It is of value to have several AP views of the navicular bone to aid in evaluation of both proximal and distal borders of the navicular bone. The authenticity of bony spurs and/or lytic areas is more convincing when the lesions can be located on several views. Unfortunately, the lateral view is often overlooked as an aid in diagnosing changes in the navicular bone. Alterations in the thickness and change in

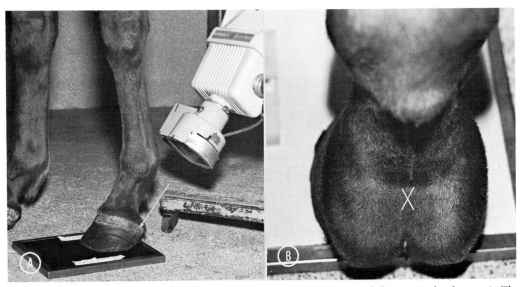

FIG. 12–53. Radiographic technique used for obtaining a DV view of the navicular bone. *A*, The horse stands on the cassette, and the central beam (arrow) is directed downward just posterior to the fetlock and between the bulbs of the heel. *B*, The point of contact of the central beam (**X**) is seen from the posterior aspect.

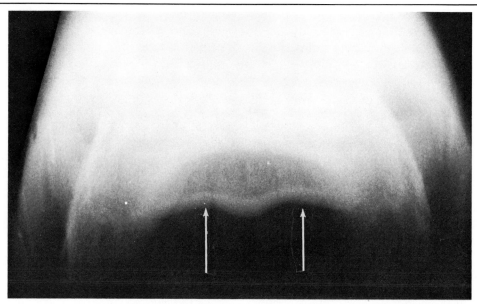

Fig. 12–54. Normal radiograph of the navicular bone taken with a DV projection. The posterior cortex (arrows) can be studied, along with the cancellous bone.

contour of the navicular bone as seen from the side can be demonstrated only on the lateral view. The dorsoventral view is the only method that permits evaluation of the posterior cortex of the navicular bone as well as providing another projection of the changes in the medullary cavity.

Radiography of the navicular bone as it lies within the intact hoof will demonstrate only major changes, including changes in vascularization that present as increased porosity of the bone, adjacent osteosclerotic changes, bony spurs, and fractures. The radiographic changes of navicular disease seem to follow the development of clinical signs. Thus, the greatest value of a radiographic study is in prognosis, notwithstanding reports that radiographic studies demonstrate pathologic change before the clinical signs are present (Wintzer, 1965). Comparison studies of the opposite leg are sometimes of value in determining whether the changes noted are of clinical significance.

As in the case of radiography of the third phalanx, it is suggested that studies of the navicular bone be made after packing the sulci as described earlier (p. 506), or using a water bath. Thorough packing will prevent a false diagnosis of fracture of the navicular bone through misinterpretation of the radiolucent lines caused by the medial sulci of the frog (Fig. 12–55).

Epiphyseal Closure

There are no normal epiphyseal lines in this area. "Fractured" navicular bones have been seen in young horses with no known evidence of trauma. In one case, a six-month-old colt had "fractures" of three of the four navicular bones. When the clinical signs do not fit the typical picture of navicular fracture, the possibility of bipartite sesamoid bone must be considered.

Metacarpal and Metatarsal Bones

Routine projections of the metacarpi and metatarsi include AP, lateral, and both oblique views. Familiarity with the radiographic appearance of the carpal and tarsal bones will eliminate the need for medial or lateral markers. However, until one gains this competence, it is suggested that the medial or lateral aspect be marked.

Views

The AP view of fore and hind limbs is taken in a weight-bearing position. The central beam is directed at the area of greatest interest, and the cassette is positioned posteriorly (Fig. 12–56). The lateral view is also taken in a weight-bearing position and is made with the tube positioned laterally and the cassette medially (Fig. 12–57).

Oblique views are made in a manner similar to oblique views of the proximal sesamoid bones. The second and fourth metacarpal and metatarsal bones require slightly different angles of projection. However, adequate studies can be obtained if the tube is placed approximately 60° from the midsagittal plane (Fig. 12–58). The *standard* technique is used for all views of the splint bones and cannon bone.

Diagnosis

The carpometacarpal (tarsometatarsal) joint and the metacarpophalangeal (metatarsophalangeal) (fetlock) joints cannot both be seen adequately on a single radiograph. It is important that at least one joint be included for purposes of orientation. Cassettes that measure 7″ × 17″ (17 × 43 cm) are excellent for studies of this area and will usually demonstrate both proximal and distal joints to some degree (Figs. 12–59 and 12–60).

The anterior cortex of the cannon bone normally is thick in the diaphyseal area; this should not be confused with an osteitis secondary to trauma.

On a lateral view of the metacarpal bones, the splint bones will appear super-

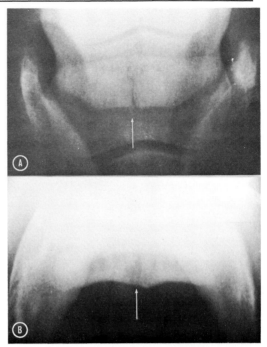

FIG. 12–55. Anteroposterior (A) and dorso-ventral (B) projections of the navicular bone with a fracture line identified in the midportion (arrows). The sulcus was not packed on the AP study. The fracture line is more clearly identified on the AP projection and closely resembles the normal shadow of the middle sulcus of the frog. The lucency in the posterior cortical shadow in the DV projection confirms pathologic change.

imposed. However, the splint bones on the hind leg are different in size and position. The fourth metatarsal bone is massive in its proximal position and is prominent as it projects farther posteriorly on the lateral view.

There is a wide variation in the appearance of the distal end of the splint bones on the radiograph. The morphology ranges from a slender tapering tip to that of a large "bulb." The tip may rest close to the cannon bone or may flare out and be up to 1 cm away from the cannon bone. Extensive separation of the splint bone from the cannon bone may suggest soft-tissue inflammation and edema secondary

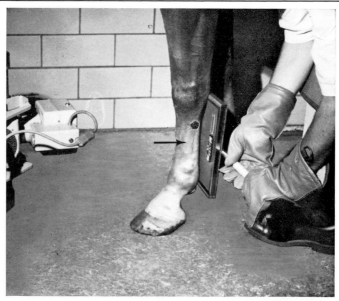

FIG. 12–56. Radiographic technique for obtaining the AP view of the metacarpal bones. The same principle is used in making the AP view of the metatarsal bones. The central beam is marked (arrow).

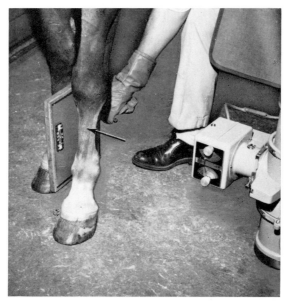

FIG. 12–57. Radiographic technique for obtaining the lateral view of the metacarpal bones. The same principle is used in making the lateral radiograph of the metatarsal bones. The central beam is marked (arrow).

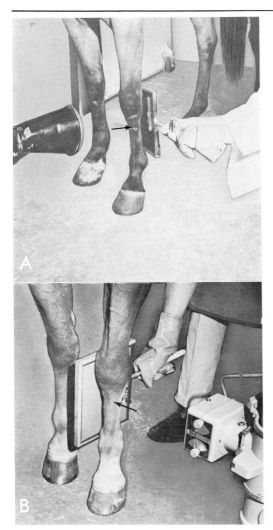

FIG. 12-58. Radiographic technique for making the medial (A) and lateral (B) oblique views of the splint bones. The same technique is used for both front and hind legs. Each splint bone requires a slightly different angle for the best projection. The central beam has been marked (arrows).

to trauma and may be an important radiographic finding.

Epiphyseal Closure

Epiphyseal lines are not seen on studies of the metacarpal or metatarsal bones of immature horses unless the examination includes the distal portion of these bones. The epiphyseal line in the distal end of the cannon bones closes by one year of age. The third metacarpal bone closes somewhat earlier than the third metatarsal bone. (See Table 12-4.) An epiphyseal line may be seen in the distal end of the second and fourth metacarpal and metatarsal bones. These bones are cartilaginous at birth and may show an epiphyseal line in their distal portions (Fig. 12-61).

Carpus

Routine radiographic examination of the carpus includes AP, flexed lateral, extended lateral, anterior-lateral/poste-

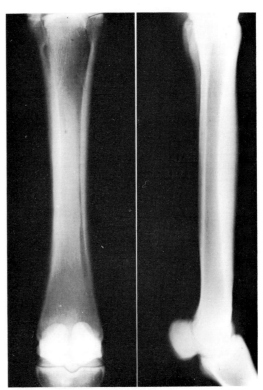

FIG. 12-59. AP and lateral views of second, third, and fourth metacarpal bones taken on a 7″ × 17″ cassette and film. This view shows the entire length of the metacarpal bones.

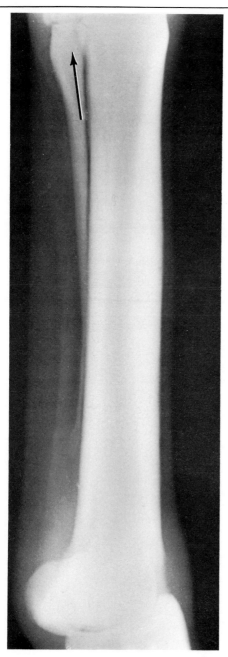

FIG. 12-60. Oblique radiograph of the metacarpal bones made on 7″ × 17″ film with the second metacarpal bone (arrow) projected free from the larger third metacarpal bone.

rior-medial oblique and anterior-medial/posterior-lateral oblique views. Proximal-distal tangential studies of the distal radius and anterior surface of the carpal bones are a necessity in determining the exact number and location of carpal fracture fragments. Since the carpus is relatively high on the leg, the horse may be allowed to stand in a normal manner regardless of the type of x-ray machine utilized. The upper portion of the leg is usually clean and little preparation prior to radiography is required unless leg paints or blisters have been applied.

Medial or lateral markers are not required on studies of the carpus because differences in morphology of the carpal bones allow positive identification. However, use of the markers is helpful until one becomes familiar with the radiographic anatomy of the area.

Views

For the AP view, the horse should be positioned to bear weight on the leg being examined. If necessary, the opposite forefoot can be raised. The central beam should be horizontal to the ground and directed at the midportion of the carpus (Fig. 12-62). Since the cassette does not rest on the ground, care must be taken to avoid motion during the exposure. Cassette holders with adjustable "legs" may be used to eliminate this problem. A well-positioned radiograph will permit visualization of the "tunnel" between the radial and intermediate carpal bones (Fig. 12-63).

Extended weight-bearing lateral and flexed lateral views are made with the x-ray tube in a similar position. The extended lateral view is made with the foot resting on the ground (Figs. 12-64 and 12-65), and in the flexed lateral view, the foot is held high off the ground (Figs. 12-66 and 12-67). In both views, but especially in the flexed lateral view, the leg

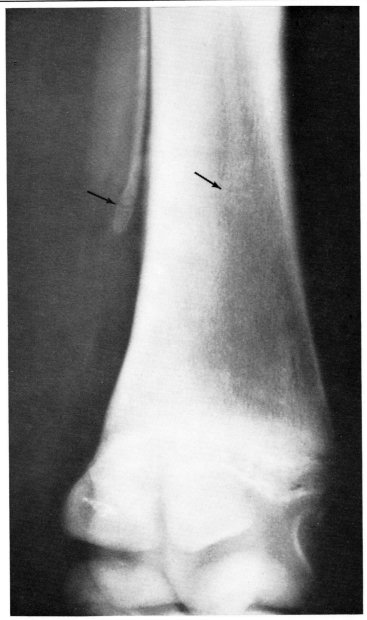

Fig. 12-61. Oblique view of the distal portion of the splint bone of a horse six months of age. The cartilaginous plate is seen in the distal end of the splint bones (arrows). This should not be confused with a fracture line. The slight bowing of the distal tip of the splint bone is normal.

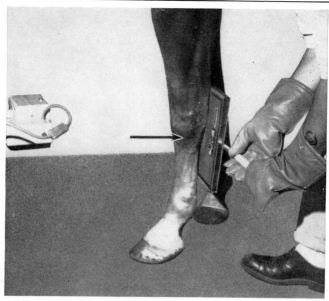

Fig. 12–62. Radiographic technique for the AP view of the carpus. A cassette holder with a "leg" is helpful for this study. The central beam is marked (arrow).

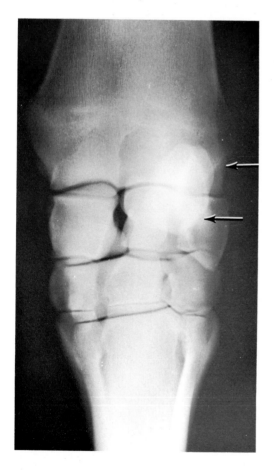

Fig. 12–63. A normal AP radiograph of the carpus of a mature horse. The accessory carpal bone is seen laterally as an area of increased density (arrows).

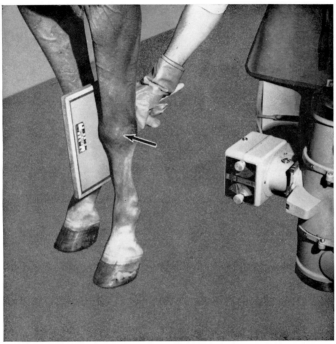

FIG. 12–64. Radiographic technique for the routine lateral view of the carpus. The central beam is marked (arrow).

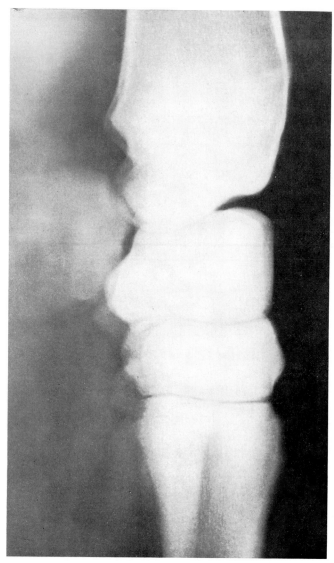

FIG. 12–65. Normal lateral radiograph of the carpus of a mature horse.

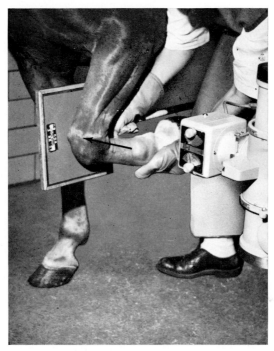

FIG. 12-66. Radiographic technique for the flexed lateral view of the carpus. The central beam is marked (arrow).

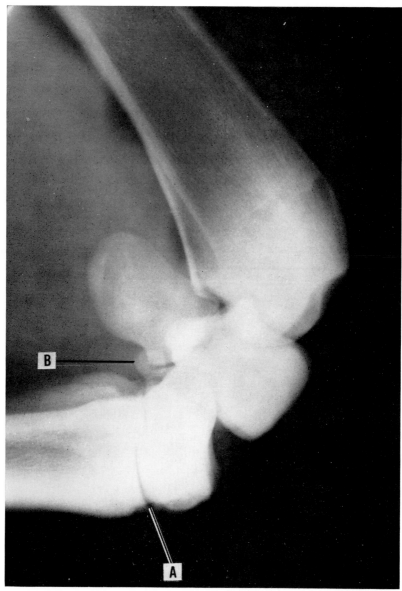

FIG. 12–67. Normal flexed lateral radiograph of the carpus of a mature horse. Note the absence of demonstrable motion in the carpometacarpal joint (*A*). The first carpal bone can be seen (*B*).

must be kept straight and not abducted at the shoulder if the joint spaces are to be accurately evaluated. The flexed lateral view can be of value in determining whether a recognized chip fracture is free or attached. Since the soft tissue is compressed when the carpus is flexed, the unattached chip will shift in position relative to its appearance on the straight lateral view. This view does provide for visualization of the articular surfaces and can be valuable for purposes of prognosis.

The oblique views are made to clearly demonstrate the anterior-medial and anterior-lateral aspects of the carpus (Figs. 12–68 and 12–69), and both oblique studies are essential in the diagnosis of carpal or radial fractures (Park *et al.,* 1970; O'Brien *et al.,* 1971; Dixon, 1969).

It is often of advantage to direct the x-ray beam in a proximal-to-distal direction to obtain a "skyline" view of the distal radius or the anterior surface of either row of carpal bones. Such a study provides a third dimension to the radiographic examination of the carpus. The examination is made with the horse standing and the carpus flexed to a maximal degree. The cassette is held beneath the knee and parallel to the floor. The x-ray tube is positioned above and in front of the horse with the beam directed at such an angle that it will project the anterior surface of the distal radius or one of the rows of carpal bones. The angle of the beam is dependent on the anatomical area of concern and the manner in which the horse is holding the leg. Usually, the cassette is held by hand, but collimation makes it easy to prevent irradiation of the gloved hand by the primary beam (Figs. 12–70 through 12–73).

The advantages of the "skyline" projections are apparent; they can demonstrate exact location of multiple chip fragments and prevent the error of noting one fracture fragment on more routine views while missing other equally important le-

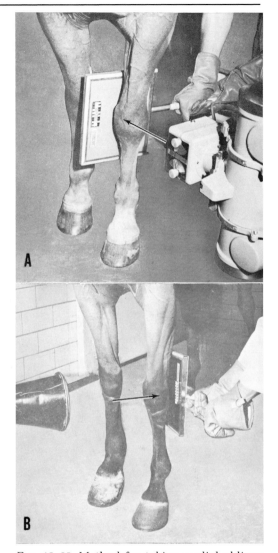

Fig. 12–68. Method for taking medial oblique (*A*) and lateral oblique (*B*) views of the carpus. (The central beam is marked by arrows).

sions. Incomplete fracture lines have been diagnosed on these views only and the horse prevented from further activity that would have led to a complete fracture with more serious complications.

Darker techniques are used for the five routine views. The lighter technique is used for the "skyline" views.

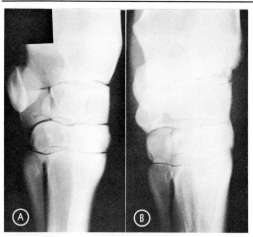

FIG. 12-69. Oblique projections of a normal carpus, demonstrating the anterior medial (A) and anterior lateral (B) aspects of the carpus.

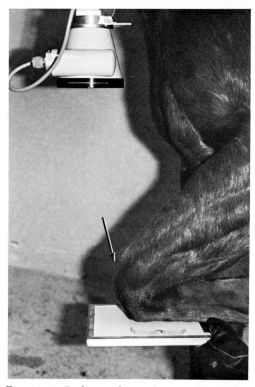

FIG. 12-70. Radiographic technique for the DV projection of the carpus that will project the anterior surface of the proximal row of carpal bones. By careful coning of the primary beam, the gloved hand can remain outside the primary beam (arrow).

Diagnosis

Several normal anatomical structures in the carpus may create problems in radiographic diagnosis. The first carpal bone, when separate, is seen on the medial side posterior to the second carpal bone. The size varies from 0.5 to 1.0 cm. On the lateral view, it is seen posterior to the distal row of carpal bones. It is differentiated from a fracture fragment by its specific location and by its smooth, round appearance (Fig. 12-74).

A small bone occasionally appearing on the lateral aspect of the carpus posteriorly is assumed to be a nonunited fifth carpal bone. It is similar in shape and size to the first carpal bone (Fig. 12-74).

The chestnut creates a soft tissue shadow just proximal to the carpus. At times, the mass of horn is dense enough to resemble soft-tissue calcification.

The medial aspect of the distal radial metaphysis is prominent and is sometimes mistakenly diagnosed as new bone secondary to trauma.

On lateral weight-bearing views, the articular surface of the distal end of the radius appears to be positioned posteriorly. The resultant "notch" on the anterior surface of the radius is normal and is not a conformational problem.

The distal end of the ulna is best seen on the lateral aspect of the distal radius on the oblique view. Its appearance is extremely variable, ranging from no apparent shadow to complete ossification (Morgan, 1965). Often there is a radiolucent line resembling a transverse fracture at the junction between two ossified portions of the distal ulna. The degree of ossification does not seem to be related to age, and the ulna on the opposite leg frequently has a dissimilar pattern.

Epiphyseal Closure

An ossification center representing the distal tip of the ulna is seen at birth, but

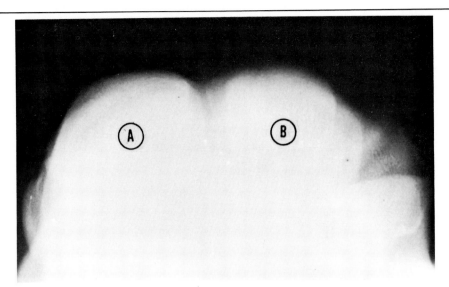

FIG. 12-71. Normal radiograph of the "skyline" projection of the anterior surface of the proximal row of carpal bones. The radial (A) and intermediate (B) carpal bones are shown.

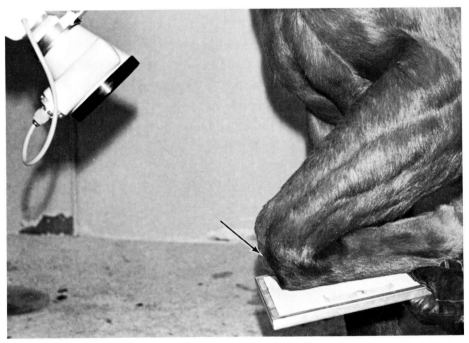

FIG. 12-72. Radiographic technique for the DV projection of the carpus that projects the anterior surface of the distal row of carpal bones. By careful coning of the primary beam, the gloved hand can remain outside the primary beam (arrow).

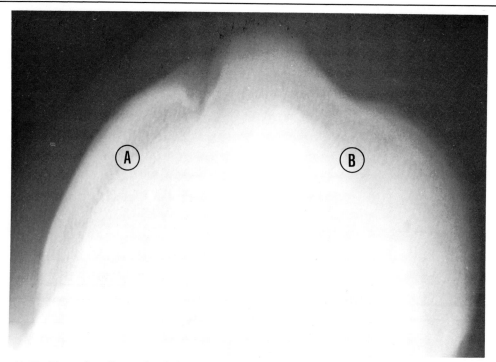

FIG. 12–73. Normal radiograph of the "skyline" projection of the anterior surface of the distal row of carpal bones. The fourth (*A*) and third (*B*) carpal bones are shown.

FIG. 12–74. AP and oblique views of the carpus of a mature horse with separate ossification centers for both the first and the fifth carpal bones (arrows). These can be differentiated from fractures because of their location and their smooth, round appearance.

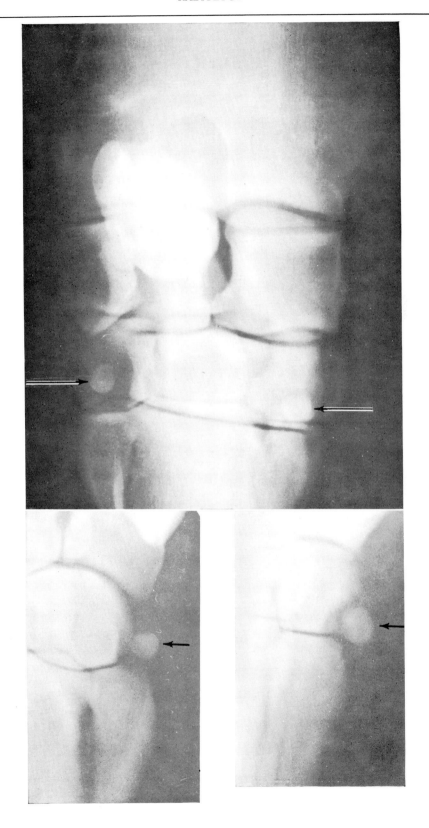

usually it fuses with the distal radial epiphysis by six to nine months of age. This union often leaves a radiolucent scar that may be visible throughout the life of the horse (Fig. 12–75).

An epiphyseal line is normally seen in the distal radius, and closure usually begins in the center by 20 months. Complete closure usually occurs between 2 and 2.5 years of age, although in certain breed lines, closure may not occur until almost 3 years of age (Figs. 12–76 and 12–77; Table 12–4).

Occasionally, an epiphyseal line is identified within the distal portion of the accessory carpal bone (Fig. 12–78). This is not a common finding, but it should not be confused with an avulsion fracture.

Elbow

Radiographic studies of the elbow are difficult because of the greater thickness of the tissue and because of difficulties in positioning the horse, cassette, and tube. The lateral view is easiest to obtain; the oblique and AP views are difficult. The thickness of the tissue requires use of a grid and much higher ma and kVp capabilities than are needed for studies of the digits.

Views

The lateral view is most easily taken with the horse standing and extending the affected limb forward. The cassette is positioned on the lateral aspect of the elbow. The tube is positioned on the opposite side of the horse, and the central beam is directed to pass cranially in front of the pectoral region. It is important to pull the affected leg forward as far as possible, placing the elbow cranial to the heavy muscle mass of the opposite leg and the pectoral region (Fig. 12–79). Because of the difficulty in visualizing both the joint space and the olecranon on the same radiograph, it is recommended that two exposures be made utilizing different exposure factors (Fig. 12–80).

The lateral exposure of the elbow may also be made with the horse recumbent, lying with the affected leg down. The radiographic technique is similar to that for the standing view: the affected leg is pulled forward and the unaffected leg is pulled backward. The cassette and grid

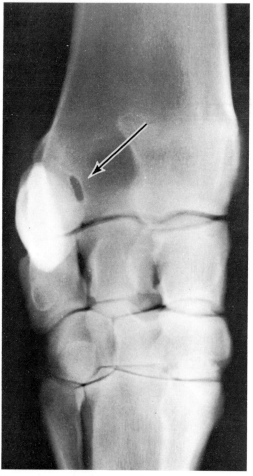

FIG. 12–75. An oblique radiograph of the carpus showing the persistent radiolucent line (arrow) that frequently remains in the mature horse and marks a cartilaginous remnant of the epiphyseal plate that once separated the distal radius and the distal epiphyseal center of the ulna.

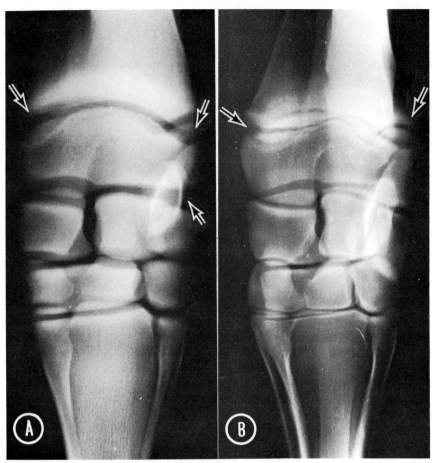

FIG. 12–76. Appearance of the epiphyseal lines in the distal radius (arrows) typical of one month of age (A) and six months of age (B). The separate ossification of the distal ulna is seen, along with the line in the distal radius. Note the apparent narrowing of the joint spaces as the horse matures.

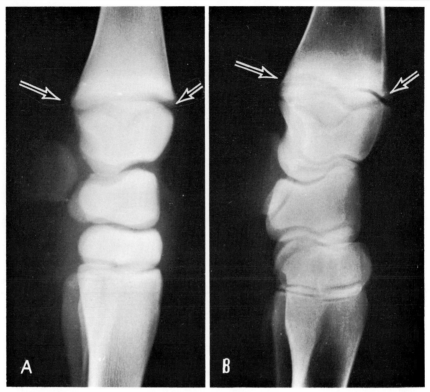

FIG. 12-77. Epiphyseal closure in the distal radius (arrows) as seen on the lateral views of the carpus. The views are typical of one month of age (A) and six months (B).

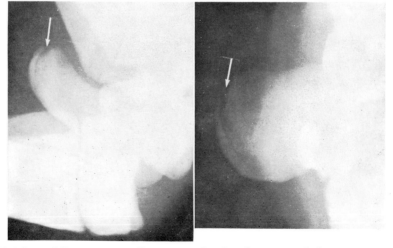

FIG. 12-78. Epiphyseal line occasionally seen in the distal portion of the accessory carpal bone (arrows).

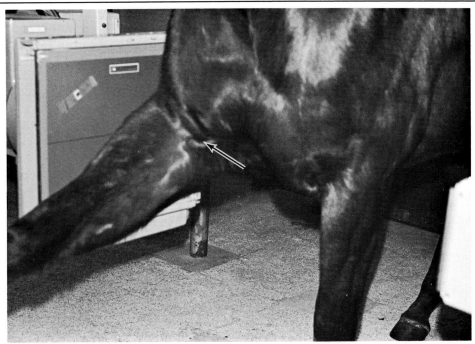

FIG. 12–79. Radiographic technique for making the lateral view of the elbow. A study of this type can usually be made with a machine of low rating if the leg can be extended sufficiently. The central beam is marked (arrow). A cassette holder of this type ensures that no one is in the primary x-ray beam.

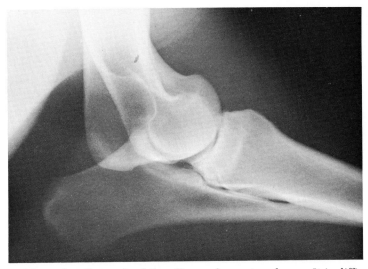

FIG. 12–80. Normal lateral radiograph of the elbow of a mature horse. It is difficult to visualize both the joint space and the olecranon on the same radiograph because of differences necessary in exposure factors.

are placed under the horse, using a tunnel device for protection.

The AP and oblique views are difficult to obtain. If the horse is standing, the cassette may be forced behind the olecranon against the rib cage (Fig. 12–81). Because the cassette must be angled, only a small portion of the humerus is seen (Fig. 12–82). If the horse is recumbent, the affected leg should be up and extended and abducted. In this way, the cassette can be placed behind the olecranon and a horizontal beam used. The radiographic technique will vary widely with the equipment and size of the horse. Either oblique view can be made with the horse standing or recumbent.

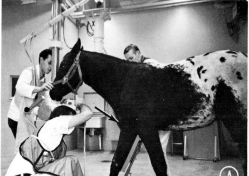
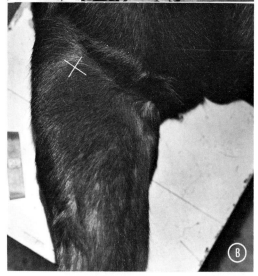

FIG. 12–81. Radiographic technique for making the AP view of the elbow, as seen from the side (A) and looking along the path of the x-ray beam (B). The central beam is marked (arrow). The cassette must be angled to fit tightly against the rib cage (B); for this reason, only a small portion of the humerus is visualized. X marks the point of contact of the central beam.

Diagnosis

Radiographic studies of the elbow are difficult to diagnose because of the inconsistency in the radiographic quality due to altered positionings and because of unique problems due to injuries that prevent the ideal positioning described above. Most studies are adequate for evaluation of the presence or absence of a fracture. The periarticular new bone growth associated with secondary joint disease is one of the easiest findings to note. Joint width may be difficult to evaluate, and early joint disease should be diagnosed with care. Too frequently, an effort is made to arrive at a diagnosis based on radiographs of insufficient quality.

Epiphyseal Closure

Epiphyseal plates are present in the immature horse in the distal humerus, olecranon, proximal radius, and medial epicondyle of the humerus (Fig. 12–83). The distal epiphysis of the humerus and the epiphysis of the medial epicondyle of the humerus are separate centers of ossification at birth. These two epiphyses unite by 6 to 12 months. Fusion of the distal epiphysis with the diaphysis occurs by 14 to 20 months. The proximal ulnar epiphysis is visible at birth and does not completely unite with the diaphysis of the ulna until 24 to 36 months. The epiphysis of the proximal radius does not close until 14 to 20 months. (See Table 12–4.)

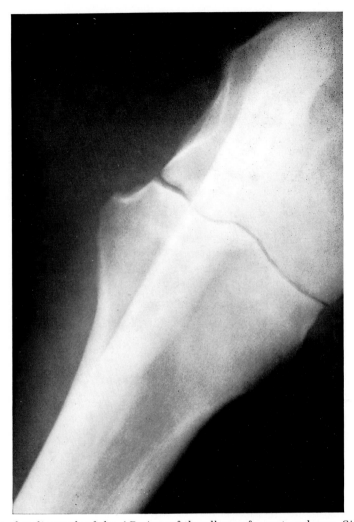

FIG. 12-82. Normal radiograph of the AP view of the elbow of a mature horse. Since the cassette must be angled, only a very small portion of the humerus is seen. This study is of value in diagnosis of joint disease.

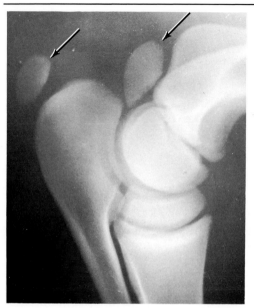

FIG. 12-83. The ossification centers near the elbow joint are easily seen on this lateral projection of a foal one month of age. In addition to the ossification centers of the proximal radius and distal humerus, the ossification centers in the medial epicondyle (arrow) and olecranon (arrow) are seen.

Shoulder

Because of its location and size, the shoulder joint is difficult to examine radiographically and impossible to examine without the use of equipment with a high ma and kVp capability. The radiographic technique will vary widely with equipment used and size of the horse.

Views

With the horse standing, it is possible to direct the central beam through the body from the opposite side and onto a cassette held against the lateral aspect of the affected joint (Figs. 12-84 and 12-85). The affected leg should be pulled slightly forward so that the shadows of the two shoulder joints are not superimposed. If the horse is recumbent, the affected leg should be placed down and the cassette and grid placed under the horse. The affected leg can then be pulled forward and the central beam directed perpendicular to the shoulder joint.

The AP, PA, and oblique views are extremely difficult to accomplish because it is not possible to extend the leg so that the joint is fully extended. Thus, the PA view is never perfect. The cassette can be placed in front of the shoulder of the standing horse and the tube placed as close to the rib cage as possible. The central beam is centered perpendicularly on the cassette. The AP view is usually not attempted because it is difficult to position the cassette posterior to the shoulder joint.

Diagnosis

Studies of the shoulder are generally limited to evaluation for fractures or severe joint diseases. The contour of the humeral head can be evaluated for osteochondritis dissecans.

Epiphyseal Closure

Two centers of ossification in the proximal humerus are present at birth. The proximal epiphysis of the humerus begins to ossify shortly after birth, and union of the proximal end of the humerus is seen to be complete by 18 to 30 months. The epiphysis of the lateral tuberosity of the humerus unites with the humerus by 2 to 3 years. (See Table 12-4.)

Two secondary centers of ossification are present at the distal end of the scapula. The center for the coracoid process and the tuber scapula fuse with the scapula before closure of the proximal humeral centers. The cranial portion of the glenoid cavity forms from a separate center. (Fig. 12-86).

Tarsus

Radiographic examination of the hock includes AP, lateral, and two oblique

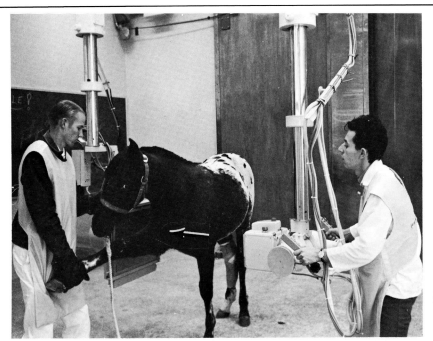

FIG. 12-84. Radiographic technique for making the lateral projection of the shoulder with the horse standing. It is important to extend the affected leg forward as far as possible to separate the shadows of the shoulder joint on the radiograph. Pulling the leg forward tends to drop the shoulder slightly. The central beam is marked (arrow).

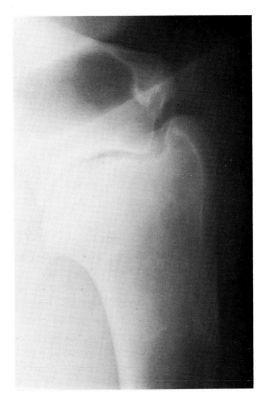

FIG. 12-85. Normal radiograph of the lateral view of the shoulder of a mature horse.

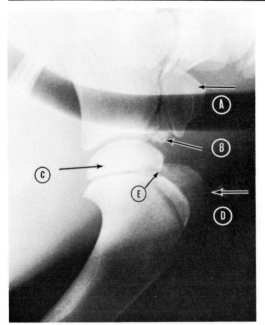

FIG. 12–86. The ossification centers near the shoulder are identified on a lateral projection made of a 14-day-old foal. The centers for the coracoid process and tuber scapulae (A) and the cranial portion of the glenoid cavity (B) of the scapula are identified. The proximal epiphysis (C), lateral tuberosity of the humerus (D), and medial tuberosity of the humerus (E) are also shown.

studies. The oblique views are made necessary by the repeated discovery of small chip fractures and minimal changes of secondary joint disease that are not detected in the more routine AP and lateral studies.

Views

The lateral view is made with the cassette positioned medially and the beam aimed at the central tarsal bone, approximately 4″ (10 cm) distal to the tip of the os calcis (Figs. 12–87 and 12–88). A common error is to center the central beam too high, causing the joint spaces to be badly obliqued on the radiograph. It may be of assistance to lift the unaffected leg

to ensure that the horse is bearing weight on the leg being examined.

The AP view is made with the cassette positioned against the back of the hock. The central beam is aimed at the central tarsal bone and is angled slightly to be perpendicular to the long axis of the metatarsal bone (Figs. 12–89 and 12–90). This is more easily done if the horse will allow the point of the hock to be rotated inward slightly. The oblique views are taken in a manner similar to the oblique views of the carpus. One study demonstrates the anterior-medial aspect (Fig. 12–91A), and the other demonstrates the anterior-lateral aspect of the hock (Fig. 12–91B). The oblique views also permit additional evaluation of the trochlear ridges of the distal tibia.

If the hock joint is severely swollen, a grid must be used to eliminate secondary radiation from reaching the film. Technique for the hock should be the *darker* technique.

Diagnosis

The majority of studies of the hock evaluate changes associated with spavin. Minimal bone and joint changes can be overlooked if positioning is not perfect, and care is needed in determining if a study is complete. Disease involving the trochlea of the tibial-tarsal bone and tibial-tarsal joint may require additional studies made with a more penetrating beam to clearly identify the pathologic change. Chip fractures and ununited bony ossicles from the trochlea of the tibial-tarsal bone have made radiographic examination of this area more important.

Epiphyseal Closure

The ossification center for the lateral malleolus of the fibula is present at birth, and unity with the distal tibia occurs within the first six months (Fig. 12–92).

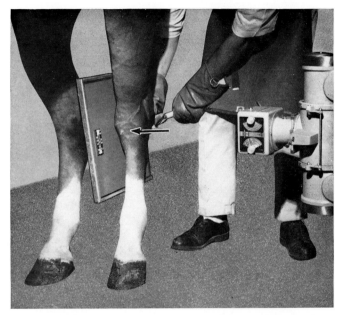

FIG. 12–87. Radiographic technique for making the lateral view of the hock joint. It is important to observe the position of the foot on this view in order to obtain a true lateral view. The central beam is marked (arrow).

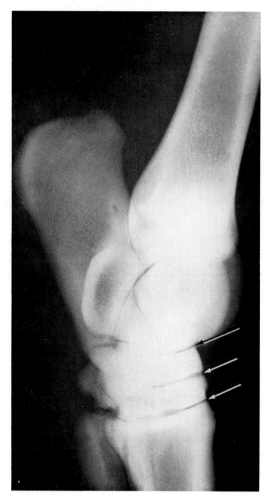

FIG. 12–88. Normal lateral radiograph of tarsus in a mature horse. The distal joint spaces (arrows) can be well evaluated. Note the proximal portion of the fourth metatarsal bone positioned posteriorly on the true lateral view.

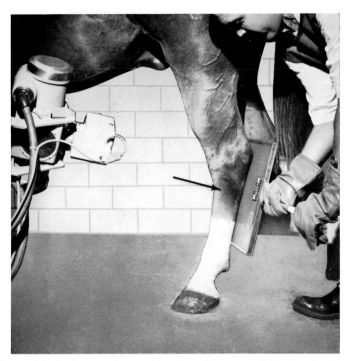

FIG. 12–89. Radiographic technique for making the AP view of the hock. The cassette is held firmly against the metatarsal bone and the central beam is angled slightly toward the ground. The central beam is aimed approximately 4″ distal to the point of the hock (arrow).

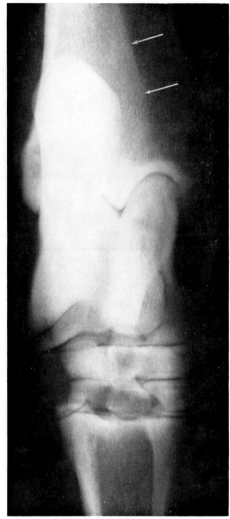

FIG. 12–90. Normal AP radiograph of the hock joint of a mature horse. The shadow created by the flexor tendons is seen across the tibia (arrows).

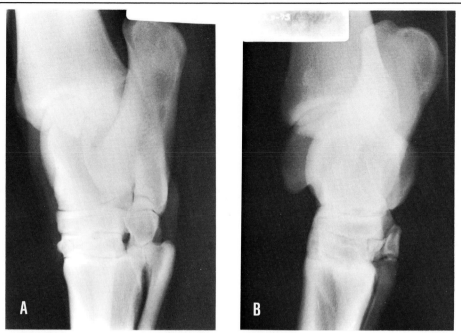

FIG. 12–91. Normal oblique radiographs of the hock joint in a mature horse. *A,* Anteriolateral/ posterior medial view; *B,* Anteriomedial/posterior lateral view.

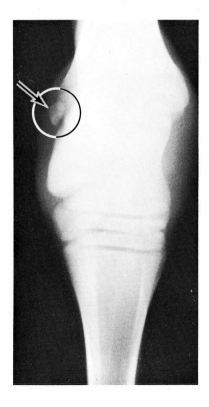

FIG. 12–92. Ossification center for the lateral malleolus of the fibula (arrow) seen on the AP projection of a normal hock at four weeks of age.

The epiphysis of the distal tibia unites with the diaphysis by two years of age. The epiphyseal plate present in the os calcis unites between 2 and 2.5 years of age (Fig. 12–93). (See Table 12–4.)

Stifle

Both AP and lateral views of the stifle should be made before the examination is considered a diagnostic one. The required studies are impossible to obtain with a portable unit. Radiographic techniques vary widely with the equipment used and size of the horse. Studies of the stifle can be made on the horse either standing or recumbent.

Views

The lateral view is the easiest and is made with the cassette placed medially and forced upward into the flank as far as possible. The central beam should be directed approximately 4″ (10 cm) distal to the patella, to permit good visualization of the joint space (Fig. 12–94). It may be necessary to use a grid for this view. Different techniques should be utilized to enhance studies of the patella, distal femur, and proximal tibia, in addition to the joint space (Fig. 12–95). If the horse is recumbent, the cassette is placed under the affected leg and the central beam is directed perpendicular to the cassette. The

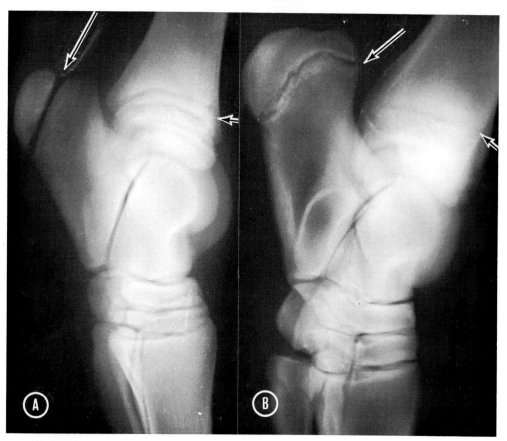

FIG. 12–93. The stages of epiphyseal closure as seen on these studies are typical for four weeks of age (A) and eighteen months of age (B). Epiphyseal plates can be identified in the os calcis and distal tibia (arrows).

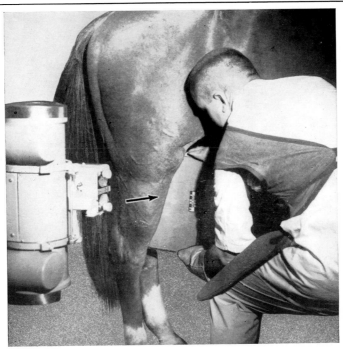

FIG. 12-94. Radiographic technique for making the lateral projection of the stifle joint. The central beam is marked (arrow).

normal leg is positioned either forward or backward, out of the primary beam.

The PA view is used in preference to AP projection, to allow the shortest possible object–film distance. The cassette is angled and pushed into the flank, as close as possible to the bony structures comprising the stifle joint. The tube is positioned posteriorly, and the central beam is directed at the stifle (Figs. 12-96 and 12-97). The PA study is more easily performed on a recumbent horse because the leg can be more fully extended, reducing the amount of soft tissue and permitting a good view of the joint space. A skyline projection of the patella is of value in diagnosis of trauma to this bone.

Diagnosis

The normal radiographic appearance of the ossification center of the tibial crest may be mistaken for aseptic necrosis or avulsion of the tibial crest. Either of these diagnoses should be embraced cautiously and only after comparison with radiographs of the opposite leg. During closure, the epiphyseal lines can create shadows that are easily mistaken for lesions unless care in interpretation is exercised. The lateral condyle of the femur as seen on the PA view does not have the smooth, round contour of the medial condyle.

A cartilaginous plate is frequently seen extending across the proximal portion of the fibula, particularly on PA views of the stifle. This has been shown not to be a fracture.

Epiphyseal Closure

The epiphyseal lines seen on radiographs of the stifle of an immature horse include the distal femur, tibial crest, and proximal tibia (Fig. 12-98). The distal femoral epiphysis fuses with the femoral diaphysis by 2 to 2.5 years of age. The tibial crest unites with the ossification center of the proximal tibia by one year of age. These combined ossification cen-

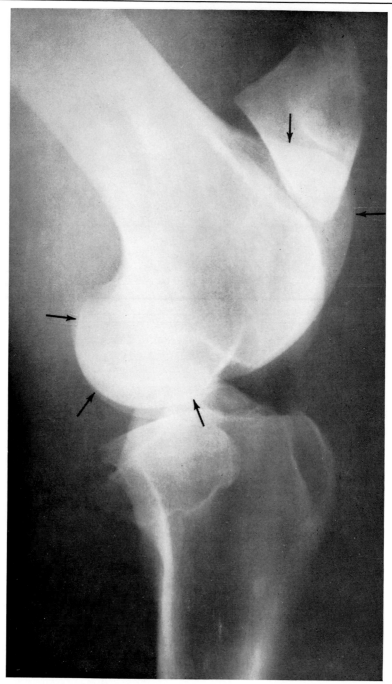

Fig. 12–95. Normal lateral radiograph of the stifle joint of a mature horse. The articular surfaces of the femoral condyles (arrows) are seen positioned farther posterior than sometimes expected. The medial portion of the trochlea is larger than the lateral (arrows).

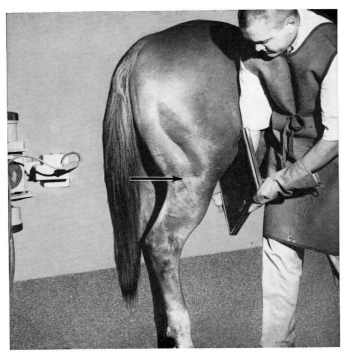

FIG. 12–96. Radiographic technique for making the PA view of the stifle. The central beam is marked (arrow).

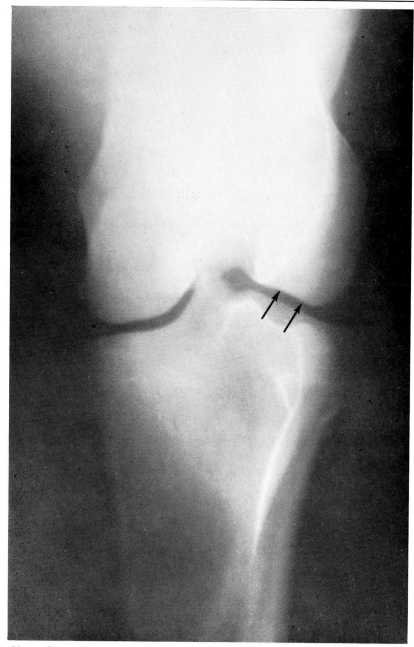

FIG. 12–97. Normal PA view of the stifle joint in a mature horse. The great difference in tissue thickness makes it difficult to see both the distal femur and the proximal tibia. The normal flattened appearance of the lateral condyle of the femur is shown (arrows).

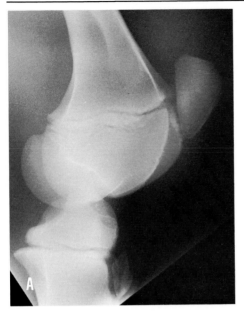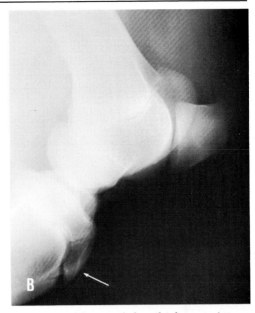

FIG. 12–98. Epiphyseal closure of the proximal tibial epiphyseal line and the tibial crest. At one week of age (A) the tibial crest and the proximal tibia both are represented by separate ossification centers. A study at two years of age demonstrates the union of the two ossification centers. The tibial crest has not completely united with the shaft of the tibia, however (arrow).

ters then unite with the shaft of the tibia by 2.5 to 3 years of age. (See Table 12–4.)

Hip Joint

Adequate studies of the hip joint can be made only if the horse is positioned on its back. Both true ventral-dorsal and oblique views are of value. Higher-rated equipment is necessary to obtain these studies.

Views

For the ventral-dorsal view, the horse is positioned on its back with the legs in a frog-leg position as described for the dog (Carlson, 1967). The actual positioning of the legs is less critical than is the fact that the limbs must be positioned identically, and the pelvis positioned symmetrically. The cassette and grid are placed under the horse, using a tunnel device, and the central beam is directed in a vertical direction (Fig. 12–99).

If a specific hip is thought to be involved, the horse can be laid on the affected side and the upper leg put into extreme abduction to remove it from the primary beam. The cassette is placed under the affected joint and the central beam is directed toward the femoral head. An identical view of the opposite hip joint should then be made for a comparison study.

It is especially important in radiographing the pelvis or hip joints that a cassette tunnel be used to protect the cassette and grid from the weight of the horse. Use of a tunnel device also permits the cassette to be inserted and removed more easily without moving the horse.

Diagnosis

Studies of the hip joint are frequently made to evaluate possible traumatic lesions. Femoral-head luxation, epiphyseal separations, and fracture of the femoral neck are frequent. Hematogenous osteo-

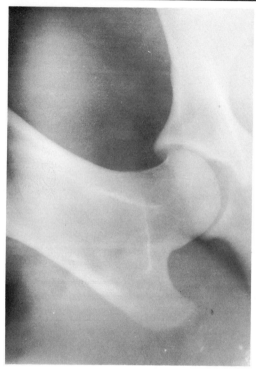

FIG. 12–99. Normal radiograph of the hip joint of a mature horse. The animal has been positioned on its back with the legs in a frog-leg position.

myelitis in the foal that occasionally leads to a suppurative arthritis is another possible diagnosis. Pelvic fractures in the adult horse may require additional radiographs centered directly over the point of suspected fracture because of the inability to include all of the pelvis on a single film.

Epiphyseal Closure

The proximal femoral epiphysis and the ossification centers for the greater and lesser trochanters are identified on the radiographs of the immature horse. Separate ossification centers in the pelvis are readily noted (Fig. 12–100).

The proximal femoral epiphysis closes between 24 and 36 months. The greater trochanter unites with the femoral shaft between 18 and 30 months. The fusion of the lesser trochanter is less consistent.

The union of the pelvic bones takes place between 18 and 24 months. Closure of the symphysis pubis is inconstant, and it often remains open after 5 years of age.

RADIOGRAPHIC DETERMINATION OF BONE MATURITY AS A GUIDE TO TRAINING HORSES

O. R. Adams, D.V.M., M.S.

A reasonable correlation between bone immaturity and increased incidence of injury during training and racing has now been established. Radiographs of the distal radial epiphyses are used most frequently for judging the degree of bone maturity. Other bones have been used, but the distal radius remains the bone of choice from the standpoints of consistent accurate interpretation, true indication of bone maturity, and ease of radiographic technique. Although this procedure is in no way a guarantee against injury, it is a valuable aid in making recommendations for training and should become a routine procedure before training of any type of horse.

The distal epiphysis of the radius is classified in A, B, and C categories. Category A is a fully mature epiphysis. Category B shows the center of the epiphysis

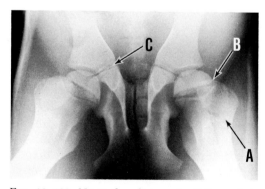

FIG. 12–100. Normal radiograph of the pelvis of an immature horse, demonstrating the epiphyseal lines in the greater trochanter (A), femoral neck (B), and in the pelvis (C).

undergoing closure while the medial and lateral aspects are not yet closed. Category C is a fully open epiphysis, meaning that growth is still proceeding. These categories can be difficult to define when they are borderline B or A categories. For this interpretation an anterior-posterior radiograph is all that is necessary. Constant distance and exposure factors must be used for comparison with earlier radiographs. Examples of A, B, and C classifications are shown in Figure 12-101.

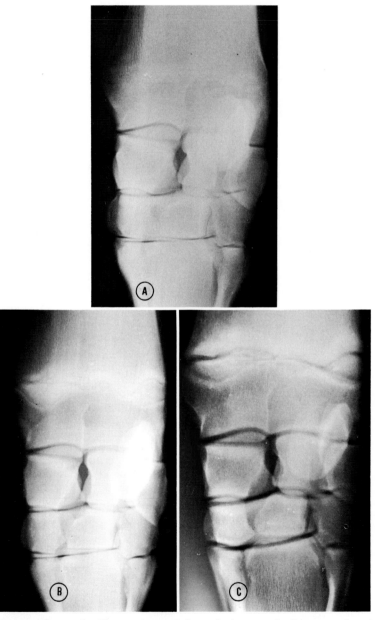

FIG. 12-101. Three radiographs illustrating epiphyseal closure. *A*, Category A epiphysis—fully closed. *B*, Category B epiphysis—closed in the center, with both medial and lateral portions of the epiphyses still open. *C*, Category C epiphysis—an example of an immature epiphysis.

For the A category horse, full race training is allowed. For the B category, it is recommended that the horse be trained and worked but allowed a limited number of starts, preferably not exceeding 10 in a season. In the C category, no heavy work should be permitted and only disciplinary training allowed. It is my experience that radiographs taken more frequently than every 60 days are probably of no value. It apparently takes at least 60 days to see enough change in the epiphyseal line to change the classification. In some blood lines, closure does not occur until as late as 33 months.

SPECIFIC REFERENCE

MASON, T. A., and J. M. BOURKE. 1973. Closure of the distal radial epiphysis and its relationship to unsoundness in two year old thoroughbreds. Aust. Vet. J. 49, 221–223.

REFERENCES

ALKSNIS, A. 1943. Röntgenaufnahmen vom becken unserer Grobtiere. Dtsch. Tierarztl. Wschr. 51:301.

BIRKELAND, R. 1963. Röntgen som diagnostisk hjelpemiddel. Nord. Vet. Med. 15:899.

CALISLAR, T., and L. E. ST. CLAIR. 1969. Observations on the navicular bursa and the distal interphalangeal joint cavity of the horse. JAVMA 154:410.

CARLSON, W. D. 1967. Veterinary Radiology. 2nd ed. Philadelphia: Lea & Febiger.

CAWLEY, A. J. 1960. Radiology: V, Navicular Disease. Can. Vet. J. 1:559.

CHAMBERLAIN, R. H., R. J. NELSON., et al. (n.d.) A Practice Manual on the Medical and Dental Use of X-Rays with Control of Radiation Hazards. Chicago: American College of Radiology.

CHRISTENSEN, E. E., T. S. CURRY III, and J. NUNNALLY. 1972. An Introduction to the Physics of Diagnostic Radiology. Philadelphia: Lea & Febiger.

DELAHANTY, D. D. 1958. Aspects of diagnosis and x-ray. Proc. 4th Ann. AAEP, 47.

DIETZ, V. O., E. NAGEL, T. KOCH, R. BERG, and O. STERBA. 1963. Zur Entslehung und zur Klinik der Sogenannten Gedeckten, Dislalen Griff elbeinfrakturen. Schweiz. Arch. Tierheilk. 105:87.

DIXON, R. T. 1969. Radiography of the equine carpus. Aust. Vet. J. 45:171.

DOUGLAS, S. W., and H. WILLIAMSON. 1972. Principles of Veterinary Radiography. 2nd ed. London: Bailliere, Tindal and Cox.

DOUGLAS, S. W., and H. D. WILLIAMSON. 1970. Veterinary radiographic facilities. Vet. Rec. 86:116.

DOUGLAS, S. W., and H. D. WILLIAMSON. 1970. Veterinary Radiological Interpretation. Philadelphia: Lea & Febiger.

DRURY, F. S., K. M. DYCE, and R. H. MERLEN. 1954. Some practical aspects of the experimental radiography of the larger domestic animals. Vet. Rec. 66:593.

E. I. du Pont de Nemours and Co., Inc. [n.d.] Darkroom Technique for Better Radiographs. Wilmington, Del. (pamphlet)

Eastman Kodak Co., Medical Division. 1968. The Fundamentals of Radiography. 11th ed. Rochester, N.Y. (pamphlet)

Gavaert Photo—Producten N.V. 1958. Processing of Medical X-Ray Films. Antwerp, Belgium. (pamphlet)

General Electric Co. [n.d.] A Look at X-Ray Film Processing, X-ray Department. Milwaukee, Wisc. (pamphlet)

GOODWIN, P. N., E. H. QUIMBY, and R. H. MORGAN. 1970. Physical Foundations of Radiology. 4th ed. New York: Harper and Row.

HABEL, R. E., R. B. BARRETT, C. D. DIESEM, and W. J. ROENIGK. 1963. Nomenclature for radiologic anatomy. JAVMA 142:38.

HICKMAN, J. A. 1954. A review of some technical aids in veterinary radiology. Vet. Rec. 66:805.

IDSTROM, L. G. 1954. X-ray machines and related physics. Vet. Med. 49:381.

JACOBSON, G. A., and D. E. VAN FAROWE. 1964. Survey of x-ray protection practices among Michigan veterinarians. JAVMA 145:793.

JOHNS, H. E., and J. R. CUNNINGHAM. 1969. The Physics of Radiology. 3rd ed., Springfield, Ill.: Charles C Thomas.

MARSHALL, J. 1969. Periarticular osteophytes: Initiation and formation in the knee of the dog. Clin. Orthop. Rel. Res. 62:37.

MILNE, F. J., D. D. DELAHANTY, D. L. PROCTOR, B. F. BRENNAN, and W. F. RILEY. 1959. X-ray technics and diagnosis. Proc. 5th Ann. AAEP, 177.

MOLE, R. H. 1961. The biological basis for precautions in veterinary radiography. Vet. Rec. 73:1140.

MONFORT, T. N. 1962. A radiographic survey of epiphyseal maturity in thoroughbred foals from birth to three years of age. Proc. 13th Ann. AAEP, 33.

MORGAN, J. P. 1972. Radiology in Veterinary Orthopedics. Philadelphia: Lea & Febiger.

MORGAN, J. P. 1965. Radiographic study of the distal ulna of the horse. J. Amer. Vet. Radiol. Soc., 6:78.

MORGAN, J. P. 1968. Radiographic diagnosis of bone and joint diseases in the horse. Cornell Vet. 58 (Suppl.).

MYERS, V. S. 1965. Confusing radiologic variations at the distal end of the radius of the horse. JAVMA 147:1310.

MYERS, V. S., and J. K. BURT. 1966. The radiographic location of epiphyseal lines in equine limbs. Proc. 12th Ann. AAEP, 21.

MYERS, V. S., and M. A. EMMERSON. 1966. The age and manner of epiphyseal closure in the forelegs of two Arabian foals. J. Amer. Vet. Radiol. Soc. 7:39.

National Bureau of Standards Handbooks, available from Superintendent of Documents, U.S. Government Printing Office, Washington, D.C.

No. 50—X-Ray Protection Design, 20¢.

No. 51—Radiological Monitoring Methods and Instruments, 25¢.

No. 54—Protection against Radiations from Radium, Cobalt 60 and Cesium 137, 25¢.

No. 59—Permissible Dose from External Sources of Ionizing Radiation, 30¢.

No. 60—X-Ray Protection, 20¢.

O'BRIEN, T. R., J. P. MORGAN, R. D. PARK, and J. L. LEBEL. 1971. Radiography in equine carpal lameness. Cornell Vet. 61(4): 646.

OLSSON, S-E. 1954. On navicular disease in the horse. Nord. Vet. Med. 6:547.

OXSPRING, G. E. 1935. The radiology of navicular disease, with observations of Its pathology. Vet. Rec. 15:1433.

PARK, R. D., J. P. MORGAN, and T. R. O'BRIEN. Chip fractures in the carpus of the horse: A radiographic study of their incidence and location. JAVMA 157:1305.

REID, C. F. 1962. Large animal radiography. Proc. 13th Ann. AAEP, 233.

REID, C. F. 1965. Radiographic film identification and positioning. Proc. 11th Ann. AAEP, 167.

REYNOLDS, J. A. 1955. Factors affecting radiographic quality. Vet. Med. 50:187.

RYAN, G. D., and H. J. DEIGL. 1969. Safety in large animal radiography. JAVMA 155:898.

SCHEBITZ, H. 1964. Podotrochlosis in the horse. Proc. 10th Ann. AAEP. 49.

SCHEBITZ, H., and H. WILKENS. 1968. Atlas of radiographic anatomy of dog and horse. Berlin: Paul Parey.

SPURRELL, F. A., L. V. BAUDIN, and W. J. L. FELTS. 1965. Radiography of the foreleg and selected cases. Proc. 11th Ann. AAEP, 181.

TAVERNOR, W. D., and L. C. Vaughan. 1962. Radiography of horses and cattle. Brit. Vet. J. 118:359.

TROUT, E. D., J. P. KELLEY, and G. A. CATHEY. 1952. The use of filters to control radiation exposure to the patient in diagnostic roentgenology. Amer. J. Roentgen. 67:942.

UNWIN, D. D. 1970. Radiation protection in a veterinary practice. J. Small Anim. Pract. 11:523.

VAN DER PLATTS, G. J. 1961. Medical X-ray Technique. 2nd ed. Eindhoven, The Netherlands: N. V. Philips' Gloeilampenfabrieken.

VAN KRUININGEN, H. J. 1963. Practical techniques for making injections into joints and bursae of the horse. JAVMA 143:1079.

VAN PELT, R. W. 1962. Intra-articular injection of the equine carpus and fetlock. JAVMA 140:1181.

VON SALIS, B. J. U. 1961. Uber Strukturveranderungen an den distalen Fortsatzen der Hufbeinaste und ihre differentialdiagnostische Bedeutung fur chronische Lahmheit beim Pferd. Schweiz. Arch. Tierheilk. 103:631.

WATSON, J. C. 1954. Considerations in formulating x-ray exposure factors. Vet. Med. 49:435.

WILLIAMS, F. L. 1957. Cassette holders for large animal radiography. JAVMA 130:28.

WILLIAMS, F. L., and D. Y. CAMPBELL. 1961. Tendon radiography in the horse. JAVMA 139:224.

WILLIAMSON, H. D. 1964. Veterinary radiography—Some aspects and problems. Radiography 30:2.

WINTZER, H. J. 1965. Zur Podotrochlitis Chronica Aseptica des Pferdes. Utrecht: Schotanus and Jens.

ZESKOV, B., J. MAROLT, E. VUKELIC, and U. BEGO. 1963. Investigations on the radiographical examination of spinous processes in the area of the withers in the horse. Zbl. Veterinaermed.

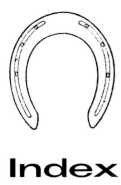

Index